Shiatsu

CORINNA SOMMA

The natural force within each of us is the greatest healer of all.

—Hippocrates, the father of Western medicine
(circa 460–377 B.C.)

Out of your belly shall flow rivers of living water.

—Jesus Christ

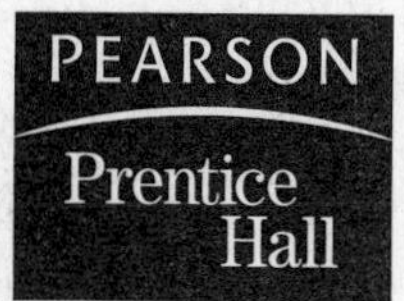

Upper Saddle River, New Jersey

Library of Congress Cataloging-in-Publication Data
Somma, Corinna.
Shiatsu/Corinna Somma. — 1st ed.
p. ; cm.
Includes bibliographical references and index.
ISBN 0-13-118419-9
1. Acupressure. 2. Medicine, Chinese.
[DNLM: 1. Acupressure—methods. 2. Medicine, Chinese Traditional—methods.
3. Meridians. WB 369.5A17 S697s 2007] I. Title.
RM723.A27S6 2007
615.8'222—dc22 2005036532

Publisher: Julie Levin Alexander
Executive Editor: Mark Cohen
Associate Editor: Melissa Kerian
Director of Production and Manufacturing: Bruce Johnson
Managing Editor: Patrick Walsh
Production Liaison: Christina Zingone
Manufacturing Manager: Ilene Sanford
Manufacturing Buyer: Pat Brown
Design Director: Maria Guglielmo-Walsh
Cover Designer: Anthony Gemmellaro
Marketing Manager: Harper Coles
Composition: GGS Book Services
Printer/Binder: Edwards Brothers, Inc.
Cover Printer: Phoenix Color

Credits and acknowledgments borrowed from other sources and reproduced, with permission, in this textbook appear on appropriate page within text.

Notice: The author and the publisher of this volume have taken care that the information and technical recommendations contained herein are based on research and expert consultation, and are accurate and compatible with the standards generally accepted at the time of publication. Nevertheless, as new information becomes available, changes in clinical and technical practices become necessary. The reader is advised to carefully consult manufacturers' instructions and information material for all supplies and equipments before use, and to consult with a health-care professional as necessary. This advice is especially important when using new supplies or equipment for clinical purposes. The author and publisher disclaim all responsibility for any liability, loss, injury, or damage incurred as a consequence, directly or indirectly, of the use and application of any of the contents of this volume.

Pearson Education Ltd., *London*
Pearson Education Australia Pty. Limited, *Sydney*
Pearson Education Singapore, Pte. Ltd.
Pearson Education North Asia Ltd., *Hong Kong*
Pearson Education Canada, Ltd. *Toronto*
Pearson Educación de Mexico, S.A. de C.V.
Pearson Education—Japan, *Tokyo*
Pearson Education Malaysia, Pte. Ltd.
Pearson Education, Upper Saddle River, New Jersey

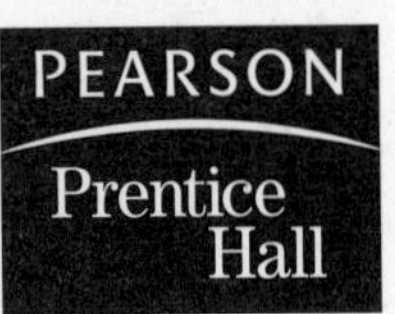

10 9 8 7 6
ISBN 0-13-118419-9

To Ryan

Two are better than one.
Ecclesiastes 4:9

CONTENTS

Preface

> People must have high spiritual development to do this Shiatsu technique, because healing disease is not only by fingertip pressure. You have to have spiritual power to do healing by hand.
>
> —Tamai Tempaku, *Shiatsu Ho*, 1919

So wrote the founder of modern Shiatsu, Tamai Tempaku, in his groundbreaking book *Shiatsu Ho*, published in 1919, and thereby affirmed the spiritual dimension of a highly manual art (Dubitsky, 1992). In my experience, most practitioners of Shiatsu and other forms of manual therapy are attracted to bodywork because it is a ministry of compassion that fosters wholeness, and this is a spiritual matter as much as a physical matter. Nevertheless, though we respond to a spiritual call, most of us invest considerable time, money, and effort in studying and mastering technique, in perfecting the form of the practice, which is what books like this are designed to support. Only much later, and perhaps by grace, we might discover our healing gift, the supernatural side of healing and the substance, heart, or spirit of the practice. In recognition of this and with an earnest desire for this for myself and others, I humbly quote Michaelangelo: "Ancora Imparo" (Latin meaning "I am still learning").

> In attending to the human body, the Chinese believe that the superior doctor prevents sickness; the mediocre doctor attends to impending sickness; the inferior doctor treats actual sickness.
>
> —Chinese proverb

Clearly, the Chinese esteem prevention above intervention in health care. This by no means disparages Western medicine, which has radically cured many, including my mother, whose breast cancer was cured through seemingly miraculous and drastic means—drugs and surgery. Rather, the quote points to the differences in priority and approach between Western and Eastern medicine. Traditional Chinese Medicine (TCM), to which Shiatsu traces its lineage, values a preventive approach to health care above crisis intervention, pain management or damage control: The aim is to keep the body and soul well through healthy lifestyle practices and thereby avert disease. The implication is rather tremendous: Shiatsu practitioners are, at least in the Eastern tradition, "superior doctors," inasmuch as bodywork is part of a health maintenance regimen. This sort of thinking is what initially prompted me to entitle the book *Shiatsu: Piercing the Sickness with Bare Hands*.

From a Western perspective, however, the assertion that healing can be accomplished with bare hands, as if some sort of bloodless surgery were taking place during a Shiatsu session, is a rather audacious claim. Nevertheless, some practitioners have certainly lived up to this claim—Tokujiro Namikoshi, who was suspected of having a healing gift, comes to mind, especially in curing his mother's rheumatism, a government official's chronic back pain, and Marilyn Monroe's deadly illness, which eluded Western medicine (Dubitsky, 1992). In any case, healing with bare hands is not an outlandish notion in the Asian tradition. Before 2205 B.C.,when stone, bone, and thorn probes were used in China to "pierce the sickness" (Jwing-Ming, 1992), the hands were used as medical instruments to apply manual pressure or acupressure. Perhaps as the United States embraces preventive medicine, as indeed it is beginning to, and perhaps as more practitioners use not only their skill but also their innate healing gift, my original title will be appropriate for future editions.

The experienced Shiatsu practitioner may note that most of the protocols in this book demonstrate a very Yang style practice. This is due to the fact that the author has a Yang temperament and constitution (Wood element type), has grown up in a Yang culture (the United States), and has adopted a version of Shiatsu that draws on the Chinese original—Tui Na, a kind of "push grab" style of bodywork (Jwing-Ming, 1992). This is an admitted departure from the Yin approach of many excellent Shiatsu texts currently on the market, but it has a definite place in America and anywhere else where the lifestyle and people tend to be Yang. A Yang treatment style will mellow a Yang client, according to the law of transformation of Yin Yang theory, which could be mathematically expressed as Yang + Yang = Yin (Esher, 2001; Kaptchuk, 2000; Maciocia, 2001).

Although the book is technical in nature and at times academic in tenor, I have tried to make it approachable, appealing, and interesting to the general public. To this end, I have drawn analogies from Western science, philosophy, and psychology to explain the more esoteric concepts. I have told human interest stories and created fanciful mnemonic devices to simplify the more difficult concepts. Examples include profiles of real people who exemplify the Five Element types; literary characters who represent stereotypical Five Element imbalances, including Ichabod Crane, Frankenstein, Don Quixote, Hamlet, and Scrooge. For instructors, this book contains helpful pedagogical tools that support teaching, including study questions and answers that can be assigned as homework, or used to facilitate class Q & A or discussion, or as alternate testing method; tests and answers to evaluate student progress, and sample Shiastu protocols to guide student practice. For students, the book promotes learning through diagrams and line drawings, tables and bullet points that summarize lessons, practice exercises, study questions and answers for review of test material, and a photographic glossary of acupressure points.

One reviewer of the rough draft of this book anticipated my intention for a future revised edition by recommending that at least one Shiatsu protocol be adapted to a massage table. The practical reality is that many, if not most, professional venues do not dedicate sufficient space to accommodate full stretches on a futon on the floor and that some practitioners have knee and back injuries or have difficulty crawling on all fours. Thus, adapting Shiatsu to the table is an important option for Western practitioners. This will be addressed in a future edition.

This book follows the precedent of reputable sources in the capitalization of the names of organs (e.g. Spleen, Liver, Kidney, etc.), conditions of the body or etiological factors in illness and disease (Cold, Wind, Damp, Heat, Dryness), as well as other medical concepts (Phlegm, Wei Qi) peculiar to TCM, and by bequest, Shiatsu. Capitalization reinforces the distinction between Eastern and Western concepts where the names are identical and would otherwise lead to the mistaken impression that Eastern and Western concepts are synonymous and interchangeable. The Eastern view of organs, for example, includes psychological capacities. Capitalization also points to the uniqueness and significance of Eastern concepts, and especially where no exact Western corollary exists: for example, Qi, Meridians, Yin Yang, the Five Elements, and Kyo Jitsu. In short, capitalization alerts the reader to a paradigm shift in the medical model, and indeed reality.

For the sake of consistency and currency, this book uses the revised standard acupuncture abbreviations as adopted by the World Health Organization in Geneva in 1989. The Geneva abbreviations uniformly and systematically designate two letters for each Meridian, whereas, the former 1982 Manila abbreviations designate one, two, or three letters (Institute of Acupuncture, 2000). This book only departs from the Geneva abbreviations on TE (Triple Energizer). Instead of TE, this book uses the older term TH (Triple Heater), which is a more accurate translation of the "three burning spaces" of the ancient texts and which retains the association of TH with body heat through its function of transmitting Source Qi to other organs to ignite their functions.

My earnest desire is that this book will edify many, serve as a repository of knowledge to which the reader can turn again and again, support a rich Shiatsu practice, and generate Shiatsu sessions that will promote compassion and wholeness for the practitioner as well as the recipient.

REFERENCES

Dubitsky, C. (1992). History of Shiatsu Anma. *Massage Therapy Journal, 31*(4), 109–110, 112, 114.

Esher, B. (2001). Asian healing arts: Got Yin/Yang? *Massage Today, 1*(12), 18–19.

Institute of Acupuncture and Moxibustion of the China Academy of Traditional Chinese Medicine & Kelin Technology Development Co. (2000). *Charts of Chinese standard location of acupoints*. Beijing China: Morning Glory Publishers.

Jwing-Ming, Y. (1992). *Chinese Qigong massage: General massage*. Boston: YMAA Publication Center.

Kaptchuk, T. (2000). *The web that has no weaver: Understanding Chinese medicine* (2nd ed.). Chicago: Contemporary.

Maciocia, G. (2001). *The foundations of Chinese medicine: A comprehensive text for acupuncturists and herbalists*. Edinburgh: Churchill Livingstone. (Original work published 1989.)

ACKNOWLEDGMENTS

Thanks to all my sources, whose work I highly esteem.

Thanks to the reviewers and copy editor who critiqued rough drafts of this book and gave me very helpful feedback for revision.

Thanks to my editors at Prentice Hall, Melissa Kerian and Mark Cohen, for their confidence in my potential, their encouragement, and their assistance.

Thanks to the Shiatsu models for lending me their bodies with patience:
Christine Allgeier, supine lower body protocol (Chapter 12)
Hether Hollenbach, supine upper body protocol (Chapter 13)
David Leighton, prone upper body protocol (Chapter 10)
Donna Luzzi, sidelying protocol (Chapter 15)
Carlos Ruiz, abdominal protocol (Chapter 14)
Jason Akira Somma, Gua Sha protocol (Chapter 17)
Rachelle Somma, practice preliminaries (Chapter 9) and tonifying Kyo exercise (Chapter 6)
Hayden Woodward, prone lower body protocol (Chapter 11)
Charley Yancey, seated protocol (Chapter 16)

Thanks to the Five Element temperament type models for their transparency:
Linda Bennington, Fire element
Diane Husson, Earth element
Ryan Somma, Metal element
Darin Somma, Water element

Thanks to the photographers for their creative labors:
Hether Hollenbach, Qi Gong exercises (Chapter 18) and moxa protocol (Chapter 17)
Joanna Seitz, Gua Sha protocol (Chapter 17)
Ryan Somma, Shiatsu protocols (Chapters 10–16)

Thanks to Linda Bennington for notifying me of Prentice Hall's interest in massage therapy authors.

Thanks to my mother, Ursula Kraft-Guy, for paying for my massage therapy education.

Thanks to those who read, study, and practice what is in this book.

Thanks to God for sustaining and empowering me through this very challenging labor of love.

Reviewers

Tom Adams
Omega Institute
Pennsauken, New Jersey

Sandra K. Anderson, BA, NCBTMB
Former Chair and Instructor
Desert Institute of the Healing Arts
Tucson, Arizona

Cheryl Siniakin-Baum, Ph.D.
Associate Professor, Director
Massage Therapy Program
Community College of Allegheny County
Pittsburgh, Pennsylvania

Linda Brecker, BS
Instructor
Phoenix College
Phoenix, Arizona

Nancy Waltz Dail, BA, LMT, NCTMB
Director, Owner, Teacher
Downeast School of Massage
Waldoboro, Maine

Cora Jacobson
Instructor
Desert Institute of the Healing Arts
Tucson, Arizona

Todd J. Koch
Director
Massage & Neuromuscular Therapy
CAPPS College
Mobile, Alabama

Margaret Avery Moon, BA, NCTMB
President
Desert Institute of the Healing Arts
Tucson, Arizona

Theresa Patterson
Blue Cliffs College
Metairie, Louisiana

Linda Sola
Maui School of Theraputic Massage
Makawao, Maui, Hawaii

INTRODUCTION

This book is divided into two parts: theory and practice. Realistically, theory cannot be separated from practice because theory informs practice: For example, theory guides the selection of areas of the body to emphasize, techniques to apply, and manner of delivery. However, this division is a convenient artifice to organize a great deal of material into a form readers can comprehend.

THEORY: INTRODUCTION TO TRADITIONAL CHINESE MEDICINE

Part 1 covers the basic concepts of Traditional Chinese Medicine (TCM)—the theoretical foundation for Shiatsu—and its major Japanese extrapolations and adaptations. Included are descriptions and explanations of the concept of vital energy flowing through the body (Qi and Meridian theory), the dynamic tension and interplay between reciprocal opposing forces (Yin Yang theory), the processes or stages in the cycle of nature and life (Five Element theory), and the state of imbalance or disharmony in energy (the Eight Principle Patterns and Kyo Jitsu), among others. These concepts all have practical applications to Shiatsu, especially in terms of assessing a client and customizing a session accordingly. All concepts progressively build on each other and are mutually intertwined.

Initially, the Western student or beginning practitioner may find the metaphysical aspects of TCM strange, the geological allegories curious, and the multilayered, cross-referential nature of TCM daunting, frustrating, and perhaps even overwhelming. Care and effort have been taken to make these concepts accessible by using Western analogies from science, psychology, and literature, as well as examples from everyday life. The good news is that the reader can begin the practice of Shiatsu before the theory is understood, just as a person can embark on and benefit from an exercise regimen without understanding what is happening on a physiological level. In time, practice will make the theory clearer, and theory will make the practice better.

PRACTICE: INTRODUCTION TO SHIATSU PROTOCOLS

Part 2 of this book presents Shiatsu protocols or practice sessions. In a broad sense, a protocol is any formal procedure for conducting human affairs in an orderly fashion. Within the medical field, a protocol is a treatment plan or regimen. In this book, the protocols are prescribed formats for giving Shiatsu, outlining a series of techniques. As prescribed formats, they are much like a judo or karate kata (a pattern of martial arts exercises) or a choreographed dance that links individual steps into a sequence of movements of strategic or artistic design.

The protocols are designed for the entry-level practitioner. As such, they serve several purposes: They provide the practitioner with a predesigned Shiatsu session, they introduce a basic repertoire of techniques, they increase the practitioner's comfort with and proficiency in techniques through repetition, and they familiarize the practitioner with Meridian routes and key acupressure points on each Meridian.

An entry-level practitioner will probably want to look at the protocol once or twice or practice it on a fellow classmate once or twice before practicing it on a client or mock client (coworker, friend, relative, or significant other who has volunteered to be a recipient). During a session, the practitioner may want to lay the book open by the client as a quick visual reference. However, the practitioner should strive to maintain the continuity and momentum of the work and avoid interrupting the session too often or too long, which may make the experience disjointed for the recipient.

The protocols follow a certain logic and consistency of approach. As in Zen Shiatsu, the direction of movement is downward and outward, that is, from a superior to an inferior aspect (head to foot) and from a medial to a lateral aspect (center to extremity). Several techniques are applied to each Meridian, progressing from general to specific (from broad, soft body tools to narrow, sharp body tools) and from moderate to intense (from shallow, static pressure to deep, dynamic pressure). Meridians in the arms and legs are usually stimulated in their entirety before a few key acupressure points are stimulated.

As much as possible, economy of effort and effectiveness of delivery have been considered in the design of the protocols. Stretches and body mobilization techniques (BMTs) are generally applied in an order of natural progression and ease: for example, a series of stretches that gradually lower a leg to the floor rather than raising it against gravity, which is far more difficult. For delivering perpendicular pressure, practitioner positioning directly over the client's midline is preferred to the more traditional positioning alongside the client, which entails twisting the torso and which places the practitioner's hara (power center) at an oblique angle relative to the client. Thus, kneeling on the client's hamstrings to work the Bladder Meridian in the lower back and straddling the client's waist to work the Conception Vessel and Stomach Meridians in the abdomen are demonstrated.

Finally, the Shiatsu protocols tackle one client position and one section or surface area of the body at a time:

- prone: back and posterior arms;
- prone: hips and posterior legs;
- supine: anterior legs;
- supine: chest, anterior arms, neck, and face;
- supine: abdomen;
- sidelying; and
- seated.

GROWING BEYOND THE PROTOCOLS

Because the protocols are learning tools, they are limited and need not be followed militantly. Instead, they should be viewed as a support structure that can be dispensed with in part or in its entirety as the practitioner grows in technical competence, discovers what feels best for his or her own body, learns how to adapt the work to different body types, and learns how to customize a session to address the client's specific needs. After practicing each protocol several times and studying the principles of application in the theory section of this book, practitioners should have had enough hands-on experience and enough time to assimilate theory to begin designing full-body Shiatsu sessions. Some practitioners are naturally more inclined to experiment and innovate than others. Using the protocols as a springboard to find a personal style is encouraged.

Understanding how the protocols are limited may help the practitioner outgrow them faster. Quite obviously, the protocols parse the body into sections to limit the scope of the surface area covered. In a learning context, this fosters mastery of a particular area of the body and prevents learning overload. In actual practice, however, unless there is a good reason for focusing exclusively on a particular section of the body, a Shiatsu session should be a full-body experience that promotes a sense of integration of body parts and mind-body holism.

In the protocols, some Meridians are worked in excess of the standard three passes to give the practitioner an opportunity to become proficient in a variety of techniques, such as palms, thumbs, fists, knuckles, forearms, elbows, knees, feet, and sides of the hands, with static and dynamic variations. In actual practice, however, three passes along a Meridian should be sufficient. Moreover, under the time constraints of a professional session, overworking one Meridian in the body would probably necessitate underworking or totally neglecting another Meridian. Therefore, once the practitioner has become adept in a number of techniques and has developed a repertoire from which to choose, he or she can select a few techniques to apply to a Meridian. Ultimately, a balanced treatment that neither overstimulates nor understimulates any Meridian should be the goal.

For the sake of uniformity and simplicity, the protocols feature certain default methods of applying Shiatsu. The first is the Zen Shiatsu method of applying compression techniques in a downward and outward direction. On Meridians that traverse the body in the same direction (downward and outward), this direction is concurrent with Meridian flow and constitutes a nourishing or tonifying treatment suitable for Kyo or deficiency conditions (see "Direction of Movement" in Chapter 6). On Meridians that traverse the body in the opposite direction (upward and inward), this direction is countercurrent to Meridian flow and constitutes a sedating or dispersing treatment suitable for Jitsu or excess conditions. As the practitioner becomes better able to assess the client's presenting condition and integrate theory into practice, the practitioner may want to reverse the default direction of the protocols. For example, the practitioner may want to work up rather than down the Bladder, Gallbladder, or Stomach Meridian to sedate excess. He or she may want to work up rather than down the Spleen, Liver, or Kidney Meridian to tonify deficiency.

The second default method is the two-handed compression technique, in which both hands travel along a Meridian simultaneously, reinforcing pressure and stimulating a larger surface area than can be stimulated with only one hand. Two-handed compression is very Yang in style and is preferable if the client likes deep, vigorous treatment; needs to discharge tension; and desires a strong effect. However, this technique may not be ideal and may even be inappropriate for some clients, especially those who present systemic deficiency conditions and those who present localized excess conditions (see "Interior/Exterior," "Deficiency/Excess," "Cold/Heat," and Qualities of Kyo and Jitsu in Chapter 6). Some clients may prefer a softer, gentler treatment style overall or may need a milder, more soothing approach in a particular area where the tissues are hypersensitive and skittish. In either case, the practitioner should feel free to depart from the default two-handed technique and opt for the Zen Shiatsu Mother/Son hand technique, in which one hand stays planted on the core of the body while the other hand performs traveling compressions (see the discussion of the Mother/Son hand technique in Chapter 9).

From a safety perspective, certain techniques may not be appropriate for the practitioner and/or the client. Some BMTs require strength, flexibility, or structural integrity that the practitioner may currently lack or never acquire due to genetic makeup, conditioning, prior injury, or some other reason. In such case, the technique should be omitted and another more user-friendly technique substituted, if possible. Some techniques, for example, require hoisting and maneuvering part of the client's body. Even with good body mechanics, such techniques should be omitted if the client is substantially heavier and larger than the practitioner or if the practitioner is otherwise concerned about a risk of strain or injury.

The same caution applies for the client. Obviously, everybody has a different capacity for bodywork, which should be respected. Most of the models in the protocols are in good health, athletic, and capable of receiving fairly intense work. For instance, the model for the supine lower body protocol is a triathlete and power Yoga instructor. Her body will flex, extend, twist, and bend in ways that are impossible for other clients. Although her body demonstrates the human potential for movement and shows what the stretches look like at their end range, she is not representative of the average client. The average client has a much narrower range of motion, which should be honored by cultivating a listening touch and encouraging client feedback. Additionally, observing general cautions and contraindications for special populations (see "The Elderly" and "Pregnant Women" in Chapter 9) and becoming adept at different methods of client assessment will help the practitioner tailor the work for the client (see the discussion of Yin and Yang types in Chapter 3, "Five Element Types" in Chapter 4, and "Deficiency/Excess" and Kyo and Jitsu types in Chapter 6).

One other drawback is that the Shiatsu protocols follow the Asian tradition of performing bodywork on the floor on a futon (a thick mat filled with cotton batting). From a professional standpoint, the floor may not be a desirable or feasible location due to cleanliness issues and space restrictions. Unless special custodial care is taken, the floor tends to be a dirty place, especially in the West, where shoes are not removed before entering a home or office. Unfortunately, at the time of this writing many professional settings that offer massage therapy do not yet dedicate a space to traditional Asian bodywork, in part because floor work takes more space than table work and the average room dimensions are not spacious enough for floor work.

For some practitioners, the floor may not be the optimal place to give Shiatsu. The practitioner may find floor work awkward, burdensome, and uncomfortable. This may be due to the practitioner's height, weight, debility, or other factor. Tall or overweight practitioners tend to have more difficulty, as do those who have sustained knee and back injuries. Westerners in general are unaccustomed to and tend to be ill at ease with the Asian custom of sitting and working on the floor. Westerners tend to have tight foot and ankle extensor muscles, which make sitting in seiza (the Japanese kneeling position) painful; their quadriceps (on the front thigh), iliopsoas (hip flexors), and adductors (on the inner thigh) tend to be tight, which makes kneeling lunges and squats difficult. Overall tightness can make floor work stressful and maladroit.

Some measures can be taken to improve the quality of the experience for the practitioner. Using sufficient floor padding or wearing nonrestrictive, flexible knee pads will cushion the knees. Engaging the abdominal muscles—especially the transverse abdominus, which sucks or draws the gut in—will support the lower back. Gaining leverage over the client and initiating movement from the hara (power center) rather than the extremities will reduce strain on the lower back ("Principles of Proper Body Mechanics" in Chapter 9). Wearing a wraparound lower back support can provide additional support for those who need it. Stretching and exercising to promote ease and adeptness in the crawling, kneeling, squatting, and lunging positions will improve the practitioner's comfort level and execution of the work. Warming up before giving Shiatsu will prepare the muscles, reducing the risk of strain. Modifying or omitting techniques that are onerous will prevent injury.

When these measures are not sufficient, Shiatsu can be adapted to a massage table. The massage table should be lowered so that the principles of proper body mechanics can be observed: maintaining a low center of gravity (standing lunge); using leverage to lean into the client; and moving from the hara, not the extremities. Most compression, stretch, and BMTs can be done on a massage table without any special adaptation. Some, however, such as knee compression of the gluteals (hips) and hamstrings (backs of thighs), require climbing on the table. Other techniques, such as foot compression of the hamstrings with the client's leg tractioned in extension and treading on the client's feet and shoulders cannot be done for logistical or safety reasons. A future edition of this book will show how to adapt most floor techniques to the table.

Please note that for the sake of visual clarity, the photographs in the protocols do not always comply with the general instructions to complete one side of the body before commencing on the other side. Also, photographic angles may change to present an alternate perspective of the same technique or a different technique.

1

HISTORY OF SHIATSU

OBJECTIVES

- To discuss the historical development of Traditional Chinese Medicine
- To describe how Shiatsu incorporates aspects of various traditional Chinese medical modalities, including Qi Gong, Tao-Yin, An Mo, Tui Na, Dian Xue, and moxabustion
- To trace the evolving status of Shiatsu in Japan over the centuries: its prominence, decline, and reinstatement to medical status
- To identify the major contributions of leading practitioners of Shiatsu, including Tempaku, Namikoshi, Masunaga, and Serizawa, and to describe other contemporary styles of Shiatsu
- To define Qi Gong and explain its importance to the practitioner

KEY TERMS, CONCEPTS, AND NAMES

Shiatsu
Acupuncture/Acupressure
Traditional Chinese Medicine (TCM)
Huang-di Nei-Jing (Nei Jing)
Moxabustion
Tao-Yin/Do-In/Qi Gong
An Mo/An Ma/Anma/Amma
Tui Na
Dian Xue
Ampuku
Tempaku
Namikoshi
Masunaga
Serizawa
Tsubo Therapy

WHAT IS SHIATSU?

Shiatsu is a Japanese form of massage therapy that incorporates traction, joint mobilization, passive stretches, and a tremendous variety of compression techniques, including **acupressure**, which is a manual version of acupuncture. The word *Shiatsu* means "finger pressure," though fingers are not the only tools used: Fists, knuckles, forearms, elbows, knees, and feet are also used when appropriate. Pressure techniques might be static or dynamic, slow or fast, superficial or deep, depending on the client's condition. Although Shiatsu stimulates physical structures of the body, such as the muscular, circulatory, lymphatic, and nervous systems, its primary purpose is to balance the flow of vital energy or life force in the body. In this respect, the goal of Shiatsu is much the same as the goal of acupuncture, though the instruments of treatment and the therapeutic experience are significantly different. Unlike **acupuncture**, which stimulates isolated points or clusters of points on limited sections of the body via needles, Shiatsu stimulates entire sequences or series of connected points all over the body via manual manipulation. These sequences or series of connected points are known as Meridians, channels or pathways of energy that traverse the whole body like a great highway system.

TRADITIONAL CHINESE MEDICINE, THE ORIGIN OF SHIATSU

Shiatsu is part of the rich legacy of **Traditional Chinese Medicine** (**TCM**), whose origin lies in Chinese oral tradition and predates the keeping of written medical records. Acupuncture, one of several TCM modalities, is thought to have originated in China about 4,000 years ago, and acupressure—a forerunner of Shiatsu—may even predate acupuncture, since the manual manipulation of the body most likely preceded the use of instruments to treat the body (Beresford-Cooke, 2000).

Interestingly, the 1991 archeological discovery of a well-preserved 5,300-year-old corpse in the Alps at the Austro-Italian border has stimulated speculation and perhaps a little controversy about how old acupuncture is and whether it originated exclusively in China (Discovery Channel, 2002). The corpse, better known as Otzi the iceman, presented 59 tattoo-like markings on his back, legs, and ankles that correspond exactly or very closely to classical acupuncture treatment points and that were probably used to treat the pain of his osteoarthritis, a degenerative condition revealed by X-rays. Because of these tattoos, some scientists now suggest that acupuncture may be much older and more widespread than previously hypothesized, having arisen in different cultures that independently discovered its benefits.

Whatever the facts may be regarding the provenance of acupuncture, it was certainly used in China four millennia ago. Archeologists have exhumed rudimentary medical paraphernalia, such as stone, bone, and thorn probes dating back to the Xia dynasty (2205–1766 B.C.) (Jwing-Ming, 1992). These probes were the predecessors of today's acupuncture needles and were used to "pierce the sickness," according to a Han dynasty expositor. Later, during the Shang dynasty (1766–1122 B.C.), bronze probes replaced stone and bone probes, and medical observations correlating certain diseases with certain organs began to be recorded through engravings on turtle shells and animal bones.

During the Han dynasty (206 B.C.–220 A.D.), when the northern and southern regions of China united, medical knowledge passed down over the centuries through the oral tradition was compiled in the ***Huang-di Nei-Jing*** (translated as *The Yellow Emperor's Classic of Internal Medicine*). The ***Nei-Jing*** is the oldest extant text on TCM—and the classic on which exegetical treatises written during subsequent dynasties were based (Kaptchuk, 2000). In it, the legendary Yellow Emperor, who ostensibly lived between 2696 and 2598 B.C., asks his minister why there are so many different methods of treating ailments (Liechti, 1998). His minister replies at length:

> In the eastern part of this country, the people live near the oceans, eat more fish and protein, and tend to develop skin diseases. In this case, acupuncture is the most effective treatment. The western part of the country is characterized by mountains and desert. [There] the people eat more animal protein and tend to be fat. This, in turn, causes internal organ malfunctioning, which is best remedied with herbal medicine. The northern part of the country is extremely cold [and there] the people have . . . pastures for dairy farming. [Their] internal organs tend to be cold [so they] develop coughing and mucus problems. In this case, moxibustion [heat therapy] is most effective. The southern part of the country is hot and damp, where people generally eat more sour and ripe foods. They are prone to get spasms. Acupuncture is very effective in treating such conditions. In the center of the country, which is flat, the people enjoy eating without hard labor. A problem of general weakness is prevalent. So, therefore, Do-In [movement and breathing exercises] and An Mo [massage therapy] are effective. (Masunaga & Ohashi, 1977/1997, p. 10)

The minister's response reveals an important point about TCM: Environmental factors influenced the development of medicine in China. Both the kinds of illnesses and the kinds of resources available in certain regions determined the kinds of treatments that were developed and prescribed. **Moxabustion**—a heat therapy—was prescribed for people in the north, where the climate was cold and cold disorders prevailed. Moxabustion entails the smoldering of mugwort, an herb that grows like a weed in China, over acupressure points, penetrating the points with heat in order to warm the body and stimulate blood, lymph, and energy flow. Acupuncture was prescribed for people on the eastern seaboard, whose fish and salt diet generated internal heat that could be dispelled by acupuncture, and also for people in the south, whose sour/ripe diet and hot/damp climate predisposed them to spasms that could be relaxed by acupuncture. Herbalism was prescribed for the animal farmers in the western mountains, whose animal product diet induced organ dysfunction. **Do-In** or **Tao-Yin**, a type of physical conditioning, was prescribed for people of the central region, whose sedentary lifestyle and overindulgence in food contributed to infirmity. Do-In/Tao-Yin are subspecialties of **Qi Gong**. Qi Gong is a broad term that encompasses several physical disciplines and practices that cultivate vital energy and promote health, including massage, martial arts, and breathing and movement exercises.

All of these modalities, practiced in different regions, were finally integrated into the comprehensive system of medicine presented in the *Nei Jing*. Thus, moxabustion, acupuncture, herbalism, and Qi Gong became the four cornerstones of TCM. Shiatsu incorporates all of these modalities to a lesser or greater degree, though it is primarily a type of Qi Gong or physical conditioning in that it promotes health through the manual manipulation and mobilization of the body. Yet Shiatsu also resembles acupuncture when the practitioner pauses and lingers over specific vital points, providing prolonged localized stimulation, though in Shiatsu the hermetic seal of the body is not pierced because manual pressure is used rather than needles. Some Shiatsu practitioners also incorporate moxabustion into their practice or recommend a particular diet, such as the macrobiotic diet, in keeping with the herbalist tradition.

MODERN MEDICINE IN CHINA

Until the mid-twentieth century, Chinese medicine remained rooted in traditional practices. After the Chinese Revolution in 1949, the communist government strove to modernize China, much of which was underdeveloped. In conjunction with its goal of modernization, the communist government reevaluated the efficacy of TCM by comparing its clinical results to those of Western medicine. During the 1950s, the Chinese conducted thousands of experiments and clinical studies and issued numerous medical reports confirming the therapeutic benefits of Chinese medicine. In 1958, motivated by economic and cultural factors as well as positive clinical results, the government officially recognized TCM as a valuable legacy to be fostered alongside Western medical practices. Since that time, there has been a parallel development in China of both Chinese and Western medicine.

CHINESE MASSAGE

Shiatsu integrates several different forms of Chinese massage, including An Mo, Tui Na, Dian Xue, and Qi massage. These forms were developed and continue to be practiced by different vocations for different purposes (Jwing-Ming, 1992).

An Mo, which literally means "press rub," is a general relaxation form of massage practiced by laymen on the public to relieve muscle tension, reduce psychological stress, and boost the immune system (Jwing-Ming, 1992).

Tui Na, which literally means "push grab," is a therapeutic form of massage developed by medical doctors and martial artists to improve blood, lymph, and energy flow in the body and to disperse stagnation and release blockages that can lead to disorders and diseases (Jwing-Ming, 1992). Martial artists use Tui Na to recover from the soreness and fatigue caused by martial art practice and to rehabilitate injuries incurred by falls or strikes. Medical doctors use Tui Na to treat illnesses in children, since most children are too skittish and hyperactive to receive acupuncture, which requires the patient to lie still for a period of time.

Dian Xue, which literally means "cavity press" or acupressure, was also developed by doctors and martial artists to propel the flow of vital energy through the body (Jwing-Ming, 1992). Dian Xue is sharper and more penetrating than An Mo and Tui Na. Although both doctors and martial artists use Dian Xue to heal, only martial artists use Dian Xue to wound or kill. While at first it may seem strange that the same modality can be used to kill or heal, the result depends on the amount of force applied, according to a neurological law articulated by Rudolph Arndt, a German psychiatrist (1835–1900): "Weak stimuli excite physiological activity; moderately strong ones favor it; strong ones retard it, and very strong ones arrest it" (St. John, 1990–1996, p. 16). In other words, the light, moderate, and firm pressures of massage improve physical functioning, whereas the extreme pressure of martial art strikes and kicks thwarts or arrests physical functioning.

Qi massage, or energy work, technically is not massage at all, since it does not involve manual manipulation but rather the transmission of healing energy through the laying on or hovering of hands over the recipient's body (Jwing-Ming, 1992). Admittedly, this is the most mysterious of the healing arts, but it nonetheless produces demonstrative results, since bioelectricity has the capacity to regenerate tissues (see Chapter 2, which focuses on Qi). Qi massage is the precursor to all energy work, including Japanese Reiki.

THE MIGRATION OF CHINESE MEDICINE TO JAPAN

Chinese philosophy, the theoretical basis for Chinese medicine, was introduced to Japan sometime during the sixth century (538–552 A.D.), when China and Japan were engaged in reciprocal diplomatic and trading missions (Liechti, 1998). Chinese medicine was disseminated soon thereafter, though accounts vary on how and when this happened. One account suggests that a Buddhist priest accompanying a Chinese trade retinue brought Chinese medicine to Japan around 552 A.D. (Dubitsky, 1992), while another account suggests that a Japanese prince commissioned a delegation of Japanese students to China around 608 A.D. to study its culture and medicine (Liechti, 1998).

In any case, by the seventeenth century, An Mo (also known as **An Ma**, **Anma** and **Amma**), general relaxation massage, and Tao-Yin (or Do-In), Chinese breathing and movement exercises, were firmly established as a core curriculum in the study of medicine. Japanese medical students were required to practice Amma to gain proficiency in palpatory skills and anatomy, the Meridian system, and acupressure points (Dubitsky, 1992). In short, mastery of Amma became a prerequisite to advanced medical practice, including acupuncture and herbalism, as it had previously been in China.

THE CHANGING STATUS OF MASSAGE THERAPY IN JAPAN

During the Edo period (1603–1867), the Shoguns jealously guarded their heritage against Dutch and Portuguese cultural influences, purposefully shunning European traditions and cultivating Asian traditions (Liechti, 1998). As a result, oriental medicine flourished. Toward the end of the seventeenth century, a blind acupuncturist who subsequently earned the honorific title of "Father of Japanese Acupuncture" cured a Shogun of an intractable and excruciating abdominal disorder, and the Shogun, in turn, ordained Amma as a special calling for the blind (Dubitsky, 1992). As a side note to this unusual incident, in Asian countries the blind have historically enjoyed preferred entry into and status in bodywork because their lack of the dominant sense of sight is assumed to enhance their tactile sensitivity and palpatory skill, and a blind practitioner offers the additional advantage of preserving client modesty.

During the Meiji period (1867–1911), European traders introduced Western medicine to Japan, including surgical procedures and methods of controlling contagious diseases, which the ruling class adopted to the exclusion of Asian healing arts (Dubitsky, 1992). Because of the aristocracy's ban on Asian medicine, Amma was loosed from its medical moorings and downgraded to a luxury service. It gradually declined in terms of technical standards and esteem until eventually it was relegated to bathhouse status, incurring some of the same sensual, nonclinical connotations as massage parlors in the West (Sasaki, 2005). In spite of this, one form of Amma, **Ampuku**, or abdominal massage, continued to be practiced within its medical context, especially for obstetric and gynecological conditions (Liechti, 1998).

In 1919, Tamai **Tempaku,** a serious practitioner of Amma, Ampuku, and Do-In who also studied Western anatomy and physiology, published an influential book entitled *Shiatsu Ho*. In it, he integrated Asian healing arts with Western anatomy and physiology, catalyzing a renaissance in the profession (Liechti, 1998; Dubitsky, 1992). This spurred others who practiced Amma as a medical modality to rename it *Shiatsu,* meaning "finger pressure," to distinguish their therapy from pleasure services, to increase their credibility, and to circumvent the restrictive regulations of the bathhouse "shampoo" massage. Two of Tempaku's students, Tokujiro Namikoshi and Katsusuke Serizawa, became prominent Shiatsu educators in their own right, and another student was mother to Shizuto Masunaga, who also became a renowned Shiatsu instructor (Dubitsky, 1992).

CONTRIBUTIONS OF MODERN PRACTITIONERS OF SHIATSU

Shiatsu came to be officially recognized and disseminated worldwide largely due to the effort of **Namikoshi** (1905–2000), a very gifted healer. He established a training institute in Hokkaido in 1925 and another in Honshu in 1940 after a famous and wealthy patient of his insured Namikoshi's thumbs (Figure 1-1) for 100,000 yen—an

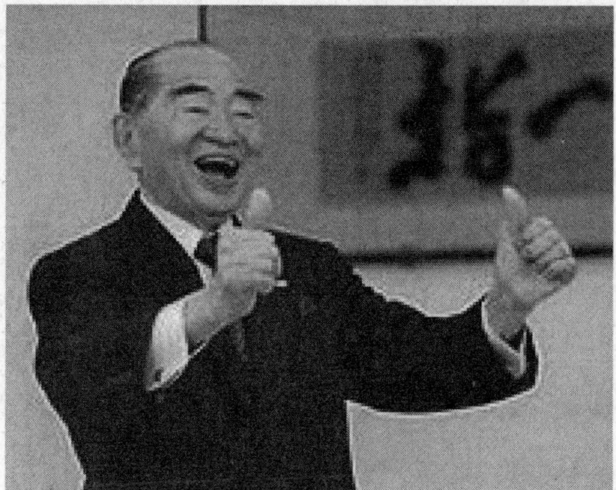

FIG 1-1 Tokujiro Namikoshi presenting his unusually large thumbs. With kind permission from Japan Shiatsu College.

astronomical sum in those days, equivalent to about $10 million—in gratitude for healing his chronic back pain, a condition that almost prevented him from keeping a public engagement (Dubitsky, 1992; Saito, 2004). Namikoshi had studied Amma for the sole purpose of obtaining a license to practice, but he also experimented with techniques and developed his own style of bodywork, and he persistently petitioned the government to recognize Shiatsu throughout his career.

An unexpected publicity boon came in 1953, when Namikoshi healed American movie star Marilyn Monroe of a life-threatening illness that defied Western medical treatment while she was in Japan on her honeymoon (Dubitsky, 1992). News of the healing spread throughout Japan, and the following year the government recognized Shiatsu as a valid and legitimate therapy, albeit as a subspecialty of Amma, which still had the reputation of folk medicine and which lacked the scientific rigor that Namikoshi hoped to establish for his modality.

In his efforts to disassociate Shiatsu from Amma and to obtain independent recognition for Shiatsu as a modern therapy corroborated by science, Namikoshi Westernized Shiatsu. He eliminated all references to the Chinese medical model and cast Shiatsu within a Western theoretical framework, explaining its benefits in terms of Western anatomy and physiology—the muscular, skeletal, nervous, and endocrine systems—not in terms of vital energy flowing through Meridians. This can be observed in the book *The Complete Book of Shiatsu Therapy*, written by his son, Toru, who carried on his father's work (T. Namikoshi, 1981/1987).

According to one source, Namikoshi's version of Shiatsu may have influenced Dr. Janet Travell's formulation of Trigger Point Therapy, which, in turn, influenced British and American forms of neuromuscular therapy (Dubitsky, 1992). Certainly, Namikoshi's version of Shiatsu has had a major influence on chiropractic, particularly in the use of pressure point therapy to release muscle tension, reduce pain and dysfunction, and facilitate and maintain skeletal adjustments. However, this influence may well have been reciprocal. In 1953, Dr. Bartlett Joshua (B. J.) Palmer invited Namikoshi to his school of chiropractic in Iowa to share his expertise (Figure 1-2). Namikoshi's son Toru accompanied him and remained there for another seven years, studying chiropractic and anatomy, after which he returned to

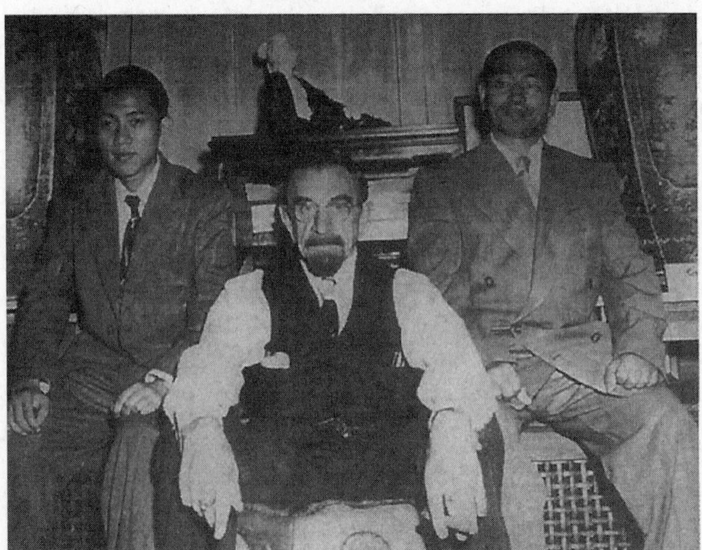

FIG 1-2 Namikoshi at the Palmer School of Chiropractic in Iowa, 1953. Pictured from left to right are Namikoshi's son Toru, who continued his work; Dr. Bartlett Joshua (B. J.) Palmer; and Namikoshi himself. With kind permission from Japan Shiatsu College.

Japan to supplement the curriculum at the Japan Shiatsu College (M. Namikoshi, 2004; Ikenaga, 2004).

In 1964, Namikoshi's lobbying finally succeeded when the Japanese Ministry of Health and Welfare recognized Shiatsu as a distinct medical modality, not just to comfort, soothe, and give pleasure, as in general relaxation massage, but also to heal bodily dysfunctions and treat particular maladies (T. Namikoshi, 1987) according to this official statement:

> Shiatsu therapy is a form of manipulation administered by the thumbs, fingers, and palms, without the use of any instrument, mechanical or otherwise, to apply pressure to the human skin, to correct internal malfunctioning, to promote and maintain health, and to treat specific diseases. (Masunaga & Ohashi, 1977/1997, p. 17)

Shizuto **Masunaga** (1925–1981), a graduate of and later a professor of psychology at Namikoshi's school, eventually opened his own school and restored Shiatsu to its Asian heritage (Henderson, 2004; M. Namikoshi, 2004). In contrast to Toru Namikoshi's book, Masunaga's book *Zen Shiatsu: How to Harmonize Yin and Yang for Better Health* is based on the Chinese medical model, emphasizing the flow and balance of Qi in the body and the physiological and psychological associations of Meridians (Masunaga, & Ohashi, 1977/1997). Supplementing thumb, finger, and palm pressure (Figure 1-3 and 1-4), Masunaga's style incorporates forearm, elbow, and knee pressure (Figure 1-5), as well as Meridian stretches and the Mother/Son hand technique, in which one hand applies stationary pressure while the other hand applies dynamic pressure through a series of traveling compressions. In giving Shiatsu, Masunaga emphasized the subtle, energetic connection between the practitioner and the recipient, and the goal of a sense of oneness. Masunaga propounded concepts and skills derived from TCM, including the concept of Kyo/Jitsu (literally "empty/full") energetic imbalances and tonification and sedation techniques used to treat these imbalances. Finally, he charted additional Meridians to supplement the classical ones.

Interestingly, Namikoshi's style is more popular in Japan, reflecting the general trend toward Westernization, and especially scientific empiricism, whereas Masunaga's style is more popular in the West, reflecting an interest in Eastern philosophy and medicine. In Japan, the term *Shiatsu* primarily refers to Namikoshi's style of Shiatsu, also known as Nippon-style Shiatsu; in the Western world, the term *Shiatsu* primarily refers to Masunaga's style, or any style anchored in TCM.

Another important practitioner in the development of Shiatsu is Katsusuke **Serizawa**, who was awarded a Doctor of Medicine degree in 1961 in honor of his experimental research during the 1950s. Serizawa used modern electrical equipment to confirm the location and function of acupressure points, empirically proving their existence as loci of high electrical conductivity and low electrical resistance relative to the rest of the body. In his book *Tsubo: Vital Points for Oriental Therapy,* he covers a variety of modalities, including acupressure, moxabustion, magnets, and even simple domestic treatments using bristle brushes, blow dryers, hot packs, and paraffin baths to treat specific ailments (1976/2000). He explains the benefits of his Tsubo Therapy using the nerve reflex arc theory. **Tsubo Therapy** is the forerunner of modern acupressure, which focuses on stimulating individual points or clusters of points rather than entire Meridians, as in Shiatsu.

One modern version of acupressure is Jin Shin Do® Bodymind Acupressure™, developed by psychotherapist Iona Marsaa Teeguarden, which applies Reichian segmental theory to the practice of acupressure for the purpose of releasing chronic emotionally-charged tension patterns known as body armoring.

One last event in the history of Shiatsu and Japanese medicine bears recounting, both for its historical significance and for its social ramifications. After World War II, when the U.S. military began repatriating American prisoners of war, rumors

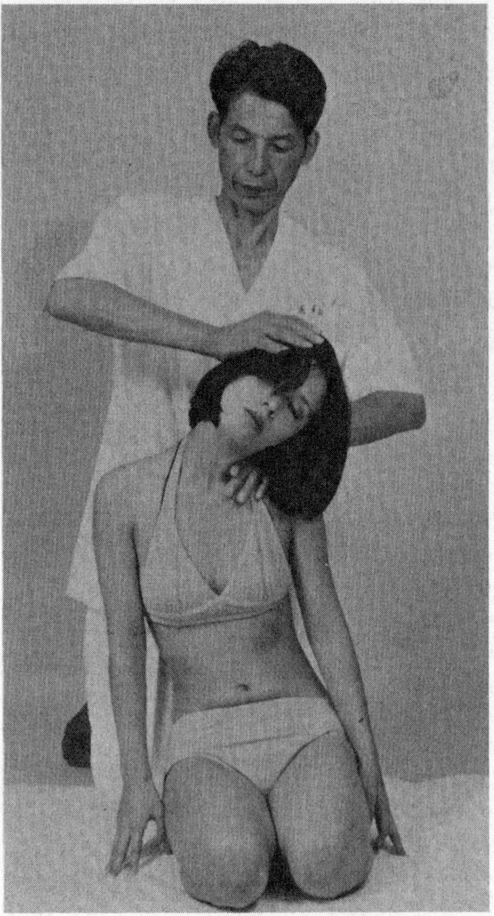

FIG 1-3 Shizuto Masunaga applying lateral flexion to the neck. With kind permission from Ido no Nihonsha, the original publisher of the Japanese language version of *Zen Shiatsu*.

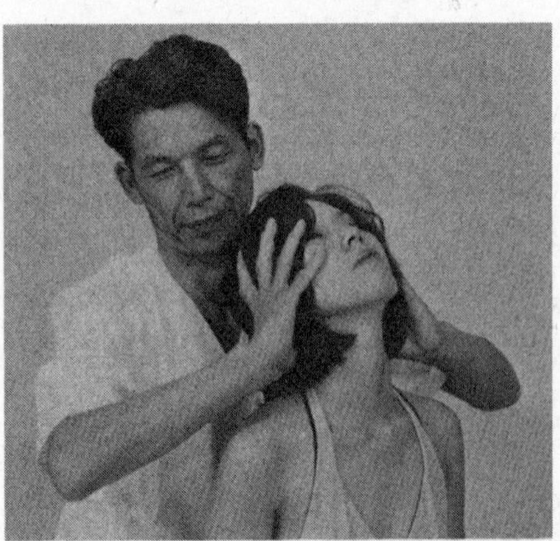

FIG 1-4 Masunaga applying extension to the neck. With kind permission from Ido no Nihonsha, the original publisher of the Japanese language version of *Zen Shiatsu*.

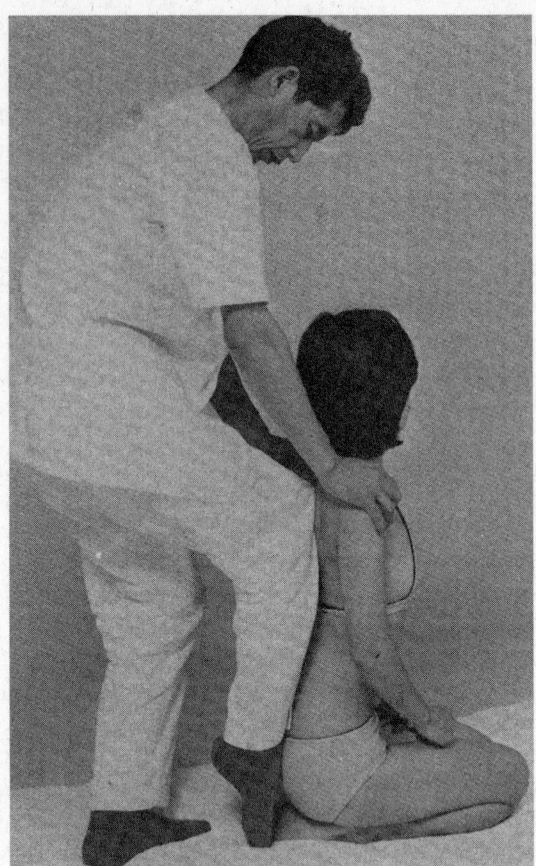

FIG 1-5 Masunaga applying a knee technique. With kind permission from Ido no Nihonsha, the original publisher of the Japanese language version of *Zen Shiatsu*.

circulated of sick soldiers who had been burned and stuck with needles (Dubitsky, 1992). In fact, these soldiers had received moxabustion and acupuncture treatments to make them well, but due to the cultural rift and postwar paranoia and hostility, these treatments were misconstrued as bizarre forms of torture. On account of this grave misunderstanding, General Douglas MacArthur outlawed the practice of traditional medicine, including Shiatsu. However, public protest secured its reinstatement. Because so many blind practitioners depended on Shiatsu to earn a living and because some committed suicide over the ban, the Japanese Blind Association entreated Helen Keller, a famous blind American and activist, to petition President Harry Truman on their behalf to rescind MacArthur's ban on Shiatsu, which he did (Henderson, 2004; Ohashi, 2001).

The Migration of Shiatsu to the West

Although Shiatsu was introduced to Europe and the United States earlier in the twentieth century, it started becoming better known during the 1970s and is perhaps just now entering public awareness through the mainstream media, which often flamboyantly depict Shiatsu as a form of massage in which the client is trampled underfoot. Today, several different styles are practiced in addition to Namikoshi's Nippon-style Shiatsu, Masunaga's Zen Shiatsu, and Serizawa's Tsubo Therapy or acupressure: These include Macrobiotic Shiatsu, Five Element Shiatsu, and Ohashiatsu, as well as some modern derivations (Jarmey & Mojay, 1999).

Macrobiotic Shiatsu, propounded by George Ohsawa, Michio Kushi, and Shizuko Yamamoto, incorporates barefoot compression techniques and advocates a balanced lifestyle and the macrobiotic diet, featuring whole grains, fresh produce, and certain Japanese food products like soybean curd, seaweed, pickled ginger, and salted plum. Five Element Shiatsu, based on the Five Element Theory of TCM, emphasizes the body-mind connection and the necessity of treating the whole person, especially the psychological imbalances associated with energetic or physiological dysfunctions. Ohashiatsu, closest to Masunaga's style, was developed by Masunaga's student Wataru Ohashi and instills a sense of practitioner poise, especially through good posture, proper body mechanics, and continuity in transitions (Ohashi, 1991).

Two modern derivations of Shiatsu are Watsu® and Ashiatsu®. Watsu®, or aquatic Shiatsu, was developed by Harold Dull at Harbin Hot Springs in northern California (Osborn, 2003). Watsu® is Shiatsu performed in warm water, with a particular emphasis on supporting and stretching the body while it is floating in a buoyant element. Although originally developed in a spa environment, Watsu® is also being used as a form of recreational therapy to rehabilitate children with brain and spinal cord injuries or congenital defects (Osborn, 2003). Ashiatsu Oriental Bar Therapy®, a hybrid of Shiatsu and Swedish massage, was developed by Ruthie Hardee. The practitioner hangs from overhead parallel bars and delivers gliding strokes with the feet, for the purpose of working deeply while conserving the practitioner's hands and lower back (Hardee, 2000–2003). Although Watsu® and Ashiatsu® arguably deviate from traditional Shiatsu, they demonstrate the continual adaptation and evolution of bodywork. Undoubtedly, more innovations on Shiatsu will follow.

Qi Gong

As mentioned previously, Shiatsu is one form of Qi Gong. In the broadest sense, Qi Gong is the study of vital energy circulating in the body (Jwing-Ming, 1992). The term encompasses many related fields, including acupuncture, herbalism, martial arts, massage therapy, energy work, breath-work, and exercise. The suffix *gong* means "effort and time" and thus implies any discipline that cultivates vital energy and requires serious dedication over a lifetime. In common parlance, Qi Gong refers to any physical discipline or exercise that develops energy and focuses the mind through movement and breath control, such as Tai Chi and Yoga.

Qi Gong is so integral to the Asian healing arts and so essential to good health and personal development that it deserves an introduction here, though a comprehensive treatment would exceed the scope of this book. The poses shown in the Qi Gong protocol (see Chapter 18) are designed to stimulate the Meridians, thereby dispersing stagnation, releasing blockages, and enhancing energy flow.

Every practitioner should cultivate a regular Qi Gong practice to maintain health, promote fitness, boost vitality, avert injury, ward off malaise, sharpen the mind, and focus and direct innate healing energy. Regular Qi Gong practice develops the strength, stamina, flexibility, balance, coordination, concentration, lung capacity, and vital energy essential for a high quality of life and a long career. Shiatsu is, after all, manual labor that can be strenuous and requires a good deal of vigor. Practitioners who abide by the life dictum of "Physician, heal thyself" will be better able to heal others.

REFERENCES

Beresford-Cooke, C. (2000). *Shiatsu theory and practice: A comprehensive text for the student and professional*. Edinburgh: Churchill Livingstone.

Discovery Channel. (2002, February). *Ultimate guide: Iceman*. Retrieved October 27, 2003, from http://www.dsc.discovery.com/convergence/iceman/evidence/tattoos.html.

Dubitsky, C. (1992). History of Shiatsu Anma. *Massage Therapy Journal, 31*(4), 109–110, 112, 114.

Hardee, R. (2000–2003). *About the author*. Retrieved August 5, 2004, from http://www.deepfeet.com/contact.html

Henderson, J. (2004). *What is Shiatsu?* Retrieved September 10, 2004, from http://www.balanceflow/BAshiatsu.htm.

Ikenaga, K. *Shiatsu and its overseas diffusion*. Retrieved September 13, 2004, from http//www.oyayubi.com/newsletter.html.

Jarmey, C., & Mojay, G. (1999). *Shiatsu: The complete guide*. (Rev. ed.). London: Thorsons.

Jwing-Ming, Y. (1992). *Chinese Qigong massage: General massage*. Boston: YMAA Publication Center.

Kaptchuk, T. (2000). *The web that has no weaver: Understanding Chinese medicine* (2nd ed.). Chicago: Contemporary. (Original work published 1982.)

Liechti, E. (1998). *The complete illustrated guide to Shiatsu: The Japanese healing art of touch for health and fitness*. New York: Barnes & Noble.

Masunaga, S., & Ohashi, W. (1997). *Zen Shiatsu: How to harmonize Yin and Yang for better health*. Tokyo: Japan Publications.

Namikoshi, M. (2004). About Shiatsu therapy. Retrieved September 13, 2004, from http//www.oyayubi.com/aboutshiatsu.html.

Namikoshi, T. (1987). *The complete book of Shiatsu therapy*. Tokyo: Japan Publications. (Original work published 1981.)

Ohashi, W. (Director). (1991). *Art of Ohashi: Volumes 1–4*. [Videocassettes].

Ohashi, W. (2001). *Do-it-yourself shiatsu: How to perform the ancient Japanese art of acupressure*. New York: Penguin.

Osborn, K. (2003 Feb/Mar). Sea of calm: Water therapy touches young spirits. *Massage & Bodywork*, 18(1), 44–46, 48.

St. John, P. (1992). *The St. John method of neuromuscular therapy: Its science and philosophy, Part 1*. Largo, FL: St. John Neuromuscular Therapy Seminars [Videocassette].

St. John, P. (1990–1996). *St. John neuromuscular therapy pain relief seminars: NMT 3 shoulder, upper torso, spinal column, and extremities*. Largo, FL: St. John Neuromuscular Therapy Seminars.

Saito, K. The Shiatsu story. Retrieved September 10, 2004, from http://www.oyayubi.com/newsletter.html.

Sasaki, P. (2005). Zen Shiatsu: An overview. In P. Benjamin & F. Tappan (Eds.), *Tappan's handbook of healing massage techniques: Classic, holistic, and emerging methods* (4th ed.) pp. 350–362. Upper Saddle River, NJ: Pearson Prentice Hall.

Serizawa, K. (2000). *Tsubo: Vital points for oriental therapy*. Tokyo: Japan Publications. (Original work published 1976.)

Teeguarden, I. (2006). Jin Shin Do® Foundation for Bodymind Acupressure™. Retrieved January 24, 2006 from http://jinshindo.org.

STUDY QUESTIONS

1. In which country did Shiatsu originate, and in which country was it further developed?
2. What does the acronym TCM stand for?
3. How old is TCM?
4. What is the *Nei Jing*?
5. How did environmental factors influence the development of TCM?
6. Identify the four main healing modalities of TCM.
7. What does Shiatsu have in common with these four main healing modalities?
8. What are Tui Na and An Mo?
9. For what purpose do martial artists practice Tui Na?
10. For what purpose do medical doctors practice Tui Na?
11. What is Dian Xue?
12. Doctors stimulate acupressure points to heal, while martial artists strike acupressure points for what purpose?
13. How can the same pressure points be used to heal or to wound and kill?
14. How does Qi massage differ from the other types of massage?
15. When was TCM introduced to Japan?

16. What role did Anma (massage) and Do-In (breathing and movement exercises) have in the study of medicine in seventeenth-century Japan?

17. Why did a Shogun ordain Anma as a special province of the blind?

18. What ultimately happened to the medical stature of Anma?

19. What is Ampuku?

20. Why was Amma (press rub) renamed Shiatsu (finger pressure)?

21. What status does Shiatsu have in contemporary Japanese society?

22. What was Tempaku's contribution to Shiatsu?

23. What was Namikoshi's contribution to Shiatsu?

24. What distinguishes Namikoshi's style?

25. What was Masunaga's contribution to Shiatsu?

26. What distinguishes Masunaga's style?

27. What was Serizawa's contribution to Shiatsu?

28. What modern form of massage is based on Serizawa's Tsubo Therapy?

29. What is the difference between acupressure and Shiatsu?

30. What is Qi Gong?

31. Why should a practitioner have a Qi Gong practice?

HISTORY TEST (20 POINTS)

SHORT ANSWER/FILL IN THE BLANK

1. The literal translation of Shiatsu is ______________________________.

2. TCM stands for ______________________________.

3. The practice of Shiatsu can be traced back to which country?
____

4. How ancient is TCM? ______________________________

MATCHING

A. Moxabustion
B. Acupuncture
C. Herbalism

D. Qi Gong
E. Qi Massage
F. An Mo, Tui Na, and Dian Xue
G. Ampuku
H. Tsubo Therapy

_____**5.** The stimulation of energy flow apart from manual manipulation or other devices, with little or no contact.

_____**6.** The stimulation of vital points with needle probing to promote energy flow.

_____**7.** The stimulation of vital points with heat penetration to promote blood, lymph, and energy flow.

_____**8.** The stimulation of energy flow through breathing and movement exercises.

_____**9.** Japanese abdominal massage used primarily for diagnosis and for gynecological and obstetric purposes.

____**10.** The stimulation of vital points with finger pressure; the precursor to acupressure.

____**11.** The stimulation of energy flow through the consumption of botanical products.

____**12.** Chinese massage modalities; the precursors to Shiatsu.

MATCHING

A. Tempaku
B. Namikoshi
C. Masunaga
D. Serizawa

____**13.** His experimental research verified the existence of acupressure points.

____**14.** He was primarily responsible for gaining government endorsement of Shiatsu.

____**15.** He reintegrated Shiatsu with TCM, reinstating concepts like Qi flow in Meridians, Kyo/Jitsu energetic imbalances, and psychological aspects of diagnosis and treatment.

____**16.** His style stimulates isolated points or clusters of points rather than entire Meridians.

____**17.** He divested Shiatsu of its Asian heritage and used the Western medical model to inform his practice.

____**18.** His style incorporates forearm, elbow, and knee pressure; stretches; the Mother/Son hand technique; and tonification and sedation.

____**19.** In addition to acupressure, he promoted the use of simple domestic remedies.

____**20.** He is considered the founder of Shiatsu and was the first person to integrate Asian bodywork with Western anatomy and physiology.

2

Qi and Meridians

OBJECTIVES

- To describe the nature of Qi: its dual manifestation as energy and matter; its ubiquitous, perpetual existence and continual transformation
- To compare Qi or energy-based healing with common diagnostic and treatment methods in Western medicine
- To identify pre- and postnatal sources of Qi; describe the five functions of Qi in the body; disharmonies of Qi; and psychological manifestations of Qi
- To locate Meridians; match Yin Yang Meridian pairs; trace the direction of energy flow in each Meridian; and describe disruptions in energy flow
- To identify the time of peak energy flow in each Meridian and correlate the regular recurrence of a disorder at the same time every day with a Meridian imbalance

KEY TERMS AND CONCEPTS

Qi/Chi/Ki
Original/Prenatal/Pre-Heaven Qi
Postnatal/Post-Heaven Qi
External Pernicious Influences/External Pathogenic Factors
Wei Qi/Defensive Qi
Deficient Qi
Sinking/Collapsed Qi
Stagnant/Excess Qi
Rebellious Qi
Jing/Essence
Shen/Spirit/Mind
Twelve Main Meridians
Jing Luo
Conception/Directing Vessel/Ren
Governing Vessel/Du

The Nature of Qi

The Chinese medical model that informs the practice of Shiatsu is very different from the Western medical model, primarily because it is premised on the concept of **Qi/Chi** (Chinese) or **Ki** (Japanese). In general terms, Qi is any kind of energy or power, including electricity, magnetism, heat, sound, and light. With respect to the human body, Qi is variously translated as vital energy, life force, electromagnetic energy, and bioelectricity.

According to the Chinese, Qi is both the matrix and the motive force of life. It gives the human body solidity and shape, and it empowers all physiological and psychological processes. Qi thoroughly permeates, animates, and constitutes a person. Thus, Qi has a dual existence as both form and phenomenon—it manifests as the stuff or substance of life and the impetus behind all movement or activity.

If this paradox seems perplexing, quantum mechanics (a subspecialty of physics) offers the particle-wave theory of light as a helpful analogy. The particle-wave theory posits that light has a dual nature: it behaves sometimes like a concrete thing having a particular locus in space and sometimes like an ongoing motion spreading across space (Columbia Encyclopedia, 2001–2005; Department of Physics, NUS). Depending on the experiment, light exhibits properties of particles, which manifest as discrete units having mass, or waves, which manifest as a continuous undulation. The particle theory is used to explain some experimental results, especially those involving particle collision and rebound, such as the photoelectric effect, in which particles are emitted or ejected when light contacts metal. The wave theory is used to explain other effects involving the reinforcement, neutralization, or deflection of waves, such as refraction, in which light changes direction when passing obliquely through an opaque object like a lens or prism; and diffraction, in which light bends around an object. These are not alternative models but rather complementary aspects of a more comprehensive, inclusive model. Hence, light is regarded as both matter and energy.

Just as light is both matter and energy, so, too, Qi is both matter and energy or, as Ted Kaptchuk, Doctor of Oriental Medicine, so aptly put it, "matter on the verge of becoming energy, or energy at the point of materializing" (2000, p. 43). When Qi condenses and consolidates, it materializes or forms matter, and when Qi disperses, it becomes energy (Maciocia, 2001). Hence, physical form is an aggregate of Qi, and energy is rarefied Qi. In the human body, Qi manifests tangibly as organs and tissues and intangibly as their functions. When the body dies, Qi is released.

Another helpful analogy for understanding the fluid behavior or versatility of Qi is the first law of thermodynamics or energy conservation, articulated in 1850 by Rudolf Clausius: "In any process, energy can be changed from one form to another, including heat and work, but it is never created or destroyed" (*Academic American Encyclopedia*, 1981, vol. 19, p. 163). This law aptly describes the continual metamorphosis of Qi. Just as matter is neither created nor destroyed but simply converted from one form to another form, likewise Qi is neither created nor destroyed but simply transformed from one thing or activity to another. For example, the food we eat and the air we breathe are converted into bodily tissues, bodily functions, physical movement, and even mental activity, or thought.

BIOELECTRICITY

While Western biologists have known for over two centuries that nerve impulses are propagated and conducted electrically (Martindale, 2004), the Chinese have taken a much broader view for several thousand years. From antiquity, Chinese medicine, and Shiatsu by extension, has asserted that the entire human body, not just the nervous system, is an energy-based system. Contemporary research is now beginning to corroborate this view that the body is buzzing with electrical fields: "Researchers have measured naturally occurring electric fields in organisms ranging from microbes to humans, and in biological systems ranging from cultured cells to embryos" (Martindale, 2004, p. 39). These naturally occurring, internally generated electrical fields appear to orchestrate, by spatial design and motive force, the growth and development of the embryo, as well as the regeneration of injured tissues. Moreover, the integrity of these electrical fields seems essential to health, since aberrations or disruptions in the fields presage the onset of dire diseases, such as cancer and AIDS, and the restitution of the fields can arrest or even reverse the progress of disease (Oshman, 2000).

In the Chinese view, the body's tissues are formed and sustained and their functions are driven and directed by metabolic processes that are electrochemical in nature. The body itself is composed of electrically conductive substances and generates an electromagnetic field and circuit through biochemical reactions of food and air (Jwing-Ming, 1992). This electromagnetic energy can be detected through various means, such as Kirlian photography, which registers electrical charges emitted by the body as phosphorescent colors (Williams, 1996).

Because the body generates and circulates electromagnetic energy and is, at least on one level, energetic in nature, it can and does respond to interventions using electromagnetic energy. Numerous research studies have confirmed that externally applied electromagnetic fields influence the way cells migrate, develop, and grow (Martindale, 2004). More precisely, electromagnetic fields outside the body induce electromagnetic fields within the body, which, in turn, catalyze, augment, or inhibit cellular and molecular processes in a cascade effect (Oshman, 2005).

Since cells do respond to electrical fields emitted by electrical devices, it seems logical that they would also respond to more subtle interventions, such as the energetic input of another human body, whether through manual techniques like massage or through the simple laying on of hands, as in faith healing (Jwing-Ming, 1992; Oshman, 2005). After all, the giver's body is itself an electromagnetic instrument capable of transmitting energy to facilitate healing. The bioelectricity in the giver's body is like a jump-starter that boosts the bioelectricity in the receiver's body, activating the process of self-regeneration.

BIOELECTRICITY IN WESTERN MEDICINE

While the idea of energetic intervention may seem strange, it is really not that alien to Western medicine. Western medicine uses many diagnostic instruments that are electromagnetic in nature, including the computerized axial tomography (CAT) scan; the magnetic resonance imager (MRI); the electrocardiogram (ECG) and the magnetocardiogram (MCG), which measure the electrical output of the heart muscle as it contracts; the electroencephalogram (EEG) and the magnetoencephalogram (MEG), which measure the electrical output of brain activity; and the electromyogram (EMG) and the magnetomyogram (MMG), which measure muscle response to nerve stimulation (Lipton, 2001; Oshman, 2005).

Western medicine also uses many electromagnetic treatments, including the defibrillator, an electroshock device that synchronizes the contractions of heart muscle cells; the cardiac pacemaker, which regulates the timing of the heartbeat; the transcutaneous electrical nerve stimulator (TENS), which controls chronic pain; and electromagnetic bone-healing instruments (Lipton, 2001), which succeed in healing difficult bone fractures when conventional treatment regimens, such as bone grafting, fail (McDonald & Bonneau, 2000; Brighton & Pollack, 1985; Scott & King, 1994). In addition, injured cartilage, ligaments, and nerves respond well to electromagnetic treatment. Preliminary research also indicates that electromagnetic therapy expedites the healing of skin wounds, though more research is needed to determine the optimal frequency, direction, and intensity of the therapy.

Aside from treatments that are electromagnetic in form and function, all medical treatments have an energetic component and could be considered fundamentally energetic in nature (Oshman, 2005). For example, ultrasound is a type of sound energy used in rehabilitative physical therapy, and laser pulses and shock wave lithotripsy are two kinds of light therapies—the former is used to treat skin disorders and dissolve blemishes, and the latter is used to shatter calcified kidney stones and gallstones so that they can pass through their respective ducts. Even prescription drugs are energetic in function, generating electrochemical reactions in the body to produce desired effects, though Western medicine has focused on the biochemical rather than the bioelectrical effects of drug therapy.

THE CHINESE IDEOGRAM FOR QI

The symbol for Qi used in Chinese medical documents has changed over the centuries, emphasizing different aspects of Qi, including the ideal state of Qi in the body, the dual nature of Qi as material and immaterial, and the two main postnatal sources of Qi. The ancient Chinese ideogram for Qi means "no fire" (Jwing-Ming,

1992). This signifies a state of energetic balance in which there is no excess, or fire, and, by implication, no deficiency. "No fire" represents a state of good health or homeostasis in Western terms.

The modern Chinese ideogram for Qi is composed of two ideograms, one meaning "space," "air" (Jwing-Ming, 1992), "vapor," "steam," or "gas" (Maciocia, 2001) and the other meaning "rice." The compound form embodies two key concepts. First, the juxtaposition of something intangible and rarefied like "air" or "gas" with something substantial and solid like "rice" expresses the dual nature of Qi as it manifests in both material and immaterial forms (Maciocia, 2001). Second, the ideogram represents the two primary postnatal sources of Qi for living beings: "space" or "air" or "gas" energy and "rice" or food energy. Obviously, the quality of the air we breathe and the food we eat affects our vitality, the quality of energy in our body.

SOURCE OF QI

According to the Chinese, human beings derive Qi from three main sources: parents who bequeath their biological heritage, air that is breathed, and food that is eaten. At conception, parents contribute **Original Qi**, also known as **Prenatal** or **Pre-Heaven Qi**, which is roughly equivalent to genetic makeup or inherited constitution. The quality of a person's Original Qi determines his or her vigor and fortitude. Original Qi can be depleted and exhausted through hard living or conserved through clean living, and especially through a good diet and therapeutic exercise like Tai Chi and Yoga, which cultivate energy flow through movement and breathing. In addition to Original Qi, a person assimilates Space Qi from air and Grain Qi from food. The Qi from these two sources is called **Postnatal** or **Post-Heaven Qi**. All together these three forms of Qi coalesce to animate and empower a person.

FUNCTIONS OF QI

In the body, Qi has five main functions: to move, protect, transform, stabilize, and warm (Kaptchuk, 2000). The movement function encompasses voluntary movement, including gross and fine motor actions, such as running and keyboarding; involuntary movement, such as respiration, heartbeat, digestion, assimilation, and elimination; and developmental processes that span a lifetime, including birth, growth, maturation, decline, and death. In a healthy body, Qi is dynamic, not static, and moves in certain directions—up, down, in, out—depending on the bodily function. Illness or disease results when Qi stagnates or is obstructed, when Qi is insufficient or excessive in quantity, or when Qi moves in the wrong direction or in the wrong way.

The protective function of Qi refers to the body's defense against deleterious environmental agents and climatic variables, such as Wind, Cold, Heat, Dampness, and Dryness, called **External Pernicious Influences** or **External Pathogenic Factors**. The body's protective mechanisms include the physical barrier of skin, an energetic barrier or armor known as **Wei Qi** or **Defensive Qi**, and other defenses such as the immune response.

The transformative function refers to the conversion of air and food into bodily substances, such as tissues and blood, or into activities, such as exercise and thought. The stabilizing function addresses the structural integrity and cohesiveness of the body and the retention of things in their proper place, such as organs in their respective locations and blood within vessels, as well as the conservation of bodily fluids like sweat. The warming function regulates body temperature in both the core and the extremities.

DISHARMONIES OF QI

Several disharmonies of Qi can arise, including deficient, sinking, stagnant, and rebellious Qi (Kaptchuk, 2000). **Deficient Qi** occurs when there is not enough Qi to form bodily substances or carry out bodily functions. For example, when deficient Qi affects the digestive organs, the result is lack of appetite, loose stools, tiredness, and weak limbs (Maciocia, 2001). In this pattern, the Stomach and Spleen are not properly digesting and assimilating food, so the body is not receiving the nutrition it needs. When deficient Qi affects the Lungs, the result is shortness of breath during exertion, cough, copious catarrh, profuse perspiration, weak voice, reluctance to speak, aversion to cold, and the tendency to catch a cold (Maciocia, 2001). In this pattern, the Lungs are not properly performing their function of extracting and dispersing Air Qi, regulating water metabolism, and resisting the elements—hence, the constellation of symptoms.

Sinking or **collapsed Qi** occurs when there is not enough Qi to hold, retain, or contain bodily substances or parts where they belong. Examples of sinking Qi include diarrhea, hernias, hemorrhoids, hemorrhaging, varicose veins, and organ prolapse.

Stagnant Qi, also known as **excess Qi**, occurs when Qi flow is impaired in some way. Rather than moving fluently, Qi becomes sluggish or stuck. An obstruction may cause Qi to accumulate and stagnate, as when a big boulder slows or blocks the flow of a stream, causing water to pool and stagnate. Stagnant Qi manifests differently depending on the organ that is affected. If Heart Qi stagnates, blood does not circulate properly, and angina pectoris symptoms arise, including heart palpitations, a feeling of pressure or tightness in the chest, a prickling or stabbing chest pain that radiates to the shoulder or down the inner aspect of the left arm, purple lips and nails, and cold hands (Maciocia, 2001). If Liver Qi stagnates, the reproductive organs are affected, and premenstrual syndrome arises, including abdominal bloating, swollen breasts, painful or irregular periods, tension, moodiness, and irritability. If Stomach Qi is in excess—usually caused by overindulging in food, eating hastily, or eating while upset—food stagnates in the Stomach, leading to a full feeling in the Stomach, acid reflux or belching, halitosis, and disturbed sleep (Maciocia, 2001).

Rebellious Qi occurs when Qi flows in the wrong direction. For example, Stomach Qi should flow downward toward the Intestines. If reversed, Stomach Qi flows upward, causing nausea, acid reflux, hiccups, belching, and vomiting. Lung Qi normally flows downward. If reversed, Lung Qi flows upward, causing sneezing and coughing.

QI AS JING AND SHEN

In addition to its five main physical functions in the body, Qi manifests as Jing and Shen. According to the Chinese, **Jing**, translated as **Essence**, resides in the Kidneys, determines a person's general physical condition, and controls developmental processes that span a lifetime, including gestation, birth, growth, maturation, decline, and death (Kaptchuk, 2000). Thus, Jing influences both the quality and the quantity of life as measured by a person's vitality, fertility, and longevity. Because of Jing's broad impact on well-being, Jing dysfunctions can affect a person's basic constitution, physical or mental development, reproductive ability, and aging process. Jing dysfunctions include hereditary infirmities and diseases, susceptibility to illness and infection, physical disabilities, developmental and learning disorders, infertility, impotence, premature aging, and age-related diseases. As a nonrenewable, limited resource, Jing can be diminished, depleted, or exhausted through an abusive lifestyle and conserved through a conscientious one, especially through regularly engaging in disciplines that cultivate Qi.

According to the Chinese, **Shen**, translated as **spirit** or **mind**, resides in the Heart and is roughly equivalent to the psyche. Shen encompasses consciousness and awareness, as well as the psychological and social aspects of personality, including the will, intellect, and emotions, which influence social interactions and relationship dynamics (Kaptchuk, 2000). The importance of Shen, the psychosocial component in health, has long been recognized by the Chinese but has only just recently been recognized in the West. As research into stress-related and psychosomatic disorders continues, more Western health practitioners are acknowledging the body-mind connection, or the role of mental and emotional factors in disease. The wisdom of Chinese medicine is that it considers the person as a whole—body and soul—in both diagnosis and treatment, and Shiatsu partakes of that legacy.

MERIDIANS

Although Qi permeates the entire body, it is more densely concentrated along certain invisible channels, pathways, or routes called **Meridians**. Unlike blood vessels or nerves, Meridians do not comprise any physical structure in the body. The concept of a conduit that has no physical structure is best understood by considering the analogy of a shaft of light or a laser beam (Jarmey & Mojay, 1999). The shaft or beam does not exist apart from light; it is, in fact, light in a highly delineated form. Likewise, Meridians do not exist apart from Qi; they are Qi in a highly concentrated, flowing form. Qi flow or Meridians are a sign of life. They exist only in a living body, just as blood and lymph flow only in a living body, not in a corpse.

Collectively, Meridians form an energy system in the body. In Chinese medicine, this system is called **Jing Luo**. Jing means "to go through," "to steer through," "to direct," or "a thread in a fabric," and Luo means "a net," "a network," or "something that connects or attaches" (Kaptchuk, 2000). Thus, Jing Luo refers to a system that transmits energy to different parts of the body, just as the circulatory system transports blood to different parts of the body and the nervous system transmits impulses to different parts of the body.

Meridians are like power lines that supply their respective organs with the energy necessary to function properly. If energy flow in a Meridian is deficient, the associated organ will be hypoactive or sluggish, and its function will be disrupted or impaired. Conversely, if energy flow in a Meridian is excessive, the associated organ will race hyperactively, eventually blowing up or burning out.

Not surprisingly, Meridians run parallel to major blood vessels and nerves in the body. Meridians, blood vessels, and nerves have a reciprocal effect on each other. Hence, where Qi flow is reduced or blocked, there is often a corresponding reduction of or blockage in blood flow, leading to ischemic (blood-malnourished), hypoxic (oxygen-deprived), hypertonic (spastic) tissues, and pathological conditions of the nerves, such as numbness, tingling, prickling, or sharp jolting sensations. Conversely, where blood flow is sluggish or stagnant and where nerve conduction is abnormal, there is often a corresponding sluggishness, stagnation, or irregularity in Qi flow.

TWELVE MAIN MERIDIANS

There are 12 main Meridians, running bilaterally on the right and left sides of the body (see Figure 2-1 and the color version of the Flow of Qi Chart at the back of the book). Each Meridian is designated as Yin or Yang, depending on such related factors as its location in the body, the direction of its flow, and the corresponding physiological and psychological functions. Yin indicates a negative polarity or feminine quality, and Yang indicates a positive polarity or masculine quality. Every

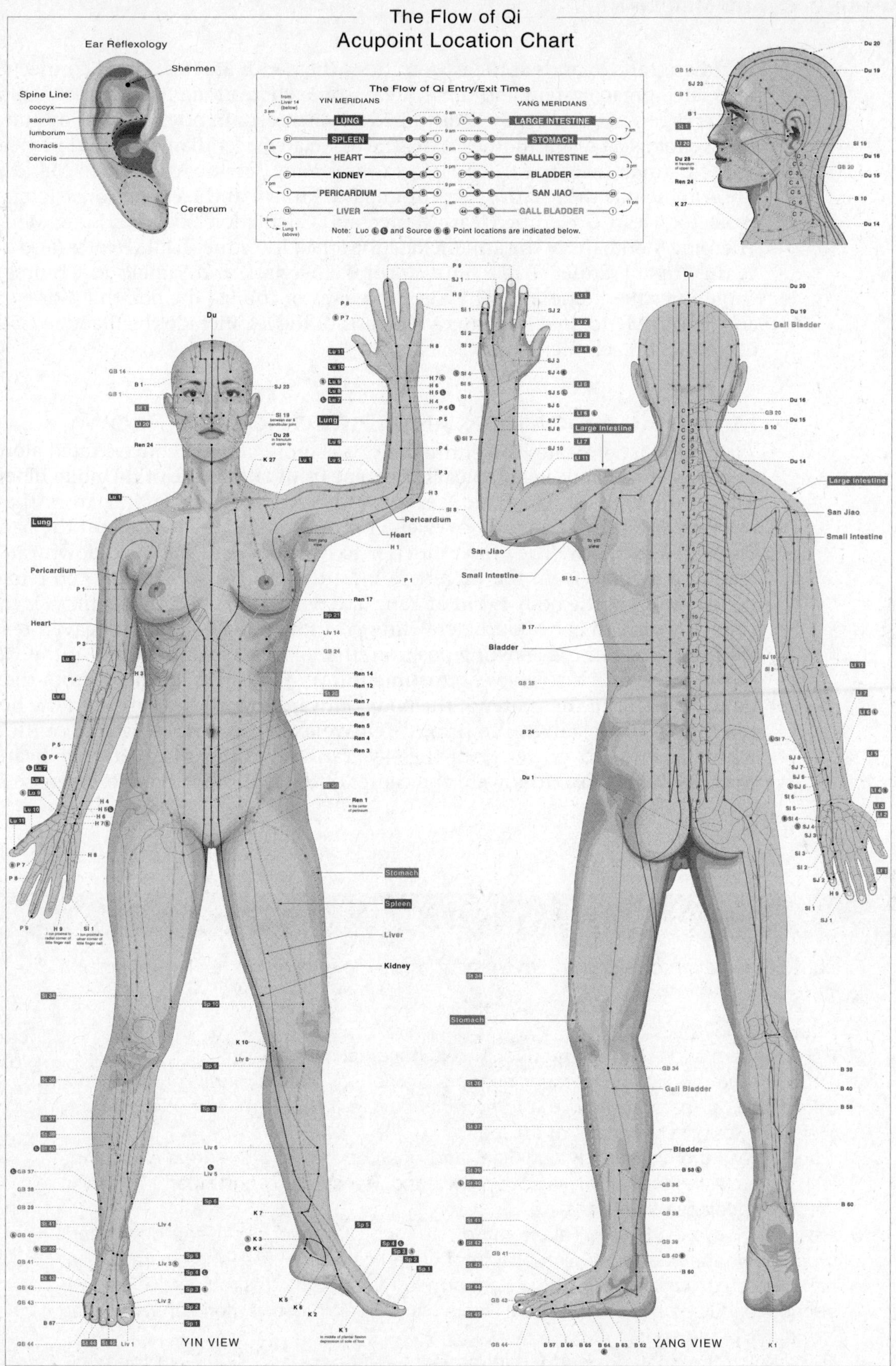

FIGURE 2-1 Meridians

With kind permission from Valentin Popov. A full size version of The Flow of Qi Chart can be obtained at www.flowofqi.com. (See Color Plate 1.)

Meridian starts or ends at the extremities—the hands and feet—and connects to an associated organ system and sense organ somewhere along its course. When a particular organ or sense organ is disturbed or when certain physiological dysfunctions or psychological disharmonies arise, the associated Meridian(s) should be treated.

Each arm and leg has three Yin and three Yang Meridians. The Yin Meridians of the arm include the Heart, Pericardium (also known as the Heart Constrictor, Heart Protector, Heart Governor, Heart Master, and Circulation Sex), and Lung Meridians. The Yang Meridians of the arm include the Small Intestine, Triple Heater (also known as the Triple Warmer, Triple Burner, Triple Energizer, and Sanjaio in Chinese), and Large Intestine Meridians. The Yin Meridians of the leg include the Kidney, Liver, and Spleen Meridians. The Yang Meridians of the leg include the Bladder, Gallbladder, and Stomach Meridians.

MERIDIAN LOCATION AND DIRECTION OF FLOW

In general, Yin Meridians are located on the front and inside of the body. They flow inferior to superior, from the feet upward, and medial to lateral, from the torso outward to the fingertips. Conversely, Yang Meridians are located on the back and outside of the body. They flow superior to inferior, from the head downward, and lateral to medial, from the fingertips inward to the torso. One way to remember which aspect of the body is Yin or Yang and which direction the Qi flows is to associate Yin with an earthbound, crawling position and Yang with a heaven-reaching warrior stance. In the crawling position, the soft, vulnerable interior is the Yin side of the body, which receives nourishment from the earth. Yin flows from the earth upward and from the center of the body outward toward the hands. In the heaven-reaching warrior stance, the firm, defensive exterior is the Yang side of the body, which receives its power from the sky. Yang flows from heaven downward and from the hands inward toward the center of the body. (See Practice Exercise 2-1.)

PRACTICE EXERCISE 2-1: MERIDIAN TRACING

To learn the direction of Meridian flow, repeat this simple Meridian tracing exercise a few times:

1. Stand in a neutral position.
2. Bend forward and touch the ground. This is the great Yin of earth.
3. Trace up the medial and anterior aspects of the legs corresponding to the inner thighs and up the midline of the torso. This covers the Spleen, Liver, and Kidney Meridians, the Yin Meridians of the legs.
4. Trace across the chest and shoulders, and open and extend the arms and hands with palms facing forward. This covers the Lung, Pericardium, and Heart Meridians, the Yin Meridians of the arms.
5. Reach up toward the sky. This is the great Yang of heaven. With the right hand, brush down the back of the left arm from fingertips to shoulder; then, with the left hand, brush down the back of the right arm from fingertips to shoulder. This corresponds to the Large Intestine, Triple Heater, and Small Intestine Meridians, the Yang Meridians of the arms.
6. Trace down the posterior and lateral aspects—the back and sides—of the neck, back, and legs, wrapping slightly around the anterior aspect of the thighs. This covers the Bladder, Gallbladder, and Stomach Meridians, the Yang Meridians of the legs.

YIN YANG MERIDIAN PAIRS

The 12 main Meridians are paired as Yin Yang couples or counterparts that share associated organs and functions. The Yin Yang Meridian pairs are best located using the seated teddy-bear position with arms and legs outstretched (Figure 2-2). In the arms, the uppermost Meridians on the radial aspect or thumb side of the arms form a Yin Yang pair: Lung on the inside of the arm and Large Intestine on the outside of the arm. The middle Meridians between the radius and ulna form another Yin Yang pair: Pericardium on the inside and Triple Heater on the outside. The lower Meridians on the ulnar aspect or little finger side form a third Yin Yang pair: Heart on the inside and Small Intestine on the outside.

In the legs, the uppermost Meridians on the front of the thighs corresponding to the quadriceps form a Yin Yang pair: Spleen and Stomach. The middle Meridians on the inner and outer thighs corresponding to the adductors and abductors form another Yin Yang pair: Liver and Gallbladder. The lower Meridians on the back of the thighs corresponding to the adductors and hamstrings form a third Yin Yang pair: Kidney and Bladder.

EXTRA MERIDIANS

In addition to the 12 main Meridians, there are 8 Extra Meridians, the most important of which are the **Conception Vessel**, also known as the **Directing Vessel** or **Ren**, running up the midline of the front of the body, and the **Governing Vessel**, or **Du**, running up the midline of the back of the body, wrapping around the crown of the head, and ending above the upper lip. The Conception and Governing Vessels function as reservoirs, regulating Qi flow in the Yin and Yang Meridians,

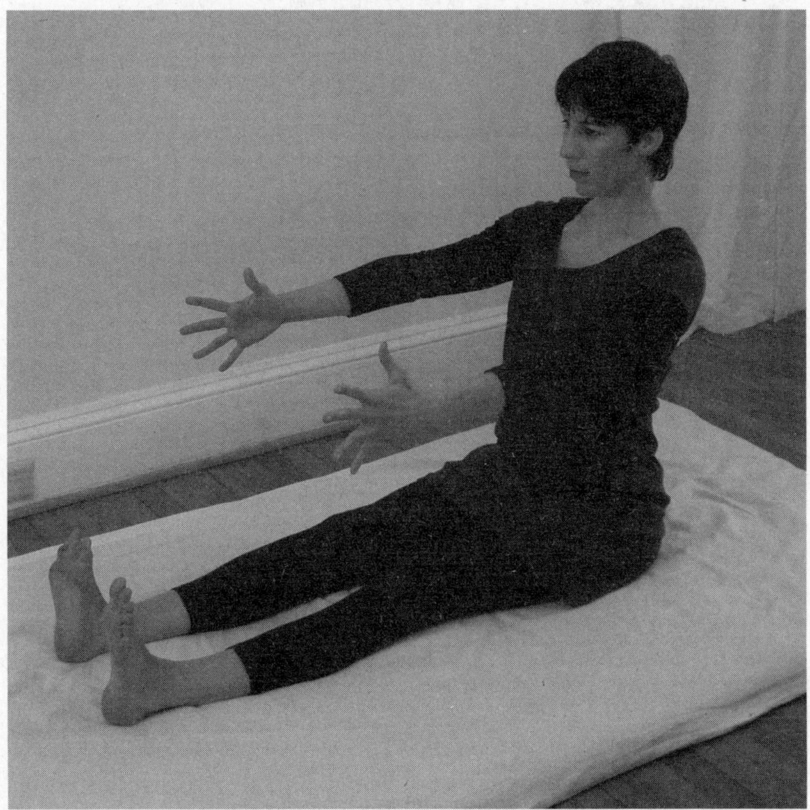

FIGURE 2-2 Teddy-bear position

respectively. These vessels drain Qi where there is excess, hold Qi in reserve where there is sufficiency, and supply Qi where there is deficiency. The Conception Vessel is associated with reproduction, while the Governing Vessel is associated with the spine and brain.

THE CHINESE MERIDIAN CLOCK CYCLE

Just as blood flows in a never-ending circuit from the heart throughout the body and back to the heart, Qi flows through the 12 main Meridians in one continuous loop during a 24-hour period. Qi flows in an orderly sequence of successive Yin Yang Meridian pairs, peaking in each Meridian at a certain time of day or night (see Table 2-1 and Figure 2-3). For a specific 2-hour interval each day, each Meridian

TABLE 2-1 The Chinese Meridian Clock Cycle

Meridian	Time of Peak Qi Flow
Lungs	3 A.M. to 5 A.M.
Large Intestine	5 A.M. to 7 A.M.
Stomach	7 A.M. to 9 A.M.
Spleen	9 A.M. to 11 A.M.
Heart	11 A.M. to 1 P.M.
Small Intestine	1 P.M. to 3 P.M.
Bladder	3 P.M. to 5 P.M.
Kidneys	5 P.M. to 7 P.M.
Pericardium	7 P.M. to 9 P.M.
Triple Heater	9 P.M. to 11 P.M.
Gallbladder	11 P.M. to 1 A.M.
Liver	1 A.M. to 3 A.M.

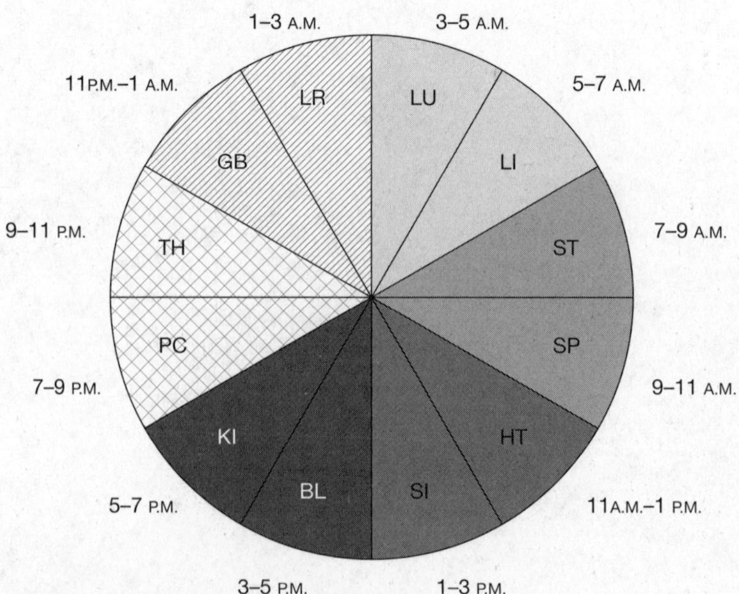

FIGURE 2-3 Chinese meridian clock cycle. (See Color Plate 2.)

supplies its associated organ with more vital energy and life force than at any other time of day. During this interval, the function of this organ is more effective and more efficient than at any other time (Demuth, 2001).

The implications of this energy flow are twofold. First, life has natural rhythms, which, if observed, promote vitality but which, if habitually violated, eventually result in distress and disease (Demuth, 2001). For example, energy flow to the Lungs culminates between the hours of 3 and 5 A.M., stimulating respiration and the capacity to receive. This is an ideal time both to engage in breathing and movement exercises to take in Air Qi and to engage in meditation and prayer to take in the divine. A stunning cultural phenomenon that takes advantage of this rhythm is the Chinese custom of performing Tai Chi very early in the morning in public parks. Literally millions of Chinese participate. Historically, in the Western world, monks and nuns arose early in the morning to commune with the divine, to receive revelation and inspiration in worship services.

As another example, energy flow to the Large Intestine culminates between the hours of 5 and 7 A.M., stimulating colon function. This is the natural time to purge wastes—to void the bowels, to scrub the body in the shower, to let go of mental baggage—in short, to empty and cleanse oneself for new input in the new day (Demuth, 2001). Energy flow to the Stomach culminates between the hours of 7 and 9 A.M. and to the Spleen between 9 and 11 A.M., stimulating digestive function. This is the best time, when the digestive organs are functioning optimally, to eat a substantial meal to fuel the day's exertions (Demuth, 2001). One "should have breakfast like a king, lunch like a prince, and dinner like a pauper," advises J. R. Worsley, but he notes that instead most Americans skip or eat a scanty breakfast, which leads to various maladies, such as headaches, irritability, fatigue, poor circulation, and cold hands and feet; conversely, many Americans typically gorge themselves before bedtime, which disturbs sleep (Demuth, 2001).

The second implication of this cycle of energy flow is that symptoms of illness, distress, or irregularity that appear at approximately the same time every day indicate a disharmony in the Meridian and the organ whose flow peaks at that time or, conversely, in the Meridian and the organ whose flow ebbs at that time, the latter being located on the opposite end of the cycle (Jarmey & Mojay, 1999). The problematic Meridian may then be given Shiatsu to promote organ function.

For example, a client who is nauseous every morning between 7 and 9 A.M. may have a Stomach Meridian disharmony that could be allayed by having the Stomach Meridian treated. A client whose energy plummets every day between 3 and 5 P.M. may have a Bladder Meridian deficiency that could be revitalized by Shiatsu on the Bladder Meridian. A client who becomes abnormally active every night between 11 P.M. and 1 A.M. may have a Gallbladder Meridian excess that could be subdued by Shiatsu on the Gallbladder Meridian. And a client who wakes up with insomnia between the hours of 3 and 5 A.M. may have a Lung Meridian disharmony that could be eased by Shiatsu on the Lung Meridian.

REFERENCES

Academic American Encyclopedia (vol. 19). (1981). Thermodynamics. Princeton, NJ: Arete.

Brighton, C. T., & Pollack, S. R. (1985). Treatment of recalcitrant non-union with a capacitively coupled electrical field: A preliminary report. *Journal of Bone and Joint Surgery, 67*(4), 577–585.

The Columbia Encyclopedia (2001–2005) (6th ed.), *S. V.* "Light"; "Interference"; "Refraction"; "Diffraction." Columbia University Press. Retrieved November 14, 2005, from www.bartleby.com/65/li/light.html.

Demuth, Sharon (Producer). (2001). *An introduction to classical five-element acupuncture: A public talk by Professor J. R. Worsley*. [Videocassette.]

Department of Physics, National University of Singapore (NUS). "Lecture 12: Waves vs. Particles." Retrieved November 14, 2005, from www.physics.nus.edu/sg/einstein/lect12.ppt.

Jarmey, C., & Mojay, G. (1999). *Shiatsu: The complete guide* (Rev. ed.). London: Thorsons.

Jwing-Ming, Y. (1992). *Chinese Qigong massage: General massage*. Boston: YMAA Publication Center.

Kaptchuk, T. (2000). *The web that has no weaver: Understanding Chinese medicine* (2nd ed.). Chicago: Contemporary.

Lipton, B. (2001). Biomagnetism and energy-medicine. *Uncovering the Biology of Belief*. Retrieved Sept. 28, 2003, from http://www.brucelipton.com.

Maciocia, G. (2001). *The foundations of Chinese medicine: A comprehensive text for acupuncturists and herbalists*. Edinburgh: Churchill Livingstone. (Original work published 1989.)

Martindale, D. (2004, May 15). The body electric. *New Scientist*, 38–41.

McDonald, M. K., & Bonneau, M. (2000). *Clinical experience with capacitively coupled electric fields*. West Vancouver, B.C., Canada: North Shore Bone Density Clinic & Biotronics Research Corp.

Oshman, J. (2000). The electromagnetic environment: Implications for bodywork; Part 2: Biological effects. *Journal of Bodywork and Movement Therapies, 4*(2), 137–150.

Oshman, J. (2002). Clinical aspect of biological fields: An introduction for health care professionals. *Journal of Bodywork and Movement Therapies, 6*(2), 117–125.

Oshman, J. (in press). Energy and the healing response. *Journal of Bodywork and Movement Therapies, 9*(1), 3–15.

Scott, G., & King, J. B. (1994). A prospective double blind trial of electrical capacitive coupling in the treatment of non-union of long bones. *Journal of Bone & Joint Surgery, 76*(6), 820–826.

Williams, T. (1996). *The complete illustrated guide to Chinese medicine: A comprehensive system for health and fitness*. Shaftesbury, England: Element Books.

STUDY QUESTIONS

1. Shiatsu is based on which medical model?
2. What unique concept informs this medical model? Describe it.
3. What is the Japanese word for energy?
4. What is the Chinese word for energy?
5. Aside from energy, which we might think of as a subtle or rarefied force, in what other way does energy manifest itself?
6. Does this energy have a beginning or end in time and space?
7. In what ways does this energy manifest in humans?
8. What happens when the smooth flow of energy in the body is disrupted?
9. Does the body respond to electromagnetic therapies? Why or why not?

10. Can massage therapy in general and Shiatsu in particular be considered electromagnetic therapy? Why or why not?

11. What does the ancient Chinese character for energy mean, and what does it suggest about the ideal state of health?

12. What does the modern Chinese character for energy mean?

13. Identify and describe the three primary sources of energy in humans.

14. Identify and describe the five basic functions of energy in humans.

15. Identify and describe the four disharmonies of energy in humans.

16. Give an example of sinking Qi.

17. Give an example of rebellious Qi.

18. What is Jing?

19. What aspects of life does Jing govern?

20. Give some examples of Jing dysfunctions.

21. Explain how various lifestyles affect Jing.

22. What is Shen?

23. What aspects of life does Shen govern?

24. How does Shen factor into health or illness and disease?

25. What are Meridians?

26. Are Meridians physical structures like blood vessels and nerves?

27. Explain how Meridians, blood vessels, and nerves influence one another.

28. Do Meridians exist in a corpse? Why or why not?

29. How many Meridians are there?

30. How are Meridians structured and paired?

31. With what are Meridians associated in addition to particular organs?

32. In general, what surface area of the body corresponds to Yang Meridians?

33. In which direction do Yang Meridians flow?

34. In general, what surface area of the body corresponds to Yin Meridians?

35. In which direction do Yin Meridians flow?

36. When Qi reaches the end of one Meridian, where does it go?

37. How does Qi flow vary during a 24-hour period?

38. Symptoms of distress, illness, or irregularity that occur at approximately the same time every day indicate what?

39. When a pattern of disharmony in Meridian flow becomes apparent, what should the Shiatsu practitioner do to address it?

40. Which Meridians does the Conception Vessel influence and how? What other associations does it have?

41. Which Meridians does the Governing Vessel influence and how? What other associations does it have?

QI TEST (45 POINTS)

SHORT ANSWER/FILL IN THE BLANK

1. When referring to the human body, the word *Qi* is translated as ____________.

2. The Japanese term for Qi is ____________.

3. Just as light behaves as both a particle and a wave, Qi manifests as both ____________ and ____________. (2 points)

4. Does Qi ever cease to be? Why or why not? (2 points) ____________.

5. What is the overall function of Qi with respect to the body-mind? ____________.

6. Identify the three primary sources of Qi for humans. (3 points) ____________.

7. Describe the moving function of Qi in the body. ____________

8. Describe the transforming function. ____________

9. Describe the protective function. ____________

10. Describe the stabilizing function. ____________

11. Describe the warming function. ____________

12. Qi manifests as Jing. What is Jing? ____________

13. What three aspects of life does Jing govern? (3 points) ____________.

14. To what extent is Jing a depletable or renewable resource? ____________

15. Qi also manifests as Shen. What is Shen? ____________

16. What two aspects of life does Shen govern? (2 points) ____________

17. How does Shen influence health? ____________

TRUE OR FALSE. CIRCLE THE CORRECT ANSWER.

True False **18.** Traditional Chinese Medicine recognizes the interdependence of body and mind in health and disease.

True False **19.** Like Western medicine, Shiatsu focuses exclusively on the body.

True False **20.** Nausea, acid reflux, hiccups, belching, and vomiting are all examples of rebellious Lung Qi.

True False **21.** Hemorrhoids are an example of a failure in the stabilizing function of Qi.

True False **22.** Weakness and frailty, mental retardation, the inability to conceive, and premature balding, graying, and senility are all examples of Jing disharmonies.

True False **23.** The ancient Chinese character for Qi means "no fire," indicating a state of energetic balance in the body, with neither excess nor deficiency.

True False **24.** Like blood vessels and nerves, Meridians are actual physical structures in the body.

True False **25.** Just as a shaft or beam of light cannot exist apart from light, so also Meridians cannot exist apart from Qi.

True False **26.** Meridians exist in a corpse.

True False **27.** In general, Meridians run parallel to the routes of major blood vessels and nerves.

True False **28.** Where Qi flow is compromised (e.g., reduced or blocked), there is often a corresponding compromise in blood flow or in nerve conduction.

True False **29.** All 12 main Meridians are unilateral, running on one side of the body.

True False **30.** Meridians are coupled in Yin Yin and Yang Yang pairs.

True False **31.** In Chinese medicine, each of the 12 main Meridians is associated with a particular organ or organ system.

True False **32.** Meridians are associated only with physiological functions.

True False **33.** In general, Yang Meridians are located on the front and inside of the body, whereas Yin Meridians are located on the back and outside of the body.

True False **34.** The flow of Qi along Yin Meridians is from the feet upward and from the torso outward to the hands, whereas the flow along Yang Meridians is from the head downward and from the hands inward toward the torso.

True False **35.** Symptoms of a disorder that regularly appear at the same time every day indicate an imbalance or disharmony in the Meridian whose Qi flow peaks or ebbs at that time.

True False **36.** Sanjaio is the Chinese name for the Triple Heater, Triple Burner, or Triple Warmer Meridian.

True False **37.** Sanjaio corresponds to an organ in Western medicine.

True False **38.** Other names for the Pericardium Meridian are Heart Constrictor, Heart Protector, and Heart Governor.

3

YIN YANG

OBJECTIVES

- To explain the meaning of the *Tai Chi* symbol of Taoist philosophy
- To describe the basic nature of Yin and Yang
- To correlate qualities and phenomena in nature and the human body-mind with Yin or Yang
- To contrast the Western analytical, causal view of polar opposites with the Eastern holistic view of complementary, dependent opposites
- To discuss the relative nature of Yin Yang within a larger context or framework and at a more refined level of analysis
- To explain Yin Yang dynamics: how they create, control, and transform into each other

KEY TERMS AND CONCEPTS

Taoism	Tai Qi (Tai Chi)	Yang
Wu Qi	Yin	The five principles of Yin Yang

TAOISM: THE PHILOSOPHICAL FOUNDATION FOR SHIATSU

As noted in Chapter 1, Shiatsu is based on Chinese medicine. In turn, Chinese medicine is based on Chinese philosophy, and specifically on Taoism. Chinese medicine and Shiatsu can be better understood by studying Taoism, and especially the concept of Yin Yang. **Taoism** was developed in the context of an agrarian culture and was inspired by observations of nature. *Tao*, translated as "the Way," can refer to several related concepts: the creation process, the cyclical interaction of natural forces, the law governing transformation, and the art of balanced, harmonious living. Taoist philosophy draws extensively on nature imagery to illustrate principles of life.

Similarly, the language of Chinese medicine is highly metaphorical, incorporating the nature theme of Taoism. In fact, the language of Chinese medicine, and by extension the language of Shiatsu, can be considered one grand environmental allegory that depicts the human body as a microcosm embodying macrocosmic dynamics. For example, the Chinese and Japanese often view the body as a landscape manifesting certain energy patterns that correspond to the Yin Yang paradigm or manifesting certain climatic conditions that correspond to the Five

Element paradigm. Ultimately, all diagnoses and treatments can be reduced to the basic concept of Yin Yang.

The Taoist symbol, which resembles two paisleys folding into each other, or two tadpoles chasing each other round and round, or two waves merging into each other, is an apt depiction of Taoist principles. The empty circle devoid of contents represents **Wu Qi** (Figure 3-1). Wu Qi has been variously translated as the emptiness, void, or nothingness that precedes all manifest phenomena (Lundberg, 1992) and as "primordial unity," which is "the state before the separation of polar opposites [Yin Yang] occurs" (Dunn, 1990). The circle filled with contents represents **Tai Qi** (Tai Chi) (Figure 3-2), the "Great Ultimate Source" of the universe and its manifold expressions of existence (Lundberg, 1992).

The dark half represents **Yin**, the feminine principle, while the light half represents **Yang**, the masculine principle. The curved line bifurcating the circle indicates that Yin and Yang are relative qualities that are in dynamic flux. Finally, the light dot inside the dark half is the seed of Yang within Yin: it represents the potential of Yin to turn into Yang. Conversely, the dark dot inside the light half is the seed of Yin within Yang: it represents the potential of Yang to turn into Yin.

As a whole, the Taoist symbol illustrates the interaction of complementary opposites. This interaction of complementary opposites produces the infinite variety of things, or as the ancient Taoist philosopher Lao Tzu said, "The two beget infinity." A biological example of this concept is the coupling of male and female to beget the unique and limitless variety of individual creatures within and among species. A technological example is the permutation of two binary numbers—one, representing Yang, and zero, representing Yin—to produce countless digital images and texts.

The Yin Yang paradigm of complementary, interdependent opposites was first recorded in the *I Ching* (*The Book of Changes*), an ancient text whose earliest formulation dates to around 2000 B.C.; Confucius later analyzed and annotated the *I Ching* around 500 B.C. (Lundberg, 1992). In the *I Ching*, Yang is designated by an extended solid line (Figure 3-3), indicating direction and motion, whereas Yin is designated by a breach or gap within a line (Figure 3-4), indicating space and stillness.

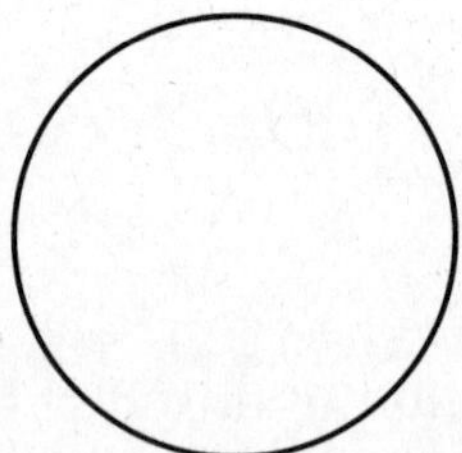

FIG 3-1 Wu Qi: The void or primordial unity

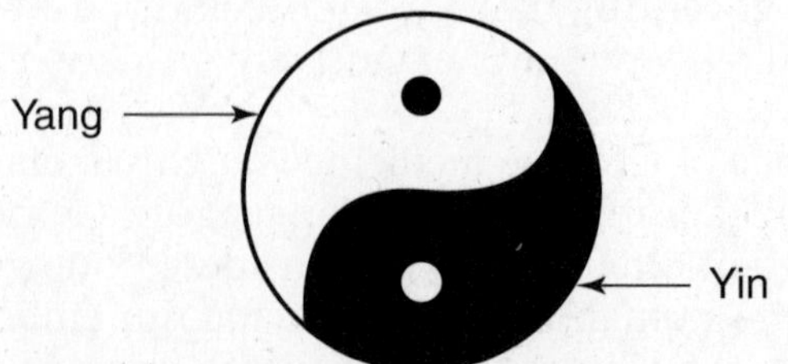

FIG 3-2 Tai Qi (Tai Chi): The great ultimate source

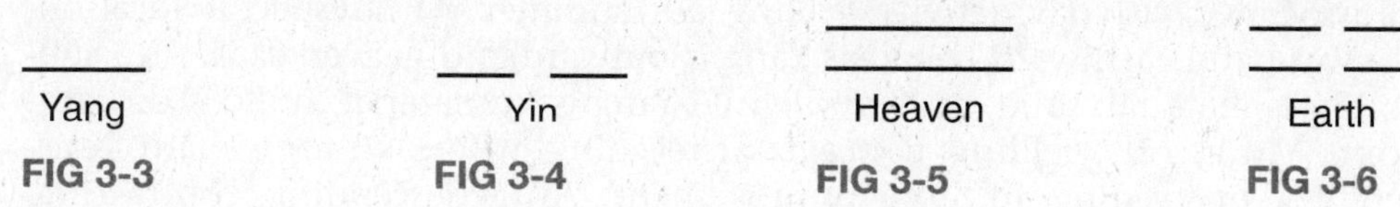

FIG 3-3 FIG 3-4 FIG 3-5 FIG 3-6

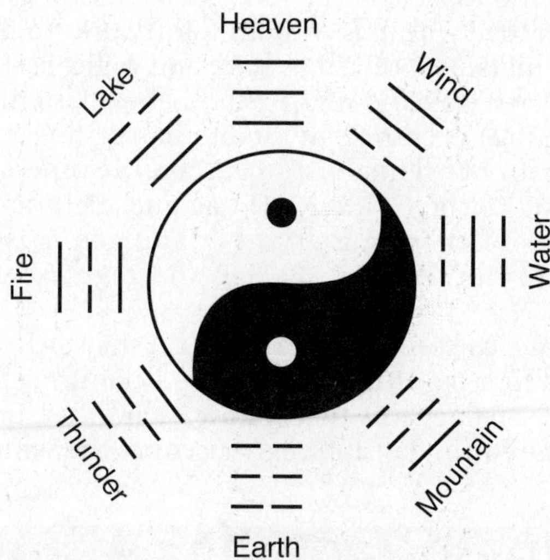

FIG 3-7 **The eight trigrams of the *I Ching***

These two lines are arranged in various triadic configurations. For instance, three parallel Yang lines stand for heaven (Figure 3-5), the creative, active, masculine principle, whereas three parallel Yin lines stand for earth (Figure 3-6), the receptive, passive, feminine principle (Lundberg, 1992). In Chinese thought, heaven and earth embody the most extreme manifestations of Qi: Heaven is the most diffused expression of Qi, and earth is the most condensed expression of Qi (Maciocia, 2001).The eight triadic configurations, or trigrams, found in the *I Ching* represent the myriad of natural phenomena in the universe (see Figure 3-7). The interplay of Yin and Yang and their material and nonmaterial expressions is the source of creation. Indeed, life and health depend on the balanced, harmonious interaction of Yin and Yang.

THE NATURE OF YIN YANG

The Chinese ideograms for Yin and Yang are emblems for the shady and sunny slopes of the same hill, suggesting the dichotomy of polar opposites within an organic whole, as well as countless correspondences of contrary pairs (Liechti, 1998). For example, the shady slope of the hill is dark, cool, moist, still, and silent, whereas the sunny slope of the hill is light, warm, dry, active, and noisy.

Using these emblems, pairs of opposites can be endlessly extrapolated. Thus, with respect to time, Yin is associated with night, rest, sleep, and winter, while Yang is associated with day, activity, waking, and summer. With respect to location, Yin is inward and earthward, whereas Yang is outward and heavenward. As a substance, Yin is material, solid, or heavy, while Yang is immaterial, hollow, or light. As a form, Yin is soft, yielding, concave, or receding, whereas Yang is hard, resistant, convex, or swelling. In terms of movement, Yin is descending, contracting, ponderous, or lumbering; Yang is ascending, expanding, buoyant, or sprightly. In terms of body zones, Yin is interior, anterior, and inferior; Yang is exterior, posterior, and superior. Manifesting as illness, Yin is pale, cold, weak, lethargic, and chronic; Yang is red, hot, strong, agitated, and acute. And so on (see Table 3-1).

The concept of opposites is certainly accessible to Western analytical thinking, which tends to dichotomize and compartmentalize. However, there are aspects of the Yin Yang paradigm, and especially the more holistic Chinese way of thinking, that are not as readily grasped within a Western framework. To illustrate the difference, let's return to the metaphor of Yin as dark and night and Yang as light and day. Westerners tend to view day and night as (1) being existentially separate, distinct, isolated events and (2) occurring in an alternating linear progression like a causal, chronological chain of events: first one, then the other, ad infinitum. The Chinese view is different. To the Chinese, (1) day and night are mutually dependent: They cannot exist apart from each other and can exist only in relation to each another. Also, to the Chinese, (2) day and night arise simultaneously, concurrently.

The Western perspective corresponds to a point on the earth, while the Chinese perspective corresponds to a point in space. From a point on the earth, day and night do appear to be discrete events that follow each other, but from a point in space, looking back at the earth, day and night occur at the same time: The side of

TABLE 3-1 Yin Yang Qualities in Nature and Humans

Quality	Yin	Yang
Time	Night, Dark, Dusk	Day, Light, Dawn
Seasons	Winter, Fall	Summer, Spring
Activity	Sleep, Rest, Dormancy	Work, Play, Productivity
Substance	Material, Solid, Heavy	Immaterial, Hollow, Light
Form	Soft, Yielding, Recessive	Hard, Resistant, Protruding
Direction of Movement	Descending, Contracting	Ascending, Expanding
Speed of Movement	Slow, Lethargic, Lingering	Fast, Frenetic, Shifting
Body Layer	Deep, Internal	Superficial, External
Body Zone	Inferior, Anterior, Medial	Superior, Posterior, Lateral
Physique	Short, Delicate, Frail	Tall, Stout, Muscular or Fat
Constitution	Weak, Infirm	Strong, Robust
Muscles	Spongy, Lax, Atrophied	Firm, Tense or Tight, Hypertrophied
Skin	Pale, Damp	Ruddy, Dry
Bladder	Frequent, Copious, Pale Urine	Scanty, Dark, Pungent Urine
GI Tract	Loose Stools or Diarrhea	Constipation
Energy Level	Hypoactive, Fatigued, Tired	Hyperactive, Restless, Agitated
Temperature	Cold, Desires Heat, No thirst, Curls Up	Hot, Desires Cold, Thirsty, Sprawls
Illness	Chronic, Malingering	Acute, Severe but Transient
Psyche	Contemplative, Intuitive	Explorative, Empirical
Social Disposition	Introverted, Sedate	Extroverted, Animated
Response	Passive, Inert, Dull	Interactive, Reactive, Sharp

the earth facing the sun is light at the same time that the side facing away from the sun is dark. Just so, Yin and Yang are not separate, distinct, isolated entities that arise and exist apart from one another. Rather, they arise together, define each other, and exist only in relation to each other.

A helpful Western analogy for the Yin Yang paradigm is Sir Isaac Newton's (1643–1727) third law of motion: "To every action, there is an equal and opposite reaction" (The Planetary System, 1987, p. 21). This law captures well the type of concurrent, dynamic activity inherent in Yin Yang: As the apple falls from the tree branch to the earth, the earth rises up to meet the apple; however, the enormous disparity in their masses makes the movement of the apple perceptible but the movement of the earth imperceptible. Essentially, this law expresses the same concept as the Yin Yang paradigm does: There is no such thing as an isolated force; forces occur in complementary and opposing pairs.

THE DYNAMICS OF YIN YANG

A full exposition of the Yin Yang paradigm includes the **five principles of Yin Yang**:

1. Everything contains both Yin and Yang qualities.
2. Every Yin or Yang quality can be further reduced into Yin and Yang qualities.
3. Yin and Yang engender one another: They are cocreative.
4. Yin and Yang limit one another: They are coregulative.
5. Yin and Yang transform into each other.

Everything contains both Yin and Yang qualities (Kaptchuk, 2000; Maciocia, 2001). Every person manifests Yin and Yang qualities physically as well as psychologically. Physically, the human body contains both Yin and Yang organs and Yin and Yang zones. In general, Yin organs are solid and produce and store vital substances, while Yang organs are hollow—food passes through them in the process of digestion, assimilation, and elimination. Yin zones of the body include the anterior (front), inferior (lower), and internal aspects (organs), while Yang zones include the posterior (back), superior (upper), and external aspects (superficial tissues) (Kaptchuk, 2000). Psychologically, a person experiences Yin emotions like sorrow and Yang emotions like anger; Yin mental states like meditation and Yang mental states like cogitation; and Yin social conditions like solitude and Yang social conditions like family gatherings, parties, and business meetings.

Every Yin or Yang quality can be further reduced into Yin and Yang qualities (Kaptchuk, 2000; Maciocia, 2001). This means that what initially appears as Yin is found at a more refined level of analysis to embody Yang and vice versa. For example, consider the zones of the torso: The front is Yin compared to the back, but the top is Yang compared to the bottom (Kaptchuk, 2000). So the chest is Yang relative to the abdomen, and the upper back is Yang relative to the lower back.

Yin and Yang create one another. This means that one arises and exists only in relation to the other. Nothing is intrinsically Yin or Yang. Something is Yin or Yang only when compared to something else. For example, hot water is Yang compared to warm water, but it is Yin compared to scalding water, and scalding water is Yin compared to steam (Kaptchuk, 2000). Cool water is Yin compared to lukewarm water, but it is Yang compared to cold water, and cold water is Yang compared to ice. In Chinese medicine and Shiatsu, determining the nature of any particular thing requires one to study the larger context or global pattern in which it occurs. The quality of a part is determined only by comparing it to other parts and to the whole.

As another example, consider height. Theoretically, tall and short fix the outer boundaries for height as a human measurement (Kaptchuk, 2000). However, taken out of context, the terms lose meaning. What is tall for a child is not tall for an adult. What is tall for a woman may not be tall for a man. What is tall in one country, Zaire, is not tall in another, Sweden. What is tall in one era, the seventeenth century, is not tall in another, the twenty-first century. The terms acquire practical meaning only in a social context where comparisons can be made. Among basketball players, tall is the norm, not a deviation from the norm, so tall is not tall but rather average in height. Yet if a few horse jockeys are introduced to the basketball team, suddenly short and tall spring into existence and acquire meaning by contrast.

The third principle—that Yin and Yang create each other—can be understood more deeply by considering how the form and function of the body are interdependent. Form, which is material in nature, is quintessentially Yin, and function, which is active in nature, is quintessentially Yang. In the body, form and function have a mutually beneficial relationship: They nourish and sustain one another (Kaptchuk, 2000). The physical form of the body engages in activity, and that activity fosters the form. For example, as organs (Yin), the Stomach and Spleen digest food, and the activity of digestion (Yang) nourishes the Stomach and Spleen with nutrients. As tissue (Yin), a muscle contracts to create movement, and that exercise (Yang) shapes the muscle.

Yin and Yang control each other (Kaptchuk, 2000; Maciocia, 2001). This means that Yin and Yang exist in a state of dynamic tension, each one counteracting or neutralizing the other. Ideally, Yin and Yang act as coequals or coregents. When Yin and Yang are in balance or proper proportion, they moderate each other's extremes, and a state of equilibrium or health results. A good example of this is the balance of Fire and Water in the body: Fire is any activity that warms and dries, and Water is any substance that cools, moistens, and lubricates.

However, when either Yin or Yang is extreme or their relative ratios are disproportionate, disorder results. If Yin is deficient, Yang even at a normal level will be in relative excess (Maciocia, 2001), and Yang symptoms, such as "Empty Heat," will arise. For example, a deficiency of Yin body fluids will result in such Yang symptoms as a sensation of heat; thirst; dry, cracked skin; scanty, dark, pungent urine; constipation, and a red complexion. Similarly, if Yang is deficient, Yin even at a normal level will be in relative excess (Maciocia, 2001), and Yin symptoms, such as "Empty Cold," will arise. For example, a deficiency in the Yang warming function of Qi will result in such Yin symptoms as cold hands and feet; blue lips and nails; frequent, copious, pale urine; loose stools or diarrhea, and a pale complexion.

Yin and Yang transform into each other (Kaptchuk, 2000; Maciocia, 2001). This principle refers to natural cycles of change, as well as to reversals of extremes. Natural cycles of change common to the rhythms of nature, such as the succession of day and night, tend to occur smoothly and gradually. But reversals of extremes in which either Yin or Yang is too dominant tend to occur abruptly and violently because an extreme imbalance in forces creates an unstable and volatile state. For example, acute illnesses, such as the flu, are often marked by violent reversals of such Yin Yang symptoms as chills and fever (Kaptchuk, 2000).

In life, a violent reversal often follows an attempt to disregard a natural cycle. Disregarding a natural cycle, such as the cycle of work and rest, always creates an unsustainable condition. For instance, if a person works incessantly (Yang), neglecting rest (Yin), the person will at some point collapse from exhaustion (Yin). The failure to respect the body's needs for alternating periods of activity and repose leads to the traumatic reversal from hyperactivity to total inactivity. Similarly, psychological rhythms, such as stress buildup and release, must also be respected. If a person does not discharge stress therapeutically, anger (Yang) may turn into depression (Yin), or continued suppression of anger (Yin) may abruptly turn into a fit of rage (Yang).

REFERENCES

Dunn, T. (Director/Producer). (1990). *Tai Qi for health: Yang short form.* [Videocassette].

Kaptchuk, T. (2000). *The web that has no weaver: Understanding Chinese medicine* (2nd ed.). Chicago: Contemporary.

Liechti, E. (1998). *The complete illustrated guide to Shiatsu: The Japanese healing art of touch for health and fitness.* New York: Barnes & Noble.

Lundberg, P. (1992). *The book of Shiatsu: A complete guide to using hand pressure and gentle manipulation to improve your health, vitality, and stamina.* New York: Fireside.

Maciocia, G. (2001). *The foundations of Chinese medicine: A comprehensive text for acupuncturists and herbalists.* Edinburgh: Churchill Livingstone. (Original work published 1989.)

Morrison, D., & Owen, T. (1987). *The planetary system.* Reading, MA: Addison-Wesley.

STUDY QUESTIONS

1. From which philosophy is the Yin Yang paradigm derived?
2. What do the dark and light halves of the Yin Yang symbol represent?
3. What do the dark and light dots represent?
4. What does the curved line dividing the two halves represent?
5. Explain the pictographic significance of the Chinese characters for Yin and Yang. (What do they mean, and what correspondences do they suggest?)
6. What temporal and spatial correspondences are associated with Yin?
7. What temporal and spatial correspondences are associated with Yang?
8. How does Yin manifest in form and substance?
9. How does Yang manifest in form and substance?
10. What kind of movement characterizes Yin?
11. What kind of movement characterizes Yang?
12. Which parts or zones of the body are associated with Yin?
13. Which parts or zones of the body are associated with Yang?
14. What symptoms are typical of a Yin illness?
15. What symptoms are typical of a Yang illness?
16. How does Western thought differ from Chinese thought in terms of the relationship of individual parts to the whole?

17. Explain why Newton's third law of motion is a good analogy for the Yin Yang paradigm.

18. Does everything contain both Yin and Yang?

19. Give an example of the aforementioned principle.

20. Is a Yin or Yang quality or aspect exclusively and absolutely Yin or Yang?

21. Give an example of the aforementioned principle.

22. Why is it necessary to view something in context to determine whether it is Yin or Yang?

23. Give an example of the aforementioned principle.

24. What keeps the influence of Yin or Yang in check?

25. What relationship between Yin and Yang indicates health?

26. What relationship between Yin and Yang indicates illness?

27. What is likely to happen when Yin or Yang has reached its maximum fullness or is too dominant?

28. Is a change from Yin to Yang necessarily a sign of disorder?

29. Give an example of transformation.

YIN YANG TEST (40 POINTS)

SHORT ANSWER/FILL IN THE BLANK

1. Yin Yang is based on ______________philosophy.

2. The Chinese character for Yin means the ______________ slope of the hill, while the Chinese character for Yang means the ______________ slope of the hill. (2 points)

3. In the Yin Yang symbol, the dark half represents ______________, while the light half represents ______________. (2 points)

4. In the Yin Yang symbol, the light dot inside the dark half represents the potential of ______________ to turn into ______________. (2 points)

5. The curved line bifurcating the two halves represents ______________.

CHOOSE YIN OR YANG. CIRCLE THE CORRECT ANSWER

Yin Yang 6. active/reactive masculine principle

Yin Yang 7. passive/impassive feminine principle

Yin Yang **8.** dark, cool, moist, still, silent

Yin Yang **9.** light, warm, dry, active, noisy

Yin Yang **10.** day, work, waking, summer

Yin Yang **11.** night, rest, sleeping, winter

Yin Yang **12.** interior, anterior, inferior

Yin Yang **13.** exterior, posterior, superior

Yin Yang **14.** immaterial substances, hollow organs, vapors

Yin Yang **15.** material substances, solid organs, solids

Yin Yang **16.** form

Yin Yang **17.** function

Yin Yang **18.** soft, yielding, concave, receding

Yin Yang **19.** hard, resistant, convex, protruding

Yin Yang **20.** ascending, expanding, light

Yin Yang **21.** descending, contracting, heavy

Yin Yang **22.** pale, cold, weak, lethargic, chronic

Yin Yang **23.** red, hot, strong, agitated, acute

TRUE OR FALSE. CIRCLE THE CORRECT ANSWER.

True False **24.** Every Yin or Yang quality is absolute; there is no Yin within Yang, nor is there Yang within Yin.

True False **25.** A woman is entirely Yin, whereas a man is entirely Yang.

True False **26.** Yin and Yang arise separately in chronological order—first one arises, then the other.

True False **27.** The Yin or Yang nature of any particular thing can be determined by examining it in isolation.

True False **28.** Newton's third law of motion—"For every action, there is an equal and opposite reaction"—is a good analogy for the simultaneous emergence of Yin and Yang.

True False **29.** A balance of Yin and Yang corresponds to good health or wellness, whereas an imbalance corresponds to illness.

True False **30.** Yin and Yang modify each other.

True False **31.** Yin and Yang are fixed, stable entities.

True False **32.** When Yin is full, it will turn into Yang, and vice versa.

True False **33.** The metamorphosis of Yin into Yang or Yang into Yin occurs abruptly.

True False **34.** The skin and hair are Yang relative to the internal organs.

True False **35.** The chest is more Yin than the abdomen.

True False **36.** A Yang psychological state, such as anger, can turn into a Yin state, such as depression.

True False **37.** A Yang physiological condition, such as fever, can turn into a Yin condition, such as chills.

4

THE FIVE ELEMENTS

OBJECTIVES

- To define Five Element theory as a dynamic, process-oriented model
- To associate each element with a particular quality of Qi, season, and stage of life
- To describe the generative, nurturing role of the elements in the Creative Cycle and to explain how Mother/Child disharmonies arise
- To describe the regulative, limiting role of the elements in the Control Cycle and to explain how humiliation/insult disharmonies arise
- To explain the significance of the Water, Fire, and Earth elements in the Cosmological sequence and its application to practice
- To identify the salient features of each element type and to correlate clinical signs with particular element imbalances
- To compare and contrast Five Element theory and Yin Yang theory in terms of historical development and theoretical significance

KEY TERMS

Wu Xing
Wood
Fire
Earth
Metal
Water
Shen/Sheng/Creative Cycle
Mother
Child
Ko/Ke/Control Cycle
Humiliation
Insult
Cosmological Sequence

DISTINGUISHING FIVE ELEMENT THEORY FROM GREEK PHILOSOPHY

The standard translation of Wu Xing as "Five Elements" is somewhat misleading because it implies that the elements are fixed forms. This connotation of fixity conflicts with the literal translation of **Wu Xing**, which is "five walk" or "five move," implying a dynamic process, not a static condition (Kaptchuk, 2000). Moreover, the resemblance of the Five Elements of Chinese medicine—Wood, Fire, Earth, Metal, and Water (Figure 4-1)—to the four elements of ancient Greek philosophy—earth, fire, air, and water—tends to compound this misconception. Greek philosophy defines its four elements as fixed material entities that are fundamental constituents of matter. Because of the similarity in terms, the Greek concepts of concreteness and permanence are easily misapplied to the Five Elements of Chinese medicine, which are not so much things as movements or progressions of nature.

Although the Five Elements can and do represent some basic components of life, inasmuch as organic life is composed of minerals and water, more accurately they represent life processes, especially cycles of change or transitions. In other words, the Five Elements point to phenomena, not things, though things certainly do

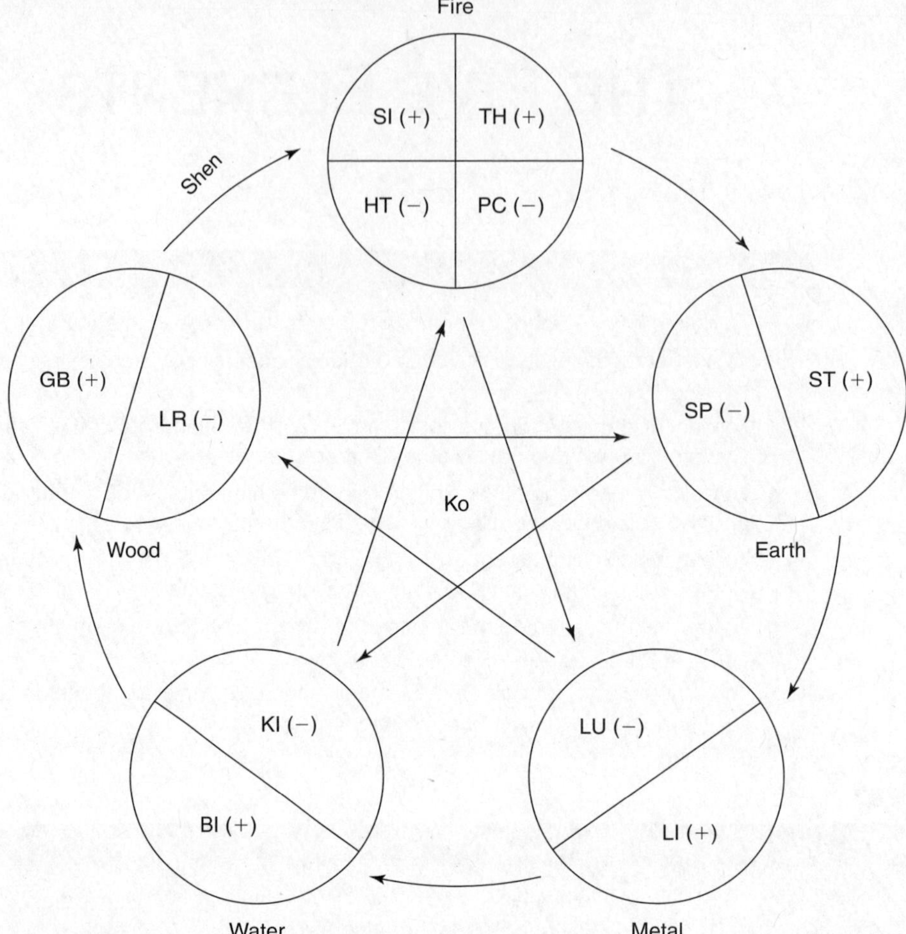

FIGURE 4-1 The Five Elements. (See Color Plate 2.)

embody particular stages or phases of development and transformation. Thus, Wood, Fire, Earth, Metal, and Water are emblems for developmental stages or phases, each of which characterizes a different quality of energy or Qi. Hence, a more accurate translation for Wu Xing than Five Elements is Five Transformations, Processes, Phases, Stages, or Transitions.

FIVE ELEMENT THEORY

Although the elements appear stable in form, like all things they are essentially mutable—subject to change. As emblems, the Five Elements capture permanence within transience, fixity within mutation. A good analogy is a photo album chronologically documenting a person's life. Each photo freezes the person at a particular stage of development—infant, child, youth, adult, senior—but the person is actually changing constantly, albeit imperceptibly. The individual is in transit, passing through each stage, transforming before the very lens shutter that immortalizes him as he is for a brief moment. The snapshot of how he appears is accurate in that it represents his energetic profile at any given time but inaccurate in that it does not reflect what his energetic profile was or will become, the full range of his energetic being. In this way, the Five Elements are freeze-frames or snapshots of energetic states that are actually in flux, waxing or waning within a cycle of change.

Another good analogy from the field of science is the first law of thermodynamics, which was introduced in the discussion of Qi in Chapter 2: "In any process, energy can be changed from one form to another (including heat and work), but it is never created or destroyed" (*Academic American Encyclopedia*, 1981, vol.19, p.163). This law summarizes the operation of the Five Elements in the Creative Cycle: Qi transforms from one element to another, from one energetic state or quality to another, in an orderly sequence, but it is never diminished or destroyed. For example, the energy in the sun is converted into plant life through the process of photosynthesis; a plant grows, matures, declines, dies, returns to the soil to nourish another plant, and so on, ad infinitum. At every stage in the life cycle of the plant, its energy manifests in a different form: a seed, a sprout, a leaf, a bud, a flower, a fruit, and back to a seed. Each of the Five Elements depicts the quality of energy in a particular stage of the life cycle.

THE SHEN (CREATIVE) CYCLE

Wood represents the growth phase and is associated with spring and childhood. **Fire** represents the culmination of growth and is associated with summer and adolescence. Both Wood energy and Fire energy are kinetic, ascending, and centrifugal—they expand upward and outward. However, Wood is growing Yang, Yang that is increasing, while Fire is utmost Yang, Yang that is maximal or full (Kaptchuk, 2000). **Earth** represents maturity and is associated with Indian summer or the end of each season and adulthood. Earth energy is neutral, balanced, centered, and stable. It is poised or suspended between the upward and outward energy of Wood and Fire and the downward and inward energy of Metal and Water. **Metal** represents decline and is associated with autumn and middle age. **Water** represents the dormant phase and is associated with winter, old age, and death or the afterlife. Water energy is latent, held in reserve like stored potential. Both Metal energy and Water energy are descending and centripetal—they contract downward and inward. However, Metal is growing Yin, Yin that is increasing, while Water is utmost Yin, Yin that is maximal or full (Kaptchuk, 2000).

This sequence is called the **Shen (Sheng)** or **Creative Cycle** (Figure 4-2) and is often illustrated using the seasons of nature or the seasons of life. In the Shen Cycle, each element fosters and generates the next. Thus, the Shen Cycle depicts the elements in nourishing or supportive relationships. The element that plays a supportive role is called the **Mother**, while the element that is nourished is called the **Child** (Kaptchuk, 2000). Just as a mother pours her life into her child—sustains the child with her own flesh during pregnancy and supports the child physically and psychologically long thereafter—so, too, each element pours its energy into and yields its life to the next element. A helpful mnemonic device for remembering the order of the elements in the Shen Cycle is as follows: Wood fuels Fire; Fire's ashes furnish Earth; Earth's minerals condense into Metal; Metal melts into Water, a liquid state, or alternatively, Metal cools and condenses Water; and Water irrigates Wood. The phases of the Shen Cycle are not necessarily equal in duration; a phase may be prolonged or brief.

Dysfunctions in the Shen Cycle can occur, usually resulting in deficiency but sometimes in excess. When an element is imbalanced, the source of the problem may be the element itself or the Mother element. For example, when the Mother element is deficient, the Mother cannot properly nourish the Child, and the Child element will become deficient, too (Kaptchuk, 2000). In cases of deficiency, then, it may be necessary to treat not only the Child element, but also the Mother element, which is not fulfilling its nurturing role. For instance, if the Wood element is deficient because its Mother, the Water element, is deficient, the practitioner should

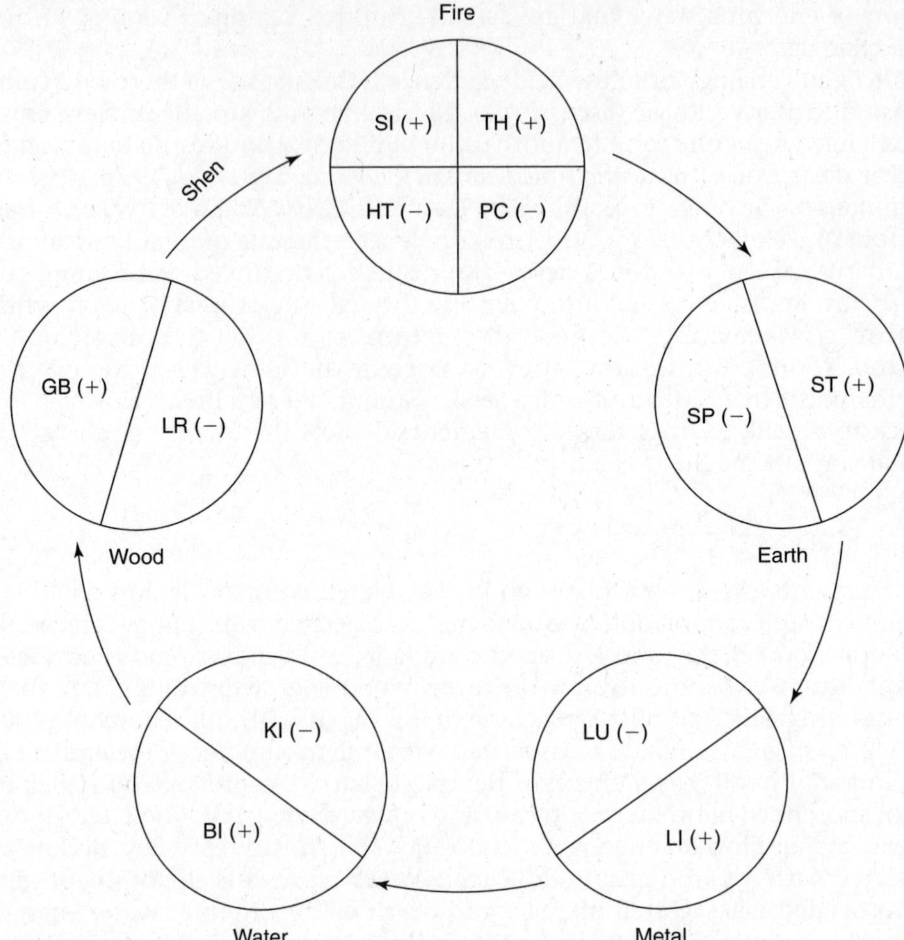

FIGURE 4-2 **The Shen or Creative Cycle.** (See Color Plate 2.)

tonify—use nourishing techniques on—the Meridians associated with Wood and Water. An example of this disharmony is a Liver Yin deficiency caused by a Kidney Yin deficiency (Maciocia, 2001). Conversely, if the Child element is deficient and needy, it may burden and drain energy from the Mother element, making the Mother element deficient also. In this case as well, the practitioner should tonify both Child and Mother.

Less common in the Shen Cycle is the dysfunction that results in excess. When the Mother element is excessive, it will transfer its excess to the Child element, and the Child element will become excessive, too. In this case, both Mother and Child should be sedated or calmed. This treatment principle comports with the "problem parent, problem child" syndrome in psychology and counseling, which recognizes that some family dysfunctions are not individual but relational in nature. Giving therapy to the problem child is not sufficient when the problem parent is instrumental in precipitating or perpetuating the crisis. To effectively treat one, both must be treated.

THE KO (CONTROL) CYCLE

Moderating or counteracting the Shen Cycle is the **Ko (Ke)** or **Control Cycle** (Figure 4-3). The Ko Cycle depicts the elements in regulatory or antagonistic relationships. Newton's third law of motion provides a useful scientific analogy: "To

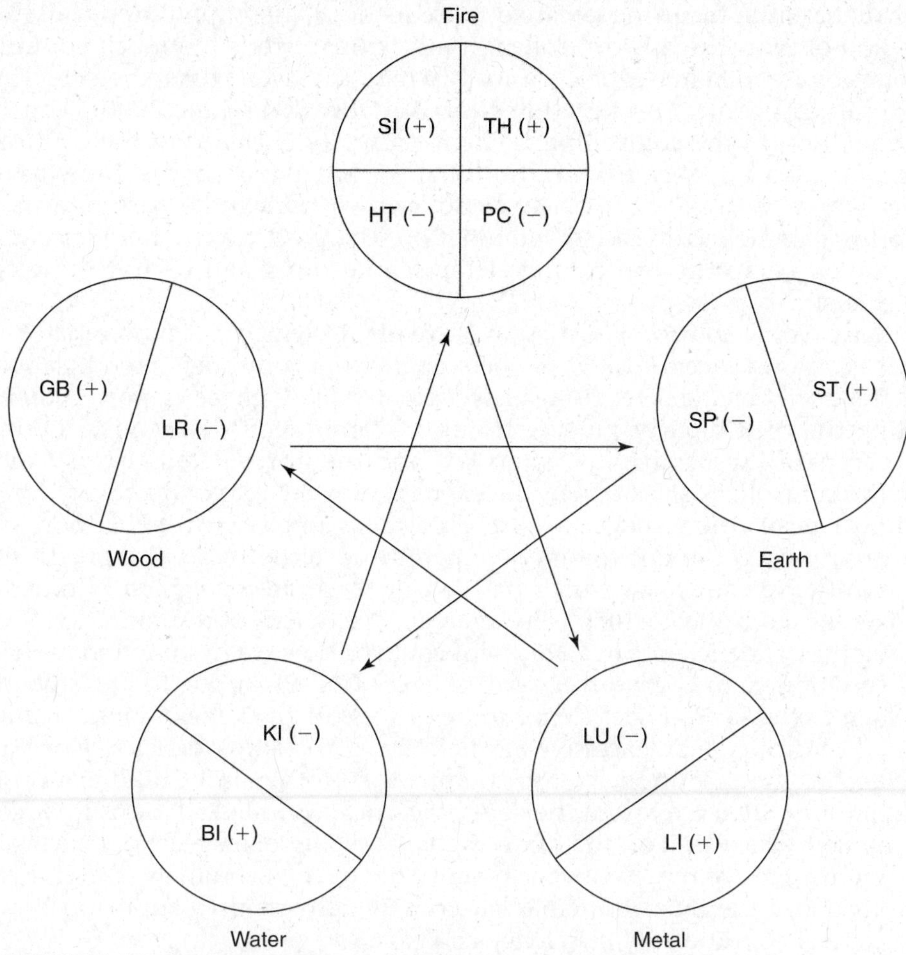

FIGURE 4-3 The Ko or Control Cycle. (See Color Plate 3.)

every action, there is an equal and opposite reaction" (*The Planetary system*, 1987, p. 21). This law of reciprocal resistance provides stability; without it, forces would be unbridled.

Another analogy for the necessity of counteractive forces is the principle of checks and balances of political power in a republic—the vertical separation of political power into federal and state governments and the horizontal separation of federal power into legislative, executive, and judicial branches so that power does not "accumulate in the same hands," leading to "tyranny" (Hamilton, Madison, & Jay, 1787/1961, no. 47). Just as people are set against each other to balance political power, so, too, the elements are set against each other to balance natural power. Each element restrains the operation of another and is, in turn, restrained so that the whole system functions well.

The restraining or limiting function of the elements in the Ko Cycle is necessary to maintain balance or equilibrium among the elements in the Shen Cycle, ensuring that no element is overgenerated, becoming too dominant and suppressing the others (Kaptchuk, 2000). A helpful mnemonic device for remembering which element controls which is as follows: Wood penetrates, pries apart, or holds together Earth; Earth blocks, dams, or channels Water; Water extinguishes Fire; Fire melts Metal; and Metal cuts or chops Wood.

The Ko Cycle can develop dysfunctions. Control, like any form of power, must be exercised in moderation to be beneficial. Both excessive control and lack of control are harmful, incurring negative consequences—the suppression, cessation, or rebellion of that which is controlled. If an element exerts too much control, it may compromise, debilitate, or even incapacitate the overregulated element; the Chinese call this control dysfunction **humiliation** (Kaptchuk, 2000). Thus, an excess condition in the controlling element causes a deficiency in the controlled element. A good analogy for the humiliation imbalance is the brow-beaten teenager whose personality is meek, timid, and withdrawn because of a harsh, overbearing parent. In the case of humiliation, the practitioner should sedate or reduce the excess in the controlling element and tonify and reinforce the controlled element.

Another possible control dysfunction is **insult**, in which the subordinated element rebels against its controller. In one scenario, the controller is too harsh, and the overregulated element rebels against the controller's abuse of power, thereby inhibiting the controller or putting it out of commission (Kaptchuk, 2000). In another scenario, the controller is too lax, and the unregulated element rebels against the controller's slackness in the exercise of power. A good analogy for the insult imbalance is the teenager who rebels against an overly strict, authoritarian parent or an overly lenient, permissive parent. In either case, the practitioner should tonify the controller, which has become weak in its regulatory function, and sedate the controlled, which is hyperactive due to lack of restraint.

To recapitulate, deficiency in an element could be due to a dysfunction in the Ko Cycle—specifically, an overbearing, excessive controller—or due to a dysfunction in the Shen Cycle—a weak, deficient Mother. Excess in an element could be due to a deficient controller or an excessive Mother. Hence, to address deficiency or excess in an element, the practitioner must examine the Mother and Child relationship according to the Shen Cycle and the controller and controlled relationship according to the Ko Cycle. Based on the findings, how the Meridians feel, and what signs and symptoms the client presents, the practitioner treats accordingly (see Chapter 6 on Kyo Jitsu and the Eight Principle Patterns for further instructions on how to assess and treat conditions of deficiency and excess).

THE COSMOLOGICAL SEQUENCE

In addition to the Shen and Ko Cycles, there is yet another sequence—the **Cosmological sequence** (Figure 4-4)—to consider. The relative positions of the elements in this sequence highlight important concepts in Chinese medicine that are not apparent in the other cycles. In the Cosmological sequence, Water forms the base, Fire the apex, and Earth the center. Ascribing a direction to each element in the diagram, Water is below; Wood is to the left; Fire is above; Metal is to the right; and Earth is in the center.

What this arrangement reveals is that Water is the root of life (Maciocia, 2001). Water is associated with the Kidneys, and in Chinese medicine, the Kidneys store our Prenatal Qi or Essence—our basic vitality or constitutional integrity. They are also the basis for the cooling, moistening, and nourishing Yin functions of all the other organs and the warming and active Yang functions of all the other organs. The clinical ramification is that a deficiency in the Water element or Kidneys often leads to deficiencies in other elements and their respective organs—hence, the importance of treating the Water element, the Kidney and Bladder Meridians. In practice, every Shiatsu session should include a good treatment of the back, thoroughly working the Bladder Meridian that runs parallel to the spinal column.

Opposite Water on a vertical axis is Fire. The Fire element is the seat of the psyche, as Fire is associated with the Heart and the Heart houses Shen—that which governs our consciousness and psychosocial being, according to Chinese medicine. The placement of Water as the foundation and Fire as the capital demonstrates the

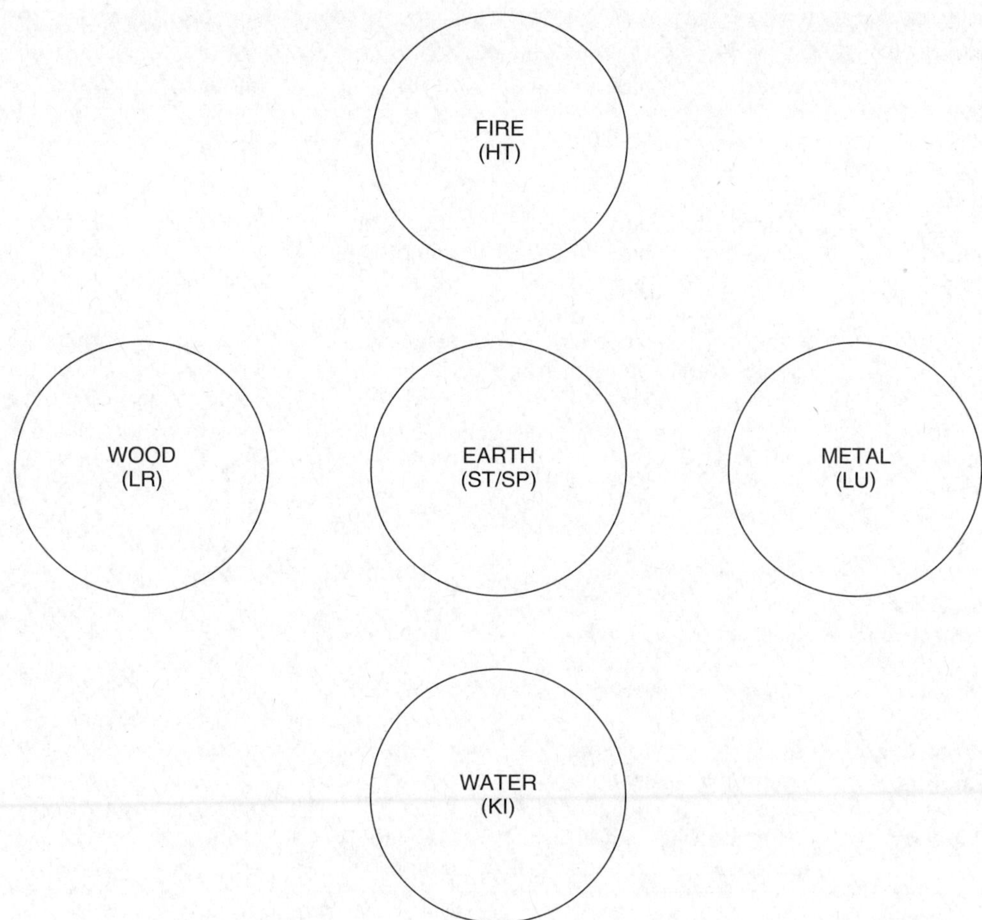

FIGURE 4-4 The Cosmological Sequence. (See Color Plate 4.)

reciprocal influence of the body-mind, as the condition of one affects the other (Maciocia, 2001). The clinical ramification here is that giving Shiatsu to the body positively affects the mind. In practice, if the client is distressed or disturbed by emotional or mental patterns, the practitioner should focus treatment on the relevant Meridians to ease or relieve the psychological condition.

Finally, the position of Earth in the center reinforces the concept that Earth is the source of our Postnatal Qi (Maciocia, 2001). Earth is associated with the Stomach and Spleen—the two digestive organs that nourish and energize the whole body, forming blood and Qi. Hence, tonifying the Earth element and its respective organs by working the Stomach and Spleen Meridians indirectly tonifies all the other elements and their respective organs.

FIVE ELEMENT CORRESPONDENCES

Beyond the Cosmological sequence and the Shen and Ko Cycles, which illustrate principles of generation and regulation found in nature and in human physiological, psychological, and social processes, the Five Element theory systematizes countless correspondences. A standard Five Element chart establishes correlations between various qualities and the Five Elements by identifying those qualities that share the same kind of energy or Qi as a particular element (see Table 4-1).

The most important correspondences for purposes of clinical practice are the following: the client's preference for, sensitivity to, or aversion to a particular climate;

TABLE 4-1 Five Element Correspondences

	Wood	Fire	Earth	Metal	Water
Season	spring	summer	Indian summer/ end of each season	autumn	winter
Phase	childhood	adolescence	adulthood	middle age	old age
Climate	windy	hot	damp/humid	arid	cold
Color	green	red	yellow/ brown	white/ silver	blue/black
Sound	shouting/ punctuated/ clipped	laughing/ tremulous	singing/ lilting	weeping/ whining/ complaining	groaning/ droning/ raspy/ hoarse
Tactile	itchy	hot	moist	dry	cold
Odor	rancid/ goatish	scorched/ burnt	fragrant/ sickly sweet	rank/ acrid	putrid/ rotten
Flavor	sour/ astringent	bitter	sweet	spicy/ pungent	salty
Yin Organ	Liver	Heart	Spleen	Lungs	Kidneys
Yang Organ	Gallbladder	Small Intestine	Stomach	Large Intestine	Bladder
Tissue	sinews	blood vessels	flesh	skin	bones/ marrow
Sense Organ	eyes	tongue	mouth	nose	ears
Emotion	irritability/ anger	joy/elation/ agitation	pensiveness/ worry	sadness/ grief	anxiety/ fear
Capacity	direction/ purpose	spirituality/ communication	cognition/ support	taking in/ letting go	will/ drive

the subtle hue of the client's skin, often seen around the mouth or eyes; the sound of the client's voice; the tactile quality of the client's skin; the smell of the client's body; the predominant taste in the client's mouth or the client's craving for a certain flavor; disorders or dysfunctions in the associated Yin and Yang organs, tissues or sense organs; sensitivity in the associated Meridians, and the client's psychological disposition. The presence of a significant number of factors correlated to a particular element not only points to the element itself, but also suggests a predisposition to develop certain element disharmonies, disorders, and diseases. Long before the manifestation of a disease, its precursor signs are apparent to the perceptive observer, including changes in the color of the face, the tone of the voice, and so on, according to the Five Element correspondences (Demuth, 2001).

FIVE ELEMENT TYPES

In addition to the element correspondences, the Five Element paradigm posits certain element types with characteristic features, body type, patterns of movement, and modes of doing, being, or relating. Most people are a hybrid of several elements, though one usually prevails. Following is a brief profile of each element type:

- The Water element type has a long bone structure, especially in the torso, which is disproportionately long; has soft features; and a blue-hued complexion;

moves smoothly; is flexible and adaptable; and can be either motivated and ambitious, like a rushing river, or lazy and complacent, like a dawdling, meandering stream.

- The Wood element type is tall, lean, and muscular; has a green-hued complexion; moves decisively; and is creative, industrious, and authoritative.
- The Fire element type has delicate, pointed features; a red-hued complexion; and curly hair or relative hairlessness or baldness; moves in a quick, sprightly manner; and is emotional, communicative, sociable, and spiritual.
- The Earth element type tends toward obesity and flabbiness or solidity, especially in the hips and legs; has a large head, wide jaws, and yellow-hued complexion; moves ponderously; and is calm, practical, and nurturing.
- The Metal element type is broad-shouldered; has a triangular-shaped face, sculptured features and a pale complexion; is hairy; moves deliberately; and is rational, methodical, meticulous, and reserved.

The Five Element paradigm has useful clinical applications. Discerning a client's element type can, like the correspondences, aid in assessment, and this, in turn, can aid in determining what kind of therapeutic treatment to give the client. The element types are prone to certain psychological imbalances and physical maladies, so giving Shiatsu to the relevant Meridians and giving acupressure to the key acupoints are indicated (see Chapter 5 on the Zang Fu organ system and Chapter 7 on acupressure points). Hence, a client who exhibits characteristics of a certain element type or manifests a cluster of signs belonging to a particular element type probably has an imbalance in that element and would benefit from having the corresponding Meridians and acupressure points pressed. Following are profiles of persons who illustrate typical characteristics and imbalances of their element type.

WATER ELEMENT PROFILE: DARIN

Darin, a Water element type (Figures 4-5 and 4-6), has a long neck, sloping shoulders, and a long torso (associated physique: relatively long spine/Bladder Meridian). His favorite colors are blue and black, which he often wears (associated color: blue/black). Although he has an aversion to cold and readily wraps himself in blankets indoors, he is typically underdressed, wearing sandals all year round, even in cold and snowy weather, because, he admits, he is too lazy to put on his socks or wear shoes that requiring lacing, buckling, or any extra effort beyond slipping on (associated climate: Cold; associated temperament: laid-back or high-strung).

His indolence manifests in other ways, as when he procrastinates on chores and bills and even on projects that matter to his heart (association: inertia or, conversely, motivation). His most dormant phase was during junior high and high school, when he slept for extended periods—14 hours or more—and was unusually resistant to waking, despite television and video games blaring full blast and siblings yelling at him, jostling him, bolting over him, and bouncing on top of him like a trampoline. The only thing that could wake him at this time was ice water. His mother had him subjected to various medical tests, but the results were all negative (association: parasympathetic relaxation mode, sleep, hibernation). He now believes he hibernated because he was bored.

On the whole, Darin is a laid-back, easygoing, languid Water element type who lives a fairly relaxed life with a flexible schedule, earning just enough money as a Yoga instructor to pay his bills in a communal household (association: parasympathetic relaxation mode)—this is in contrast to the ambitious, driven, high-strung, workaholic Water element type. However, during college, he did manifest the Water element's other tendency toward overachievement, maintaining a high

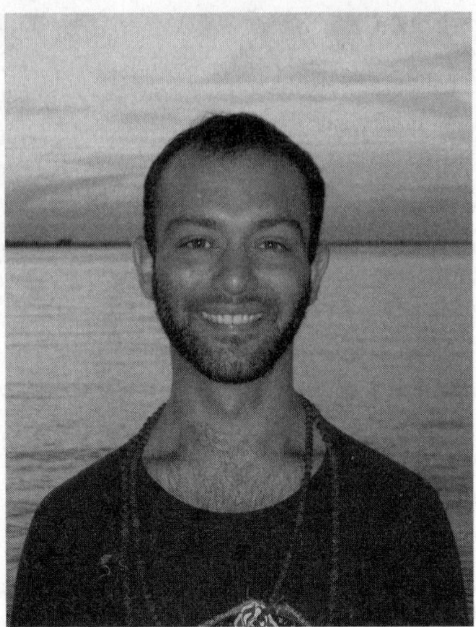

FIGURE 4-5 **Darin, Water element type.**

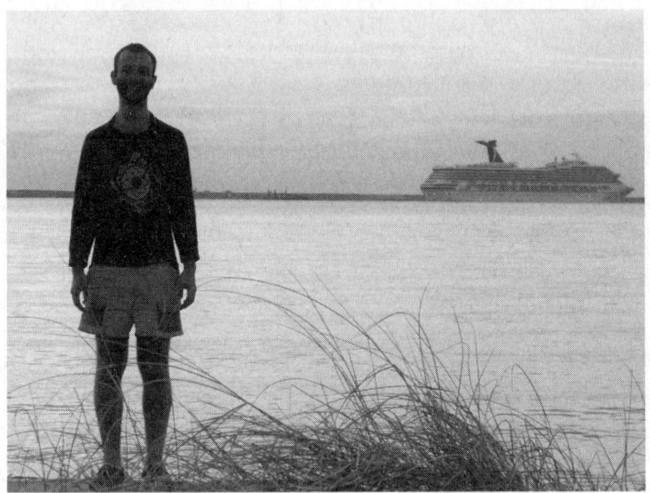

FIGURE 4-6 **Darin, Water element type.**

grade point average at Virginia Tech while triple-majoring in philosophy, psychology, and math and minoring in physics; working 15 hours per week as a tutor during his junior year and 30 hours per week as a tutor and poll-taker during his senior year; and partying as much as he could in between (association: sympathetic stress mode).

Darin enjoys traveling but often does so under less than optimal or even substandard conditions (associated psychological traits: fluid, flexible, adaptable). Without any concern for his safety or security and with little or no money and resources, he has hiked the Appalachian Trail for 2 months in the eastern United States and has hiked for 5 months around Western Europe, traveling through France, Belgium, the Netherlands, Germany, Austria, Italy, Slavonia (formerly Yugoslavia), and Egypt, toting a backpack and accepting rides, food, and lodging from total strangers or staying by invitation with home fellowship groups and friends (associated emotion: lack of fear, daring).

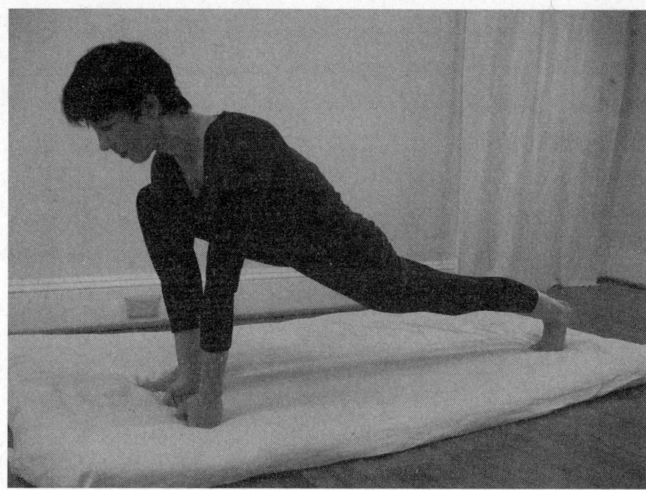

FIGURE 4-7 **Corinna, Wood element type.**

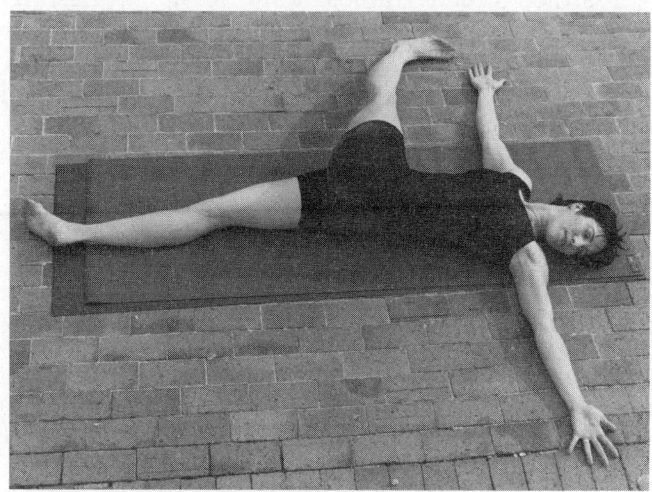

FIGURE 4-8 **Corinna, Wood element type.**

Darin's sense of hearing is not acute; he sometimes has difficulty hearing what others say, and he is susceptible to ear infections (associated sense organ: ears). Shiatsu on the Kidney and Bladder Meridians is indicated.

WOOD ELEMENT PROFILE: CORINNA

Corinna, a Wood element type (Figures 4-7 and 4-8), is svelte and sinewy looking. She loves vigorous exercise: She studied classical ballet for 10 years, performed professionally in cabaret jazz and modern dance troupes, and is currently a power Yoga instructor (associated movement: smooth and dynamic). She prefers good ventilation and circulating air, especially from fans and breezes through open windows, but in the fall and winter, she has an aversion to Cold Wind and wraps her head and neck in scarves (associated climate: Wind). She likes key lime, rhubarb, and tart berry pies; lemonade and limeade; margaritas, and especially red wine, which contributes to heat in her Liver (associated flavor: sour; associated disorder: Liver Yang rising).

Corinna has an assertive, take-charge personality (associated temperament: authoritative) and a crisp voice that projects well (associated sound: shouting, clipped).

Although she is compassionate and generally interacts harmoniously with others (associated social potential: benevolence), she is extremely prone to impatience and frustration and is often irked and vexed in traffic, in lines, and by obstacles, encumbrances, delays, or setbacks that thwart her progress, especially when due to human negligence or ineptitude or circumstances beyond her control (associated emotion: anger). In unproductive social situations, her attitude is "lead, follow, or get out of the way" and, in idle conversations, "make a point or get lost." A college teacher who saw Corinna striding across the campus quad told her later that her gait reminded her of Caesar's motto, "Vini, vidi, vici [I came, I saw, I conquered]."

Corinna is nearsighted, has poor night vision, and wears corrective lenses for these problems (associated sense organ: eyes). When she doesn't focus on anything in particular, she sees floaters—curly, crimped, or fuzzy black specks in her field of vision. Periodically, her eyes burn or sting, feel gritty or swollen, and look bloodshot. These eye flare-ups often occur in conjunction with a tension headache that lodges around her temples, forehead, and occiput. Any number of factors can precipitate a tension headache, including long hours of mental work at the computer, emotional upset, hormonal fluctuations around her menstrual period, and overindulgence in red wine (tension headaches are due to Liver Yang rising).

Corinna is often afflicted by rebellious Stomach Qi, manifesting as mild nausea and/or continuous, obstreperous belching. Alternatively, she sometimes experiences Spleen Qi deficiency, manifesting as poor appetite and loose stools. In both patterns, the Wood element is overacting on and upsetting the Earth element via the Ko cycle, resulting in a humiliation disharmony.

Although Corinna is flexible, she notices that her abductors and adductors (outer and inner thighs) are relatively tense and tight compared to other major muscle groups. Every now and then when she holds a low lunge in power Yoga, a sharp, paroxysmal sensation shoots down the outside of her leg like a lightning bolt (associated pathway: Gallbladder Meridian). Also, the stretch position that is most painful and limited for her is the side or straddle splits (associated pathway: Liver Meridian). Shiatsu to the Liver and Gallbladder Meridians, as well as to the compromised Stomach and Spleen Meridians, is indicated.

FIRE ELEMENT PROFILE: LINDA

Linda, a Fire element type (Figures 4-9 and 4-10), is petite and has fine features and wavy, auburn hair (associated features: delicate or pointy; associated hair texture and color: curly and red). She is drawn to warm colors—yellows, oranges, and reds—and often wears fabrics, buys artwork, and accents her home in these colors (associated color: red). She likes her coffee black, and she likes dark chocolate (associated flavor: bitter). Sunbathing energizes her, and whenever possible she treats herself to some form of heat therapy: sauna, whirlpool, or steam room. On a recent trip to the Dominican Republic, she hiked for 5 miles during the midday siesta in 105 degree weather. She feels hot most of the time and sweats easily and profusely, which she doesn't mind (associated climate/season: hot/summer).

Linda has a buoyant, effervescent personality (associated temperament: animated and lively), and her standard response to everything is laughter (associated emotion: joy). Events that most people consider stressful or traumatic she regards as funny or preposterous. For example, on the same day hospital staff notified her that she had received a contaminated unit of blood and was eligible for free HIV testing, she hit a car on her blind side and laughed so hard that the firefighters wondered if she had suffered head trauma.

Linda constantly multitasks, darting nimbly like a squirrel. The typical guest in her home will observe her cooking, baking, washing, clearing away a mess here or there, setting the table, relocating furniture, attending to her four cats, answering the doorbell and the telephone, and retrieving something a family member

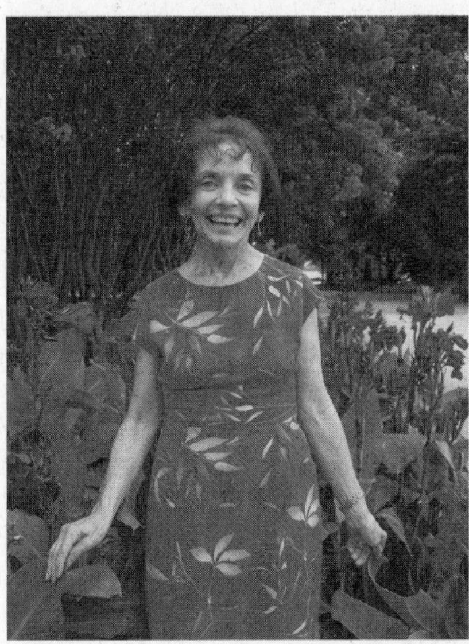

FIGURE 4-9 Linda, Fire element type.

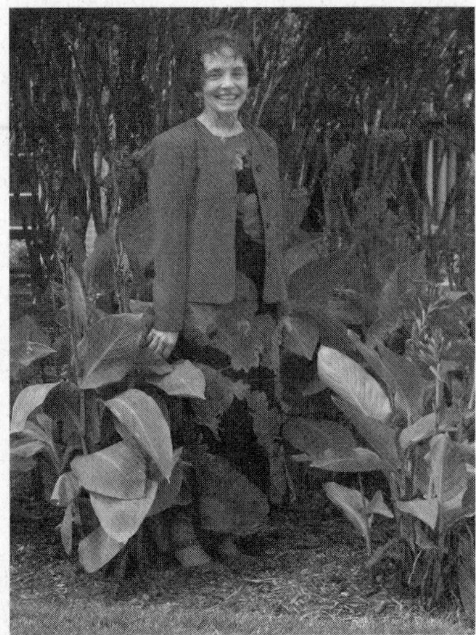

FIGURE 4-10 Linda, Fire element type.

misplaced, while carrying on a highly technical conversation (associated movement: quick and light). Linda speaks rapidly and at length, and in fact her listeners sometimes have difficulty processing all the information (associated disposition: communicative; associated sense organ: tongue). Busy is her way of life: She teaches nursing full-time at a university, works part-time as a nurse at a hospital, is pursuing a Ph.D., is remodeling her house, regularly entertains guests, provides legal or medical advocacy to friends, supports her four children in their various academic or career paths, helps manage a condominium complex, and monitors and cares for her husband's diabetes and sports-related injuries (association: high energy, hyperactivity).

From time to time, Linda has profoundly accurate prophetic dreams (dreams are the domain of Shen), and for her, the supernatural permeates all human affairs: "There's a reason for everything," she says, smiling (association: spirituality). As a doctoral student in nursing, she is exploring the relationship between spirituality and health and the integration of spirituality into medicine, particularly prenatal care. She has written several graduate papers and a research proposal on the subject of spirituality in nursing (associations: communication and spirituality). She plans to design and conduct a research study on the correlation between spirituality during pregnancy and various maternal and infant health outcomes. In one of her graduate papers, she defines spirituality as "an essential philosophy of life centered on the awareness of a pervasive universal creative force that provides a sense of interconnectedness and an awareness of purpose and meaning" (Bennington, 2003).

Linda's heart palpitates like a galloping horse all the time; she sometimes feels as if her heart is going to leap right out of her chest (associated organ: Heart). In addition, she suffers from insomnia, mental restlessness (a "vexed Heart"), and fidgetiness (Heart Shen cannot rest). As a pattern, these signs point to Heart Yin deficiency, or Empty Heat in the Heart, which implicates the Water element via the Ko cycle. The Water element is not controlling the Fire element—not cooling and moistening it—resulting in an insult disharmony.

Aside from a Fire element disharmony, Linda also presents a few signs pointing to an Earth element disharmony: She suffers from chronic morning diarrhea and abdominal cramps, and she bleeds easily and profusely (associated tissue: blood vessels), a condition known as reckless blood in TCM (the Spleen controls blood, retaining it in the vessels, but in Linda's case, this Spleen function is deficient). This pattern suggests that the Fire element is transmitting its deficiency to the Earth element via the Shen cycle (the Mother element, Fire, is failing to nourish the Child element, Earth). Occasionally, SI 12—an acupressure point on her Small Intestine Meridian—is painful, tense, and knotted. Shiatsu to the Fire element Meridians, as well as the Earth and Water element Meridians, is indicated.

EARTH ELEMENT PROFILE: DIANE

Diane, an Earth element type (Figures 4-11 and 4-12), has a large head and a stout, chubby build; she carries most of her weight around her belly, hips, and thighs (associated form: bottom-heavy, pear-shaped). For years, sweet cravings have been her nemesis, and when they overtake her, she is likely to consume several candy bars in one sitting, especially if she feels pressured (associated flavor: sweet). Sometimes she

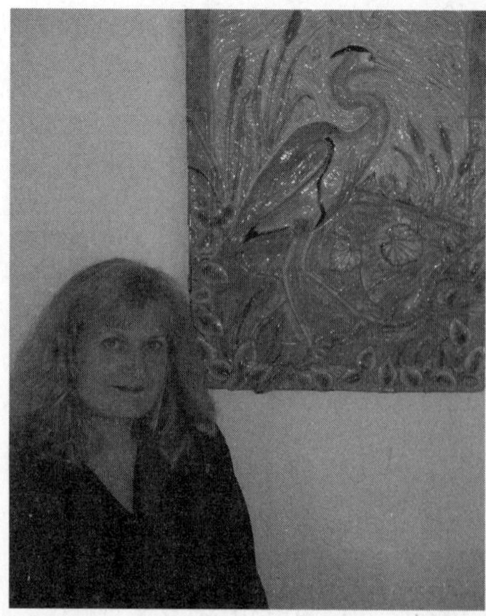

FIGURE 4-11 Diane, Earth element type.

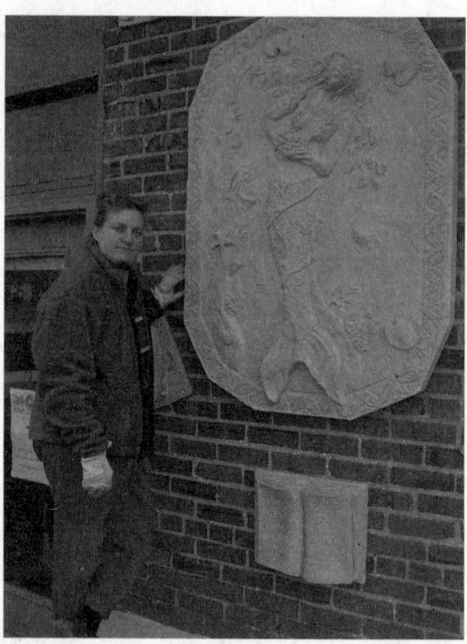

FIGURE 4-12 Diane, Earth element type.

overindulges in other foods she considers vices, like chips, red meat, and desserts. She laments at having struggled with weight control all her life; she has tried and continues to try various diets, including the Atkins and South Beach diets, and has vacillated in her motivation to exercise (associated issues: appetite and weight disorders).

Diane has a down-to-earth personality and is practical, dependable, full of common sense, and helpful (associated temperament: stable, grounded, and supportive). As a professional artist specializing in ceramic wall sculptures (Figures 4-13 and 4–14), she molds, glazes, and fires the earth into three-dimensional works that focus on such Earth-related themes as the natural world, creature comforts, maternal nurturing, fertility and abundance, and warm fellowship (associations: nature, comfort, motherhood, productivity, home, and family). Recently, she has begun to explore brick carving—another form of earth sculpting—as well.

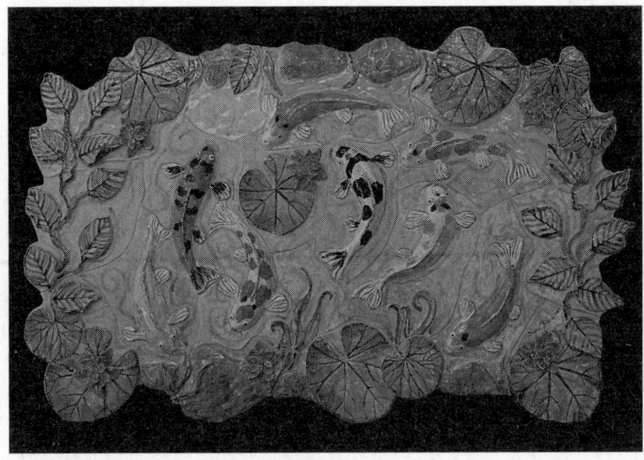

FIGURE 4-13 Koi Pond.
With kind permission from Diane Husson at www.newrelics.com.

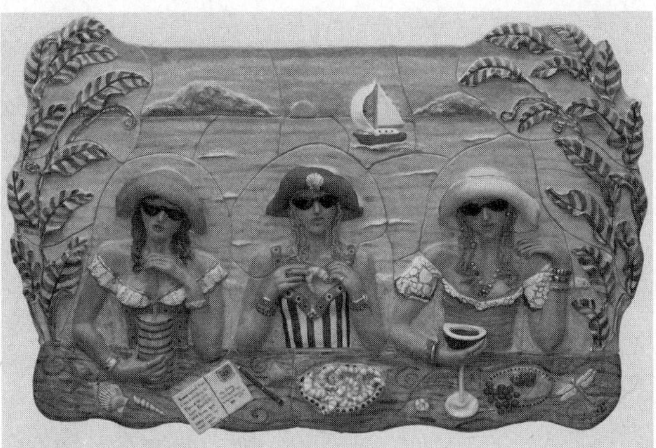

FIGURE 4-14 Three's a Charm.
With kind permission from Diane Husson at www.newrelics.com.

Diane often mulls over, broods, and frets unduly about professional and personal concerns, both small and large (associated emotion: worry, overthinking). This tendency quickly degenerates into an unhealthy fixation on or obsession with her social responsibility to others, which is always exaggerated in her own mind (association: caretaking). For example, at an art show Diane spontaneously waved to a customer of hers who was on the verge of browsing through another artist's booth. She was immediately mortified that her hand signal could have been misconstrued as a devious and malicious attempt to divert potential business to herself. When the customer walked over to her, she purged her "guilt" by begging the customer to explore the other artist's work and by apologizing profusely to the other artist, who was not in the least bit threatened. Afterward Diane agonized over the incident for days.

Diane suffers from dysmenorrhea, especially bloating and cramps before and during her menstrual period (Earth element association: reproductivity). She often experiences a strange tingling in her quadriceps, especially when she first lies down (associated pathways: Stomach and Spleen Meridians). Shiatsu to the Spleen and Stomach Meridians is indicated.

METAL ELEMENT PROFILE: RYAN

Ryan, a Metal element type (Figures 4-15 and 4-16), has a triangular-shaped face, pale complexion, well-defined features, and slightly angular frame. At Thai, Indian, and Mexican restaurants, he typically orders the hottest items on the menu, and at home, he supplements almost all of his meals with liberal dashes of hot sauce (associated flavor: pungent and spicy).

Apart from interactions with close friends and family, Ryan is introverted and quiet (associated temperament: socially reserved, reticent). Even at family gatherings, he defers to others, listening but rarely contributing much to conversation. His monastic silence at work, and especially during excruciatingly long business

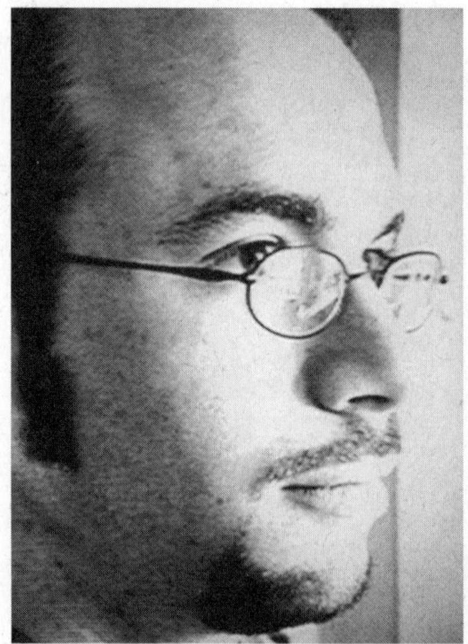

FIGURE 4-15 Ryan, Metal element type.

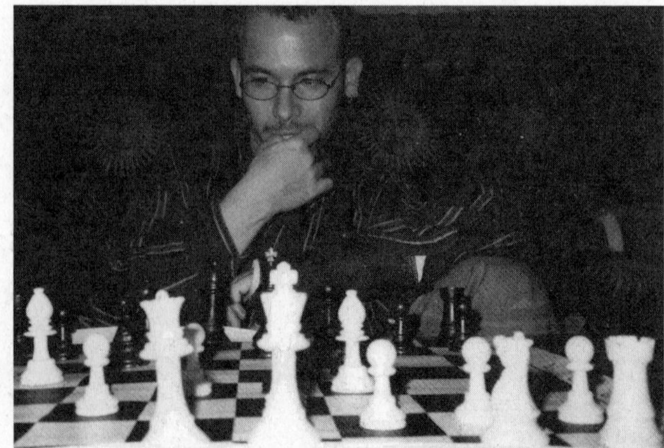

FIGURE 4-16 Ryan, Metal element type.

meetings, has become a running joke among coworkers. However, on those rare occasions when he does speak about a subject that ignites his enthusiasm, his voice sounds as if it is projected through a megaphone (associated vocal quality: in Yang fullness, loud; in Yin weakness, faint).

Ryan is reluctant to socialize, so reluctant in fact that he would rather live with a broken fixture than call a handyman, he would rather eat and pay for a meal he didn't order than complain to the wait staff, and he would rather wear a pair of sneakers with a right/left size discrepancy than return them to the store for a refund or exchange (association: socially reserved or withdrawn). Due to his retiring nature, he has never taken initiative socially: He has never proactively chosen friends and has never pursued a woman. His friends have sought him out, and his first significant relationship was with a woman who pursued him. Following that relationship, he lived like a hermit for 6 years (association: solitude, isolation), until his kinsmen orchestrated a blind date in the guise of a larger social function to place romantic opportunity in his lap.

In general, Ryan is self-controlled and self-contained, presenting a modest, well-mannered, subdued, even restrained disposition to the world. Of all emotions, sorrow and grief are the most perplexing, troubling, and alien to him. He has difficulty experiencing and expressing sorrow even when there is good cause, as when he found out that his mother almost died in the hospital (associated emotion: grief, repressed grief, or stoicism). He has cried unwillingly a few times in his life, and only when under tremendous strain, as when his Web design consulting firm went belly up during the dot-com bust.

Ryan is a typical geek in his work and play: He writes computer code for Coast Guard aviation programs all day; for pleasure, he reads and writes hard science fiction novels; plays chess and Magic—a fantasy card game requiring mental strategy; solves MENSA riddles, puzzles, and brainteasers; delights in exposing fallacies in political arguments via online discussion forums like Spin Sanity, and posts new articles on his blog every weekend (associated temperament: logical, rational, analytical, meticulous, orderly, methodical, systematic). Most of his social interactions are buffered and mediated by technology and logic (association: social isolation).

Physically, Ryan presents typical Metal element disharmonies. His sense of smell is not sharp; he has difficulty discerning fragrances and odors that others notice, such as strong essential oil blends or rank cat litter. He is often plagued with sneezing fits and bouts of nasal congestion or drainage (associated sense organ: nose/sinus disorders). Prone to respiratory illnesses, he catches colds, though not as frequently or as severely as during the decade he smoked, when he developed annual cases of bronchitis, strep throat, or pneumonia (associated organ: Lungs/respiratory disorders). He contends with pimples, boils, and yeast infections on his skin (associated sense organ: skin) and occasionally suffers from constipation or hemorrhoids (associated organ: Large Intestine). His pectoral and anterior deltoid muscles in his chest and the front of his shoulders are quite tender and sensitive, especially at Lu 1 and 2 (associated pathway: Lung Meridian). Shiatsu to the Lung and Large Intestine Meridians is indicated.

History, Strengths, and Weaknesses of the Five Element Theory

Although the Five Element theory is clinically very useful as a convenient and expedient guide to assessment, a number of prominent sources consider it subordinate to the Yin Yang theory (Kaptchuk, 2000). There are several reasons for this.

Historically, the Five Element paradigm was developed and articulated much later than Yin Yang. The earliest reference to Yin Yang occurs in the *I Ching* (*The Book of Change*), the oldest Chinese classic and the font of all Chinese philosophy, including Taoism and Confucianism (a written commentary on the *I Ching* dates back to 1144 B.C.). By contrast, the earliest allusion to the Five Elements dates to the fifth century B.C. and the earliest recorded reference to the fourth century B.C.; systemization of the Five Elements occurred even later, between 350 and 270 B.C. (Kaptchuk, 2000; Maciocia, 2001).

Another reason for the theoretical subordination of the Five Element theory is that during its development, several different and mutually exclusive versions of correspondences between the elements and their respective organ systems were formulated, suggesting that the presently accepted correlations are to some extent arbitrary (Kaptchuk, 2000). Additionally, the theory was not fully developed as a medical paradigm until around the tenth century A.D., when it was finally used to explain the origin of disease and the disease process.

In terms of peer review, the Five Element theory has failed to command unanimous support among medical scholars; detractors have contested its accuracy and applicability throughout Chinese history, even as far back as the fourth century B.C. (Kaptchuk, 2000). Among proponents in antiquity and modernity, the Five Element theory has always been explained in terms of the Yin Yang theory, and not vice versa, indicating that Yin Yang takes theoretical precedence. For example, each of the elements is described as expressing a Yin or Yang quality: Wood is growing Yang; Fire is utmost Yang; Earth is balanced between Yin and Yang and is therefore neutral; Metal is growing Yin; Water is utmost Yin. Perhaps of greatest clinical concern is the fact that strict adherence to the prescribed correspondences yields convenient, though formulaic, clinical conclusions that sometimes contradict the more sensitive Yin Yang conclusions.

Many sources regard the Five Element theory as an elaboration or extrapolation of the Yin Yang theory. While this certainly seems to be true conceptually, the Five Element and Yin Yang theories were developed independently and existed as two distinct systems until they were integrated in the *Nei Jing* during the Han dynasty, a period of political unification and ideological syncretism (Kaptchuk, 2000). The only historical connection between the two theories is that both were developed by the Yin Yang school or naturalist school of philosophy (Maciocia, 2001).

Many contemporary sources also regard the two theories as completely compatible. However, both Kaptchuk and Maciocia point out discrepancies in their views of wellness and illness. Such discrepancies are based on their different orientations: the Five Element theory stresses fixed correlations between things, whereas the Yin Yang theory stresses the importance of the whole in determining the meaning or significance of any part (Kaptchuk, 2000; Maciocia, 2001). Thus, while the Five Element paradigm relies on predetermined connections or one-to-one correspondences for diagnosis and treatment, the Yin Yang paradigm relies on context or global configuration for diagnosis and treatment. These different approaches can yield different results (Maciocia, 2001).

For example, the significance of a red complexion may be interpreted differently. A practitioner applying the Five Element theory would initially surmise that the Heart Meridian or organ was implicated, since red corresponds to the Fire element and the Fire element corresponds to the Heart Meridian and organ. A practitioner applying the Yin Yang theory would reserve judgment until more symptoms were compiled and a comprehensive view could be obtained. While red might indicate a Heart condition, it could also indicate a heat condition in any number of Meridians and associated organs, depending on other presenting symptoms (Kaptchuk, 2000).

The main point is that the Five Element theory is a quick and easy instrument, but is not as accurate or precise as the Yin Yang theory. Hence, it should be regarded as a preliminary guide to therapy and a supplement to, but not a substitute for, the Yin Yang theory. The Five Element theory is especially suited for Shiatsu practitioners who are generally expected to provide relief without elaborate medical intakes and tests and without years of advanced study. While Shiatsu practitioners are not legally permitted to diagnose or treat, the nature of their work requires them to make some kind of assessment, however rudimentary, before providing therapy.

The Five Element theory is an excellent base, since it enables a practitioner to organize signs and symptoms into a clinically significant pattern in short order. On a more analytical level, it helps the practitioner understand the complexity of deficiency and excess patterns, and especially the concept that a client's presenting symptoms are not necessarily the sole cause of disharmony and should not be the sole focus of therapy: The cause may lie elsewhere, as indicated by the Shen and Ko Cycles, and therapy may need to be directed elsewhere. Finally, the Five Element theory emphasizes the importance of a client's habitual psychological disposition—anger, excitability, pensiveness, grief, fear—as a factor in health, as well as the importance of treating the whole person, not just the body.

In Japan, Korea, and the West, the Five Element theory is commonly used to enhance the Yin Yang theory (Kaptchuk, 2000), whereas in China the Yin Yang theory is practiced almost exclusively.

REFERENCES

American Academic Encyclopedia (Vol. 15). (1981). *Physics*. Princeton, NJ: Arete.

Bennington, L. (2003). *Concept analysis of spirituality*. Unpublished doctoral essay, Virginia Commonwealth University School of Nursing.

Demuth, S. (Producer). (2001). *An introduction to classical Five-Element acupuncture: A public talk by Professor J. R. Worsley*. [Videocassette].

Hamilton, A., Madison, J., & Jay, J. (1961). *The Federalist papers*. New York: Penguin. (Original work published 1787.)

Kaptchuk, T. (2000). *The web that has no weaver: Understanding Chinese medicine* (2nd ed.). Chicago: Contemporary.

Maciocia, G. (2001). *The foundations of Chinese medicine: A comprehensive text for acupuncturists and herbalists*. Edinburgh: Churchill Livingstone. (Original work published 1989.)

Morrison, D. & Owen, T. (1987). *The planetary system*. Reading, MA: Addison-Wesley.

STUDY QUESTIONS

1. Are the Five Elements fixed entities, stable constituents of matter, or do they represent something else?

2. What is another, more accurate translation for the Five Elements?

3. How is Five Element theory related to Ki/Qi/Chi?

4. Describe the Water element. Which season, stage in a person's life, and Meridians correspond to Water?

5. Describe the Wood element. Which season, stage in a person's life, and Meridians correspond to Wood?

6. Describe the Fire element. Which season, stage in a person's life, and Meridians correspond to Fire?

7. Describe the Earth element. Which season, stage in a person's life, and Meridians correspond to Earth?

8. Describe the Metal element. Which season, stage in a person's life, and Meridians correspond to Metal?

9. What is Shen of the Five Element theory? (*note:* This differs from Shen of the Qi theory, which refers to spirit, awareness, or mind.)

10. State the sequential order in which the elements progress through the Shen Cycle.

11. In the Shen Cycle, is each stage or phase equal in duration?

12. What is meant by the Mother/Child relationship in the context of the Shen Cycle?

13. How does the "problem parent, problem child" dysfunction treated in psychological counseling relate to a disharmony in the Shen Cycle?

14. What treatment principle is implied by a problem parent, problem child diagnosis?

15. How can the practitioner resolve a Child element deficiency using the Shen Cycle?

16. How can the practitioner resolve a Child element excess using the Shen Cycle?

17. What is Ko of the Five Element theory?

18. Why is Ko necessary?

19. Which elements regulate which other elements in Ko?

20. Describe the regulatory dysfunction known as insult.

21. How can the practitioner restore balance in the case of insult?

22. Describe the regulatory dysfunction known as humiliation.

23. How can the practitioner restore balance in the case of humiliation?

24. What important TCM concepts does the Cosmological sequence convey?

25. What element type are you? Identify your primary and secondary types and any relevant associations (e.g., climate, color, taste, odor, organs, tissues, sense perception, body type and emotion).

26. How can knowing the element types aid a practitioner in formulating a suitable therapeutic session for a particular client?

27. Identify the emotional correspondence for Wood.

28. Identify the emotional correspondence for Fire.

29. Identify the emotional correspondence for Earth.

30. Identify the emotional correspondence for Metal.

31. Identify the emotional correspondence for Water.

32. How can knowing the element correspondences aid a practitioner in formulating a suitable therapeutic session for a particular client?

33. Which was developed first—the Yin Yang theory or the Five Element theory?

34. How is the Five Element theory related to the Yin Yang theory? Upon what common principle are both theories premised?

35. Does the Five Element theory always yield the same diagnostic results as the Yin Yang theory?

36. Explain some of the limitations of the Five Element theory.

FIVE ELEMENT THEORY TEST (50 POINTS)

SHORT ANSWER/FILL IN THE BLANK

1. The translation of Wu Xing as "Five Elements" is misleading because it suggests that the elements are fixed, material entities or static conditions. Wu Xing literally means "five walk" or "five move," suggesting dynamic change. Therefore, a better translation for Wu Xing would be ____________.

2. The Five Elements represent different qualities or states or manifestations of ____________.

3. In the context of the Five Element theory, to what does Shen refer? ____________

4. In Shen, the elements are in what kind of relationship? ____________

5. In Shen, the element that promotes or generates another element is called ____________.

6. In Shen, the element that is fostered or produced is called ____________.

7. Using Shen as a guide to therapy, how should a practitioner remedy a deficiency in an element? ____________

8. To what does Ko refer? ____________

9. In Ko, the elements are in what kind of relationship? ____________

10. Describe the regulatory dysfunction known as insult. ____________

11. Using Ko as a therapeutic guide, how can the practitioner remedy an insult disharmony? ____________

12. Describe the regulatory dysfunction known as humiliation. ____________

13. Using Ko as a therapeutic guide, how can the practitioner remedy a humiliation disharmony? ____________

MATCHING

A. Wood element
B. Fire element
C. Earth element
D. Metal element
E. Water element

____**14.** Represents the dormant phase; is associated with winter, old age, and death or the afterlife.

____**15.** Represents maturity; is associated with Indian summer and adulthood.

____**16.** Represents the growth phase; is associated with spring and childhood.

____**17.** Represents decline; is associated with autumn and middle age.

____**18.** Represents the culmination of growth; is associated with summer and adolescence.

____**19.** Energy expands upward and outward: lesser Yang.

____**20.** Energy reaches maximum kinetic fullness: greater Yang.

____**21.** Energy stabilizes; is centered and balanced.

____**22.** Energy contracts downward and inward: lesser Yin.

____**23.** Energy is latent, has stored potential: greater Yin.

____**24.** The root of life and source of Pre-Heaven Qi in the Cosmological sequence.

____**25.** The source of Post-Heaven Qi in the Cosmological sequence.

____**26.** Heat; red skin hue; laughing/tremulous voice; scorched odor; bitter taste.

____**27.** Cold; blue/black skin hue; groaning voice; rotten/putrid odor; salty taste.

____**28.** Wind; green skin hue; shouting/clipped voice; rancid/goatish odor; sour taste.

____**29.** Dry; white skin hue; weeping voice; rank/acrid odor; spicy taste.

____**30.** Damp; yellow skin hue; singing voice; sickly sweet/fragrant odor; sweet taste.

____**31.** Joyful; agitated.

____**32.** Irritable; angry.

____**33.** Pensive; worried.

____**34.** Melancholy; mournful.

____**35.** Anxious; fearful.

____**36.** Kidneys; Bladder; bones; ears.

____**37.** Stomach; Spleen; flesh; mouth.

____**38.** Heart; Small Intestine; blood vessels; tongue.

____**39.** Lungs; Large Intestine; skin; nose.

____**40.** Liver; Gallbladder; sinews; eyes.

TRUE OR FALSE. THE FOLLOWING STATEMENTS CONCERN SHEN. DRAWING THE DIAGRAM MAY HELP YOU ANSWER THE QUESTIONS. CIRCLE THE CORRECT RESPONSE.

True False **41.** Wood generates Fire.

True False **42.** Earth is the Child of Fire.

True False **43.** Earth is the Mother of Metal.

True False **44.** Metal is the Child of Water.

True False **45.** Water generates Wood.

FILL IN THE BLANK. THE FOLLOWING STATEMENTS CONCERN KO. DRAWING THE DIAGRAM MAY HELP YOU ANSWER THE QUESTIONS.

46. Wood regulates ______________.

47. Metal regulates ______________.

48. Earth regulates ______________.

49. Fire regulates ______________.

50. Water regulates ______________.

5

THE ZANG FU ORGAN SYSTEM

OBJECTIVES

- To distinguish TCM from Western medicine
- To describe the physiological functions of each organ and to identify the sense perception and tissues associated with each organ
- To give examples of typical disorders and diseases afflicting each organ
- To describe the psychological capacities, social dynamics, and emotions associated with each organ
- To give examples of typical emotional extremes, psychological imbalances, and social disharmonies associated with each organ
- To discuss the interconnectedness of the Zang Fu system, especially the mutual sharing of functions and the transference of an imbalance or dysfunction from one organ to another

KEY TERMS AND CONCEPTS

Zang
Fu
Marrow
Jing/Essence
Ming-Men/Life Gate Fire/Gate of Vitality/Original Qi/Source Qi
Shen/Mind/Spirit
Pericardium/Heart Constrictor/Heart Master/Heart Governor/Heart Protector
Triple Heater/Triple Burner/Triple Warmer/San jaio
Wei Qi/Defensive Qi/Protective Qi
Nutritive Qi
Postnatal Qi/Post-Heaven Qi

THE ZANG FU ORGAN SYSTEM

After reading about Qi, Yin Yang, and the Five Elements, the theoretical differences between TCM and Western allopathic medicine should be striking. This difference extends further to the view of organs and treatment approaches. Overall, TCM is process-oriented: It emphasizes the flow of vital substances, especially Qi; and it views organs primarily as interactive functions, disease as an imbalance in Yin Yang energies of the body, the role of medicine primarily as preventive and secondarily as restorative, and treatment as a balancing of energy through acupuncture, herbs, massage, and exercise. In contrast, Western allopathic medicine is structure-oriented: It emphasizes anatomy; and it views organs primarily as discrete physical entities, disease as organ malfunction, the role of medicine as curative, and treatment as a mechanical or chemical intervention—a repair of parts through surgery and/or drugs. Other differences are also readily apparent: The Chinese view of organ functions is broader and includes psychological functions; organ functions often overlap or reinforce one another rather than being distinct, as they are in Western medicine; and there are two "organs" that have no Western corollary, namely, the Pericardium and Triple Heater.

The Chinese categorize organs into Zang or Yin and Fu or Yang counterparts. Each Zang organ is paired with an elementally related Fu organ. In general, the **Zang** or Yin organs are solid, with the exception of the Heart/Pericardium, and their function is to generate, convert, regulate, and store substances such as Qi, blood, Essence, and fluids (Kaptchuk, 2000). The Yin organs include the Heart, Pericardium, Lungs, Spleen, Liver, and Kidneys. The **Fu** or Yang organs are hollow, and their function is to digest food, assimilate nutrients, and eliminate waste. The Yang organs include the Stomach, Gallbladder, Triple Heater, Small Intestine, Large Intestine, and Bladder.

In oriental medical practice, the Yin organs are considered more important because of their role in producing substances necessary to life. For example, the Lungs produce Air Qi, the Spleen produces Grain Qi, and the Kidneys store and distribute Source Qi. However, for the Shiatsu practitioner, all organs and Meridians, both Yin and Yang, are equally important because their energetic functions and psychological associations influence the whole person.

Although the attribution of psychological associations—especially emotions—to organs may seem strange, traces of this understanding exist in the Western worldview. For example, fear is associated with loss of bladder control, worry with an upset stomach, grief with convulsive suspiration of the lungs, and joy with a merry heart. Some idiomatic expressions reveal a familiarity with the temperament imbalances and energetic disorders identified by Chinese medicine. For example, the term *hothead*, used to denote an easily angered person, depicts the Wood element imbalance of Liver Yang rising; the Elizabethan term *lily-livered*, used to denote a timid or cowardly person, depicts the Wood element imbalance of Liver Qi deficiency; and to be *beside oneself* depicts the Fire element imbalance of scattered Qi or a state of shock.

Although Western medicine does not assign psychological states to organs as Chinese medicine does, it nonetheless recognizes the body-mind connection and the reality of psychosomatic disorders. In fact, the impact of stress, a psychological factor, in the development of pathologies such as asthma, cancer, and heart disease is now widely acknowledged, and treatments incorporating stress management therapies are becoming more and more prevalent. Western medicine also recognizes that psychological states and disorders have a distinct physiological signature or biochemical component: For example, stress-related emotional states such as anger, depression, and anxiety are correlated with low levels of serotonin and high levels of adrenalin and cortisol. In short, Western medicine is beginning to corroborate the centuries-old body-mind view of Chinese medicine.

The sections below describe the main physiological functions and psychological capacities of each Zang Fu organ pair, its associated tissue and sense organ, and typical disharmonies that suggest the need for Shiatsu on the corresponding Meridians.

THE WATER ELEMENT: KIDNEYS AND BLADDER

The Water element is associated with life and motive force of the body and mind. The body expresses life and motive force as vigor and vitality, while the mind expresses them as willpower and determination. In the natural world, water varies in its volume and rate of flow: It can manifest as a rushing river or a lolling brook, as a torrential waterfall or a stagnant pond. So, too, Water element types vary in their physical and mental impetus: Some are aspiring, enterprising, ambitious, or extremely driven, while others are mellow, languid, unmotivated, or even lackadaisical.

This variance is related to the Water element's influence on the central and autonomic nervous systems. The central nervous system controls conscious action such as the movement of voluntary skeletal muscle, while the autonomic nervous system controls unconscious or nonvolitional action such as heartbeat, respiration, and alimentary processes. Both the central and the autonomic nervous systems jointly determine a person's overall state of excitation or calm, and the Water element influences their condition and function in several ways.

The first influence of the Water element on the nervous system is through its associated tissue, bone. In TCM, bone includes not only teeth, but also **Marrow**, which includes the brain, spinal cord, and nerves (Maciocia, 2001). Hence, the tissue of the Water element is closely identified with the central nervous system (CNS). Since the CNS translates conscious decision into action, executing the individual will, the overall state of the CNS is determined by a person's significant and habitual choices in life, choices that constitute a dominant or default mode of being, doing, and relating. These choices, which include personal initiative and personal response, affect a person's general state of excitation or calm. Insofar as these choices are voluntary, a person's experience of life as hectic or laid back is self-generated and self-imposed. To a certain extent, however, such choices may be socially or environmentally conditioned, as when, for example, a person lives in a big city like New York rather than a rural town in West Virginia.

The second influence of the Water element is through the path of the inner Bladder Meridian. Because the inner Bladder Meridian runs parallel to the spinal cord, its energy flow affects the spinal cord, its nerve branches, and the internal organs. The quality of energy flow in the Bladder Meridian is due to lifestyle choices, as well as environmental conditions.

The third influence of the Water element is through its associated organ, the Kidneys. The Kidney organ complex affects the autonomic nervous system (ANS) through the adrenal glands. The ANS has two branches, a sympathetic branch, which governs the "fight or flight" stress response, and a parasympathetic branch, which governs the "rest and digest" relaxation response. The Kidneys' adrenal glands trigger the "fight or flight" stress response through the secretion of norepinephrine (adrenalin) into the bloodstream. Adrenalin is a hormone that accelerates the heart and respiratory rates and increases blood flow to the skeletal muscles in preparation for action. It concurrently inhibits housekeeping functions like alimentation. This state of stress can be self-induced, as, for example, by drinking a double espresso, riding a roller-coaster, watching a horror movie, reading a thriller, or failing to leave early enough to arrive somewhere on time. On the other hand, such a state of stress can be a response to circumstances beyond a person's control such as deadline pressure at work, a family crisis, an encounter with a hostile dog or mugger, or a Murphy's law day (a day characterized by an uncanny series of mistakes, malfunctions, mishaps, and misfeasance).

Because of the Bladder Meridian's broad influence on the nervous system, Water element imbalances can manifest as two diametrically opposed states or types. These states are aptly described by Newton's first law of motion: "[A]n object in motion tends to stay in motion and an object at rest tends to stay at rest unless acted upon by an external force" (*Academic American Encyclopedia*, 1981, vol. 15, p. 280). An object in motion depicts the ANS disharmony of a person perpetually on the go, whereas an object at rest depicts the ANS disharmony of a person prone to or relegated to inertia.

The "object in motion" Water element type lives in a sympathetic state of heightened arousal marked by hyperactivity, psychological stress, and physical tension. Such a person is a zealous striver who tends to be characterized by others as a workaholic or overachiever (Maciocia, 2001). This person may react to stimuli as threats or potential threats. He or she may habitually take stimulants such as caffeinated sodas, coffee, tea, antisoporifics, or thermogenics (metabolic enhancers) to tap into the Kidney Essence to fuel a hectic pace, which can eventually deplete Kidney Essence (Beresford-Cooke, 2000). The upward-bound urban professional and the self-employed businessperson who average 60 to 80 hours of work per week are classic examples.

By contrast, the "object at rest" Water element type lives in a parasympathetic state of relative inertia or hibernation. Such a person may lack motivation or may be suffering from burnout. He or she may be idle by choice (lazy) or by necessity (exhausted) and may be characterized by others as an underachiever or work casualty. This person may regard effort or exertion as taxing because it would disturb the preferred state of repose or because it would further deplete already diminished reserves. The laid-back hippie and the crashed workaholic are typical examples.

Aside from its unique dichotomy of types, the Water element is unique among the elements in another way: It is considered the foundation for the other elements (Maciocia, 2001). It forms the basis of Yin and Yang in the body, the Yin and Yang of all other organs. This is because the Kidneys are the keepers of our ancestral inheritance, storing and dispensing Jing and Ming-Men. **Jing**, or **Essence**, resides in the hara, the abdominal power center, and is the source of Water and form in the body. Jing is the root of Yin in the body, the basis of fluids, bodily substances, and all supportive, nourishing, and moistening functions (Beresford-Cooke, 2000). Interestingly, the Chinese view of the Water element as the basis for Yin in the body comports with the fact that water constitutes about 60 to 70 percent of the body's mass.

Kidney Jing controls long-term developmental processes spanning an entire life, including gestation, birth, growth, maturation, reproduction, decline, and death (Maciocia, 2001). Thus, the Kidneys are a blueprint for a person's physical life: They are roughly equivalent to a genetic code that determines a person's constitutional fortitude or robustness, the rate at which a person develops and passes through the stages of life, the quality of those stages, and the capacity to pass that physical blueprint on to progeny. In short, Kidney health affects vitality, fertility, and longevity. Because Essence orchestrates the unfolding of life phases, disruptions in Kidney function can cause developmental disorders, such as stunted growth or retardation; reproductive disorders, such as infertility or impotence; and premature aging, including degeneration of the skeletal structure, graying or thinning of the head hair, baldness, deafness, and senility.

Ming-Men, the other aspect of a person's ancestral inheritance, resides between the Kidneys at the level between the second and third lumbar vertebrae, where the acupuncture point known as Governing Vessel 4 is located. Variously translated as **Life Gate Fire**, **Gate of Vitality**, **Original Qi**, and **Source Qi**, Ming-Men is the root of Yang in the body, the source of Fire and activity, and the basis for all physiological processes and transformations—all active, dynamic, heating, and converting functions (Beresford-Cooke, 2000). Thus, the Kidneys store and dispense to each organ its form and animating power, its Yin substance and Yang energy. Hence, Chinese medicine regards the Kidneys as vital to the health of the whole body and refers to the Kidneys as "the root of life . . . the mansion of Fire and Water, the residence of Yin and Yang . . . the channel of death and life" (Kaptchuk, 2000, p. 84).

As the source of Yin and Yang in the body, the Kidneys supply and regulate the body's Water and Fire. Although other organs are involved in processing Water—for example, the Spleen extracts Water from food, the Lungs disperse Water to the skin, the Small Intestine purifies Water, and the Bladder excretes waste water or urine—the Kidneys "rule" or control Water, and by derivation all fluids, including sweat and urine. Similarly, although the Triple Heater is involved in regulating the body's temperature, it merely acts as an intermediary, transmitting Kidney Fire to other organs to ignite their functions. Kidney Fire is like a pilot light in a gas stove that is always burning, enabling various units to be lit as necessary (Beresford-Cooke, 2000), or like an ignition or engine starter, initiating and empowering the coordinated functions of the other organs.

Because Water and Fire counteract and neutralize each other, the Kidneys must balance the body's Water and Fire, ensuring that Water does not extinguish Fire and Fire does not evaporate Water. If the Kidneys fail to balance Water and Fire,

Kidney dysfunctions occur that involve disproportionate ratios of Water and Fire. When Kidney Fire is deficient, Kidney Water is in relative excess, and Water and Cold symptoms manifest not only in the Kidneys, but in other organs as well. Conversely, when Kidney Water is deficient, Kidney Fire is in relative excess, and Heat symptoms manifest not only in the Kidneys, but also in other organs.

For example, in a condition called Kidney Yang deficiency, or weak Life Gate Fire, Kidney Fire is too weak to control Kidney Water, resulting in Water and Cold symptoms (Maciocia, 2001). Various Lower Burner—genital and urinary tract—disorders develop that are overflowing in nature, such as frequent, pale, copious urination; nighttime urination or bed-wetting; incontinence; seminal discharge, vaginal discharge; and edema of the legs. Cold symptoms also arise, such as cold, sore lower back; cold, weak knees; low or no libido/sexual fire; and a subdued, apathetic disposition or lack of willpower. Because the Kidneys are foundational to health, they can transfer this dysfunction to other organs, most notably the Spleen. If the Spleen is adversely affected, related digestive symptoms will occur, including poor appetite; abdominal bloating, gurgling, and rumbling; loose stools or diarrhea; physical lassitude; and mental listlessness.

In an opposite condition known as Kidney Yin deficiency or Kidney Water exhausted, Kidney Water is too weak to control Kidney Fire. Consequently, various Heat symptoms arise, such as thirst; hot palms and soles; low-grade afternoon fever or hot flashes; night sweating; dark, scanty urine; and dry stools or constipation (Maciocia, 2001). Other symptoms affecting the tissue, sense organ, or body zones associated with the Water element also occur, such as dizziness, vertigo, and poor memory; ringing in the ears, poor hearing, tone deafness, and deafness; sore, weak lower back; and achy bones. Again, because the Kidneys are foundational to health, they can transfer this dysfunction to other organs, especially the Liver and Heart. If the Liver is adversely affected, related Liver symptoms will arise, including headaches, dry inflamed eyes, blurred vision, and scanty menstrual periods. If the Heart is adversely affected, related Heart symptoms will arise, including mental restlessness (experiencing uneasiness, fidgetiness, and agitation); insomnia (waking up several times during the night); and palpitations (having a rapid, fluttering, or throbbing heartbeat).

Psychologically, the Kidneys are associated with the will, which includes both a Yin and a Yang aspect (Kaptchuk, 2000). The Yang aspect of the will is volition, motivation, and drive, especially as expressed in major personal and professional investments that shape a person's life, such as career path and significant relationships. The Yin aspect of the will is a soft yet intentional surrender to the inevitable, to "fate" or "destiny," such as the graceful acceptance of circumstances beyond one's control or of the prospect of aging or dying. When Kidney function is compromised, a person may develop insecurities, phobias, or angst about life, the aging process, or mortality. In fact, the emotion associated with the Water element is fear. Although fear is a normal response to a serious risk or threat, an emotional imbalance exists when a person fears without good cause or fears inordinately. A less obvious and less common imbalance occurs when a person has no fear in spite of good reason to fear. Extreme fear, such as the kind evoked by a near scrape with death, can lead to loss of Bladder control.

A literary character that illustrates the Water element imbalance of fear is Ichabod Crane, from the nineteenth-century horror story *The Legend of Sleepy Hollow*, by Washington Irving (1820/1992). As a country schoolmaster, Crane is preoccupied with the mundane duties and social perks that attend his post as a local pedagogue. However, he is addicted to horror stories and their "frightful pleasure[s]." Every day after dismissing his students, he commits passages of the "History of New England Witchcraft" to memory until dusk. Then on the walk home, Crane is mortified by nebulous shapes and eerie shadows on the path, startled by collisions with insects, alarmed by the moaning of whippoorwills and the hooting of screech owls, and aghast at the crunching of his own footsteps. Despite his dread, he repeats this ritual daily and eagerly swaps witch stories for old wives' tales about ghosts and goblins.

One night after a community shindig, Crane has an ominous feeling that he will encounter the headless horseman, a baleful spirit that haunts the locality. Crane's teeth chatter, his knees knock against his saddle, and his hair stands on end: Fear has deranged his physiological functions, especially those associated with the Water element—teeth, an outgrowth of bone; knees, a body zone affected by the Kidneys, and head hair, governed by the Kidneys. When the headless horseman appears, Crane's horse misbehaves and bolts in the wrong direction. Crane panics, loses the saddle, and winds up riding bareback until the horseman hurls his decapitated head at Crane, knocking him out. In the denouement, the narrator implies that the headless horseman was really a mischievous rogue, Crane's rival in disguise, and that the head was really a pumpkin. This closing revelation about Crane's fear points to the self-inflicted nature of an inveterate temperament imbalance.

THE WOOD ELEMENT: LIVER AND GALLBLADDER

Psychologically, Wood element energy expresses the fruitfulness of life: creativity, productivity, individual self-expression, and growth. Growth in the Wood element tends to be disciplined, orderly, and focused. Hence, the Wood element is associated with a sense of direction or purpose in life, a long-term plan or vision, and in the short run, task or goal orientation. From these spring the character qualities of initiative, resolve, decisiveness, boldness, and authoritativeness. In a state of psychological harmony, the Wood element's pursuit of personal aspirations is marked by smooth progress, adaptability, social harmony, and cooperation. In a state of disharmony, the Wood element type may get stuck in a recursive loop of excessive planning or preoccupation with details or may have control issues that manifest as micromanagement or the brusque dismissal of other people as obstructions on the path to self-actualization (Beresford-Cooke, 2000).

Because the urge to grow, create, and express is so strong, a Wood element type who feels thwarted or blocked in personal or professional life will become frustrated, and this frustration may manifest as anger or depression—internalized, repressed anger (Beresford-Cooke, 2000). When excess Liver and Gallbladder energy cannot find an adequate creative outlet, it accumulates and eventually leads to a psychological explosion or implosion. Hence, among the main signs of Liver/Gallbladder imbalance are anger and derivations of anger: impatience, irritability, frustration, resentment, indignation, rigidity, rash or reckless behavior, antagonism, hostility, aggression, fury, rage, and so on.

Because Wood energy rises upward, anger often manifests physically as a unilateral temporal headache, usually right-sided, or a headache around the eyes—a condition known as Liver Yang rising; other symptoms, such as thirst and redness of the face and eyes, indicate a related condition known as Liver Fire blazing (Maciocia, 2001). If anger is suppressed, it may manifest as blockages at horizontal junctures of the body, such as the throat, chest, diaphragm, or pelvis, often with symptoms of pain and distention. Signs of Wood imbalance that are deficient rather than excessive in nature include lack of direction and purpose, lack of creativity, indecisiveness, and timidity.

Physiologically, the Liver's main functions are to detoxify and store blood and to distribute blood and Qi. These functions are similar to those of Western medicine, which also attributes blood filtration and energy reserves to the Liver: The Liver controls blood nitrogen levels by filtering out chemicals, pesticides, drug deposits, and other pollutants, and the Liver produces and stores glycogen, a form of energy, for release when blood glucose levels fall.

According to Chinese medicine, the Liver stores blood during periods of rest; releases it during periods of physical or biological activity, such as exercise and menstruation; and ensures the mellifluous movement of Qi throughout the body (Maciocia, 2001). Disturbances in Liver function can impair the circulation of Qi or blood, causing Qi to stagnate or blood to congeal (Kaptchuk, 2000).

Stagnant Qi and congealed blood are characterized by pain and distension, but distension is the more prominent feature of stagnant Qi, and pain is the more prominent feature of congealed blood (Maciocia, 2001). Stagnant Qi is distinguished by internal pressure, an inflated or bloated feeling that migrates around the body, whereas congealed blood is distinguished by a spiked or drilling pain that remains fixed in one location. In other respects, symptoms differ. Stagnant Qi produces transient abdominal masses that materialize and dematerialize, but congealed blood produces permanent abdominal masses. Tissue discoloration does not occur with stagnant Qi but may be conspicuous with congealed blood, as in ecchymosis (bruising), purple nails, purple lips, or a purple complexion. A common example of stagnant Qi is premenstrual syndrome, characterized by sore and swollen breasts, bloated loins, irritability, and moodiness, while a common example of congealed blood is dysmenorrhea, a painful menstrual period characterized by cramps and dark, burgundy blood clots.

While the two previous conditions are patterns of Liver excess, Liver deficiency can also occur. If Liver blood is deficient, the associated sense organ, the eyes, and the associated tissues, the nails and the sinews, will be malnourished, engendering various maladies such as dry gritty eyes, floaters, blurred vision, poor night vision, nearsightedness, color blindness, or blindness; dry, cracked, corrugated nails; and muscle cramps or tremors (Maciocia, 2001). Also, the associated function, menstruation, will be underactive, and scanty periods or no period will result.

Because the Wood element controls the Earth element, Liver dysfunction can disrupt Stomach and Spleen functions, resulting in digestive disorders, most notably Liver invading Spleen and Liver invading Stomach. Liver invading Spleen is characterized by abdominal churning, erratic bowel movements, and low energy. Symptoms include abdominal bloating, rumbling and gurgling, flatulence, loose stools or diarrhea alternating with constipation, and tiredness (Maciocia, 2001). Liver invading Stomach is characterized by fullness and a reversal of Stomach energy. Symptoms include abdominal bloating and pain, queasiness, belching, sour regurgitation, and vomiting.

As an accessory organ to the Liver, the Gallbladder converts waste products of the Liver into one of the components of bile—a bitter, yellow fluid that is secreted into the Small Intestine to digest fats. Liver disharmonies may adversely affect the Gallbladder's secretion and cause regurgitation of bile. Aside from its distinct function of storing bile, the Gallbladder is energetically the same as the Liver and the two organs reinforce one another.

The tissues associated with the Wood element are nails and sinews, which include tendons and ligaments. The Liver fortifies the nails and maintains the tensile strength and elasticity—the contractile and extensible quality—of the sinews. When Liver blood is ample, the nails are rosy and shiny, and the sinews are strong enough to provide joint stability yet supple enough to permit joint mobility (Kaptchuk, 2000). However, when Liver blood is deficient, the nails become pallid, thin, brittle, or dented, and the sinews become tense (Maciocia, 2001). Tense sinews impair mobility and sensation, resulting in painful obstruction syndrome—stiffness, rigidity, and numbness—or in spasms, tremors, and weakness.

The sense organ associated with the Liver is the eyes. When Liver blood is ample, the eyes feel moist and see well. But when Liver blood is deficient, the eyes feel dry and gritty like sandpaper; vision is impaired, and various eye disorders occur, such as nearsightedness, hazy vision, color blindness, poor night vision, and floaters (Maciocia, 2001). Rising Liver Heat makes the eyes look bloodshot, feel hot and sandy, and sting.

A literary character that exemplifies the main Wood element imbalance of Liver/Gallbladder excess is the monster in Mary Shelley's early science fiction novel *Frankenstein* (1818/1996). Because his creator, Dr. Frankenstein, created him out of dead body parts, the monster's form is hideous and grotesque. His skin is green, the color of the Wood element, and his eyes are bloodshot, a sign of Liver Yang rising, which inflames the Liver's sense organ, the eyes. Due to his shocking appearance, the monster unintentionally frightens, alarms, and repulses people he wants to befriend. Ultimately, he realizes that his desire for companionship will be forever thwarted. Fueled by the pain of social rejection, the monster's mounting frustration transmogrifies into a single, undeviating purpose—the goal-oriented Liver drive—to kill his creator, Dr. Frankenstein, the man who doomed him to social isolation and misery. In film adaptations of the story's climax, the monster is often depicted as marching toward his master with outstretched arms to throttle him. His motor movements are stiff, rigid, jerky, and halting, an example of Liver excess impeding the smooth movement of the associated tissues, the sinews. Tragically, the monster's mission to murder his maker is born of rage—a destructive distortion of the productive and kind Wood element energy.

THE FIRE ELEMENT: HEART/PERICARDIUM AND SMALL INTESTINE/TRIPLE HEATER

The Fire element, especially the Heart, influences the quality of a person's psychological and social life. As when friends talk to one another around a campfire or hearth, the Fire element is associated with vibrant, animated expression: excitement, exuberance, light-heartedness, alacrity, personal warmth, and responsiveness. The Fire element also inclines a person toward the spiritual dimension of life. Like tongues of fire and radiant halos set upon the head of Christ and saints, Buddha and bodhisattvas, the Fire element is associated with spiritual awakening and inspiration. And just as fire in a crucible transforms substances, the Fire element catalyzes change on many levels, personal and professional, individual and collective.

The main emotion of the Fire element is joy or elation. When balanced, joy manifests as a sunny, upbeat disposition; an effervescent, buoyant humor or mood; and pleased contentment or an optimistic expectation of good. When excessive, joy becomes excitable and volatile. This excitability has an overstimulated, hyperactive, agitated quality that can turn into manic behavior: extremely fast speech and motor movement; exaggerated or inappropriate enthusiasm, euphoria, and laughter; and in extreme cases, hysteria. When deficient, joy—or any emotion, for that matter—is notably absent, conferring a flat, dead quality to social interactions. This lack of joy in the Fire element can be altered, at least temporarily, through stimulation and good cheer, unlike in the Metal element.

While the psychological strength of the Heart is outgoing liveliness, the physical strength of the Heart is outgoing, life-giving blood distribution. In Chinese medicine, the Heart is the last organ in the process of transforming Grain Qi into blood, so it plays a role in producing the substance that supports life (Maciocia, 2001). As in Western medicine, the Heart also regulates blood circulation throughout the body. In fact, the blood vessels—the tissue associated with the Fire element—are considered an extension of the Heart. The quality of blood and circulation can to some extent be observed in the complexion or felt in the hands. A pink, shiny complexion suggests ample blood and good circulation; a pale or white complexion suggests blood deficiency or poor circulation; a bluish or purplish complexion suggests blood stagnation; and a red complexion and skin eruptions suggest Heat in the blood. If the hands are warm, circulation is good, but if the hands are cold, circulation is impaired.

Disorders and diseases of the Heart are cardiovascular in nature and include the following: high blood pressure; thickening, hardening, narrowing, and occluding of the arteries; localized weakening and expansion of artery walls; enlarged and engorged veins whose nonreturn valves no longer function properly; inflammation of deep veins, especially in the legs; blood clots attached to blood vessel walls; and Heart attack and stroke, both of which are caused by a blocked or hemorrhaging artery that impairs blood flow to the Heart or brain, depriving that organ of oxygen and leading to tissue death. Symptoms of these cardiovascular crises correlate in surprising ways to Chinese medicine. For example, the classic sign of a Heart attack—chest pain that radiates down the inner arm—follows the path of the Heart Meridian. Some symptoms of stroke, especially speech difficulties, paralysis, and loss of consciousness, correspond to pathological impairment or disruption of various Fire element capacities, including the tongue, the associated sense organ of the Fire element and its activity of speech; celerity, the associated quality of movement; and Shen, the associated psychological capacity for awareness and interactiveness.

Despite the serious nature of Heart maladies, Chinese medicine emphasizes the psychological functions of the Heart more than the physiological. The Heart enshrines **Shen—spirit** or **mind**—which governs our consciousness and awareness, psychological adjustment to the world, social dynamics, short-term memory, and sleep. Signs of a healthy Shen include normal waking consciousness, awareness of self and others, appropriate emotional responses and social interactions, good short-term memory, and refreshing sleep. Conversely, signs of a disturbed Shen are usually manic in nature and include frenetic thoughts, agitation, nervous excitability, inappropriate or immoderate emotional responses and social interactions, hysteria or shock, delirium or unconsciousness, forgetfulness or absentmindedness, and insomnia—especially the inability to fall asleep and dream-disturbed sleep or nightmares.

As for interpersonal relations, the Heart is responsible for ensuring the appropriateness of behavior within a particular social context, especially with respect to time, place, and manner issues (Kaptchuk, 2000). When Shen is disturbed, a person will think, say, or do something at the wrong time or in the wrong place or in the wrong way, such as wearing sweats to a business meeting or a sexually provocative outfit to church, cracking jokes and clowning around at a funeral, laughing hysterically about a serious accident or illness, discussing bowel movements at the dinner table, or mulling over bills at bedtime. Other manifestations of disturbed Shen are social or situational angst and eccentric behavior. Corresponding physiological symptoms include "sweating, blushing, being flustered, and [heart] palpitations" (Kaptchuk, 2000, p. 89).

The sense organ associated with the Heart is the tongue, and the Heart's radiance and vitality are expressed in the face. Consequently, the ability to communicate well—to express meaning and to engage socially—is a function of the Heart, as are congeniality and appropriate facial expressions (Katpchuk, 2000). Often, Fire element types talk rapidly and extensively; in fact, they might be accused of having a motor mouth (Maciocia, 2001). Heart disturbances of the tongue can result in pathological conditions, such as tongue sores or ulcers, speech impediments, stuttering, stammering, aphasia (loss of the ability to speak or understand spoken or written language), and muteness.

A literary prototype for manic disorders of the Heart appears in Cervantes' *Don Quixote* (1605/2004). Don Quixote, a relatively poor and socially defunct nobleman, explores the lore of chivalry in his personal library. What begins as an interest soon turns into an obsession, then a compulsion, then full-blown mania, illustrating by degrees the zealous distractibility of a Fire element imbalance. Inflamed by the idealism in these chivalrous novels, Don Quixote sells acres of his farmland to expand his book collection and fill his imagination with more tales of knights. His frenzied studies deprive him of sleep and wit, contributing to a floating, ungrounded Shen. Eventually, his literary fanaticism, insomnia, and irrationality culminate in a decision to roam the world in rusty armor as a pseudo-knight-errant in a single-handed attempt to right the world's wrongs.

Although Don Quixote's journey can be viewed as a quest for social redemption or a crusade against social injustice, it is also clearly an allegory for a disturbed Shen and the absurd and outlandish way it manifests socially. Among his many misadventures, Don Quixote assaults a band of itinerant merchants for refusing to compliment a peasant girl's beauty and winds up severely battered. Mistaking an inn for a castle, Don Quixote denounces the innkeeper as rude for presenting him with a bill and is forcibly ousted. While sharing dinner with illiterate goatherds, Don Quixote waxes eloquent, delivering a long, erudite lecture on the Golden Age of Mythology, the meaning of which totally escapes them. Topping off his flamboyant escapades in Book One are his duels against windmills, which he erroneously identifies as giants.

Don Quixote's misguided efforts to treat ordinary people like literary characters and to do chivalrous deeds at a time when chivalry is out of vogue, in places where such deeds are ill suited, and in a manner that is ridiculous, exemplify a distortion of the Fire element's usual sensitivity to social context and to time, place, and manner appropriateness. Don Quixote's inappropriateness and eccentricity spring from misperceptions or delusions about social reality: for example, proclaiming himself a "knight" and a manual laborer his "squire," defending a "lady's" (peasant girl's) honor, repudiating a "nobleman's" (innkeeper's) lack of hospitality, amusing "genteel" guests (goatherds), and slaying "giants" (windmills). Ultimately, his eccentricity creates a serious disconnect between himself and others, reflecting the maladjusted, and at times almost farcical, behavior of a disturbed Shen.

Although the Heart is featured prominently as the primary organ of the Fire element, the other Fire organs—Small Intestine, Pericardium, and Triple Heater—reinforce and supplement the Heart in different ways. Notably, the Fire element is the only element associated with four organs and two pairs of Meridians: the primary pair is the Heart and Small Intestine, while the secondary pair is the Pericardium and Triple Heater.

While the pairing of the Heart and Small Intestine may seem incongruous at first, certain observations can help reconcile the seeming mismatch. During embryonic development, the Heart and Small Intestine develop from the same layer of cells, the most internal germ layer of cells, called the endoderm (Beresford-Cooke, 2000). The Heart and Small Intestine are also somewhat similar in form and function: Structurally, they are both hollow receptacles—one is a four-chambered vessel and the other a long tube—that by muscular contraction propel substances through to other parts of the body. Further, the Heart and Small Intestine work, albeit in conjunction with other organs, to supply the body with nutrient-rich blood: The Small Intestine assimilates nutrients and water from partially digested food, which the Heart ultimately delivers throughout the body. Last, but perhaps most important from a TCM perspective, the Small Intestine serves the Heart through its psychological function of discernment or discriminatory judgment (Maciocia, 2001).

Physiologically, the Small Intestine's main function is to assimilate partially digested food received from the Stomach or, as the classical texts say, to "separate the pure from the impure or turbid" (Kaptchuk, 2000, p. 95). The Small Intestine extracts what is beneficial to the body, passing it on to the Spleen for further processing, and disposes of the rest, passing the solid and liquid wastes on to the organs of elimination, the Large Intestine and Bladder. Because the Small Intestine works under the direction of the Spleen to process food and the Kidneys to process fluids, Small Intestine disorders often implicate the Spleen or Kidneys (Maciocia, 2001). Small Intestine disorders include abdominal bloating and pain; gurgling and rumbling; flatulence; changes in bowel patterns, especially sudden alternations of diarrhea and constipation; anemia; and low energy.

Just as the Small Intestine separates pure from impure on a physical level, so, too, it separates pure from impure on a psychological level, serving the Heart. The Small Intestine divides sensory, emotional, and mental input into beneficial and detrimental categories. This psychological capacity is known as clarity, discernment, or discriminatory judgment: the ability to identify relevant issues; to distinguish between good and bad, right and wrong, true and false, just and unjust, effective and ineffective; and—refining further—to identify the best among several alternatives or the least harmful among several evils. If the Small Intestine fails in this filtering, screening, or quality control function, the Heart will integrate input that is "impure"—psychologically damaging—leading to psychological distress and confusion (Beresford-Cooke, 2000).

Like the Heart, the Small Intestine can be disturbed by shock, which scatters Qi (Beresford-Cooke, 2000). Shock is a psychological state in which a person blocks unacceptable, deeply traumatic, or life-threatening information. This corresponds to the Small Intestine's function of rejecting harmful wastes in the process of "separating the pure from the impure." Paradoxically, the state of shock also renders a person peculiarly susceptible to the power of suggestion (Olness, 1993), which corresponds to the Small Intestine's function of absorbing nutrients. Victims of severe trauma, such as those incurred by electrocution or chemical explosion, demonstrate remarkable powers of regeneration when given positive input while in a state of shock. A medical doctor and hypnotherapist who treats burn victims, Dr. Dabney Ewin, always reassures his patients while they are in a state of shock that their skin feels "cool" and that their prognosis is good, despite medical signs to the contrary, and accordingly, his patients manifest remarkable recoveries in remarkable time (Kennard, 1993).

The **Pericardium**—variously known as the Heart Constrictor, Heart Protector, Heart Governor, and Heart Master, depending on which of its functions is emphasized—shares and reinforces Heart functions. Because the Pericardium supplements Heart functions, Heart disorders can be treated by working both the Heart and the Pericardium Meridians. The Pericardium is a type of fascia, a bandage or sheath of connective tissue that encloses the Heart. This fibrous membrane enables the Heart to pump blood by providing firm resistance against which the Heart muscle can contract. The name **Heart Constrictor** best emphasizes this function. As a protective outer covering, the Pericardium also defends the Heart against physical and psychological harm. The name **Heart Protector** best emphasizes this function. Finally, the names **Heart Governor** and **Heart Master** both convey the meaning of an official or ministerial agent acting for or on behalf of the Heart by assisting in circulation.

Physical disorders of the Pericardium are cardiovascular in nature and include all the previously mentioned disorders affecting the Heart. Psychological disorders of the Pericardium are social in nature: A person with an energetic imbalance in the Pericardium tends to be either underprotective or overprotective. A person who is underprotective may be unduly open and vulnerable to violations of personal boundaries, whereas a person who is overprotective may be shy or socially guarded, armored, distant, or aloof, usually as a result of having been hurt in the past. Like the Pericardium, the **Triple Heater** reinforces the Heart in the context of social interactions, ensuring harmonious social relations. As with Pericardium imbalances, a person with a Triple Heater imbalance may be socially vulnerable or, more often, socially defensive; this defensiveness may aggregate as tension in the forearms, indicative of holding others at arm's length (Beresford-Cooke, 2000).

Physically, the Triple Heater is not an organ but rather a system of organs that regulate water. The Chinese characters for Triple Heater signify "three that burn" or "three that scorch," indicating the function of the body's Fire in controlling the body's Water (Maciocia, 2001, p. 118). Other names for the Triple Heater are **Triple Burner**, **Triple Warmer**, **Triple Energizer**, and **Sanjaio**. The *Nei Jing* describes the Triple Burner as "the official in charge of irrigation and control of water passages" and likens the Upper Burner to a mist, the Middle Burner to a foam, and the Lower Burner to a swamp. The Lungs of the Upper Burner vaporize and disperse the body's Water, moistening the tissues; the Stomach and Spleen of the Middle Burner churn the body's Water in digestion like a "bubbling cauldron" or "maceration chamber," and the Kidneys, Bladder, and Small and Large Intestines of the Lower Burner dredge waste from the body's Water like a "drainage ditch" (Maciocia, 2001, pp. 119–120).

Alternatively, a complementary model assigns physical zones to each of the three burning spaces. The Upper Burner extends from the chest to the diaphragm, corresponds to the thorax, and includes the Heart and Lungs; the Middle Burner extends from the diaphragm to the navel, corresponds to the solar plexus, and includes the Stomach and Spleen, and the Lower Burner extends from the navel to the groin, corresponds to the hara, and includes the Kidneys, Small and Large Intestines, and Bladder (Maciocia, 2001).

As a distribution system, the Triple Heater transmits various types of Qi to various parts of the body and thereby protects, energizes, and warms the body (Maciocia, 2001). In the Upper Burner, the Triple Heater distributes **Wei Qi**, also known as **Defensive Qi** or **Protective Qi**. Wei Qi is an invisible armor or bodysuit of vital energy between the skin and muscles that deflects or wards off invasion by pathogens and Pernicious Influences, such as Cold, Wind, and Heat. Because of this protective function, the Triple Heater is sometimes likened to the body's immune and lymphatic functions.

In the Middle Burner, the Triple Heater distributes **Nutritive Qi**, biologically processed food, from the Stomach and Spleen to all the organs, nourishing them and fueling their functions (Maciocia, 2001). In the Lower Burner, the Triple Heater distributes Original Qi from the Kidneys to the other organs, thereby igniting their functions and warming the entire body. Because the Triple Heater is integrally involved in the transmission of Defensive Qi, Nutritive Qi, and Original Qi, the Triple Heater is implicated in immune, digestive, and thermal disorders, including allergies, susceptibility to infections, lack of resistance to Pernicious Influences and other pathogens, hypoactivity of the digestive organs, and chilliness, especially in the lower body.

THE EARTH ELEMENT: SPLEEN AND STOMACH

The Earth element is associated with home and family, security, physical nourishment, emotional nurture and support, receptivity, and fertility. Just as the earth enfolds and decomposes vegetable matter and subsumes and deconstructs mineral matter, returning things to itself and reconstituting things as itself, so the theme of the Earth element is absorption and transformation into the self, physically and psychologically.

The psychological disposition associated with the Earth element has been variously identified as cognition, analytical reasoning, rumination, and reflective thought: It is a digesting of ideas, a mental chewing of the cud that often includes an emotional component of sympathy or concern (Beresford-Cooke, 2000). When the Earth element is imbalanced, this capacity turns into mulling, brooding, and worrying or, as the Chinese say, overthinking. Overthinking has an obsessive quality, like a mother catastrophizing over the whereabouts of her absent family members at dinnertime. Overthinking can degenerate further into a paralysis of analysis, in which thought is so ponderous, torturous, and convoluted that it cripples action. When directed inward toward the self, the sympathetic aspect of overthinking can turn into self-pity. Other Earth element disharmonies related to cognition include the inability to concentrate; muddled, confused, and irrational thinking; and mental apathy, lethargy, boredom, and disinterest.

A literary character who exemplifies the Earth element imbalance of overthinking is Shakespeare's character Hamlet, whose tragic flaw, according to some literary critics, is "thinking too precisely." This character defect is revealed during many of Hamlet's private ruminations, including the famous "To be or not to be" soliloquy, in which he admits to himself that his mental qualms are delaying and even arresting his moral imperative to avenge his father's murder: "And thus the native hue of resolution is sicklied o'er with the pale cast of thought, and enterprises of great pith and moment with this regard their currents turn awry and lose the name of action" (3.1. 92–96).

To a great extent, the play's plot is driven by Hamlet's mental agonizing and vacillations. In the beginning, Hamlet broods over his father's death and nurses suspicions that his uncle murdered his father. Although he intuits foul play, he is not fully persuaded until he meets his father's ghost, who divulges the details and makes him swear vengeance. At this point, Hamlet's conviction and resolve are strong. Yet not long afterward he begins to doubt the ghost and decides he needs another confirmation of his uncle's guilt. To entrap his uncle, Hamlet orchestrates an evening of entertainment that features a play that reenacts the murder. As expected, his uncle betrays his own guilt. In spite of this incriminating evidence and an opportunity to kill his uncle during a private confessional, Hamlet postpones because he reasons that killing his uncle during an act of repentance would absolve his uncle's soul, whereas true vengeance would require killing him in the midst of an act that has "no relish of salvation" in it.

Toward the play's end, Hamlet castigates himself again for this paralysis of analysis as he observes an army of men preparing to die for a cause that lacks merit, while he himself has just cause but is immobilized: "Surely [God] that made us with such large discourse . . . gave us not that . . . godlike reason to fust in us unused. Now, whether it be . . . some craven scruple of thinking too precisely on the event, . . . I do not know why yet I live to say, 'This thing's to do,' [since] I have cause, and will, and strength, and means to do it. . . . O, from this time forth, my thoughts be bloody, or be nothing worth!" (4.4. 38–48, 67–68).

In addition to this capacity for careful reflection, which sometimes bogs the Earth element down, another psychological capacity of the Earth element is the ability to give and receive in social contexts (Beresford-Cooke, 2000). When the Earth element is balanced, a person tends to cultivate relationships that are mutually beneficial and supportive, relationships characterized by reciprocity in giving and receiving. But when the Earth element is imbalanced, a person either gives without receiving or receives without giving. Stereotypical examples of these extremes are the caretakers or martyrs who devote themselves to and sacrifice themselves for others and the freeloaders or social drains who neglect or shirk personal responsibility and depend on the services and financial and emotional support of others.

Caretaker Earth element types feel validated and empowered by giving but often have difficulty receiving (Beresford-Cooke, 2000). These people may opt for a professional role that defines them as a giver, such as a social worker, psychologist, minister, physical therapist, nurse, doctor, teacher, or handyman. In their personal lives, they may gravitate toward codependent relationships in which they financially support other adults and become socially and legally responsible for them, even to the point of rescuing others from the negative consequences of their own irresponsible behavior—for example, discharging somebody's credit card debt or bailing somebody out of jail.

Conversely, recipient Earth element types seek relationships in which they are supported. These people somehow find themselves or render themselves perpetually needy, relying on others to compensate for their shortcomings or failings—these are, for example, the housemates who never pay their share of the rent or mortgage on time; who through neglect allow the water, gas, electric, or cable service to be interrupted; whose slovenly habits require others to perform custodial services for them; and who continually impose, by eating others' food, borrowing others' belongings, and expecting rides and favors and free pet- or baby-sitting service.

Either extreme of giver or receiver can be depleting and demoralizing. Sometimes, however, these roles cannot be avoided, either because they are the very nature of a relationship, as when the role of a mother is giver and that of a child is receiver, or because they result from circumstances beyond one's control, as when a loved one takes on the role of caring for a family member who is injured, ill, or elderly. In all these situations, Shiatsu to the Stomach and Spleen Meridians is indicated.

Physiologically, the Spleen and Stomach produce **Post-Heaven** or **Postnatal Qi**, the nutrients and energy extracted from ingested food and drink that form the basis for blood and Qi in the body. In Chinese medicine, the Stomach plays a subordinate role, assisting the Spleen in digestion. The Stomach initiates the process of digestion by receiving food and drink for "rotting and ripening," or decomposition and fermentation, passing the pure portion to the Spleen for transformation into blood and Qi and the impure down to the Small Intestine for further separation (Maciocia, 2001). Stomach disorders are often a reversal of the normal direction of descent to the Small Intestine. Such reversals or upheavals are called rebellious Stomach Qi and can manifest as queasiness and nausea, burping and belching, hiccups, acid reflux, and vomiting (Kaptchuk, 2000).

In Chinese medicine, the Spleen—not the Stomach—is considered the primary digestive organ. The Spleen rules "transformation and transportation," that is, the conversion of food and drink into an assimilative form for distribution throughout the body (Kaptchuk, 2000). The Spleen extracts nutrients from the Stomach's partially processed food and drink and transforms these raw materials into a substance compatible with and absorbable by the body, sending it up to the Lungs for conversion into Qi and blood. Blood and Qi circulate throughout the body, providing the building blocks for tissues and the impetus for movement. In health, Spleen energy ascends toward the Lungs. In disharmony, this upward direction is reversed, resulting in sinking Spleen Qi or various kinds of physical sagging and collapse, such as hemorrhoids, hernias, and organ prolapse (Beresford-Cooke, 2000).

Because of its instrumental role in producing Postnatal Qi, the Spleen is the main organ (in conjunction with the Lungs) responsible for building and nourishing the flesh, the tissue associated with the Earth element, and for energizing the activities of the flesh. The Spleen's Western counterpart, the pancreas, has similar functions: to produce digestive enzymes that catabolize carbohydrates, fats, proteins, and acids, thereby creating nutrients for cell and tissue growth, maintenance, and repair; and to produce the hormones insulin and glucagon, which regulate blood sugar levels, thereby affecting energy levels.

Since the Spleen is essential in creating blood and Qi, Spleen disorders can result in deficient blood or anemia, deficient Qi or chronic fatigue, and malnourished or emaciated flesh (Maciocia, 2001). Robust flesh and vitality indicate a healthy Spleen, whereas flaccid or wasted flesh, weakness, fatigue, and exhaustion indicate Spleen deficiency. In contrast, fat, lumpy, and congested flesh indicates Dampness or Phlegm affecting the Spleen. In TCM, Dampness and Phlegm are conditions of excess moisture. Phlegm manifests either substantially as masses like lipomas, cysts, polyps, and tumors or insubstantially as numbness or paralysis along a Meridian (Beresford-Cooke, 2000). Dampness of the Spleen (or Kidneys) manifests as edema in the lower half of the body, indicating that the Spleen is not properly processing fluids, resulting in fluid retention, whereas edema in the upper half of the body implicates the Lungs.

Besides creating blood, the Spleen "governs" the retention of blood, ensuring that it stays within the vessels. Hence, various blood disorders—especially reckless blood or hemorrhaging (Kaptchuk, 2000)—indicate Spleen dysfunction, including nosebleeds; blood in stools, sputum, or urine; spider and varicose veins; and excessive or prolonged menstruation (Beresford-Cooke, 2000).

In general, Spleen and Stomach disorders center on the theme of eating and span the full range of alimentary tract issues, including mouth, appetite, digestive, and weight disorders. The mouth is, of course, the sense organ associated with the Earth element. Mouth disorders include cold sores, inflamed and bleeding gums, foul breath due to Stomach Fire, and dull taste or lack of taste due to Spleen deficiency. Appetite disorders include poor appetite or lack of appetite due to Spleen deficiency, ravenous or insatiable appetite due to Stomach excess, and cravings for sweets or sugar addiction. Digestive disorders include poor or upset digestion due to Spleen malfunction, ulcers due to Stomach stress, and abnormal bowel conditions or movements, such as abdominal bloating and diarrhea, due to Spleen deficiency. Weight disorders include anorexia (self-starvation), bulimia (binging and purging), and habitual or compulsive overeating (Beresford-Cooke, 2000). Appetite and weight disorders usually involve an emotional or social component. As such, these disorders are often compensatory in nature and point to unsatisfied emotional or social needs.

Lastly, the Earth element is associated with maternal functions. The Stomach and Spleen Meridians traverse the lower abdomen, where the reproductive organs are located, and the chest, where the breasts are located. Stomach disorders can adversely affect the ovaries, uterus, and breasts, and Spleen disorders (as well as Liver disorders) can adversely affect menstruation.

THE METAL ELEMENT: LUNGS AND LARGE INTESTINE

The theme of the Metal element is best summarized as "vitality through exchange" (Beresford-Cooke, 2000). In exchange, one thing is traded for another of comparable value. This process of continual exchange is vital to life and common to commerce. Before the invention of modern currency, one means of exchange, aside from bartering goods and services, was payment by precious metals, the most valuable of which was gold. Interestingly, the Chinese ideogram for the Metal element is white gold, indicating value through exchange or the power to sustain life through exchange (Beresford-Cooke, 2000). Continual exchange connects a person to the environment, gives a person a sense of belonging, and is necessary for a person's physical, emotional, and social well-being. On a biological level, for example, the body must eat food (intake) in order to work (output) and then must discharge waste (output) to clear space for more food (intake).

Physiologically, the Lungs and Large Intestine—along with their associated tissue, the skin, and their associated sense organ, the nose—constitute the boundaries of a person's physical being and give a person the sense of a separate physical and psychological identity. The entrance into the body is through the nose and Lungs, while the exit from the body is through the Large Intestine. The skin is the barrier that encloses and separates a person from the environment. Yet the skin also joins a person to the environment by being the medium through which contact with the environment is made. By defining a person's physical parameters, the Lungs, Large Intestine, and skin also define the sense of self, and by engaging in exchange with the environment, they give a person a dynamic sense of belonging or bonding (Beresford-Cooke, 2000).

The Lungs engage in exchange through respiration, inhaling pure Air Qi and exhaling "dirty" Air Qi—carbon dioxide and stale energy. Because the Lungs directly contact the environment through the opening of the nose, they are particularly susceptible to invasion by pathogens and Pernicious Influences—Cold, Wind, Heat, Dampness, and Dryness—and are therefore called the "tender Organ" (Maciocia, 2001). Lung disorders can manifest as olfactory, sinus, and respiratory disorders. Olfactory disorders include a dull sense of smell, lack of smell, and hypersensitivity to natural or normal odors. Sinus disorders include nose bleeds due to Lung Heat; an itchy, tickly nose; sneezing; sinus congestion or blockage, and sinus drainage. Respiratory disorders include colds and flu, coughing, Lung and nasal congestion, difficult or labored breathing, allergies, and asthma.

Because Air Qi combines with Grain Qi to form the Qi of the body that empowers all physiological processes and movement, Lung disorders can cause deficient Qi anywhere in the body, resulting in substandard organ functioning and lethargy (Kaptchuk, 2000). Normally, Lung Qi descends and facilitates downward movements in the body, such as the "grasping and anchoring" of Air Qi, the descent of bodily fluids, and the evacuation of wastes, both solid and fluid. When Lung Qi fails to descend, various upward-bound maladies may arise, such as a feeling of stuffiness and pressure in the chest that restricts breathing; the reversal of Lung Qi in the form of coughing and sneezing; edema in the upper body and face; constipation; and less commonly, urinary retention (Maciocia, 2001).

In addition to respiration, the Lungs disperse fluids throughout the body and control the function of the sweat glands and the quality of the skin and body hair (the head hair is governed by the Kidneys). The skin engages in exchange through the pores, absorbing Air Qi and emollient nutrients, dissipating excess Heat or fluids in the form of sweat, and excreting poisons and wastes in the form of pus. When the Lungs are healthy, the pores function properly, and the Lungs diffuse a "mist" of body fluids around the periphery of the body between the muscles and skin, making the skin smooth and glossy and the body hair thick and lustrous (Maciocia, 2001). But when the Lungs are impaired, the skin is rough and dry; the body hair is thin, dull, and brittle; and the pores are blocked, obstructing sweat, or lax, allowing too much sweat to escape.

The Lungs also form the basis for Defensive Qi and work in conjunction with the Triple Heater to circulate Defensive Qi throughout the periphery of the body. When the Lungs are healthy, Defensive Qi shields the body from Pernicious Influences, but when the Lungs are impaired, Defensive Qi cannot circulate, and inclement environmental agents penetrate and lodge in the body, producing illness.

The Large Intestine engages in exchange by absorbing water from the fecal mass and expelling the residue as solid waste. This expulsion of waste material is also essential to vitality, since without it, the body would putrefy from toxicity. The Lung descending function assists the Large Intestine in defecation. If the Lung descending function is impaired, the Large Intestine will lack the power to evacuate, and constipation will result (Maciocia, 2001). Most Large Intestine disorders, such as abdominal pain, gurgling and rumbling, constipation, and diarrhea, arise in conjunction with disorders of other organs, especially the Spleen.

Psychologically, the Lungs and Large Intestine are associated with a sense of self-worth, receiving, and releasing (Liechti, 1998). Disharmonies of the Metal element can result in low self-esteem and the inability to open up, take in, or let go. On a minor level, a person may have difficulty introducing himself to others or chatting with others, asking for favors or help, accepting gifts and acts of kindness, shedding grievances, or disposing of junk. On a major level, a person may have trouble communicating his or her needs and desires, may feel that he or she has nothing of value to offer others or that he or she is a mere burden to others; and may be unable to forge or sustain close relationships and enjoy intimacy or may be unable to end relationships that are no longer viable.

The man who lacks confidence to ask a woman out on a date or who cannot quit an unsatisfactory job because of a psychological block against leaving or applying elsewhere and the woman who pines and languishes in a prolonged depression after a breakup with an ill-matched suitor or who stays indefinitely in an unsatisfactory relationship with a philandering or physically abusive lover because she thinks no one else would want her are examples of possible Metal element imbalances affecting the psyche and, in turn, the social life. These scenarios revolve around poor self-image and the inability to accept something good or reject something bad.

In general, Metal element types tend to be introverted, reserved, reticent, and socially retiring. However, a Metal disharmony can compel a person to reduce or avoid social exchange to an unhealthy degree, resulting in physical withdrawal and seclusion or social isolation and alienation.

Sadness and grief born of loss or unfulfilled longing are the emotions associated with the Metal element (Kaptchuk, 2000). Although sadness and grief are natural and normal responses to loss or disappointment, a Metal element disharmony can render sorrow or bereavement disproportionately intense or prolonged relative to the event that precipitated it. Grief as a habitual state of mind can manifest as a gloomy, downbeat, or melancholy temperament; perpetual negativity; pessimism; or cynicism (Liechti, 1998). Conversely, a Metal element disharmony can also result in stoicism or repressed grief—the inability to feel or express sorrow when appropriate, as, for example, when a person seems unaffected by a divorce or the death of a loved one.

A literary prototype of a Metal element disharmony is Ebeneezer Scrooge from Charles Dickens' *A Christmas Carol*. As a banker, Scrooge is in the business of circulating and compounding money, a form of value, through exchange. But Scrooge is extremely miserly, hoarding money and begrudging himself and others necessities like coal for a fire in winter and alms to feed the poor. His hoarding and miserliness are forms of Metal element statis or "constipation," a reluctance to share what he has with others. This reluctance extends to sharing himself in social relationships as well. Scrooge is a bitter old man who lives alone, according to the Metal element tendency toward sullenness, withdrawal, and seclusion.

Over the years, Scrooge has failed to forge close bonds with other people: the fiancée of his youth, whose devotion he neglected because she didn't have a dowry; his business partner and friend, whose death he didn't mourn and whose presence he seems not to miss; his clerk, a very loyal employee, whom he has taken for granted and treated austerely over the years; his nephew, whose invitations to hospitality he has repeatedly refused; and his community, whose philanthropic appeals he has repeatedly rebuffed. Scrooge's failure to form close romantic, platonic, professional, and civic relationships points to a Metal element unwillingness or inability to open up, take in, and put out. His stoicism over his partner's death and indifference toward any form of human suffering also indicate an emotional void or block, an unwillingness or inability to experience and express the full spectrum of emotions, especially grief and sorrow.

The ghosts of Christmas past, present, and future show Scrooge the error and consequences of his ways: that his morose attitude and antisocial temperament will doom him not only to a gloomy life, but also to a morbid end. Fortunately, he repents. In the end, Scrooge anonymously gives gifts, donates to charity, raises his clerk's salary, and accepts his nephew's invitation to celebrate Christmas, an annual invitation that he has spurned for years. This turnabout presages a new life of meaningful relationships and meaningful exchange.

REFERENCES

Academic American Encyclopedia (vol. 15). (1981). *Physics*. Princeton, NJ: Arete.

Beresford-Cooke, C. (2000). *Shiatsu theory and practice: A comprehensive text for the student and professional*. Edinburgh: Churchill Livingstone.

Cervantes, M. (2004). *The history of Don Quixote: Volume 1. Complete* (J. Ormsby, Trans., & G. Dore, Ill.). Retrieved from Project Gutenberg at http://www.gutenberg.org. (Original work published 1605.)

Dickens, C. (2004). *A Christmas Carol* (J. Menendez, Ed.). Retrieved from Project Gutenberg at http://www.gutenberg.org (Original work published 1843.)

Irving, W. (1992). *The Legend of Sleepy Hollow* (I. Newby, G. Newby, & J. Menendez, Eds.). Retrieved from Project Gutenberg at http://www.gutenberg.org (Original work published 1820.)

Kaptchuk, T. (2000). *The web that has no weaver: Understanding Chinese medicine* (2nd ed.). Chicago: Contemporary.

Kennard, D., Institute of Noetic Sciences, & Turner Original Productions (Producers). (1993). *The heart of healing: Remarkable stories of how we heal ourselves.* [Videocassette].

Liechti, E. (1998). *The complete illustrated guide to Shiatsu: The Japanese healing art of touch for health and fitness.* New York: Barnet & Noble.

Maciocia, G. (2001). *The foundations of Chinese medicine: A comprehensive text for acupuncturists and herbalists.* Edinburgh: Churchill Livingstone. (Original work published 1989.)

Olness, K. (1993). Hypnosis: The power of attention. In D. Goleman & J. Gurin (Eds.), *Mind body medicine: How to use your mind for better health* (pp. 277–290). Yonkers, NY: Consumer Reports Books.

Shakespeare, W. (1958). *The tragedy of Hamlet, Prince of Denmark: The Folger Library General Reader's Shakespeare* (L. Wright & V. ZaMar, Eds.). New York: Washington Square Press Simon & Schuster. (Original work published 1602.)

Shelley, M. (1996). *Frankenstein: The 1818 text, contexts, nineteenth century responses, modern criticism* (P. Hunter, Ed.). New York: Norton. (Original work published 1818.)

STUDY QUESTIONS

1. What are Zang organs?
2. What features and functions distinguish Zang organs?
3. What are Fu organs?
4. What features and functions distinguish Fu organs?
5. Which organs and Meridians are more important to the Shiatsu practitioner—Zang or Fu?
6. Which tissue is associated with the Water element and what does it encompass?
7. How does the Water element influence the autonomic nervous system?
8. Describe the physiological effects of a sympathetic nervous system Water element disharmony.
9. Describe the psychological characteristics of a sympathetic nervous system Water element disharmony.
10. Describe the physiological effects of a parasympathetic nervous system Water element disharmony.
11. Describe the psychological characteristics of a parasympathetic nervous system Water element disharmony.
12. Why is the Water element considered the foundation of the other elements?

13. What is Ming-Men?

14. What does Ming-Men do?

15. What is Jing?

16. What does Jing do?

17. How do the Kidneys influence the body's Water?

18. How do the Kidneys influence the body's Fire?

19. Kidney dysfunctions usually entail a disproportion of what?

20. What major signs indicate a deficiency of Kidney Fire?

21. What kinds of disorders arise from Kidney Fire deficiency?

22. Which other organ may be affected by Kidney Fire deficiency?

23. What major sign indicates a deficiency of Kidney Water?

24. What kinds of disorders arise from Kidney Water deficiency?

25. Which other organs may be affected by Kidney Water deficiency?

26. What sense organ is associated with Water?

27. Identify a few disorders that can arise with Water's associated sense organ.

28. Identify the main psychological capacity of the Water element.

29. What emotions and emotional imbalances are common to Water?

30. What psychological qualities are associated with the Wood element?

31. What is the main emotion associated with excess Wood energy?

32. What psychosomatic disorder can develop from Wood energy rising upward?

33. How does deficient Wood energy manifest psychologically?

34. What are the Liver's main physiological functions?

35. In what way do disturbances in Liver function manifest?

36. A disharmony in the Wood element can adversely affect which other element?

37. What is the Gallbladder's main function?

38. What tissues are associated with Wood?

39. Identify a few problems that can arise with the associated tissues.

40. What sense organ is associated with Wood?

41. Identify a few problems that can arise with Wood's associated sense organ.

42. What is unique about the Fire element in terms of its Meridians and organs?

43. More than any other organ, the Heart influences what aspect of a person's being?

44. What is the main emotion associated with the Fire element?

45. Describe the psychological distortions of Fire that occur with excess.

46. Describe the psychological distortions of Fire that occur with deficiency.

47. What are the main physiological functions of the Heart?

48. Which tissue is associated with the Fire element and what is its relationship to the Heart?

49. Identify the nature of Heart disorders and give a few examples.

50. What does the Heart enshrine?

51. What aspects of being does Shen govern?

52. Describe a few manifestations of a disturbed Shen.

53. Explain how issues of time, place, and manner relate to Heart function.

54. What sense organ is associated with Fire?

55. Identify a few pathological conditions of the tongue.

56. What distinctive communication qualities are associated with Fire?

57. What is the Small Intestine's main physiological function?

58. Which other organ is implicated in Small Intestine disorders?

59. What is the Small Intestine's main psychological function?

60. Identify other names for the Pericardium.

61. Explain how the Pericardium assists, shares, and reinforces Heart functions.

62. What aspect of one's being does the Pericardium influence?

63. How do psychological imbalances of the Pericardium manifest?

64. What sphere of influence do the Triple Heater and the Pericardium share?

65. Identify other names for the Triple Heater.

66. Describe the *Nei Jing*'s view of the Triple Heater.

67. What three physical zones correspond to the three burning spaces?

68. What are the Triple Heater's main physiological functions?

69. Identify a few Triple Heater disorders.

70. What is the psychological capacity of the Earth element?

71. In what way does an imbalance in the Earth element distort this psychological capacity?

72. What other psychological disharmonies are associated with the Earth element?

73. Identify the psychological capacity of the Earth element in a social context.

74. What relational dysfunctions can arise when this capacity is imbalanced?

75. Describe the giving Earth element type.

76. Describe the receiving Earth element type.

77. What is the Earth element's role with respect to Post-Heaven/Postnatal Qi?

78. What is the Stomach's main physiological function?

79. What is rebellious Stomach Qi?

80. According to TCM, which digestive organ is considered primary, and which is considered secondary?

81. What is the Spleen's main physiological function?

82. In which direction does Spleen Qi normally flow?

83. Give a few examples of sinking Spleen Qi (reversal in flow of Spleen Qi).

84. In conjunction with the Lungs, the Spleen is credited with producing what and providing what for the body?

85. Give a few examples of Spleen disorders.

86. Which tissue is associated with the Earth element?

87. What is Phlegm in TCM?

88. What is reckless blood?

89. Elaborate on Earth element disorders that center around the theme of eating.

90. In what way is the Earth element associated with female or maternal functions?

91. Why is the Metal element associated with a sense of self?

92. Describe how the Lungs engage in exchange.

93. Why are the Lungs called the "tender Organ"?

94. Give examples of Lung disorders.

95. What sense organ is associated with the Metal element?

96. Explain how the Lungs affect the energy level of the body.

97. In which direction does Lung Qi normally flow?

98. What disorders indicate a reversal of Lung Qi flow?

99. What part of the body do the Lungs moisten?

100. Give examples of Lung disorders that adversely affect water metabolism.

101. Both the Lungs and the Spleen can cause edema, but they affect different parts of the body. Which organ affects which part?

102. What tissue is associated with the Metal element?

103. Describe how the skin engages in exchange.

104. Describe how the Large Intestine engages in exchange.

105. What other organs are implicated in Large Intestine disorders?

106. Identify the psychological associations of Metal.

107. What psychological problems might a Metal element type suffer?

108. Explain how a Metal element imbalance could impact a person's social life.

109. What emotion is associated with Metal?

110. What outlook is associated with a Metal element imbalance?

111. Although Metal element types naturally tend to be private, solitary types, how might a Metal element disharmony exacerbate this tendency?

ZANG FU ORGAN TEST (50 POINTS)

MATCHING. ORGAN PAIRS, BASIC FUNCTIONS

A. Lungs and Large Intestine
B. Spleen and Stomach
C. Heart and Small Intestine
D. Kidneys and Bladder
E. Pericardium and Triple Heater
F. Liver and Gallbladder

____1. Circulation, protection, thermal regulation.

____2. Center of being, circulation, assimilation.

____3. Respiration and elimination, exchange across borders.

____4. Digestion, transformation, satisfying needs.

____5. Storage and distribution of blood, free-flowing blood and Qi.

____6. Genetic inheritance/constitution, autonomic nervous system.

SHORT ANSWER. INDICATE WHICH ORGAN HAS THE FOLLOWING PHYSIOLOGICAL FUNCTIONS AND ASSOCIATIONS.

7. Supplements and reinforces the Heart's function. ____________

8. "Separates pure from impure" and absorbs nutrients. ____________

9. Detoxifies, stores, and distributes blood, distributes Qi, governs sinews (tendons and ligaments); associated with the eyes. ____________

10. Stores and secretes bile. ____________

11. Eliminates liquid waste; associated with bones, teeth, and ears. ____________

12. Houses Shen, regulates circulation. ____________

13. Regulates body temperature, associated with immune function, transmits Source Qi from Kidneys to various organs. ____________

14. Decomposes and ferments ("rots and ripens") food (secondary organ of digestion); associated with breasts, ovaries, uterus. ____________

15. Processes and distributes Air Qi; associated with skin and nose. ____________

16. Transforms and distributes Grain Qi (primary organ of digestion); associated with menses. ____________

17. Eliminates solid waste; associated with skin and nose. ____________

18. Houses Jing, which controls long-term developmental processes, vitality, fertility, and longevity; associated with bones and teeth and ears. ____________

MATCHING. MATCH THE ORGAN WITH THE APPROPRIATE PSYCHOLOGICAL FUNCTIONS AND ASSOCIATIONS, WHETHER POSITIVE OR NEGATIVE.

A. Lungs and Large Intestine
B. Spleen and Stomach
C. Heart
D. Small Intestine
E. Kidneys and Bladder

F. Pericardium and Triple Heater
G. Liver and Gallbladder

____19. Willpower, impetus.

____20. Receiving and/or releasing; general outlook (positive or negative).

____21. Reflective thought, concentration; home and family.

____22. Social relations and emotional protection.

____23. Social relations, emotional tenor, communication, memory, sleep.

____24. Control, planning, initiative, authority.

____25. Discriminating judgment (distinguishing good from bad or good from better, best).

____26. Overcontrolling or out of control, indecisiveness or rashness, impatience, irritability, frustration, resentment, anger, fury, rage.

____27. Shyness, social phobia, inappropriate or eccentric behavior, nervous excitability, agitation, hysteria, delirium, shock, lack of emotion, speech impediments, insomnia, nightmares.

____28. Lack of judgment, shock.

____29. Socially overprotective (defensive and armored) or underprotective (vulnerable, lacking personal boundaries).

____30. Inability to concentrate; muddled, confused thinking; overthinking: mulling, brooding, worrying, fretting, obsession, paralysis of analysis, self-pity.

____31. Inability to open up, take in, or let go; negativity; pessimism; depression; exaggerated or prolonged grief.

____32. Lack of willpower, lack of impetus, insecurities, fears, phobias.

MATCHING. MATCH THE TEMPERAMENT TYPE WITH THE ELEMENT.

A. Water
B. Wood
C. Fire
D. Earth
E. Metal

____33. Extroverted, sociable, talkative.

____34. Introverted, reserved, quiet.

____35. Sympathetic, concerned.

____36. Hyperactive, manic, frenzied.

____37. Withdrawn, isolated.

____38. Bold, decisive, enterprising.

____39. Timid and indecisive or overbearing and impulsive.

____40. Ambitious, driven, workaholic.

____41. Easy-going, laid-back, lazy.

____42. Practical, supportive.

MATCHING. MATCH THE THEME WITH THE ELEMENT.

A. Water
B. Wood
C. Fire
D. Earth
E. Metal

____43. Ambition, drive.

____44. Comfort and security.

____45. Being, repose.

____46. Self-worth and exchange.

____47. Self-expression, personal growth, professional development.

____48. Spirituality and synergy.

____49. Caretaking.

____50. Direction and purpose.

6

THE EIGHT PRINCIPLE PATTERNS AND KYO JITSU

OBJECTIVES

- To categorize clinical symptoms using the Eight Principle Patterns as an organizational model
- To explain the difference between actual and relative deficiency or excess
- To define Kyo and Jitsu and to describe how each manifests physically, psychologically, and socially
- To identify possible causes of a Kyo Jitsu imbalance and to distinguish between temporary and permanent imbalances
- To assess the client's condition using various diagnostic techniques and to adapt the session accordingly
- To apply tonifying techniques to nourish Kyo, dispersal techniques to sedate Jitsu, and the even touch the rest of the time

KEY TERMS AND CONCEPTS

The Eight Principle Patterns
Interior/Exterior or Internal/External
Deficiency/Excess or Empty/Full
Cold/Heat
Full Cold vs. Appearance of Cold or Empty Cold
Full Heat vs. Appearance of Heat, Empty Heat, or Empty Fire
Kyo/Jitsu
Even Touch
Tonify/Nourish
Sedate/Disperse
Kenbiki

The Eight Principle Patterns are a clinical extrapolation of the Yin Yang paradigm. In essence, they describe physiological and psychological disorders as basic patterns of Yin Yang imbalance or disharmony. The *Nei Jing*, as well as other ancient classical medical texts, refers to the Eight Principle Patterns as distinguishing features of diseases (Maciocia, 2001). As the most comprehensive and inclusive method of clinical analysis, the Eight Principle Patterns are the cornerstone of TCM diagnosis. Masunaga's Kyo Jitsu paradigm is a modern application of the Eight Principle Patterns, though his paradigm focuses on energy levels rather than levels of vital substances, such as fluids and blood, or levels of organ activity (Beresford-Cooke, 2000). A basic understanding of these medical paradigms enables the practitioner to assess the client's condition and customize Shiatsu to meet the client's needs.

THE EIGHT PRINCIPLE PATTERNS

The Eight Principal Patterns consist of four pairs of polar opposites as applied to the human body-mind: Yin/Yang, Interior/Exterior, Deficiency/Excess, and Cold/Hot (Kaptchuk, 2000). Yin/Yang is the primary pair from which the others are derived. Yin conditions are characterized by Interior, Deficiency, and Cold symptoms, while Yang conditions are characterized by Exterior, Excess, and Heat symptoms. These symptoms can be observed through the four classical examinations of looking, listening and smelling (TCM groups these together), asking, and touching (Kaptchuk, 2000). Oriental medical doctors (OMDs) and acupuncturists primarily rely on tongue (looking) and pulse (touching) diagnosis, but the average Shiatsu practitioner relies on different methods of assessment: noting the client's concerns; observing the client's physique or figure, general physical condition, and other physical attributes; observing the client's posture, gait, and other movement patterns; observing the client's psychological demeanor and social interaction; smelling the client's odor; listening to the quality of the client's voice and respiration; and palpating the client's tissues.

INTERIOR/EXTERIOR

The Interior/Exterior pair refers to the location of the disorder or malady, whether deep inside the body, afflicting the internal organs, or on the periphery, afflicting the superficial tissues—skin, subcutaneous tissues, muscles—and Meridians (Maciocia, 2001). **Internal** disorders are chronic in nature, slow in onset, and lingering and are usually the result of constitutional infirmities or prolonged emotional disturbances. The pattern of presenting symptoms for an Internal disorder depends on which organ is affected and whether the condition is also Hot or Cold and Full or Empty. Treatment of Internal disorders usually requires a medical regimen or intervention beyond the purview of a Shiatsu practice. Nevertheless, healthy lifestyle changes and Shiatsu to the associated Meridians and key acupressure points may prove beneficial.

In contrast, **External** disorders are acute, sudden in onset, severe in symptom, and relatively brief in duration. They are caused by External Pernicious Influences, including inclement climatic conditions, such as Cold, Heat, Wind, Dampness, and Dryness; virulent environmental agents, such as pathogenic microbes and poisonous plants and insects; and other external factors, such as mechanical injuries from auto collisions and sport-related activities (Maciocia, 2001). In general, these disorders correspond to infectious illnesses, contagious diseases, or trauma (Kaptchuk, 2000). External disorders usually respond well to therapeutic dispersal techniques that facilitate the body's expulsion of pathogenic agents or propel stagnant Qi and blood at the injury site (Beresford-Cooke, 2000).

DEFICIENCY/EXCESS

The Deficiency/Excess pair—also known as Empty/Full— refers to a lack or a surplus of Qi, blood, or other bodily substance or to the hypoactivity or hyperactivity of an organ or other bodily function (Kaptchuk, 2000). **Deficiency** disorders are characterized by lack—insufficient substance and inadequate activity—while **Excess** disorders are characterized by abundance—superfluous substance and immoderate or extreme activity.

Symptoms of Deficiency include a gray, white, or pale yellow complexion; faint voice; superficial respiration or breathlessness; feeble movement; physical lassitude or inertia; emotional listlessness or apathy; dull pain alleviated by pressure; perspiration unprovoked by physical exertion; an acrid odor; and a flaccid abdomen (Kaptchuk, 2000). Symptoms of Excess include a red complexion; strident voice; bellowing respiration; heavy or forceful movement; physical and emotional intensity or agitation; sharp pain aggravated by pressure; a putrid odor; and a distended abdomen (Kaptchuk, 2000). Several factors may precipitate a pattern of Excess, such as a Pernicious Influence that invades the body, a bodily function that launches into overdrive, or a blockage that causes Qi and blood to stagnate.

When a Pernicious Influence invades the body, it may settle in the joints, causing painful obstruction syndrome: Cold causes severe pain that is relieved by Heat; Heat causes severe pain and inflammation that is relieved by Cold; Dampness causes swelling; and Wind causes pain that migrates from joint to joint (Maciocia, 2001). When a blockage obstructs the free flow of Qi, Qi accumulates and stagnates. Stagnant Qi then manifests as "distention and/or soreness and pain . . . and the [psychological] feeling of being blocked, frustrated, tense, or moody" (Kaptchuk, 2000, p. 241). Mechanical stress, such as strenuous exercise, hard manual labor, and repetitive movement, can also cause blockages (Maciocia, 2001). So, too, can lifestyle factors, such as habitually poor posture or faulty body mechanics, a sedentary lifestyle, an unhealthy diet, or poor stress-management skills.

COLD/HEAT

The Cold/Heat pair refers to thermal imbalances. **Cold** symptoms include a white complexion; cold limbs, and especially cold hands and feet; aversion to cold and preference for warmth; discomfort alleviated by heat; no thirst or the desire for hot drinks; profuse, pale urine and fluid stools; slow movement; and a passive, introverted disposition (Kaptchuk, 2000). Causes of Cold include invasion by Cold, excess Yin, and deficient Yang that results in the relative predominance of Yin, also known as the Appearance of Cold or Empty Cold (Maciocia, 2001).

Heat symptoms include a red complexion; hot body; aversion to heat and preference for cold; discomfort alleviated by cold; thirst or the desire for cold drinks; scanty, dark urine and dry stools; brisk or restless movement; and a boisterous, extroverted disposition (Kaptchuk, 2000). Causes of Heat include invasion by Heat, excess Yang, and deficient Yin or fluids that result in the relative predominance of Yang, also known as the Appearance of Fire or Empty Fire (Maciocia, 2001).

MIXED PATTERNS

Few clients exhibit a classic Yin or Yang pattern of Deficiency plus Cold or Excess plus Heat. Instead, most clients present a combination of seemingly contradictory symptoms: Excess plus Cold or Deficiency plus Heat (Kaptchuk, 2000). This apparent inconsistency can be best understood by analyzing the difference between an actual Deficiency versus a relative Deficiency and between an actual Excess versus a relative Excess.

For example, a Cold condition can be caused by too much Yin (Cold/Water) or not enough Yang (Heat/Fire). In the case of excess Yin, an abnormally high level of Yin overpowers the normal level of Yang, resulting in a condition known as **Full Cold** (Maciocia, 2001). In the case of deficient Yang, however, an abnormally low level of Yang cannot counteract the normal level of Yin; this condition is known as the **Appearance of Cold** or **Empty Cold** to distinguish it from Full Cold (Figure 6-1).

Likewise, a Heat condition can be caused by too much Yang (Heat/Fire) or not enough Yin (Cold/Water). Again, in the case of excess Yang, an abnormally high level of Yang overpowers the normal level of Yin, resulting in a condition known as **Full Heat** (Maciocia, 2000). By contrast, in the case of deficient Yin, a lack of Yin results in the relative preponderance of Yang; this condition is known as the **Appearance of Heat**, **Empty Heat**, or **Empty Fire** to distinguish it from Full Heat (Figure 6-2).

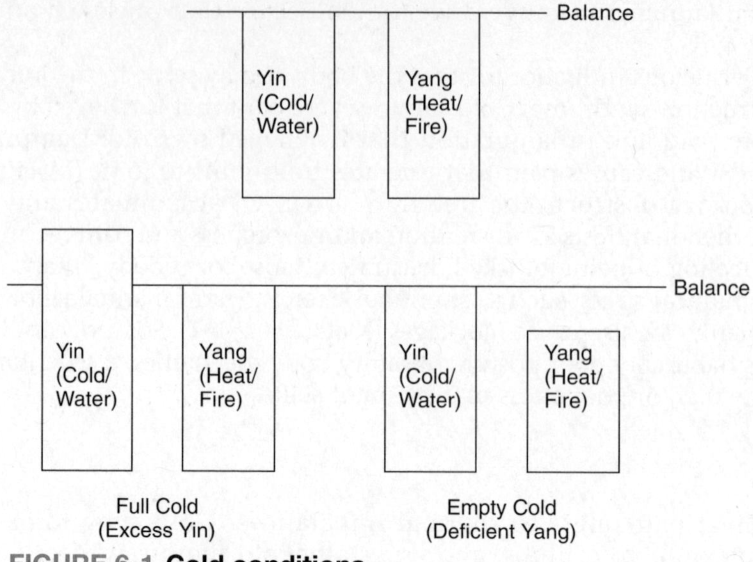

FIGURE 6-1 Cold conditions.

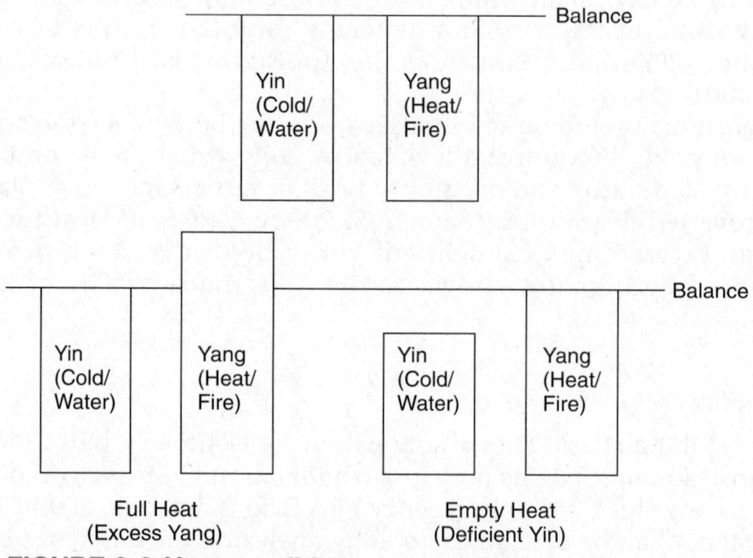

FIGURE 6-2 Heat conditions.

KYO JITSU

Like the Eight Principle Patterns, Shizuto Masunaga's Kyo Jitsu paradigm is appealing because of its simplicity in reducing clinical complexes to bare essentials. The Kyo Jitsu paradigm is a contemporary extrapolation of Yin Yang and the Eight Principle Patterns, especially Deficiency/Excess, but with a narrower emphasis. Kyo Jitsu emphasizes Qi levels in Meridians, whereas the Eight Principle Patterns emphasize levels of all vital substances—Qi, blood, fluids, Jing—as well as organ activity (Beresford-Cooke, 2000).

When the flow of Qi in the Meridian network is imbalanced, Masunaga describes this as "the condition of energy distortion" (Masunaga & Ohashi, 1977/1997, p. 139). The condition of energy distortion in the body typically manifests as one Meridian that is Jitsu or hyperactive due to a concentration of energy and another Meridian that is Kyo or hypoactive from a paucity of energy. **Jitsu** means "full" in

Japanese: It is a condition where energy is immoderately high (Beresford-Cooke, 2000). **Kyo** means "empty": It is a condition where energy is immoderately low. Hence, excess Qi is Jitsu, and deficient Qi is Kyo (Masunaga & Ohashi, 1977/1997). Like Yin and Yang, Kyo and Jitsu are mutually dependent and reciprocally related: If one exists, the other does also, and the greater the imbalance in one, the greater the imbalance in the other. Hence, the presence of Excess somewhere in the body necessarily implies Deficiency elsewhere.

TEMPORARY VERSUS PERMANENT IMBALANCES

Kyo Jitsu is an inevitable aspect of life; it arises naturally in the ongoing process of satisfying needs. Masunaga explains this using the amoeba analogy (Beresford-Cooke, 2000). The amoeba represents any living organism, but in particular, the human being. As shown in Figure 6-3, the amoeba begins in a temporary state of energy balance but then develops a need—perhaps physical, psychological, or social—that is generalized as the need for nutrients. The need, want, or emptiness is a Kyo condition of energy deficit. To satisfy the need, the amoeba projects a pseudopodium (false foot) toward the nutrients and engulfs and absorbs the nutrients, satisfying the need. The pseudopodium—the compensatory drive to satisfy the need—is a Jitsu condition of energy surplus or expenditure.

In this theoretical model, the Kyo condition of energy deficit arises first and is the cause behind the Jitsu condition of energy surplus or expenditure. Once the Kyo condition or need is satisfied, the Jitsu condition or compensatory drive automatically subsides, since the Jitsu condition arises only to resolve the Kyo condition. To humanize this example, suppose a person is hungry: She has developed a Kyo

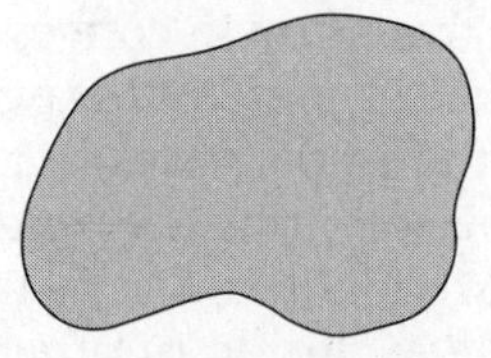

1. The amoeba is in a temporary state of balance.

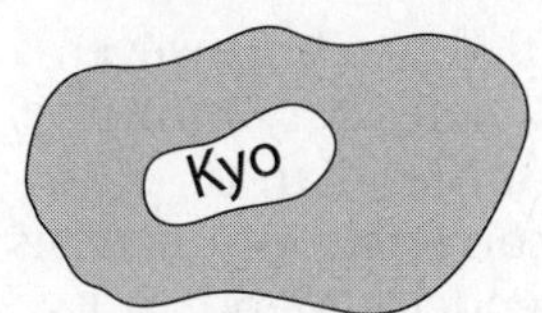

2. The amoeba develops a need for nutrients. The need, want, or emptiness is a Kyo condition of energy deficit.

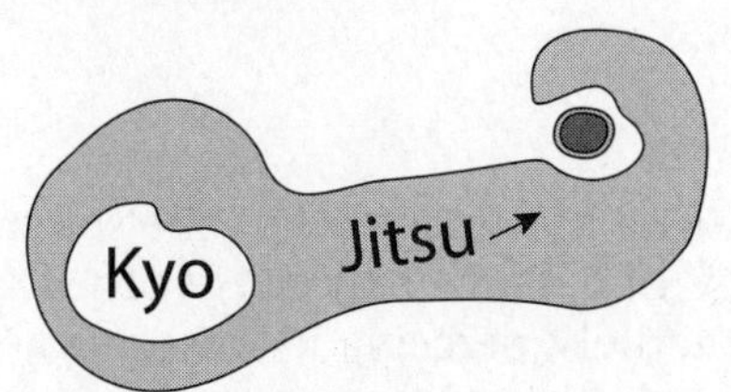

3. The amoeba projects a pseudopodium toward the nutrients. The pseudopodium is a Jitsu condition of energy expenditure, a compensatory drive to satisfy a need.

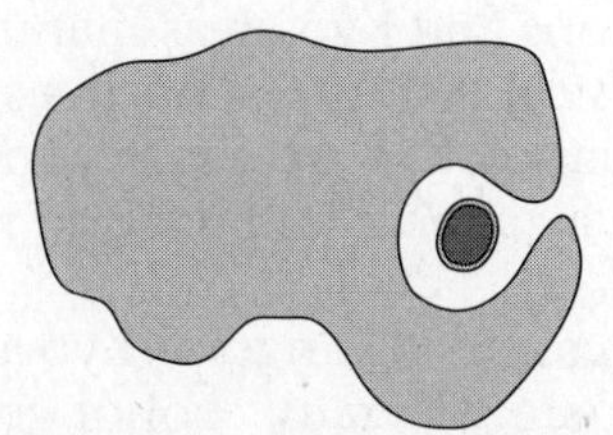

4. After engulfing the nutrients and satisfying Kyo, the amoeba gradually returns to a temporary state of balance.

FIGURE 6-3 The amoeba analogy.

need or want. She notes that her pantry and refrigerator are bare, a condition of Kyo emptiness. Her hunger, a Kyo state of energy deficit, compels her to take action, a Jitsu state of energy expenditure. So she drives to the grocery store, gathers groceries in a shopping cart, buys them at the register, drives home, unloads the car, stocks her pantry and refrigerator, cooks a meal, sets the table, and finally eats. All these actions, including the spending of money (money is Qi—it represents work, the value of which enables a person to buy goods and services), are Jitsu in nature and are aimed at satisfying the Kyo need.

Life itself is an ongoing process of satisfying Kyo needs through Jitsu drives. In this respect, temporary Kyo Jitsu conditions are natural and normal. Thus, a Kyo Jitsu condition does not necessarily imply a pathological condition, such as disease (Beresford-Cooke, 2000). It could reflect a normal fluctuation in physical energy, a brief stage in an acute illness, or a fleeting mood precipitated by some incident, such as joy at receiving a package in the mail, anger at being cut off in traffic, fear at discovering one's wallet is missing, or sorrow at seeing a homeless person. Or the Kyo Jitsu condition could reflect a psychological state centered on an event lasting a few months: starting a new job, moving to another city, or ending a relationship. Or it could reflect a habitual mode of relating: "mothering" everybody or distancing everybody. Only when a Kyo need cannot be satisfied through a Jitsu drive does a more permanent state of imbalance or disharmony set in, which could then lead to distress or disease.

CAUSES OF KYO JITSU

The causes of a Kyo Jitsu imbalance are varied. As mentioned, the most common cause of a Jitsu condition is an underlying Kyo condition for which the Jitsu is compensating. But a Jitsu condition can also arise when an obstruction or blockage causes Qi to accumulate and concentrate in a Meridian or organ, resulting in congestion and stagnation. Temperament and lifestyle factors—habitual or preferred ways of thinking, feeling, doing, and relating, and especially personal imperatives that drive a person—can also account for a Jitsu condition. When a person prioritizes and inordinately focuses on functions associated with a particular Meridian and invests tremendous personal energy in those functions, especially to the exclusion of other functions, that Meridian becomes Jitsu (Beresford-Cooke, 2000).

The most common cause of a Kyo condition is an unsatisfied need. However, a Kyo condition can also arise when a constitutional weakness, hereditary infirmity, trauma, long-term illness, or Jitsu condition depletes Qi in a Meridian or organ. Again, temperament or lifestyle factors, especially when a person neglects functions or aspects of life associated with a particular Meridian, can render a Meridian Kyo (Beresford-Cooke, 2000).

QUALITIES OF KYO AND JITSU

There are various ways to detect a Kyo Jitsu imbalance. Masunaga offers the sphere or ball model to illustrate how a Kyo Jitsu energy imbalance can cause physical distortions in the body that can be visually or tactilely perceived (Masunaga & Ohashi, 1977/1997). In this model, the healthy body is likened to a perfectly round sphere or ball, and the unhealthy body is likened to a spiked and cratered sphere in which Jitsu areas manifest as bulging, convex protrusions and Kyo areas manifest as pitted, concave depressions (Figure 6-4). These physical distortions on the surface of the body are one way to detect a Kyo Jitsu imbalance. Kyo areas may appear hollow and feel soft and spongy, whereas Jitsu areas may appear bulbous and feel firm and distended.

Aside from distortions on the surface plane, other qualities distinguish Kyo and Jitsu (see Table 6-1). The soft, spongy surfaces of Kyo are generally cool or cold, hypoactive, and impassive. When pressed, a Kyo area may elicit a dull sensation for

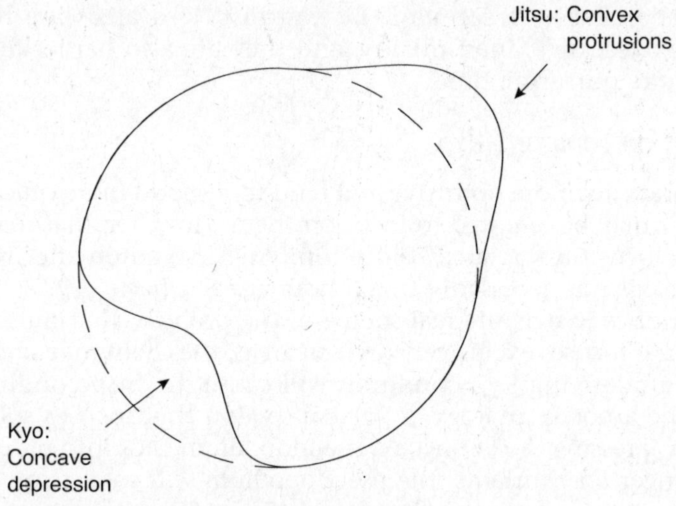

FIGURE 6-4 Surface distortions.

TABLE 6-1 Kyo Jitsu Qualities

Quality	Kyo	Jitsu
Surface	Hollow, concave depressions	Bulging, convex protrusions
Texture	Soft, spongy, flaccid	Firm, tense, tight
Hard	Stiff, rigid, board-like	Repelling, rebounding, spring-like
Energy	Low, deficient, hypoactive, sluggish	High, excessive, hyperactive, urgent
Temperature	Cool, cold	Warm, hot
Response	Inert, impassive, deadened	Responsive, reactive
Sensation	Dull or no sensation	Sharp sensation, tender, sensitive
Pain	Dull pain, feels good	Sharp pain, feels invasive

the client or no sensation if the area is deadened (Jarmey & Mojay, 1999). Pressure on a Kyo area may feel like a "good hurt" or "good pain" that soothes and relieves, especially when warmth is a component. By contrast, the firm, distended surfaces of Jitsu are generally warm or hot, hyperactive, and reactive. When pressed, a Jitsu area may elicit a sharp, lancinating sensation. Pressure on a Jitsu area that is especially stagnant may feel intrusive or invasive because the associated tissues are tender, sensitive, and irritable.

Interestingly, both Kyo and Jitsu can manifest as a hard, resistant surface, but subtle differences distinguish them. Jitsu hardness has a full, lively, outward-bound quality that repels or pushes against applied pressure like an inflated rubber ball. Moreover, Jitsu hardness is buoyant and resilient—it rebounds once pressure is released—like a spring or trampoline. Unlike Jitsu hardness, Kyo hardness is inert and unyielding: It feels stiff and rigid like a wooden board and does not respond or react to pressure the way Jitsu does (Beresford-Cooke, 2000). Kyo hardness lacks elastic give and feels unnaturally resistant, like a plate of armor that cannot be penetrated.

Jitsu areas are much easier to detect both visually and tactilely than Kyo areas because of their conspicuous qualities and responsive or reactive nature. Jitsu areas tend to jut out, repel pressure, and are tender or hypersensitive to touch: "Jitsu symptoms often have a Yang quality of urgency, because of the greater investment of energy in the Jitsu" (Beresford-Cooke, 2000, p. 92). This dynamic quality makes

Jitsu more responsive to treatment. By contrast, Kyo areas are harder to find because of their recessive, inert quality, and they are also harder to treat because they require more nurturing time.

Focus Therapy on Tonifying Kyo

Because Jitsu areas are more obtrusive and tend to respond more quickly to therapy, the practitioner may be tempted to focus on them. However, Masunaga advises the practitioner to focus on Kyo areas, since tonifying Kyo automatically sedates Jitsu, but the converse is not necessarily true (Masunaga & Ohashi, 1977/1997). In short, Masunaga identifies Kyo as the real source of the problem that must be addressed. If the practitioner focuses exclusively on Jitsu areas, the client may obtain temporary relief, but the underlying Kyo condition will cause the Jitsu condition to return. To return to the amoeba analogy, a Shiatsu session that focuses solely on Jitsu is tantamount to "pressing the [amoeba's] pseudopodium back into place" without satisfying the hunger for nutrients; the pseudopodium will soon reappear (Beresford-Cooke, 2000, p. 92). In extreme cases of depletion, a Shiatsu session that focuses on dispersing Jitsu could further exhaust a chronically Kyo client (Masunaga & Ohashi, 1977/1997).

Lifestyle Factors Perpetuating a Kyo Jitsu Imbalance

Unfortunately, a client's lifestyle often perpetuates a Kyo Jitsu imbalance, and until the client decides to change that lifestyle, the best the Shiatsu practitioner can do is provide temporary relief or damage control and tactfully recommend lifestyle reform or refer the client to appropriate specialists. Lifestyle factors that can cause a Kyo Jitsu imbalance include the familiar litany: poor nutrition (excessive consumption of devitalized, processed, irradiated foods containing white sugar, white flour, fat, salt, preservatives, conditioners, and artificial flavors and colors; excessive consumption of animal products contaminated with growth hormones, antibiotics, and pesticides; inadequate consumption of fresh fruits and vegetables and whole grains; and overeating or fasting); a sedentary lifestyle or excessive physical exercise or manual labor; bad posture and faulty body mechanics; repetitive movements that stress joints; insufficient mental and physical rest; poor quality sleep, sleep deprivation, or irregular cycles of waking and sleep; smoking; excessive consumption of alcohol, coffee, caffeinated tea, and soft drinks; overindulgence in or addiction to recreational, prescription, or over-the-counter drugs; maladaptive psychological patterns; and dysfunctional social relationships.

Assessment

Assessing the client's energy pattern is a necessary prerequisite to therapy but does not have to be an elaborate preliminary procedure. Unlike acupuncture, whose diagnosis and treatment are separate and distinct installments of an office visit, Shiatsu assessment and therapy are done at virtually the same time. There are several methods of assessment, including visual observation, Meridian diagnosis, hara diagnosis, and back diagnosis.

The first opportunity for assessment—visual observation—presents itself upon greeting the client and going through the formalities of introduction and the protocol of basic questioning: "What would you like to receive from your Shiatsu session today?" "What are your chief complaints?" "Where do you hold your tension?" Aside from any information the client volunteers concerning his condition, more information can be gathered by observing the face, body, movement patterns, and demeanor to determine whether the client is primarily Kyo or Jitsu (see Table 6-2) and whether any discrepancies exist between the upper and lower

TABLE 6-2 Kyo Jitsu Client Types

Type	Kyo	Jitsu
Energy	Fatigued, tired, depleted	Restless, nervous, explosive
Frame	Delicate, frail	Robust, stout
Tissues	Flabby, wasted	Muscular, fat
Color	Pale	Ruddy
Speech	Reticent, quiet	Garrulous, loud
Movement	Cautious, sluggish, feeble	Bold, agitated, frenetic
Disposition	Reserved, meek, bland, dull	Sociable, dramatic, demanding
Therapy	Tonification	Sedation
Techniques	Relaxing	Stimulating
Needs to Be	Soothed, lulled	Worked over, wrung out
Conditions	Client is mainly Kyo Kyo dominates body-mind Client requests relief for Kyo Repeat client with low energy	Client is mainly Jitsu Jitsu dominates body-mind Client requests relief for Jitsu First-time client with even energy
Yin Yang Theory	Add Yin to Yin: turn to Yang	Add Yang to Yang: turn to Yin
Effect	Revitalize	Tranquilize

halves, the front and back halves, or the right and left side of the body. On the basis of this information, the Shiatsu session can be designed.

Diagnosis by Observation

A client who is pale; is thin and frail or soft and flabby; speaks quietly, minimally, or not at all; walks or moves gingerly, sluggishly, or feebly; and has a reserved, timid, bland, or dull demeanor is Kyo and would probably benefit from a tonifying session, which would energize and invigorate the client. On the other hand, a client who is ruddy; is muscular, fat, stout, or robust; speaks loudly, freely, or incessantly; walks or moves boldly, haphazardly, or frenetically; and has a sociable, dramatic, or demanding disposition is Jitsu and would probably benefit from a sedating session, which would calm and relax the client. A client who presents both Kyo and Jitsu qualities would probably benefit from a moderate session emphasizing the even touch.

Discrepancies between sides or halves of the body can also be visually observed and then treated during the session (Jarmey & Mojay, 1999). Thus, if a client's upper half is more Jitsu, the practitioner should sedate the torso and tonify the hips and legs, and especially the most Kyo Meridian. This upper half Jitsu/lower half Kyo disparity is common in males, especially male weightlifters, whose exercise regimen targets the arms, chest, and back but neglects the hips and legs. Conversely, if the client's lower half is more Jitsu, the practitioner should sedate the legs and tonify the torso and arms, and especially the most Kyo Meridian. The lower half Jitsu/upper half Kyo disparity is common in women who have pear-shaped, bottom-heavy figures. The client may have issues about food and personal or professional relationships. Usually, the Stomach and Spleen Meridians are implicated in themes of physical and social nourishment.

If the client's back is Kyo and the front is Jitsu, the practitioner should tonify the back and sedate the front of the torso, especially the chest; however, even though stimulating techniques are used on the chest, they should never be used on the vulnerable abdominal area (Jarmey & Mojay, 1999). Conversely, if the client's back is Jitsu and the front is Kyo, the practitioner should sedate the back and tonify the chest and hara. Finally, if the client has a right/left discrepancy, the practitioner should tonify the Meridians on the most Kyo side, especially the Gallbladder and Liver Meridians, which may be implicated.

MERIDIAN DIAGNOSIS

Another method of assessment that is incorporated into therapy is touch diagnosis of the Meridians. During the Shiatsu session, the practitioner places the limbs in various Meridian stretch positions and palpates the Meridians to determine their quality. A Meridian can manifest both Kyo and Jitsu along its entire length, but one or the other will predominate and characterize the Meridian as a whole (Jarmey & Mojay, 1999).

A Jitsu Meridian feels firm, resistant, and buoyant in the stretch position, whereas a Kyo Meridian feels flaccid or, less often, inflexibly hard and inert (Jarmey & Mojay, 1999). Jitsu Meridians are treated with vigorous techniques to propel Qi through and beyond the area, whereas Kyo Meridians are treated with nurturing techniques to draw Qi to the area. Often the initial session is exploratory in nature: While working the whole body, the practitioner identifies which Meridian is most Kyo and which is most Jitsu. If the pattern is well established due to temperament or lifestyle, the practitioner can confirm this in future sessions, concentrating immediately on the most Kyo and Jitsu Meridians and making adjustments as the client's energy pattern changes on the basis of therapy, lifestyle, or other conditions.

HARA DIAGNOSIS

Other methods of touch diagnosis include hara diagnosis and back diagnosis, but these methods—especially hara diagnosis—require considerable sensitivity and practice. In hara diagnosis, light and relaxed fingertip pressure is applied on the abdomen to discern the nature of Qi in each of the reflex zones (see Figure 6-5), with the goal of finding the most Kyo and the most Jitsu zones so that their respective Meridians can be treated. Each organ has a reflex zone—an area between the ribcage and pelvic bowl—that corresponds to it and its associated Meridians. Jitsu areas in the hara tend to be conspicuous or obtrusive, active, and reactive, whereas Kyo areas tend to be hollow, inactive, and passively resistant or stiff (Beresford-Cooke, 2000).

The easiest way to diagnose the hara is to find the most Jitsu reflex zone first, maintain contact with one hand, and then palpate with the other hand for the most Kyo reflex zone: "The most Kyo area is that which palpably connects with the most Jitsu area" (Beresford-Cooke, 2000, p. 237). This connection is variously described as a "blip" or pulse transmitted from one hand to the other or a feeling of the Jitsu area sinking and shrinking and the Kyo area rising and ballooning.

BACK DIAGNOSIS

Back diagnosis is similar to hara diagnosis in that certain points—known as Shu in Chinese and Yu in Japanese—along the inner and outer Bladder Meridians correspond to certain organs and their associated Meridians (see Figure 6-6 and Chapter 7 on acupoints). Palpation of the back is firmer than the abdomen since the back is Yang and defensive in nature. Tenderness, sharp pain, or any other distinctive sensation in the Shu/Yu points on the inner Bladder Meridian, which runs closer to the spine, indicates an energetic imbalance that is physical in nature, such as a malady in the corresponding organ, while tenderness in the Shu/Yu points on the outer Bladder Meridian, which runs closer to the shoulder blades, indicates an energetic imbalance that is psychological or emotional in nature (Beresford-Cooke, 2000). Because the back exhibits long-term imbalances that are chronic in nature and the hara exhibits short-term imbalances that are acute in nature, diagnostic

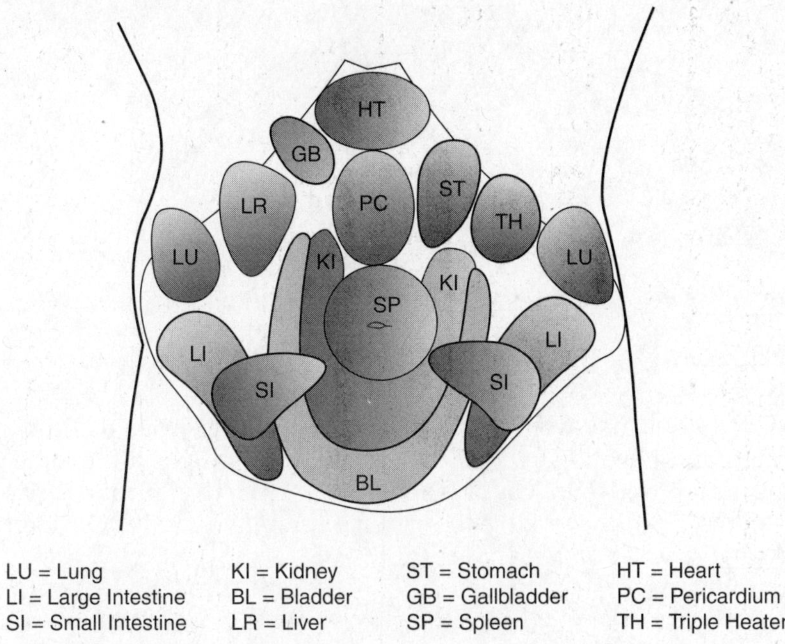

FIGURE 6-5 Hara Reflex Zones.

results from the back and hara may differ; therefore, only one method of diagnosis should be used (Beresford-Cooke, 2000).

For example, back diagnosis of a client who recently quit smoking after 35 years of smoking two packs a day will undoubtedly indicate a Lung imbalance (Lung Kyo), whereas hara diagnosis of the same person may indicate a Gallbladder imbalance (Gallbladder Jitsu) due to a serious altercation with a significant other, most likely precipitated or exacerbated by nicotine withdrawal and detoxification. The results may seem conflicting, but are not. The back diagnosis (Lung Kyo) points to a relatively permanent condition that can be improved or remedied through lifestyle changes (the cessation of smoking and the practice of breathing exercises), while the hara diagnosis (Gallbladder Jitsu) points to a temporary condition that will most likely resolve itself, unless other perpetuating factors are present. Because the assessment methods point to different therapeutic emphases, the practitioner should rely on one method of touch assessment—hara or back diagnosis—to design a session, plus additional information provided through other forms of intake. For example, if the client's anger is troubling or distracting her, emphasizing Shiatsu on the associated Gallbladder Meridian may be best, but if client is more concerned about persevering in abstaining from cigarettes, emphasizing Shiatsu on the associated Lung Meridian may be best.

THERAPY

Unless the client is very imbalanced toward Kyo or Jitsu, the even touch is used for most of the Shiatsu session, reserving dispersal techniques for Jitsu areas and tonification techniques for Kyo areas (Beresford-Cooke, 2000). The **even touch** entails applying medium pressure at a moderate rate of speed. This, of course, is relative to the client's composite energy profile and may be adapted accordingly. For instance, a Jitsu client may prefer a firmer, brisker even touch, whereas a Kyo client may prefer a gentler, slower even touch. The beginning of the Shiatsu session often sets the tone for the whole session—whether the even touch will tend toward dispersal or toward tonification.

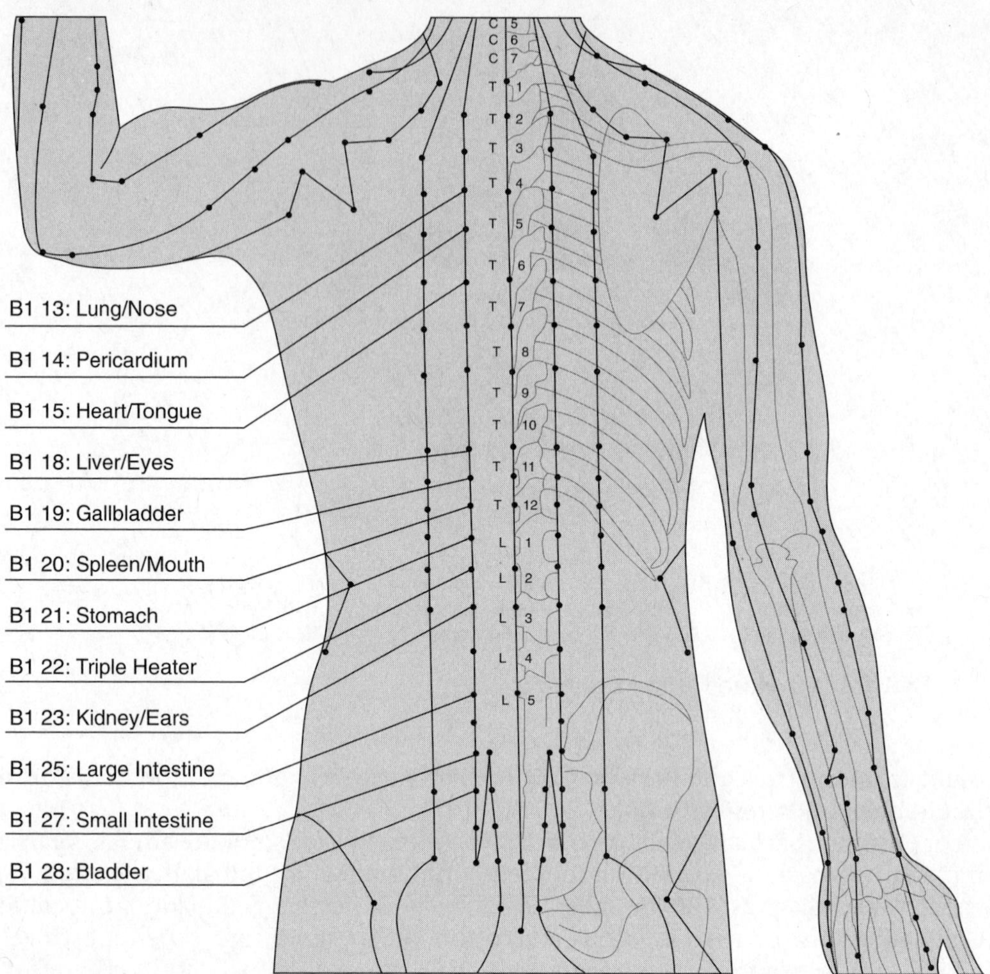

FIGURE 6-6 Back Shu/Yu Points.
Authorized Derivation of the Flow of Qi chart: Copyright 1998–2004 by Valentin Popov. www.flowofqi.com.

Although most sessions begin with the even touch, sometimes the practitioner may want to begin by dispersing Jitsu or tonifying Kyo. This is a matter of client preference and practitioner judgment. At the beginning of a session, a Jitsu client tends to be too physically tense and psychologically wound up to enjoy mild, gentle tonifying techniques. In fact, if the practitioner begins by trying to soothe or lull a Jitsu client with nurturing techniques, the client may become inwardly restless and annoyed. Therefore, sedating Jitsu first is preferable if the client is predominantly Jitsu or the Jitsu condition dominates the client's body-mind landscape. In addition, the practitioner should begin a session by sedating Jitsu if the client has specifically requested relief for a Jitsu condition. Honoring the client's request at the beginning of the session is good protocol and will set the client at ease to accept additional therapy the practitioner deems necessary. Finally, the practitioner should begin by sedating Jitsu if the client is new and a preliminary assessment indicates that the client's energy level is fairly normal, that is, not deficient. During a first session, the practitioner is becoming familiar with the client's energy patterns, and the Jitsu areas, which are more obvious than the Kyo areas, are easier to dispatch first.

The situation is reversed with a Kyo client. A Kyo client tends to be too depleted to enjoy dynamic dispersal techniques, especially at the beginning of a session before the client has had time to acclimate to therapy or experience a replenishment of energy. If a practitioner begins with intense techniques likes pumping, jostling, and pummeling, the client will recoil at the invasive treatment. Consequently, tonifying Kyo first is preferable if the client is predominantly a Kyo type, a Kyo condition dominates the client's body-mind landscape, the client has specifically requested relief for a Kyo condition, or the client is a regular client and the practitioner is familiar with the client's energy pattern, which points toward Kyo.

In general, Kyo clients tend to enjoy mild, nurturing sessions, which have the effect of revitalizing them, whereas Jitsu clients tend to enjoy intense, vigorous sessions, which have the effect of tranquilizing them (Esher, 2001, Got Yin/Yang?). These therapeutic preferences can be explained by the Yin Yang principle of transformation: When Yin is maximal, it turns into Yang, and when Yang is maximal, it turns into Yin. Thus, adding Yin energy through tonifying techniques to a Yin or Kyo client causes the client to become more Yang. Adding Yang energy through dispersal techniques to a Yang or Jitsu client causes the client to become more Yin. Interestingly, practitioners who are Yang types tend to have a Yang treatment style and attract clients who prefer Yang treatments. Conversely, Yin practitioners tend to have a Yin treatment style and attract clients who prefer Yin treatments.

Application of Techniques

Different techniques are used to sedate Jitsu and to tonify Kyo (see Table 6-3). To **tonify** and **nourish** Kyo, gentle techniques are applied. In general, broad, flat surfaces—such as all four finger pads, the palm, the heel of the hand, the thenar eminence (the fleshy pad of muscle at the base of the thumb), the pisiform (the padded bony protuberance at the outer base of the palm), and the ulnar side of the

TABLE 6-3 Kyo Jitsu Techniques

Condition	Kyo	Jitsu
Treatment	Tonify, nurture, draw Qi in	Sedate, disperse, propel Qi through or out
Style	Gentle, mild	Vigorous, stimulating
Pressure	Static, stationary	Flowing, mobile
Level	Light to medium	Medium to deep
Quality	Sustained, abiding	Dynamic, rhythmic
Pace	Still or relatively slow	Brisk or relatively fast
Body Tools	Palms Heels of hands Thenar eminences Pisiform surface of palms All four fingers Forearms Thumbs	Knife side of hands Knuckles Fists Elbows Knees Feet Thumbs
Techniques	Mother/Son Meridian stretches Traction	Two-handed compression Kenbiki: circular or cross-fiber friction, torsion wringing, compression plus rocking Jostling: shaking or vibrating Pummeling: pecking, hacking, pounding, cupping BMT: rotation and farthest ROM stretch
Direction	Inferior to superior Distal to proximal With Meridian current Clockwise	Superior to inferior Proximal to distal Against Meridian current Counterclockwise

hand—are used to apply pressure. The forearms, which are broad and fleshy, may also be used to apply pressure, especially to crawl on the client, but dynamic use of the forearm, as in the sawing or rolling pin technique, is reserved for Jitsu conditions.

To tonify Kyo, pressure is applied slowly and gradually, is light to medium in depth, and is sustained for a prolonged period of time to attract Qi to the area to warm it (Beresford-Cooke, 2000). Tonifying Kyo requires an abiding presence that cannot be rushed. According to Masunaga, one should treat Kyo like a lover patiently awaiting his beloved, "without regard to time" (Masunaga & Ohashi, 1977/1997, p. 39). The most efficient way to do this when working under professional time constraints is to use the Mother/Son hand technique, resting the stationary Mother hand on a Kyo area, such as the lower back, sacrum, or abdomen, or holding a Kyo point, while the Son hand simultaneously works the length of a Meridian (Beresford-Cooke, 2000). For a full description of the Mother/Son hand technique, see Chapter 9; for an overview of this technique, see Practice Exercise 6-1 on tonifying Kyo.

Usually, tonification techniques are still, static, and stationary. However, some techniques incorporating motion, such as rocking, vibrating, and waving, can also be calming if applied gently, as indicated for Kyo (Jarmey & Mojay, 1999). Traction and gentle static stretches involving less than the full range of motion, such as the Meridian stretch positions, are also indicated for Kyo.

To **sedate** and **disperse** Jitsu, vigorous, stimulating techniques are applied. In general, sharper, more industrial-strength body tools are used to apply pressure, such as knuckles, fists, elbows, knees, and feet. Additionally, movement is often combined with compression. For example, thumb and knuckle pressure is combined with circular friction, cross-fiber friction, or vibration of an acupressure point. Fist pressure is combined with a twisting motion. Forearm pressure is combined with a sawing motion directed transversely against the orientation of the muscle fibers, first pushing and then pulling the tissues, or it is combined with a rolling pin motion directed parallel to the orientation of the muscle fibers, repeatedly compressing and flattening the tissues. Knee pressure is combined with a clamp-like squeezing motion or a cross-country skiing motion and foot pressure with a treading motion.

In fact, any compression technique becomes dispersing and sedating in nature when combined with dynamic movement. For example, palm or heel of the hand pressure is dispersing if combined with vigorous jostling, shaking, or vibrating, as when the gluteus medius (outer hip) or middle trapezius (mid back) is pressed and shaken. Side of the hand pressure is dispersing if combined with a scooping movement that bunches and wedges the tissues together or a spreading movement that pulls them apart. Squeezing or pincer palpation is dispersing if combined with jostling, as when a muscle belly, such as the gastrocnemius (calf) or quadriceps (front thigh) is grabbed and shaken.

To disperse or sedate Jitsu, pressure is applied smoothly but fairly quickly; pressure is medium to deep, and the quality of compression is dynamic in order to mobilize stagnant or blocked Qi (Beresford-Cooke, 2000). Double-handed compression that advances fairly swiftly along a Meridian like the rhythmic plunging of an air pump is an effective treatment for a Jitsu Meridian. So also is **kenbiki**, which may be applied along the length of a Meridian or confined to a more localized area of stagnation. The literal translation of kenbiki means "pushing and pulling": It includes cross-fiber friction or strumming of a muscle or tendon, torsion wringing of a muscle belly, and compression plus rocking. Kenbiki effectively propels stagnant Qi and congested blood (Jarmey & Mojay, 1999).

Another category of stimulating techniques is *tapotement*, also known as pummeling or percussion. Tapotement involves drumming the body with various body tools, such as tapping or pecking with the fingertips, hacking or chopping with the sides of the hands, beating or pounding with the fists, and cupping or slapping with the palms. Tapotement draws stagnant Qi to the surface, where it can be brushed or stroked away (Jwing-Ming, 1992).

Practice exercise 6-1: Tonifying Kyo

Here are some protocols for tonifying Kyo. Identify which method or methods of tonification are used in each protocol. *Hint*: Determine whether the direction of treatment moves with or against the flow of the Meridian.

1. The client's Spleen Meridian is Kyo. Place the client in the supine position, and with the Mother hand, press and hold Sp 6 while the Son hand presses up the Meridian and pauses at CV 4, a lower burner point that tonifies several digestive organs (Esher, 2002).

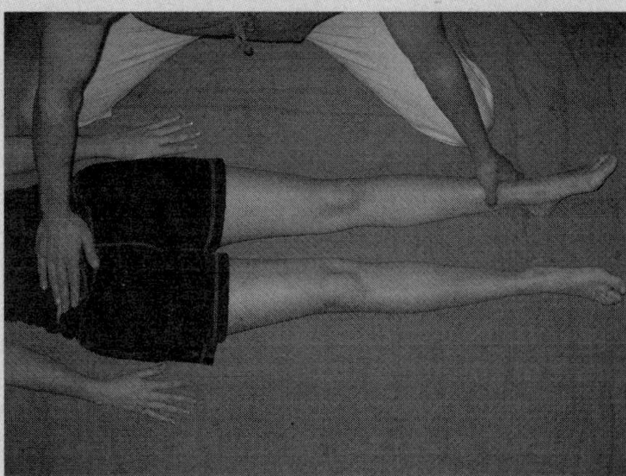

FIGURE 6-7 **CV 4 and Sp 6.**

This protocol uses the following method(s):
A) To tonify, move from an inferior to a superior aspect and from distal to proximal.
B) To tonify, move with the current of the Meridian flow.

2. The client's Kidney Meridian is Kyo. Place the client in the prone position, and with the Mother hand, press and hold Ki 3 while the Son hand presses up the Meridian and pauses at the lower back, squeezing both Bl 23, the Kidney Shu/Yu points, with a pincer grip (Esher, 2002).

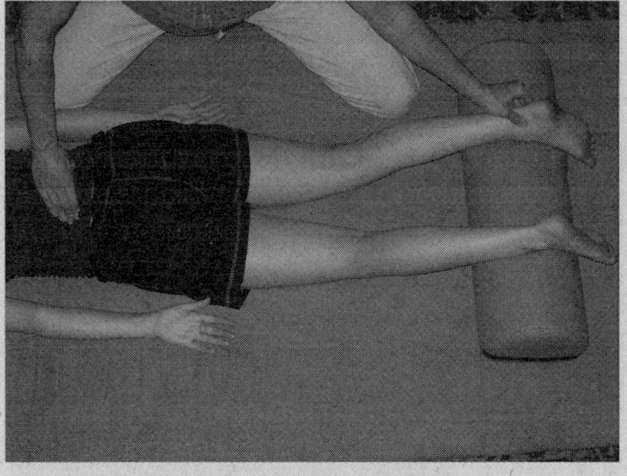

FIGURE 6-8 **Bl 23 and Ki 3.**

continued

PRACTICE EXERCISE 6-1: CONTINUED

This protocol uses the following method(s):
A) To tonify, move from an inferior to a superior aspect and from distal to proximal.
B) To tonify, move with the current of the Meridian flow.

3. The client's Lung Meridian is Kyo. Place the client in the supine position, and with the Mother hand, press and hold Lu 9 while the Son hand presses up the Meridian and pauses at Lu 1, the Lung referral point on the chest (Esher, 2002).

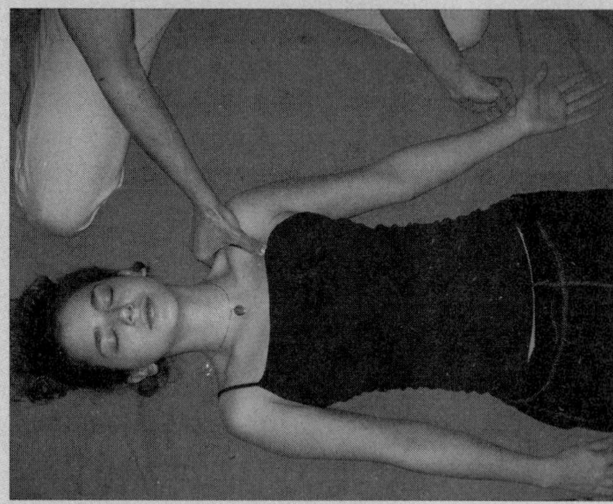

FIGURE 6-9 **Lu 1 and Lu 7.**

This protocol uses the following method(s):
A) To tonify, move from an inferior to a superior aspect and from distal to proximal.
B) To tonify, move with the current of the Meridian flow.

4. The client's Heart Meridian is Kyo. Place the client in the prone position, and with the Mother hand, press and hold Ht 7 while the Son hand presses up the Meridian and pauses at Bl 15, the Heart Shu/Yu point on the back (Esher, 2002).

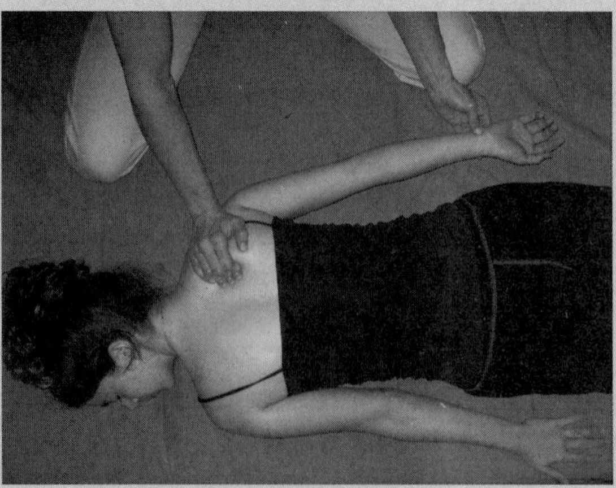

FIGURE 6-10 **Bl 15 and Ht 7.**

This protocol uses the following method(s):
A) To tonify, move from an inferior to a superior aspect and from distal to proximal.
B) To tonify, move with the current of the Meridian flow.

Answers:

1. A and B (move from foot to hara with Sp current)
2. A and B (move from foot to lower back with Ki current)
3. A (move upward and inward from hand to chest)
4. A (move upward and inward from hand to upper back)

Body mobilization techniques (BMTs), especially wide rotations, and stretches that move a limb to the outer limit of its range of motion (ROM) are also stimulating (Beresford-Cooke, 2000). BMTs and ROM stretches should be applied after an area has been warmed and loosened through compression techniques, whereas simple traction or placing a limb in a Meridian stretch position can be done before compressions.

Direction of Movement

The direction of movement also affects whether the technique is sedating or tonifying. Some differences of opinion exist as to what constitutes the right direction to sedate or tonify. Two major views are presented here, and the practitioner is encouraged to experiment and form his or her own judgment. One view holds that sedation is accomplished by driving energy downward and outward, while tonification is accomplished by drawing energy upward and inward. To release or expel Jitsu, the practitioner applies Shiatsu from the client's head to the client's feet or from a superior to an inferior aspect, and from the center of the torso outward to the extremities—that is, from the chest or upper back out along the arms to the hands or from the abdomen or lower back out along the legs to the feet (Jwing-Ming, 1992). Conversely, to tonify and nourish Kyo, the practitioner applies Shiatsu from the client's feet to the client's head or from an inferior to a superior aspect, and from the extremities in toward the center—that is, from the hands or feet in toward the torso. The rationale for this method is that the downward direction grounds excess Yang energy, which tends to flare upward, especially toward the head, and the outward direction drives excess energy out of the body, discharging Heat. The upward direction raises deficient Yin energy, which tends to sink downward, and the inward direction draws energy into the body where it is needed.

The other view holds that sedation is accomplished by moving against the current of the Meridian flow and tonification is accomplished by moving with the current of the Meridian flow (Ohashi, 1976/2001). Thus, to sedate Jitsu, the practitioner begins by pressing the last, highest-numbered point on the Meridian and works backward to the first, lowest-numbered point. For example, if the Bladder Meridian is Jitsu, the practitioner begins with Bl 67 on the little toe, works up the back of the body against the current of the Meridian, and ends with Bl 1 at the inner corner of the eye. Conversely, to tonify, the practitioner begins with the first, lowest-numbered point on the Meridian and ends with the last, highest-numbered point. Thus, if the Bladder Meridian is Kyo, the practitioner begins with Bl 1 at the inner corner of the eye, works down the back of the body with the current, and ends with Bl 67 on the little toe. The rationale for this method is that when a

Meridian is predominantly Jitsu, its energy is too Yang, too forceful and fast; hence, moving against or countering the flow of the current will decrease its force and speed. When a Meridian is predominantly Kyo, its energy is too Yin, too weak and slow; hence, moving with and reinforcing the flow of the current will increase its force and speed, ushering it along.

The direction of circular rubbing also affects whether the technique is sedating or tonifying. When applying circular rubbing techniques, the clockwise direction from the practitioner's perspective tonifies and nourishes Kyo, whereas the counterclockwise direction disperses and releases Jitsu (Jwing-Ming, 1992). When circling clockwise, the practitioner draws in Qi, which the client absorbs, but when circling counterclockwise, the practitioner draws out Qi, which the client releases.

REFERENCES

Beresford-Cooke, C. (2000). *Shiatsu theory and practice: A comprehensive text for the student and professional*. Edinburgh: Churchill Livingstone.

Esher, B. (2001). Asian healing arts: Got Yin/Yang? *Massage Today, 1*(12), 18–19.

Esher, B. (2002). Asian healing arts: Yin and Yang deficiency, part III. *Massage Today, 2*(11), 8, 19.

Jarmey, C., & Mojay, G. (1999). *Shiatsu: The complete guide* (Rev. ed.). London: Thorsons.

Jwing-Ming, Y. (1992). *Chinese Qigong massage: General massage*. Boston: YMAA Publication Center.

Kaptchuk, T. (2000). *The web that has no weaver: Understanding Chinese medicine* (2nd ed.). Chicago: Contemporary.

Maciocia, G. (2001). *The foundations of Chinese medicine: A comprehensive text for acupuncturists and herbalists*. Edinburgh: Churchill Livingstone. (Original work published 1989.)

Masunaga, S., & Ohashi, W. (1997). *Zen Shiatsu: How to harmonize Yin and Yang for better health*. Tokyo: Japan Publications. (Original work published 1977.)

Ohashi, W. (2001). *Do it yourself Shiatsu: How to perform the ancient Japanese art of acupressure*. New York: Penguin. (Original work published 1976.)

STUDY QUESTIONS

1. What are the four classical examinations used in TCM?

2. How do the methods of diagnosis used by an OMD or acupuncturist differ from the methods of assessment used by a Shiatsu practitioner?

3. To what does the Interior/Exterior pair of the Eight Principle Patterns refer?

4. Describe the characteristics of an Internal disorder.

5. What are the primary causes of Internal disorders?

6. Describe the characteristics of an External disorder.

7. What are the primary causes of External disorders?
8. What kind of therapeutic technique is beneficial for External disorders?
9. To what does the Deficiency/Excess pair of the Eight Principle Patterns refer?
10. Describe the physical symptoms of a Deficiency disorder.
11. Describe the emotional symptoms of a Deficiency disorder.
12. Describe the physical symptoms of an Excess disorder.
13. Describe the emotional symptoms of an Excess disorder.
14. What are the primary causes of Excess disorders?
15. What is painful obstruction syndrome?
16. What kind of therapeutic technique is beneficial for stagnation?
17. To what does the Cold/Heat pair of the Eight Principle Patterns refer?
18. What are the symptoms of a Cold disorder?
19. What are the primary causes of a Cold disorder?
20. What are the symptoms of a Heat disorder?
21. What are the primary causes of a Heat disorder?
22. Explain the difference between the Appearance of Cold and true Cold.
23. Explain the difference between the Appearance of Fire and true Fire.
24. Do most clients present a classic Yin (Interior, Deficient, Cold) or Yang (Exterior, Excess, Heat) condition or a hybrid of the two?
25. What is the literal translation and meaning of the word *Jitsu*?
26. What is the literal translation and meaning of the word *Kyo*?
27. Using the amoeba analogy, to what state or condition does Kyo correspond?
28. Using the amoeba analogy, to what phenomenon does Jitsu correspond?
29. Which arises first: Kyo or Jitsu?
30. Which is considered the true cause of the energy imbalance: Kyo or Jitsu?
31. What happens to Jitsu once Kyo is resolved?
32. Explain why a Kyo Jitsu energy imbalance is not necessarily abnormal.

33. Aside from a pathological condition, what other conditions could a Kyo Jitsu imbalance reflect?

34. Under what circumstance could a Kyo Jitsu imbalance lead to disease?

35. What are the primary causes of Jitsu?

36. What are the primary causes of Kyo?

37. Using the ball or sphere analogy, how does Jitsu manifest as a physical distortion?

38. Using the ball or sphere analogy, how does Kyo manifest as a physical distortion?

39. Describe the symptoms of Jitsu.

40. Describe the symptoms of Kyo.

41. Distinguish between Jitsu hardness and Kyo hardness.

42. How does pressure on a Jitsu area feel to the client?

43. How does pressure on a Kyo area feel to the client?

44. Which is easier to detect: Kyo or Jitsu?

45. Explain why one is easier to detect than the other.

46. Which should one focus on: Kyo or Jitsu?

47. Explain why the practitioner should focus on one more than the other.

48. When the client's lifestyle is causing a perpetual Kyo Jitsu imbalance, what is the best one can expect from Shiatsu?

49. Under what circumstances is it better to begin a session by sedating Jitsu?

50. Under what circumstances is it better to begin a session by tonifying Kyo?

51. What aspects of the client are assessed during visual observation?

52. Describe the profile of a Kyo client.

53. Describe the profile of a Jitsu client.

54. What kind of therapy do Kyo clients prefer?

55. What kind of therapy do Jitsu clients prefer?

56. What Yin Yang principle explains these general preferences?

57. How should a practitioner address a superior/inferior, anterior/posterior, or right/left discrepancy?

58. Which Meridians might be implicated in a bottom-heavy disparity?

59. Which Meridians might be implicated in a right/left disparity?

60. Describe Meridian diagnosis.

61. Is a Meridian either all Kyo or all Jitsu?

62. How does a Jitsu Meridian feel to the practitioner?

63. How does a Kyo Meridian feel to the practitioner?

64. What kind of pressure is used in hara diagnosis?

65. How does one distinguish a Jitsu area on the hara?

66. How does one distinguish a Kyo area on the hara?

67. What method should one use to find the most Kyo area?

68. What kind of pressure is used in back diagnosis?

69. What does tenderness or sharp pain in a Shu/Yu point on the inner Bladder Meridian signify?

70. What does tenderness or sharp pain in a Shu/Yu point on the outer Bladder Meridian signify?

71. Contrast the results of hara diagnosis with those of back diagnosis. How might they differ?

72. How should pressure be applied to tonify Kyo?

73. What is the standard tonification technique developed by Masunaga?

74. Which stretches are considered gentle enough to be tonifying?

75. How should pressure be applied to disperse Jitsu?

76. Describe kenbiki and its use.

77. What other techniques are used to disperse Jitsu?

78. Which stretches are considered stimulating enough to be sedating?

79. In which directions should one move to expel Jitsu?

80. In which directions should one move to nourish Kyo?

81. In which direction should one rotate to release energy from Jitsu?

82. In which direction should one rotate to draw in energy toward Kyo?

EIGHT PRINCIPLE PATTERNS AND KYO JITSU TEST (60 POINTS)

MATCHING. LETTERS MAY BE USED MORE THAN ONCE.

A. Interior/Exterior
B. Deficiency/Excess
C. Cold/Heat
D. Interior
E. Exterior
F. Deficiency
G. Excess
H. Cold
I. Heat

____**1.** Hyperactivity of an organ.

____**2.** Location of malady.

____**3.** Congestion and stagnation of Qi or blood.

____**4.** Low or high levels of substances or activity.

____**5.** Hypoactivity of an organ.

____**6.** Temperature imbalances.

____**7.** Caused by excess Yin or deficient Yang.

____**8.** Caused by excess Yang or deficient Yin.

____**9.** Pale complexion, whispers, sluggish, dull mood, pressure relieves.

____**10.** Chronic: slow onset, malingering, difficult to eliminate.

____**11.** Ruddy complexion, shouts, agitated, tense mood, pressure hurts.

____**12.** Curls up in fetal position under blanket near radiator, immobile, withdrawn.

____**13.** Acute: sudden onset, severe symptoms, brief duration.

____**14.** Sprawls naked and spread-eagle, desires an iced drink and an ice pack, restless or fidgety.

____**15.** Corresponds to contagious diseases or trauma.

____**16.** One type is painful obstruction syndrome.

KYO JITSU. CIRCLE THE CORRECT ANSWER.

Kyo Jitsu **17.** Immoderately high energy

Kyo Jitsu **18.** Arises first

Kyo Jitsu **19.** Caused by an obstruction or blockage that leads to congestion and stagnation

Kyo Jitsu **20.** Immoderately low energy

Kyo Jitsu **21.** Need, want, emptiness, deficit

Kyo Jitsu **22.** True cause of imbalance

Kyo Jitsu **23.** Compensatory drive, expenditure

Kyo Jitsu **24.** Caused by constitutional infirmity, trauma, or long-term illness that depletes

Kyo Jitsu **25.** Focus therapy on remedying this

Kyo Jitsu **26.** Diminishes or vanishes if the other is partially or fully resolved

Kyo Jitsu **27.** Concave depressions

Kyo Jitsu **28.** Hyperactive, excitable, hot, sharp pain

Kyo Jitsu **29.** Buoyant, resilient hardness

Kyo Jitsu **30.** Stiff, rigid hardness

Kyo Jitsu **31.** Convex protrusions

Kyo Jitsu **32.** Hypoactive, sedated, cold, dull pain

Kyo Jitsu **33.** Unresponsive

Kyo Jitsu **34.** Reactive

Kyo Jitsu **35.** Easy to detect

Kyo Jitsu **36.** Hard to treat

Kyo Jitsu **37.** Tonify and nourish

Kyo Jitsu **38.** Deep, intermittent, rapid, rhythmic pressure

Kyo Jitsu **39.** Sedate and disperse

Kyo Jitsu **40.** Moderate, gradual, slow, sustained pressure

Kyo Jitsu **41.** Tapotement, vigorous jostling

Kyo Jitsu **42.** Kenbiki

Kyo Jitsu **43.** Move from head to foot, from the center outward, or against Meridian current

Kyo Jitsu **44.** Move from foot to head, from the extremities inward, or with Meridian current

Kyo Jitsu **45.** Clockwise

Kyo Jitsu **46.** Counterclockwise

TRUE OR FALSE. CIRCLE THE CORRECT ANSWER.

True False **47.** The existence of Jitsu implies the existence of Kyo.

True False **48.** A Kyo Jitsu imbalance always indicates a pathological condition.

True False **49.** If one focuses exclusively on Jitsu and neglects Kyo, Jitsu will return.

True False **50.** The practitioner can resolve Kyo Jitsu imbalances that are due to lifestyle.

True False **51.** The general rule is to sedate Jitsu first before tonifying Kyo.

True False **52.** Begin by tonifying Kyo when the client is a Yang/Jitsu type.

True False **53.** Yin/Kyo clients prefer dispersal techniques.

True False **54.** A lower half Jitsu/upper half Kyo disparity often implicates the Stomach and Spleen Meridians.

True False **55.** A right/left disparity often implicates the Bladder Meridian.

True False **56.** Apply dispersal techniques to the chest and abdomen in case of anterior Jitsu/posterior Kyo disparity.

True False **57.** Firm pressure is used for hara diagnosis and light pressure for back diagnosis.

True False **58.** For hara diagnosis, find the most Jitsu reflex zone first, maintain contact, and then palpate for the most Kyo reflex zone.

True False **59.** Tenderness in the Shu/Yu points along the inner Bladder Meridian indicates a physical imbalance, while tenderness in the points along the outer Bladder Meridian indicates a psychological imbalance.

True False **60.** Hara and back diagnosis produce the same results and are interchangeable.

7

ACUPOINTS

OBJECTIVES

- To describe the nature, structure, and function of acupoints
- To locate acupoints using anatomical landmarks, cun as a measuring unit, and the sensation of De Qi
- To explain how acupressure works according to different theories
- To combine local/distal, superior/inferior, and anterior/posterior acupoints to achieve a synergistic effect
- To sequence the order of acupoints to clear a Meridian obstruction
- To maximize or minimize therapeutic intensity according to the client's need, preference, or vitality level
- To reinforce a therapeutic effect by stimulating complementary acupoints and Meridians according to the principle of correspondence
- To reflexively treat an inaccessible or contraindicated area of the body by stimulating alternative acupoints and Meridians according to the principle of correspondence
- To choose acupoint combinations to balance superior/inferior and right/left discrepancies
- To balance acupoint combinations, especially Yin/Yang combinations, so that the client is neither overstimulated nor understimulated

KEY TERMS

Tsubo
Ahshi
Acupoints
Cun
Shu/Yu/Back Transporting/Associated Points
Mu/Bo/Front Collecting/Alarm Points

ACUPOINTS

The Qi that flows in Meridians is particularly accessible at certain fixed locations called Qi Xue, which means "energy cavities" in Chinese (Jwing-Ming, 1992, pp. 49, 90), and **Tsubo**, which means "body points" or "pressure points" in Japanese (Serizawa, 1976/2000, p. 29). The Japanese character for Tsubo resembles a vase-shaped storage container with a slender neck and round belly that is used to store seed, suggesting that a large reserve of energy is accessible through a narrow aperture (see Figure 7-1) (Jarmey & Mojay, 1999). These energy cavities are also known as **Ahshi**—"That's it!" or "Ouch!" points—referring to the client's exclamation or startle response when the point is manipulated (Liechti, 1998, p. 89). Ahshi points elicit pain, and as with their Western correlate, trigger points, this pain may be felt as a chronic, low-grade nagging sensation that intensifies with palpation (Jarmey & Mojay, 1999). Both Ahshi and Tsubo are synonyms for acupressure or acupuncture treatment points, which may be referred to by the abbreviated term acupoints.

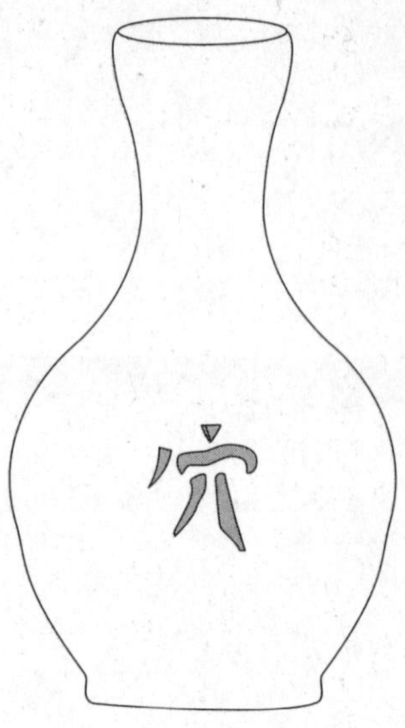

FIGURE 7-1 Tsubo.
The Chinese character for Tsubo resembles a vase with a slender neck and a round belly, indicating a large reserve of energy available through a small aperture.

According to TCM, there are 365 acupuncture points on the body, though modern research and methods have increased the number to about 2,000 (Kaptchuk, 2000). The 365 classical acupuncture points are points whose properties have been studied and recorded over the centuries, but theoretically any point along a Meridian pathway can manifest energetically and have a salubrious effect when stimulated (Jarmey & Mojay, 1999). Despite the vast repertoire of possible points, the average OMD or acupuncturist uses only about 150 (Kaptchuk, 2000), and even less can be stimulated by the fingers due to the manual inaccessibility of some points.

These **acupoints** are entrances, gateways, or portals into the body's energy system. Scientific research has confirmed the existence of acupoints by their distinctive electrical properties. Acupoints are points of low electrical resistance (Liechti, 1998) and high electrical conductivity relative to the rest of the body (Jwing-Ming, 1992). Low electrical resistance means that they are particularly susceptible to electrical charges, and high electrical conductivity means that they readily transmit these charges to elsewhere in the body through the energy network. Acupoints interface in a dynamic way with the environment and are often described and depicted as energy whirlpools or vortices—swirling funnels that draw or suck energy into the body and release or expel energy out of the body (see Figure 7-2) (Lundberg, 1992). As portals, they can be wide open, moderately open, or barely open, depending on their function and condition.

From a diagnostic perspective, acupoints are points where distortions on the body's surface—anomalies in the skin, subcutaneous tissue, or musculature—signify distress, illness, or disease in the deeper layers of the body, especially the organs (Serizawa, 1976/2000). Acupoints are often located at junctures that are physically weak or where energy flow tends to decelerate or stagnate, leading to disorders or maladies.

LOCATING ACUPOINTS

In general, acupoints are located at indentations, depressions, or hollows near bony prominences; on knots, cords, ropes, or bands of tense muscle; and near other physical landmarks, such as a nail border, hairline, sense organ, nipple, navel, or the juncture of red and white flesh on the sole of the foot. The exact location of an acupoint is measured by a unit that is relative to the physical proportions of the individual, such as the breadth of a finger, rather than some standard unit of measurement, such as an inch or centimeter (Junying & Zhihong, 1991/1997). A standard unit of measurement lacks accuracy in that an inch proportionally covers more of the total surface area available on a short or slender person than on a tall or obese person. In

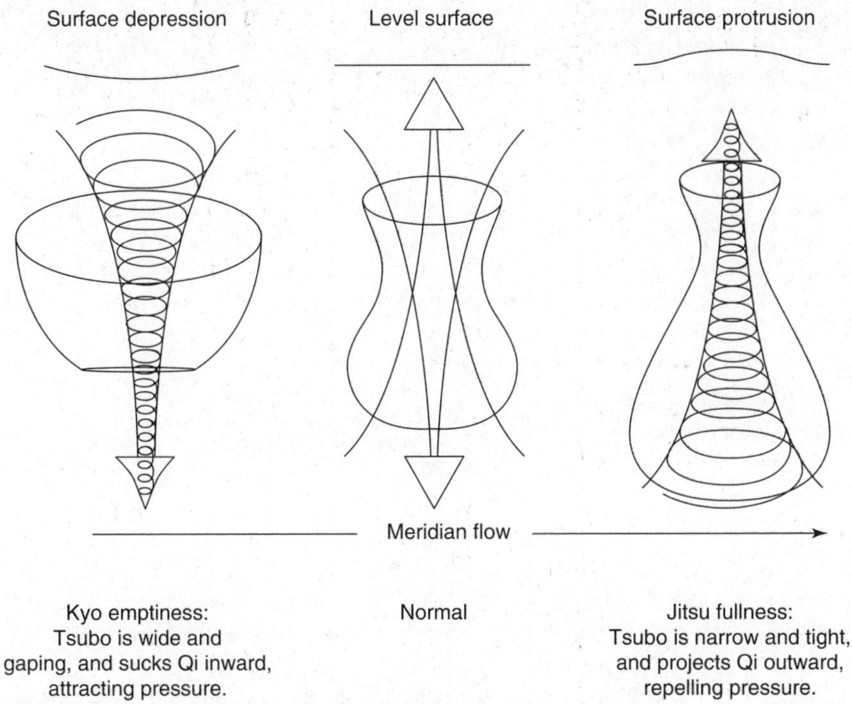

FIGURE 7-2 Acupoints as energy whirlpools or vortices.

TCM, the preferred unit of measurement that is relative to the individual is a **cun** (pronounced "chun"). One cun is equal to the breadth of the client's thumb at the middle joint or the distance between the innermost creases of the middle joint of the middle finger. Three cun are equal to the breadth of four fingers (see Figure 7-3).

In locating acupoints, the Chinese tend be more regimented and the Japanese more intuitive in their approach. The Chinese rely on precise measurements based on anatomical landmarks, whereas the Japanese rely on palpatory skill and the sensation of De Qi or contacting Ki (personal communication with Dr. Daniel Redwood, February 13, 2004). Shiatsu practitioners should cultivate both skills—technical and intuitive—in their practice. Technical mastery is attained by memorizing the directions or location formulas for finding particular points and by gaining proficiency in identifying anatomical landmarks and measuring in cun. For example, Sp 6 is located 3 cun or the width of four of the client's fingers above the medial malleous (inner ankle bone), hooking under the tibia (shin bone), and St 36 is located 3 cun or the width of four fingers below the patella (kneecap), against the tibia (shin bone).

Intuitive mastery is attained by practice in discerning an energetic response. Sometimes the search for an energetic response may lead the practitioner slightly away from the academic location, and this should not cause concern about neglecting technical accuracy (personal communication with Dr. Daniel Redwood, February 13, 2004). For instance, CV 12, an organ point for the Stomach, is technically located half way between the xyphoid process of the sternum and the navel. Finding the anatomical location is a good starting point for palpating De Qi, which may lead the practitioner to a point slightly lower or higher on the CV Meridian.

Each of the 365 classical acupoints is designated by a descriptive Chinese name, such as Leg Three Mile, as well as a standard referencing number, such as St 36, indicating where in the consecutive sequence of points a certain point lies on a particular Meridian (Gach, 1990). A low number indicates that the point lies near the beginning of a Meridian, whereas a high number indicates that the point lies near the end of a Meridian. Many of the names are environmental metaphors, such as Bubbling/Gushing Spring (Ki 1) and Joining the Valley (LI 4). Other names are

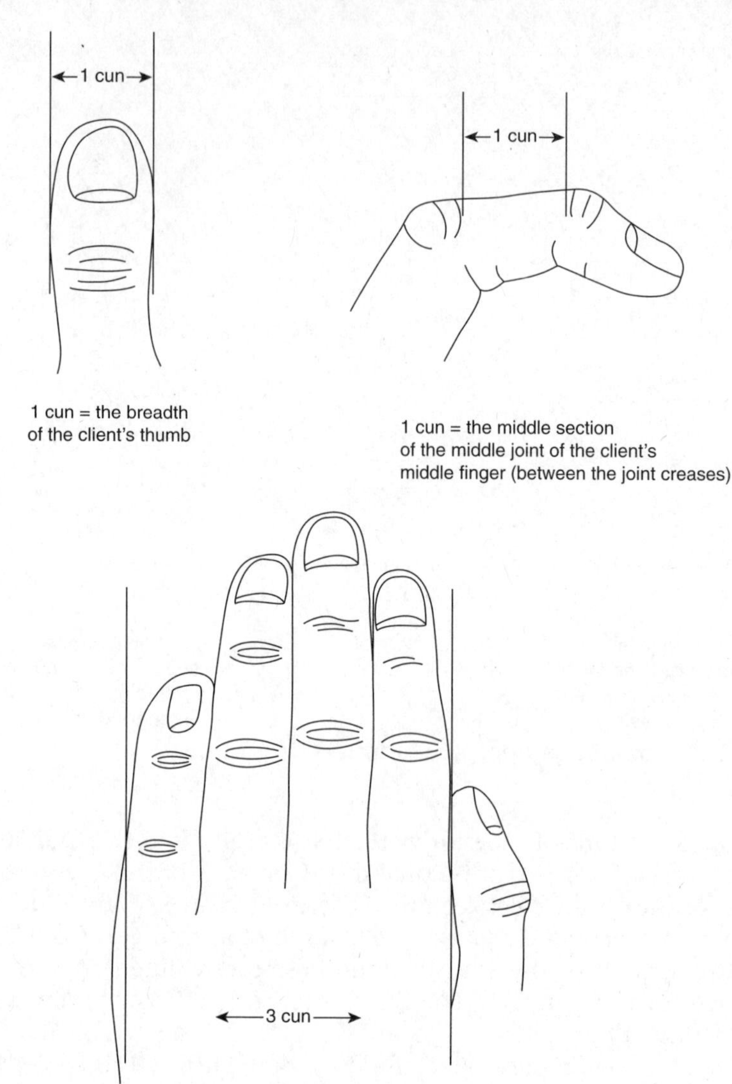

FIGURE 7-3 Cun measurements.

poetic metaphors, such as Heavenly Pillar (Bl 10) and Gates of Consciousness (GB 20). Still others suggest either a point's location, as in Shoulder Well (GB 21), or its therapeutic properties, as in Welcome Fragrance (LI 20) and Eyes Bright (Bl 1).

Some discrepancies exist in the numbering of points on charts or in texts. Some Bladder Meridian points on the posterior side of the body may be numbered differently, depending on the source. For example, the point on the buttocks at the level of the second sacral foramen is Bl 53 in the Chinese system but Bl 48 in the Japanese system; the point under the fold of the buttock at the hamstring attachment to the ischial tuberosity (sit bone) is Bl 36 in the Chinese system but Bl 50 in the Japanese system; and the point behind the knee on the popliteal crease is Bl 40 in the Chinese system but Bl 54 in the Japanese system. A few texts, such as Katsusuke Serizawa's *Tsubo: Vital Points for Oriental Therapy* (1976/2000), are based on the Japanese system, but the majority are based on the Chinese system. Because most Shiatsu texts and acupuncture charts are based on TCM, this text uses the Chinese system as well.

ACUPRESSURE

Proper manipulation of an acupoint often elicits a distinct sensation or even a startle response if the sensation is sudden and sharp enough (Nielson, 2002). When the practitioner accesses the client's energy and the connection is felt, the Chinese refer to this as De Qi, which means that the Qi of the point has been contacted (Jarmey & Mojay, 1999). The De Qi sensation can manifest in any number of ways: as a soothing or relieving soreness, ache, or pain; as a thermal sensation (usually warmth); and as a neural sensation, such as numbness, tingling, prickling, or an electrical pulse or jolt. The sensation may be confined to the local point being pressed, or it may travel distally to other associated areas as a sharply delineated radiating sensation or a diffused spreading sensation. If no sensation occurs, the acupoint is inactive; the point has not been accessed at the correct location, angle, or depth; or the client's condition is deficient. If the sensation is intolerable, energy at the point may be stagnant or blocked, or pressure may have been applied too abruptly or deeply for the client, in which case a gentler, more gradual approach is indicated.

As a therapy, acupressure can be applied to particular sections of the body or incorporated into a full-body Shiatsu session that stimulates Qi flow in all the Meridians. Acupressure promotes good health and can ease symptoms of a wide array of disorders but cannot intervene the way Western medicine can in cases of infectious diseases, cancer, and conditions requiring surgery (Serizawa, 1976/2000).

THEORIES EXPLAINING ACUPOINT THERAPIES

Various theories have been advanced to explain the therapeutic effects of stimulating acupoints, whether by acupuncture, acupressure, Shiatsu, moxabustion, Gua Sha, or some other modality. These theories view the same phenomenon from different perspectives—neural, muscular, vascular, biochemical, and energetic. Like the proverbial elephant that was described as a rope, a fan, and a wall by three blindfolded men who touched the elephant in three different places—the tail, the ear, and the flank, respectively—these theories are complementary, not contradictory. Most, however, are predicated on a Western frame of reference. As such, Western allopathic medicine focuses on the goal of symptom reduction or elimination rather than organ harmony and explains therapeutic results in terms of anatomy and physiology rather than energetic balance.

Two theories—the biochemical endorphin theory and the neurological gate theory—emerged from clinical research studies into the analgesic property of acupuncture, a property that is highly coveted by the American public and Western practitioners of medicine and that has increasingly commanded the attention of researchers, particularly as the American public has turned to complementary medicine as an alternative to the side effects of drug therapy.

While the goal of reducing or eliminating pain is certainly worthwhile, historically the Chinese have used acupuncture primarily to treat organ maladies by balancing the body's energy, thereby gradually restoring a state of wellness devoid of pain. Only secondarily have they used it as an analgesic—for example, as an anesthetic during surgery (Demuth, 2001). J. R. Worsley, a traditional practitioner of acupuncture, advises against using acupuncture merely for the purpose of killing pain unless an illness is terminal or no cure is known. Pain, Worsley notes, is a warning sign that indicates something is wrong. Disabling the pain signal without treating the underlying condition is tantamount to dismantling the warning lights on a car's dashboard without fixing the mechanical problems that triggered the warning lights. Such mechanical problems, if serious and if left unattended, will eventually destroy the car.

Although Worsley's remonstrance addresses the indiscriminate symptom-suppressing use of acupuncture rather than acupressure or Shiatsu, his point is clear: The general purpose of all Asian healing arts is to balance the body's energy, not to mask pain. In the process of balancing the body's energy, harmony is restored and symptoms of disorder, such as pain, naturally subside. The theories below shed light from different angles on the mechanisms that underlie the healing process.

NERVE REFLEX ARC THEORY

According to the nerve reflex arc theory, the inside and outside of the body communicate with and affect each other via the nervous system (Serizawa, 1976/2000). Through neural connections, an organ malady is relayed as distress signals to associated reflex areas, tissues that are neurologically connected to the organ via the spinal cord and its branches. These distress signals manifest as aberrations in the skin, subcutaneous tissues, and muscles of the reflex area (Serizawa, 2000). Symptoms vary and include tenderness, hypersensitivity, pain, or numbness of the tissues; tension, hardening, and stiffening of the muscles into a splint that braces or immobilizes the ailing part, protecting it from injurious stimulation; restricted movement or rigidity; discolorations in skin pigmentation; excessive or deficient secretions of the sebaceous (oil) glands and sudoriferous (sweat) glands; dilation or constriction of blood vessels with concomitant flushing or chilling; and contraction of the erectorpilae, causing goosebumps.

Such aberrations in the reflex areas facilitate both diagnosis and treatment. In terms of diagnosis or assessment, abnormal or pathological conditions in the body's superficial tissues suggest abnormal or pathological conditions in the body's deep tissues or organs. In terms of treatment or therapy, treating the outside of the body can benefit the inside. In other words, the principle of the nerve reflex arc is reciprocal (Serizawa, 1976/2000). Just as impulses from inside the body are transmitted via the spinal cord and nervous system to the surface of the body, causing external changes, impulses from the surface of the body are transmitted within, causing internal changes. Hence, acupressure and Shiatsu can benefit the internal organs, improving their function.

RELAXATION RESPONSE THEORY

Another neural-somatic theory is the relaxation response theory. Stimulating acupoints, especially along the Bladder Meridian on either side of the spine, promotes the relaxation response of the autonomic nervous system (ANS). The ANS regulates functions that are not usually subject to conscious control or volition, such as heartbeat, respiration, and digestion. The ANS has two branches, the sympathetic branch, which is like an accelerator and external task manager, and the parasympathetic branch, which is like a decelerator and internal task manager. The functions of these two branches are roughly inversely coordinated: When the sympathetic branch is activated, the parasympathetic branch is suppressed, and when the sympathetic branch is de-activated, the parasympathetic branch restores homeostasis.

Given a sufficient stressor, the sympathetic branch initiates the stress response, the "fight or flight" reaction to a perceived environmental threat. Overall, the sympathetic nervous system shunts blood away from the gastrointestinal tract and routes it to the heart, lungs, and skeletal muscles to support activities that expend stored energy. Specifically, the sympathetic branch stimulates the release of epinephrine (adrenaline), a hormone that excites physical activity; dilates the pupils to augment distance vision; accelerates heart rate; opens the bronchial tubes to promote respiration; releases glycogen (stored energy) from the liver and increases blood volume to the skeletal muscles to fuel physical exertion, all while inhibiting gastrointestinal and reproductive functions (Coulter, 2001).

Once the threat is over and the effects of the stress response subside, the body returns to its maintenance mode and resumes its housekeeping functions, such as digestion, assimilation, and elimination. In the absence of a stressor that precipitates the "fight or flight" mode, the parasympathetic nervous system continues unabated in this default "rest and digest" mode, routing blood to support various activities of the digestive tube from mouth to anus and, in general, conserving energy. Specifically, the parasympathetic branch constricts the pupils to augment near vision; decelerates heart rate; constricts the bronchial tubes to subdue respiration; stimulates the secretion of digestive juices and intestinal peristalsis, facilitating digestion; stimulates the conversion of glucose into glycogen, a form of stored energy held in reserve for the stress mode; and relaxes the urethral and anal sphincters, facilitating elimination (Coulter, 2001).

Acupressure to the cervical, lower lumbar (L3–L5), and sacral regions affects the parasympathetic branch, while acupressure to the thoracic and upper lumbar (L1 and L2) regions affects the sympathetic branch (Coulter, 2001). Collectively, acupressure all along the inner Bladder Meridian, where the nerves innervating the organs exit the spinal cord, soothes the ANS, harmonizing the functioning of the sympathetic and parasympathetic branches so that the overall effect is calming and relaxing (Liechti, 1998).

GATE THEORY

The gate theory explains the pain-relieving effect of acupoint stimulation as a form of "hyperstimulation analgesia" (Kaptchuk, 2000). In simplistic terms, hyperstimulation analgesia is a kind of sensory overload—a neurological crowding that blocks pain signals from reaching the brain. This anesthetic effect is due to a regulatory mechanism—a "gating mechanism"—at the spinal cord level that controls the kind and amount of sensory input that is transmitted through the spinal cord to the thalamus, a part of the brain that processes pain. As impulses from the large-diameter nerve fibers, such as the kind stimulated by acupuncture, outnumber impulses from the small-diameter nerve fibers of pain receptors, the spinal gate closes to pain signals, inhibiting sensations of pain. Acupressure and Shiatsu are manual versions of acupuncture with ostensibly similar results.

BIOCHEMICAL THEORY

Another theory explains the analgesic property of acupoints in biochemical terms. According to the biochemical theory, the stimulation of acupoints releases endogenous morphines, which are ordinarily suppressed by certain antagonists in the brain (Kaptchuk, 2000). The word *endogenous* means "generated within or produced internally," and *morphine* refers to a narcotic pain reliever and sedative. Hence, endogenous morphines, or endorphins for short, are opiates naturally synthesized by the body. These endorphins are extremely powerful painkillers that not only raise pain thresholds during and after treatment, but also regulate the body's stress response and induce a sense of well-being or euphoria. The most potent of endorphins "is 5,000 to 10,000 times more potent than morphine," according to the *New England Journal of Medicine* (Kaptchuk, 2000, p. 137). Both acupuncture and bodywork stimulate the release of endorphins, as does vigorous exercise, as evidenced in "runner's high."

TRIGGER POINT THEORY

Still another theory explains the benefits of acupressure as the manual disruption of a structural deformity in a muscle that is perpetuated by a functional derangement of its associated nerve. This theory is premised on a high degree of correlation between the location of acupoints and the location of neuromuscular trigger points. Since about 80 percent of major trigger points correspond to acupoints (Wall & Melzack, 1989), some sources equate acupoints—especially hyperirritable Ahshi—with neuromuscular trigger points. A description of the trigger point mechanism follows so that effects of manual intervention can be understood.

A trigger point is a hypersensitive, "exquisitely tender" spot inside a tense nodule within a taut band of muscle (Travell, Simmons, & Simmons, 1999). Besides local tenderness, a trigger point transmits, either spontaneously or upon pressure, a radiating or spreading sensation to a more distant location, known as its *referral zone*. Usually, the radiating sensation is steady, deep, and aching. Less commonly, it is lancinating, that is, piercing, stabbing, or jolting in quality. Neural sensations, such as numbness, prickling, and tingling, are another manifestation, and thermal sensations, such as cold, heat, burning, and stinging, are yet another. Even quirkier sensations are possible, such as itching, crawling, and tickling. The referral zone of the trigger point is an area that is often, though not always, functionally related to the muscle harboring the trigger point. Thus, a trigger point in a primary muscle can propagate satellite trigger points in associated muscles that assist its action.

Trigger point tenderness is a symptom of contracture: a chronic, pathological contraction of muscle tissue due to a faulty neural mechanism that overstimulates and hyperactivates the muscle. The dysfunctional nerve that innervates the muscle produces a kind of bioelectrical noise or static discharge that keeps the muscle in a constant state of contraction (Travell, Simmons, & Simmons, 1999). Prolonged contracture or spasm at the trigger point site creates a domino effect of problems that compound one another, beginning with vasoconstriction, a narrowing of blood vessels supplying the area.

Like a tightened fist squeezing a rubber hose, a chronically contracted muscle throttles the vascular structures that support it, impeding blood and lymph flow to and from the tissues. Reduced blood flow to the tissues results in ischemia or lack of blood in the tissues. In turn, ischemia results in hypoxia or lack of oxygen, as well as nutrient deprivation. The net result of compromised incoming blood flow is malnourished tissues. Also, because outgoing blood and fluid flow is compromised, waste removal is impaired, and fluid and waste products accumulate. Fatigue metabolites, such as lactic acid, carbonic acid, and hyaluronic acid—chemical byproducts of sustained muscle contraction—become concentrated, attracting more fluids to the area. Wastes chemically irritate tissues, causing pain, and fluid pressure mechanically irritates tissues, causing pain. Additionally, tension in the muscle itself creates mechanical stresses in the belly of the muscle and at its attachment sites that cause pain (Travell, Simmons, & Simmons, 1999).

Digital compression or acupressure on a trigger point interrupts this unhealthy state of affairs by manually flattening, spreading, and lengthening muscle fibers that are bunched, clumped, and shortened. This elongates, stretches, teases, and pries apart hypertonic, adhered muscle fibers, relaxing them. Once a contracture is released, mechanical stress is relieved, and blood and lymph flow to the tissues improves, promoting normal cell respiration. As blood and lymph flow is restored, tissues are supplied with oxygen and nutrients, and metabolic wastes and excess fluids are transported away. Then pain and other symptoms of distress subside.

GOLGI TENDON ORGAN THEORY

Another theory that is based on neuromuscular mechanisms is the Golgi tendon organ theory. Golgi tendon organs are sensory receptors located at the musculotendinous junction, the site where muscle fibers taper and converge into a tendon that anchors the muscle to its bone. These sensory organs monitor the degree of tension in a muscle or the stress load on a muscle (Coulter, 2001). When a Golgi tendon organ detects too much tension in a muscle or an excessive load on a muscle, it relays this information to neurons that inhibit muscle contraction, causing the muscle to relax. This relaxation reflex is a safety mechanism designed to protect the tissues from strain (rupture) due to excessive tension or load. A familiar and dramatic example of this occurs in an arm wrestling match when sustained muscular exertion causes the weaker opponent's arm to collapse under the pressure of an irresistible, insurmountable force. Aside from vigorous muscle contraction, deep manual manipulation at the musculotendinous junction where the Golgi tendon organs are located simulates a load on the muscle and also triggers this mechanism, inducing muscle relaxation. Hence, acupressure and Shiatsu techniques directed to muscle attachment sites elicit this reflex.

TCM THEORY

The aforementioned theories originate from a Western frame of reference and explain the benefits of acupressure and Shiatsu in terms of Western anatomy and physiology—in particular, the nervous, muscular, circulatory, lymphatic, and endocrine systems of the body. While Shiatsu positively affects these physical systems, it also affects the body's energetic system. Although acupoints and Meridians are located within physical structures, such as muscles, and follow the course of blood vessels, lymph vessels, and nerve routes, they constitute a distinct, discrete energy system that works in conjunction with these other systems of the body.

In other words, the Qi system is not just another name for these other systems. It is existentially unique, though inextricably intertwined with other systems in a symbiotic relationship. According to TCM, imbalances in the Qi system will manifest as aberrations in other systems and may even result in pathological conditions of physical structures. Conversely, abnormalities in these other systems will manifest as an energetic disharmony. Shiatsu, acupressure, acupuncture, moxabustion, and Gua Sha are primarily energetic interventions that sedate or disperse Qi where it is excessive, tonify or nourish Qi where it is deficient, release Qi where it is blocked, propel Qi where it is stagnant, and redirect Qi where it is perverse. Restoring energetic harmony is often a prerequisite to restoring physical health in the other systems.

ACUPOINT COMBINATIONS

Acupoints are usually stimulated not in isolation, but in combination with other acupoints in order to enhance the therapeutic effect and balance the overall treatment (Maciocia, 2001). Two main principles guiding point selection are the therapeutic properties of the points themselves and their collective synergistic effect. There are several methods of coordinating points, including local/distal, superior/inferior, posterior/anterior, right/left, and Yin/Yang combinations. These point combinations ensure that the treatment is harmonized so that no part of the body is neglected or overstimulated.

LOCAL/DISTAL POINT COMBINATION

The local/distal point combination is defined slightly differently, depending on the source. The Chinese State Administration for TCM and Pharmacology, a governmental authority that promulgates and disseminates official policies on TCM, defines local as being near the affected site and distal as being far from the affected site but having a salutary influence on the affected site (Junying & Zhihong, 1991/1997). Another highly respected source, Giovanni Maciocia, OMD and author of *The Foundations of Chinese Medicine,* defines local as on the torso or head and distal as on the limbs (2001).

In practice, both definitions refer to the same thing. For example, LI 4, the point on the web of flesh between the thumb and forefinger, which is stimulated by hooking and pressing under the second metacarpal bone, has a wide range of therapeutic properties and is often combined as a distal point with other local points on the head or shoulder to reinforce the desired effect: LI 4 is combined with Bl 1 and 2 for the eyes; with LI 20 for the nose; with St 6 and 7 for the jaws and teeth; with GV 16, Bl 10, and GB 20 for the neck; and with GB 21, LI 15, and TH 14 for the shoulder. Another example of a distal point that is used in conjunction with local points to treat conditions of the upper body is SI 3. SI 3 is located midway on the outside of the hand and is stimulated by hooking and pressing under the fifth metacarpal bone. It functions as a distal point when combined with several local points near the ear—TH 17, GB 2, and SI 19—to resolve ear problems and with several local points near the scapula, especially SI 11, to resolve shoulder problems.

The method of combining one or more distal points on a limb with one or more local points on the torso applies equally well to the lower body. For example, a distal point on the back of the knee, Bl 40, is often combined with local points on the lower back, Bl 23 and 25, to relieve lumbago. Distal points near the ankle, Bl 60 and GB 40, are combined with local points on the hips—Bl 53, Bl 54, and GB 30—to relieve hip tension. See Table 7-1 for more examples of local and distal point combinations.

The local/distal point combination is also used for chronic disorders or diseases. Distal points on the limbs are combined with local points on the torso that are associated with the functioning of particular organs (see the section below on posterior/anterior combinations) (Maciocia, 2001). In cases of chronic headaches, local points on the head treat symptoms due to stagnant Qi and blood, while distal points on the limbs treat the source of the problem—organ maladies. For example, chronic headaches due to Liver Yang rising can be relieved by pressing distal points on the foot and lower leg, such as Lr 3, Ki 3, and Sp 6, to treat the "root" and by working the Gallbladder Meridian and points on the head to treat the symptoms.

Principle 1: Distal Points Before Local Points to Clear Blockages

Several principles guide the use of local/distal point combinations, and some require the practitioner to exercise good judgment (Maciocia, 2001). First, the order in which points are stimulated is not arbitrary. Distal points are stimulated before local points to clear obstructions in a Meridian so that the maximum benefit can be gained from stimulating local points. An obstruction in a Meridian can

TABLE 7-1 Local/Distal Point Combinations

Problem Area	Local Points	Distal Points
Eyes	Bl 1, 2	LI 4
Ears	TH 17; GB 2; SI 19	SI 3, 5
Nose	LI 20, St 3	LI 4
Teeth, Jaws	St 6, 7	LI 4
Neck	GV 16; Bl 10; GB 20	LI 4, 11
Chest	Lu 1; CV 17	Lu 5, 7, 9
Shoulder	GB 21; LI 15; TH 14; SI 11	LI 4, 11; SI 3
Upper Abdomen	CV 12	St 36; PC 6
Lower Abdomen	CV 4, 6; St 25	Sp 6
Lower Back	BL 23, 25	Bl 40, 60
Hip	BL 53, 54; GB 30	Bl 60; GB 40

be caused by the invasion of an External Pernicious Influence, such as Cold, Damp, or Wind, or by Qi and blood stagnation due to muscle strain or tendon sprain. When energy flow in a Meridian, especially a Yang Meridian, is obstructed or blocked, as in illness or injury, distal points are opened first so that space is cleared for the movement of Qi through the channel. This is somewhat analogous to removing a barricade from an exit before ushering traffic through.

For example, TH 4 and 5 at the wrist are stimulated before LI 10 and 11 at the elbow to treat a cold or to treat sore strained arm muscles. St 41 and 42 and GB 40 on the dorsal surface of the foot are stimulated before St 36 and GB 34 on the lower leg and before St 31 and GB 31 on the thigh to treat sore strained leg muscles. Sp 3 on the arch of the foot, under the head of the first metatarsal bone, is stimulated before Sp 6 and 9 on the lower leg, and before Bl 20 and 21 on the back or CV 3 and 4 on the abdomen to resolve Dampness.

Principle 2: Distal Points on Feet for Intense Effect, on Hands for Moderate Effect

A second guiding principle is that the location of distal points, whether on the hands or the feet, alters the intensity of the sensation and therapeutic effect. For a stronger sensation and effect, distal points on the feet are best, but for a milder sensation and effect, distal points on the hands are best (Maciocia, 2001). Distal points on either the hands or the feet are chosen, depending on which is more appropriate for the client's condition. Distal points on the feet are preferable for vivacious and robust clients or in cases of acute injury, such as a sprain where strong energy is needed to clear blockages and disperse stagnation, whereas distal points on the hands are preferable for weak or elderly clients—those whose Qi is deficient and for whom a strong treatment would be depleting or exhausting.

Principle 3: Correspondence between Similar Joints and Meridians

A third guiding principle is the correspondence between similar joints and similar Meridians (Maciocia, 2001). The principle of correspondence between similar joints pairs functionally and spatially related joints for treatment purposes. A good synopsis of this principle is the aphorism "As above, so below." Hence, wrist and ankle, elbow and knee, and shoulder and hip are corresponding joints that have mutually beneficial, reciprocal effects.

The principle of correspondence also applies to Meridians that occupy similar energetic zones on the upper and lower halves of the body. Meridians are similar if they possess the same polarity—both Yin or both Yang—and if they are located on the same aspect or surface area of their respective limbs when the person is seated in the teddy-bear position with legs and arms outstretched in front (Figure 7-4) (Beresford-Cooke, 2000). This pairing of Meridians by polarity—Yin with Yin and Yang with Yang—and by relative location is referred to as the Six Divisions.

Thus, the Lung and Spleen Meridians are paired because they are both Yin and located on the inner upper aspect of their respective limbs. The Pericardium and Liver Meridians are paired because they are both Yin and inner middle Meridians. The Heart and Kidney Meridians are paired because they are both Yin and inner lower Meridians. The Large Intestine and Stomach Meridians are paired because they are both Yang and located on the outer upper aspect of their respective limbs. The Triple Heater and Gallbladder Meridians are paired because they are both Yang and outer middle Meridians. The Small Intestine and Bladder Meridians are paired because they are both Yang and outer lower Meridians. (see Figure 7-5 and Table 7-2.)

Because the Six Division Meridian pairs are energetically similar, they influence each other and are to a certain extent interchangeable in treatment (Beresford-Cooke, 2000). Thus, if one of the pair needs treatment, its counterpart can also be treated to reinforce the effect, or if one of the pair cannot be treated for some reason, its counterpart can be treated instead. The Six Division pairs also reveal the depth of

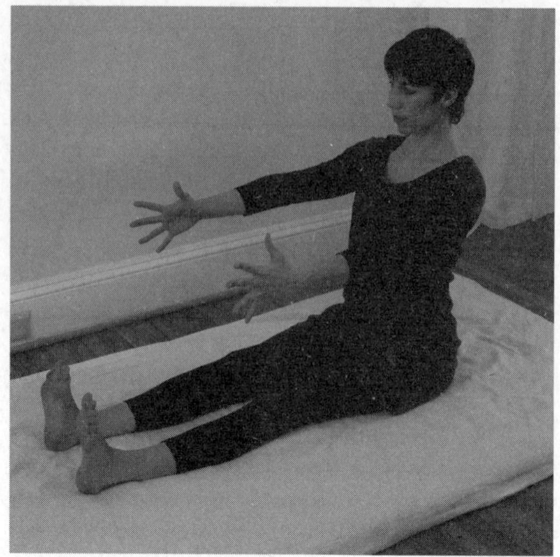

FIGURE 7-4 Teddy–bear position.

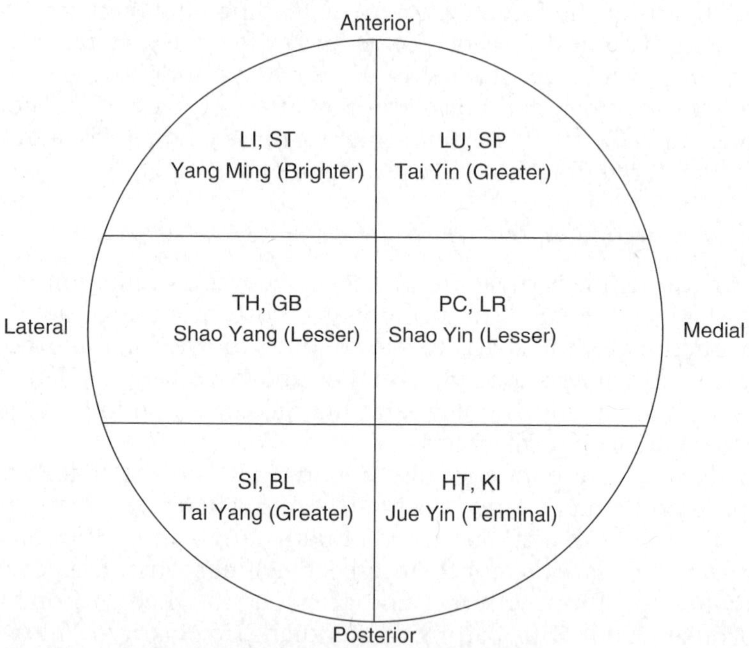

FIGURE 7-5 Relative placement of the Six Divison Meridian pairs on the left limb.

TABLE 7-2 Six Division Meridian Pairs

Pair Name	Limb Location	Polarity	Arm Meridian	Leg Meridian
Tai Yin (Greater)	Inner, upper	Yin	Lung	Spleen
Shao Yin (Lesser)	Inner, middle	Yin	Pericardium	Liver
Jue Yin (Terminal)	Inner, lower	Yin	Heart	Kidney
Yang Ming (Brighter)	Outer, upper	Yang	Large Intestine	Stomach
Shao Yang (Lesser)	Outer, middle	Yang	Triple Heater	Gallbladder
Tai Yang (Greater)	Outer, lower	Yang	Small Intestine	Bladder

a disorder or disease, how far it has progressed into the interior of the body, though this information is not generally used in Shiatsu (Jarmey & Mojay, 1999).

One way to apply the principle of correspondence is to stimulate acupoints on or near a painful or dysfunctional joint, as well as those on or near the corresponding joint, to achieve a synergistic effect. However, if the dysfunctional joint cannot be touched or moved because it is in an acute stage of injury or otherwise inaccessible (in a cast) or it is contraindicated, the practitioner can indirectly treat it by stimulating acupoints on the corresponding joint (Maciocia, 2001). For example, to generate a reflexive healing response for a lateral ankle sprain during the inflammatory phase of recovery, the practitioner first identifies the acupoint on the ankle closest to the traumatized tissues by asking the recipient to point to the site where the pain is greatest or where the injury occurred, most likely GB 40 or Bl 60. Then the practitioner stimulates the corresponding acupoint on the wrist, TH 4 or SI 5, respectively. In the case of an injured knee, the practitioner identifies the most tender or traumatized acupoint on the knee and stimulates the corresponding acupoint on the elbow. For a strained hip, the practitioner identifies the most tender or traumatized acupoint on the hip and stimulates the corresponding acupoint on the shoulder. Table 7-3 lists additional joint, acupoint and Meridian correspondences.

Another way to apply the principle of correspondence to reinforce a therapeutic effect is to press acupoints on a symptomatic Meridian, as well as on its corresponding Meridian. The treatment protocols below use the principle of correspondence to alleviate headaches that manifest in different locations on the head, implicating different Meridian pairs.

- For an occipital or Tai Yang (Bl/SI) headache that manifests at the nape of the neck, the practitioner presses and rubs Bl 10 on the posterior neck and other points along the inner and outer Bladder Meridian between the shoulder blades, and then presses SI 12, 11, 10, and 9 on the posterior shoulders, following the Small Intestine Meridian down the arms and hands (Esher, 2001).

TABLE 7-3 Joint/Acupoint/Meridian Correspondences

Leg	Arm	Six Division Meridian Pair
Ankle	**Wrist**	
Stomach 41	Large Intestine 5	Yang Ming/Brighter Yang
Gallbladder 40	Triple Heater 4	Shao Yang/Lesser Yang
Bladder 60	Small Intestine 5	Tai Yang/Greater Yang
Spleen 6	Lung 7	Tai Yin/Greater Yin
Liver 4	Pericardium 7	Shao Yin/Lesser Yin
Kidney 3	Heart 7	Jue Yin/Terminal Yin
Knee	**Elbow**	
Stomach 36	Large Intestine 11	Yang Ming/Brighter Yang
Gallbladder 34	Triple Heater 10	Shao Yang/Lesser Yang
Bladder 40	Small Intestine 8	Tai Yang/Greater Yang
Spleen 9	Lung 5	Tai Yin/Greater Yin
Liver 8	Pericardium 3	Shao Yin/Lesser Yin
Kidney 10	Heart 3	Jue Yin/Terminal Yin
Hip	**Shoulder**	
Stomach 31	Large Intestine 15	Yang Ming/Brighter Yang
Gallbladder 30	Triple Heater 14	Shao Yang/Lesser Yang
Bladder 36	Small Intestine 10	Tai Yang/Greater Yang
Spleen 12	Lung 1	Tai Yin/Greater Yin
Liver 12	Pericardium 2	Shao Yin/Lesser Yin
Kidney 11	Heart 1	Jue Yin/Terminal Yin

- For a temporal or Shao Yang (GB/TH) headache that manifests at the side of the head, the practitioner presses and rubs GB and TH points at the temple and around the ears and then GB 20 on the neck, GB 21 on the upper shoulders, and TH 14 on the outer shoulders, following the Triple Heater Meridian down the arms and hands (Esher, 2001).
- For a Yang Ming (St/LI) headache due to constipation, in addition to Ampuku, the practitioner presses and rubs LI 11 and 10 near the elbows, following the Large Intestine Meridian down to LI 4, the Great Eliminator on the hands; then the practitioner presses St 36 in the lower compartment of the legs, following the Stomach Meridian down to the feet.

SUPERIOR/INFERIOR POINT COMBINATION

Besides the local/distal point combination, there are several other methods of combining points. Use of superior/inferior point combinations entails stimulating points from the waist up along with points from the waist down (Junying & Zhihong, 1991/1997). For example, to calm rebellious Stomach Qi, a superior point on the wrist, PC 6, is combined with an inferior point on the lower leg, St 36. In general, treatment should be balanced, including points on the upper and lower halves of the body unless the client's condition indicates otherwise, as in the case of an energy disparity between the upper and lower halves (Maciocia, 2001).

For instance, if the client has deficient energy below the waist and excessive energy above, manifesting as a red complexion, hypertension, vertigo, anxiety, and insomnia, the practitioner should focus treatment on the lower half of the body, stimulating such points as Ki 1 and 3, Lr 3, and Sp 6 on or near the feet to draw energy downward (Maciocia, 2001). Conversely, if the client suffers from conditions of sinking Qi, such as hemorrhoids or prolapse of the uterus or rectum, the practitioner should focus treatment on the upper half of the body and stimulate GV 20 on the crown of the head to draw energy upward.

POSTERIOR/ANTERIOR POINT COMBINATION

Use of posterior/anterior point combinations entails stimulating points on the back of the torso along the inner and outer Bladder Meridians in conjunction with points on the front of the torso on the chest and abdomen, many of which are on the Conception Vessel but some of which are on other Meridians (Junying & Zhihong, 1991/1997). Each organ has a posterior and an anterior point associated with it (see Figure 7-6 and 7-7 and Table 7-4).

The posterior or back points are called **Shu** in Chinese and **Yu** in Japanese. They are also known as **associated points** because they are located near their respective organs and **back transporting points** because they transmit or direct Qi to their respective organs (Jarmey & Mojay, 1999). The anterior or front points are called **Mu** in Chinese and **Bo** in Japanese. They are also known as **front collecting points** because the Qi of their respective organs gathers there and **alarm points** because they are used for acute conditions.

A pathological condition in a Zang (Yin) or Fu (Yang) organ will cause an abnormal sensation, such as hypersensitivity, tenderness, or sharp pain in the corresponding Shu/Yu or Mu/Bo point (Junying & Zhihong, 1991/1997). The Shu/Yu points that run along the inner Bladder Meridian about 1.5 cun lateral to the spine are stimulated to improve the physiological functioning of the corresponding organs and sense organs. Although these Shu/Yu points may be stimulated in isolation, they are often combined with Mu/Bo points to treat chronic organ conditions, especially when Qi, blood, fluids, or Jing is depleted (Jarmey & Mojay, 1999), as in chronic fatigue syndrome. In contrast, the Mu/Bo points are

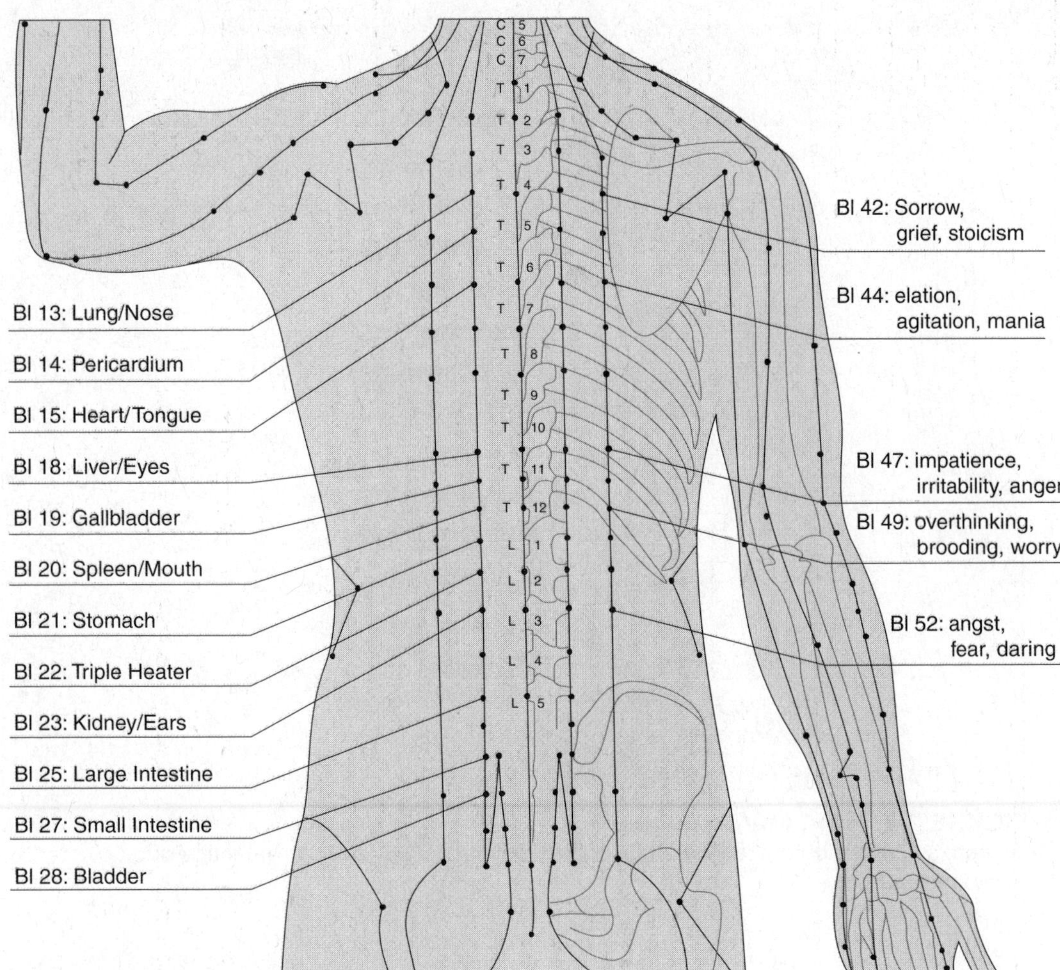

FIGURE 7-6 Back Shu/Yu points and emotional points.
Authorized Derivation of The Flow of Qi chart:
Copyright 1998–2004 by Valentin Popov.
www.flowofqi.com

stimulated to treat acute organ conditions, especially of the Yang organs, such as upset stomach, abdominal bloating, flatulence, constipation, diarrhea, and bladder infection.

While the posterior points along the inner Bladder Meridian are stimulated to improve the physiological functioning of organs and sense organs, the posterior points along the outer Bladder Meridian are stimulated to address psychological issues associated with the organs, especially emotional imbalances (Table 7-5) (Beresford-Cooke, 2000). Points on the outer Bladder Meridian are located in the intercostal spaces between the ribs about 3 cun lateral to the spine. In the upper back, points on the outer Bladder Meridian are much closer to the scapula than are points on the inner Bladder Meridian.

Right/Left Point Combination

Use of right/left point combinations entails stimulating points bilaterally—that is, on both sides of the body—for a strong, balanced effect (Maciocia, 2001). However, in certain cases points are stimulated unilaterally—that is, on only one side of the

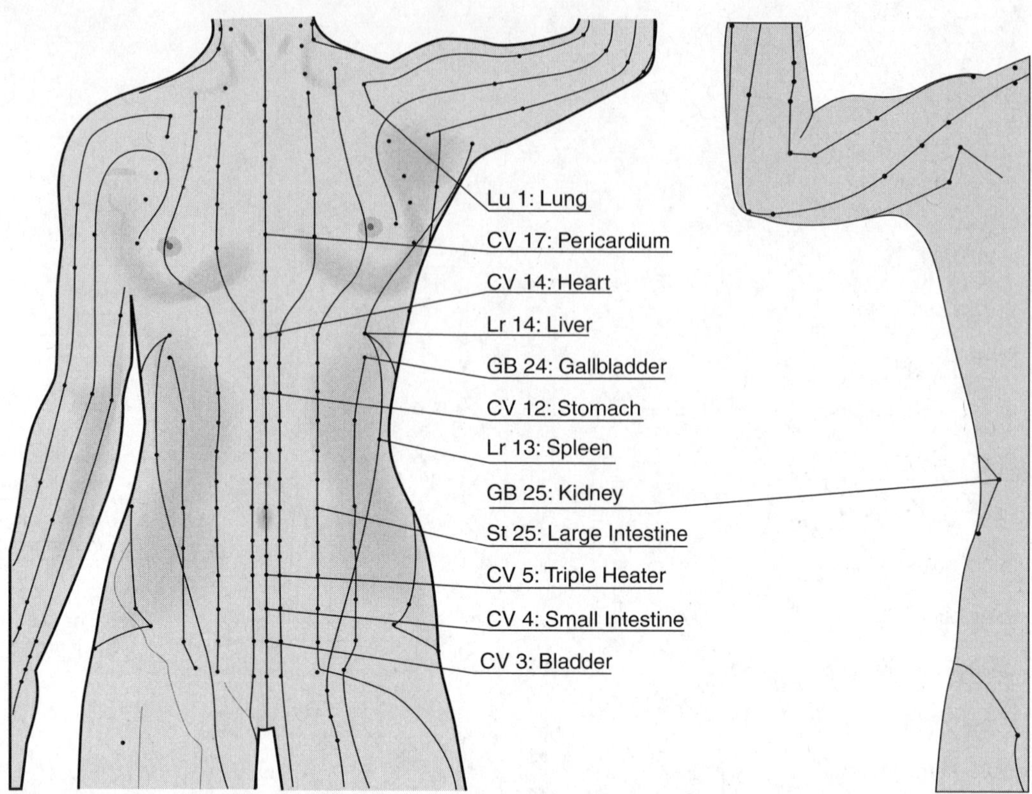

FIGURE 7-7 Front Mu/Bo points.
Authorized Derivation of the Flow of Qi chart: Copyright 1998–2004 by Valentin Popov. www.flowofqi.com

body—as when, for example, the client has a right/left discrepancy, when one side of the body is contraindicated, or when the client is nervous or deficient and a minimalist approach, using the minimum rather than the maximum number of possible points, is indicated (Maciocia, 2001). In such cases, unilateral stimulation works well because Meridians and points on the right and left sides of the body are symmetrical and mirror each other. Stimulating one side reflexively benefits the other as well (Junying & Zhihong, 1991/1997).

Thus, if an area of the body needs treatment but such treatment is contraindicated, the same area on the opposite side of the body can be worked. For example, if the client has had surgery on one side, the practitioner can work the same area on the opposite side; if one side is very deficient, as when the flesh is flaccid or wasted, the practitioner can work the same area on the opposite side to reroute energy from the stronger side to the weaker side (Maciocia, 2001). By the same principle, if the client is skittish about receiving treatment, the unilateral point approach can be used to reduce the total number of points stimulated. For example, if the client has Stomach excess, the practitioner can stimulate PC 6 on one side and St 40 on the other rather than stimulating both points on both sides.

YIN/YANG POINT COMBINATION

Use of Yin/Yang point combinations entails stimulating points of both polarities to ensure a balanced treatment (Maciocia, 2001). Using too many Yang points can agitate or unnerve a client, and using too many Yin points can fatigue or drain a client. When several Yang points are used to treat a condition, they should be

TABLE 7-4 Front/Back Points

Mu/Bo	Shu/Yu	Organ and Sense Organ	Disorders
Lu 1	**BL 13**	**Lungs and Nose/Smell**	Respiratory and sinus disorders; breathlessness; coughing; sneezing; excess sputum and phlegm or dry, itchy, tickly mouth and throat; catarrh; colds; allergies; asthma; skin disorders; sweating and night sweating; tiredness; fatigue; edema of upper body
CV 17	**BL 14**	**Pericardium**	Cardiac disorders; chest pain; arrhythmia
CV 14	**BL 15**	**Heart and Tongue/Speech**	Cardiac disorders; chest pain and constriction; palpitations; breathlessness; sweating and night sweating; listlessness and stupor; fidgetiness; jumpiness/easily startled; cold extremities and cyanosis; overheating; forgetfulness; mental restlessness; agitation; anxiety; insomnia; dream disturbed sleep; speech disorders; incoherent speech; muttering
Lr 14	**BL 18**	**Liver and Eyes/Vision**	Jaundice; hepatitis; stress; abdominal distention; abdominal twitching, pulsing, or churning; nausea; belching; hiccupping; acid reflux; vomiting; PMS; irregular, painful, scanty, or absent periods; breast distention; tension headaches, especially temporal or behind the eyes; migraines; eye disorders; nearsightedness; poor night vision; blurry vision; floaters; sore, red, strained eyes; cramps; spasms; weakness; numbness; tremors; tics; convulsions; paralysis
GB 24	**BL 19**	**Gallbladder**	Gallbladder disorders (stones); pain in upper abdomen; nausea; vomiting
Lr 13	**BL 20**	**Spleen and Mouth/Taste**	Digestive disorders; little or no appetite; indigestion; abdominal distention and pain; loose stools; diarrhea; weight disorders; weak or heavy limbs; lassitude or chronic fatigue; edema; prolapse; hemorrhoids; varicose veins; excessive bleeding during periods
CV 12	**BL 21**	**Stomach**	Digestive disorders; little or no appetite or insatiable appetite; sweet cravings; lack of taste; bleeding gums; foul breath; burning sensation in upper abdomen; abdominal distention and pain; nausea; belching; hiccupping; acid reflux; vomiting; loose stools; constipation; thirst
CV 5	**BL 22**	**Triple Heater**	Upper burner disorders: cold, flu, sneezing, runny nose, sore throat, body aches, fever, occipital headache; middle burner disorders: abdominal distention, indigestion, retention of food in stomach; lower burner disorders: dysfunctions in urination or defecation
GB 25	**BL 23**	**Kidneys and Ears/Hearing**	Soreness, pain, or coldness in low back; weakness or pain in knees; frequent, copious, or nocturnal urination; incontinence; ear disorders; poor hearing; tone deafness; deafness; tinnitus; dizziness; vertigo; amnesia; edema of lower body; reproductive disorders; chronic vaginal discharge; infertility; low libido or frigidity; spermatorrhea; nocturnal emissions; premature ejaculation; impotence; bone disorders; loose teeth; arthritis; osteoporosis; head hair loss; dull occipital or vertex headache; insomnia—waking up several times at night
St 25	**BL 25**	**Large Intestine**	Abdominal distention and pain; abdominal gurgling and churning; constipation; diarrhea; burning anus; hemorrhoids
CV 4	**BL 27**	**Small Intestine**	Abdominal distention and pain; abdominal gurgling and churning; flatulence; diarrhea
CV 3	**BL 28**	**Bladder**	Urinary disorders; frequent, copious, urgent, burning, painful, or difficult urination; nocturnal urination; incontinence; aching or heaviness in lower abdomen; low backache

TABLE 7-5 Outer Bladder Meridian Points

Point	Location	Emotion	Issues	Element	Organs
BL 42	Between T-3 and T-4	Sorrow, grief, stoicism	Loss or separation	Metal	**Lu/LI**
BL 44	Between T-5 and T-6	Elation, agitation, mania	Heartbreak	Fire	**Ht/SI**
BL 47	Between T-9 and T-10	Impatience, irritability, anger	Frustration of purpose	Wood	**Lr/GB**
BL 49	Between T-11 and T-12	Overthinking, brooding, worry	Mental stew or fog	Earth	**Sp/St**
BL 52	Between L-2 and L-3	Angst, fear, daring	Willpower	Water	**Ki/BL**

balanced with one or more Yin points, and vice versa. For example, if the client has a strained shoulder, implicating several Yang Meridian points (such as LI 15, TH 14, and SI 9, 10, 11, and 12), the practitioner can balance this Yang point combination with a Yin point like Lr 3.

REFERENCES

Beresford-Cooke, C. (2000). *Shiatsu theory and practice: A comprehensive text for the student and professional*. Edinburgh: Churchill Livingstone.

Coulter, H. D. (2001). *Anatomy of Hatha Yoga: A manual for students, teachers, and practitioners*. Honesdale, PA: Body & Breath.

Demuth, Sharon (Producer). (2001). *An introduction to classical five-element acupuncture: A public talk by Professor J. R. Worsley*. [Videocassette].

Esher, B. (2001). Asian healing arts: Using the Six Divisions. *Massage Today, 1* (3), 18, 20.

Gach, M. R. (1990). *Acupressure's potent points: A guide to self-care for common ailments*. New York: Bantam.

Jarmey, C., & Mojay, G. (1999). *Shiatsu: The complete guide*. (Rev. ed.). London: Thorsons.

Junying, G., & Zhihong, S. (1997). *Practical Traditional Chinese Medicine and pharmacology: Acupuncture and moxibustion*. Beijing: New World Press. (Original work published 1991.)

Jwing-Ming, Y. (1992). *Chinese Qigong massage: General massage*. Boston: YMAA Publication Center.

Kaptchuk, T. (2000). *The web that has no weaver: Understanding Chinese medicine* (2nd ed.). Chicago: Contemporary.

Liechti, E. (1998). *The complete illustrated guide to Shiatsu: The Japanese healing art of touch for health and fitness*. New York: Barnes & Noble.

Lundberg, P. (1992). *The book of Shiatsu: A complete guide to using hand pressure and gentle manipulation to improve your health, vitality, and stamina*. New York: Fireside.

Maciocia, G. (2001). *The foundations of Chinese medicine: A comprehensive text for acupuncturists and herbalists*. Edinburgh: Churchill Livingstone.

Serizawa, K. (2000). *Tsubo: Vital points for oriental therapy*. Tokyo: Japan Publications. (Original work published 1976.)

Travell, J., Simmons, D., & Simmons, L. (1999). *Myofascial pain and dysfunction: The trigger point manual: Vol. 1. Upper half of body* (2nd ed.). Baltimore, MD: Lippincott, Williams & Wilkins.

Wall, P., & Melzack, R. (1989). *Textbook of pain*. Edinburgh: Churchill Livingstone.

STUDY QUESTIONS

1. What are acupoints?
2. What does the term *Ahshi* emphasize about acupoints?
3. What unique electrical properties of acupoints have been confirmed by scientific research?
4. What tends to happen to the flow of energy near acupoints?
5. How are acupoints numbered on a Meridian?
6. Aside from numbers, how else are acupoints identified?
7. On what physical landmarks are acupoints generally located?
8. Describe a cun.
9. Why is cun a better unit of measurement than an inch or centimeter?
10. Describe the basic principle behind the nerve reflex arc theory.
11. According to the nerve reflex arc theory, what do distortions in surface tissues indicate?
12. According to the nerve reflex arc theory, what part of the body can acupressure benefit?
13. What happens to the body when it shifts to the sympathetic mode of the ANS?
14. What happens to the body when it shifts to the parasympathetic mode of the ANS?
15. Where (along what portion of which Meridian) is the best place to do acupressure to induce the relaxation response?
16. Explain the analgesic (painkilling) property of acupressure according to the gate theory.
17. Explain the analgesic (painkilling) property of acupressure according to the biochemical theory.
18. Explain the connection between acupressure and trigger point therapy.
19. What is a trigger point?
20. Why is a hypertonic (spastic) muscle ischemic (blood deficient)?
21. Aside from lack of nutrients and oxygen, what other detrimental effects arise from ischemia?
22. What does acupressure do to a trigger point?
23. What is the primary function of the Golgi tendon organ?
24. How does the Golgi tendon organ prevent injury?

25. Besides acupressure, what other technique triggers the Golgi tendon organ?

26. Is the energetic model of TCM just a different way of describing the functions of the muscular, nervous, circulatory, lymphatic, and endocrine systems?

27. What is the TCM view of the relationship between the body's energy system and the other systems?

28. What are the two main ways of selecting acupoints?

29. Why is stimulating point combinations better than stimulating isolated points?

30. How does the Chinese State Administration for TCM and Pharmacology define the local/distal point combination?

31. How does Maciocia define the local/distal point combination?

32. Why is it important to stimulate distal points before local points?

33. Which points are more intense and powerful—distal points on the feet or distal points on the hands?

34. In what cases is it appropriate to stimulate distal points on the feet?

35. In what cases is it appropriate to stimulate distal points on the hands?

36. Explain the principle of correspondence between joints.

37. Explain the principle of correspondence between Meridians.

38. Describe the superior/inferior point combination.

39. Give an example of a client condition that calls for stimulating points on the lower half of the body but not the upper half.

40. Give an example of a client condition that calls for stimulating points on the upper half of the body but not the lower half.

41. Describe the anterior/posterior point combination.

42. On which side of the torso are Shu/Yu points located?

43. On which side of the torso are Mu/Bo points located?

44. How do the functions of the inner and outer Bladder Meridian differ?

45. For what kind of conditions are back transporting points indicated?

46. For what kind of conditions are front collecting points indicated?

47. Which point combination relies on the fact that Meridians and points run in bilateral pairs and are mirror images of each other?

48. Under what circumstances is unilateral point stimulation more appropriate than bilateral point stimulation?

49. What could happen to a client if only Yang points are used?

50. What could happen to a client if only Yin points are used?

ACUPOINT TEST (60 POINTS)

SHORT ANSWER

1. What is an acupoint? ____________

2. What is the Japanese term for acupoint (promulgated by Serizawa)? ____________

3. The term *Ahshi* emphasizes what distinctive feature of an acupoint? ____________

4. Acupoints have unique electrical properties relative to the rest of the body. What are they? ____________

5. Distortions in the superficial tissues near acupoints indicate what about the body? ____________

6. Energy flow tends to do what near acupoints? ____________

7. Identify the two most common physical landmarks where acupoints can be found. (2 points) ____________

8. Describe the unit of measurement known as a cun. ____________

9. Why are acupoints measured in cun rather than some standard unit of measurement, such as centimeters or inches? ____________

MATCHING. LETTERS MAY BE USED MORE THAN ONCE

A. Nerve reflex arc theory
B. Relaxation response theory
C. Gate theory
D. Biochemical theory
E. Trigger point theory
F. Golgi tendon organ theory
G. TCM theory

____10. Acupressure releases endorphins in the brain.

____11. Acupressure improves internal organ functioning.

____12. Acupressure relaxes muscle spasms and enhances blood and lymph flow.

____13. Acupressure induces the parasympathetic mode of the ANS.

____**14.** Acupressure blocks pain signals to the brain.

____**15.** Acupressure balances the body's energy system.

____**16.** Acupressure triggers a mechanism that signals muscles to relax.

____**17.** Acupressure reverses the effects of ischemia: Nutrients and oxygen are delivered and fatigue metabolites and excess interstitial fluids are purged.

____**18.** An abnormal or pathological condition in the body's superficial tissues indicates internal distress or an organ malady.

____**19.** Acupressure slows heartbeat and respiration and promotes housekeeping functions such as digestion, assimilation, and elimination.

____**20.** Nerve impulses elicited by acupressure crowd the entrance to the spinal cord, barring the admission of pain stimuli.

____**21.** Acupressure is primarily an energetic intervention; it displaces or scatters Qi in areas of excess and attracts or draws Qi to areas of deficiency.

____**22.** Acupressure constitutes a stress load on muscles, which, though moderate, sets off a protective alarm that induces muscle relaxation.

____**23.** Acupressure on certain points stimulates nerve impulses to organs associated with those points.

____**24.** The energy system interacts with the muscular, neural, circulatory, lymphatic, and endocrine systems of the body.

MATCHING. LETTERS MAY BE USED MORE THAN ONCE

A. Local point
B. Distal point
C. Anterior point
D. Posterior point
E. Local/distal point combination
F. Superior/inferior point combination
G. Posterior/anterior point combination
H. Right/left point combination
I. Yin/Yang point combination

____**25.** Stimulate unilaterally when one side is contraindicated or when there is a disparity between sides.

____**26.** Stimulate points above and below the waist.

____**27.** Stimulate bilaterally for a strong effect.

____**28.** Stimulate points on the back, chest, and abdomen.

____29. Stimulate unilaterally when the client is depleted or anxious about therapy.

____30. Stimulate points of different polarities (negative and positive, masculine and feminine).

____31. Stimulate points near and far from the affected site, or stimulate points on the torso/head and points on the limbs.

____32. Stimulate Shu/Yu and Mu/Bo points.

____33. A point near the affected site.

____34. A point far from the affected site.

____35. A point used for chronic conditions of the organs or associated sense organs.

____36. A point used for acute conditions of the organs.

TRUE OR FALSE. CIRCLE THE CORRECT ANSWER

True False 37. In general, one should balance points on the upper and lower halves, front and back halves, and right and left sides of the body.

True False 38. Stimulate distal points before local points to clear Meridian blockages.

True False 39. Distal points on the hand are more intense than distal points on the feet.

True False 40. Stimulate distal points on the feet when the client is infirm.

True False 41. Stimulate distal points on the hand when the client feels lethargic (sluggish) or enervated (weary).

True False 42. The principle of correspondence refers to stimulating points on similar joints such as ankle and wrist, knee and elbow, and hip and shoulder.

True False 43. The principle of correspondence refers to stimulating points on Meridians of the same polarity, such as LI and St, TH and GB, and SI and BL.

True False 44. In cases of sinking Qi (varicose veins, hemorrhoids, hernia, organ prolapse), stimulate points on the lower extremities where the energy has pooled.

True False 45. In cases of excess Qi in the head (temporal headache; irritability; hot, red, gritty eyes), stimulate points on the lower extremities to draw energy downward.

True False 46. Hypersensitivity, tenderness, or sharp pain in a Shu/Yu or Mu/Bo point indicates a malady in the corresponding organ.

True False **47.** When the left side of the body is traumatized by injury or surgery, stimulate points on the right side instead.

True False **48.** Stimulating too many Yang points will tire a client.

True False **49.** Stimulating too many Yin points will make a client edgy.

MATCHING

A. Headaches
B. Shoulder and arm pain
C. Low back and hip pain
D. Knee pain
E. Ankle pain
F. Colds; flus; sinus disorders
G. Digestive disorders
H. Lower burner (menstrual/urinary) disorders
I. Anxiety/emotional upset
J. Pregnancy and labor

____**50.** Ht 7, 9; PC 6; CV 17; GV 24.5

____**51.** Bl 23, 25, 36, 40, 53, 54, 56, 57, 60; GB 30, 31, 34; St 27, 31

____**52.** PC 6, 7; LI 4; Sp 6; GB 21; Bl 67

____**53.** St 8; Bl 2, 10; GB 1, 20, 21; LI 4; Lr 3; Tai Yang

____**54.** St 35, 36; GB 34; B1 40; Sp 10

____**55.** LI 4, 10, 11, 14, 15; TH 14; SI 9, 10, 11, 12; GB 20, 21

____**56.** Sp 3, 6, 9, 10; CV 3, 4, 5, 6

____**57.** St 25, 36; CV 6, 12; Lr 13; B1 20, 21; Sp 3, 6; LI 4, 11

____**58.** Lu 1, 7, 9; Ki 27; LI 4, 20; TH 5; St 3

____**59.** Ki 3; B1 60; St 41; GB 40

8

COMPLEMENTARY MODALITIES

OBJECTIVES

- To describe the benefits of moxabustion, magnets, and Gua Sha
- To explain how moxabustion and Gua Sha work
- To observe the indications, contraindications, and precautions for moxabustion, magnets, and Gua Sha
- To obtain client consent for moxabustion and Gua Sha and to instruct the client in self-administration of moxa and magnet therapy
- To properly administer each modality, following general principles of application, using correct techniques, and designing the therapy to address the client's chief complaint and presenting condition

KEY TERMS AND CONCEPTS

Moxabustion/Moxibustion
Seeds
Pellets
Permanent Magnets
Pulsing Electromagnetic Fields (PEMFs)
Gauss
Bionorth
Biosouth
Gua Sha
Press and Blanch
Petechiae
Chasing the Dragon

MOXABUSTION

Moxabustion is one of the four classical healing modalities of TCM. It was developed in northern China, where the climate is cold, vegetation is sparse, and cold disorders are common. The term **moxabustion**, also spelled **moxibustion**, is a compound word composed of *moxa*, a derivation of the Japanese word *mogusa*, meaning "herb," and *combustion*, which refers to the controlled burning of a substance. Hence, moxabustion is a heat therapy that involves the controlled burning of an herb, usually Artemisia vulgaris (Latin botanical name) or mugwort (common name), a member of the sage family. This herbal heat therapy is applied directly to or over acupoints to introduce Yang energy into the body to fortify a weak area, dispel cold, or disperse stagnation.

MOXA INDICATIONS AND CONTRAINDICATIONS

In general, moxabustion is beneficial for Yin conditions, such as Cold, Dampness, chronic pain, frozen joints, weakness, tiredness, and Deficiency. However, it is contraindicated for Yang conditions, especially those characterized by Heat, such as fever and inflammation, since heat would only exaggerate the Yang imbalance and intensify the symptoms.

The radiant heat energy of moxabustion neutralizes internal Cold and Dampness by warming and drying tissues and counteracts the contraction of Cold by expanding tissues. For example, moxabustion to the lower back and abdomen can raise the body's core temperature, offsetting chilliness locally and in the extremities (Serizawa, 2000). Moxabustion to the abdomen can help resolve conditions of Dampness in the lower burner, such as abdominal bloating accompanied by a white vaginal discharge (Beresford-Cooke, 2000). Moxabustion to acupoints around a frozen joint can help unlock it by relaxing and loosening tense or spastic muscles and tendons, and moxabustion to acupoints around an arthritic joint can relieve discomfort and immobility, providing the arthritis is noninflammatory (Serizawa, 2000).

In addition to counteracting Cold and Dampness, the kinetic energy of moxabustion accelerates movement and expedites processes, dispersing the stagnation that contributes to inertia in the body. For example, moxabustion can relieve the physical distress of dysmenorrhea, a painful period caused by congealed (stagnant) blood and characterized by burgundy-black clots of blood (Beresford-Cooke, 2000). It can reduce cramping and assist the body in expelling menstrual waste. However, moxabustion is contraindicated for menorrhagia—excessive menstrual bleeding—because it could exacerbate blood flow.

Besides stimulating movement, the heat energy of moxabustion fortifies areas of weakness in the body. Areas of weakness can manifest as Deficiency disorders like hemorrhoids, chronic diarrhea, impotence, and poor immune function. Moxabustion to GV 20 on the crown of the head can raise sinking Qi, alleviating hemorrhoids. Moxabustion to Bl 23 and 25 on the lower back, CV 12 and St 25 on the abdomen, LI 11 on the forearm, and St 36 on the lower leg can alleviate chronic diarrhea (Serizawa, 2000). Moxabustion to the sacrum, Bl 23 and GV 4 of the lower back, CV 3 and 4 of the lower abdomen, and Ki 3 and 9 of the lower leg can improve virility, especially when impotence is caused by stress. Moxabustion to GV 16 and GB 20 of the neck, Bl 12 and 13 of the upper back, and Lu 1 of the chest can boost the immune system to prevent a person from catching a cold or, once a cold is caught, to expel it before it turns into something worse, like bronchitis or pneumonia.

In general, moxabustion is particularly helpful during the autumn and winter, when inclement environmental conditions, and especially cold wet weather, precipitate cold and flu epidemics, make the joints feel stiff and achy, and cause the body to feel dull and sluggish.

MOXA THEORIES

The benefits of moxabustion can be explained in various ways. The kinetic theory of matter, a subdiscipline of the physical sciences that integrates the interests of physics and chemistry, supports a basic understanding. All matter, including the human body, is composed of microscopic particles—atoms and molecules—that are not static but in perpetual motion (*Academic American Encyclopedia*, 1981, vol. 12). The quality of movement of these particles accounts for the temperature, pressure, and consistency of matter. Slower, narrower oscillations of particles correspond to lower temperatures, lighter pressure, and denser forms, such as solids and high-viscosity (thick, sticky) liquids. Faster, wider oscillations correspond to higher temperatures, greater pressure, and lighter forms, such as gases and low-viscosity (thin, fluid) liquids. When the temperature of matter rises, the movement of its particles accelerates and expands, pressure increases, and viscosity decreases.

Introducing vibrant heat energy into the body raises tissue temperature, accelerates the speed and scope of physiological activity, increases pressure differentials that promote diffusion or exchange of substances across cell membranes, and decreases the viscosity of body fluids, such as blood and lymph, so that they flow more easily and swiftly. Thus, heat from burning moxa warms internal Cold and evaporates internal Dampness; stimulates the flow of sluggish or stagnant blood, lymph, and Qi (Beresford-Cooke, 2000); counteracts local and systemic inertia; and relaxes, softens, and loosens contractures.

Shizuko Yamamoto, a proponent of Macrobiotic Shiatsu, offers another theory to explain the immune and health benefits of moxabustion. According to Yamamoto, the heat from moxabustion transforms subcutaneous protein into a chemical called histotoxin, which together with the essential oil of moxa increases the number of white blood cells, thereby boosting the immune system, and alkalizes the blood, thereby promoting good health (Yamamoto & McCarty, 1993).

Katsusuke Serizawa, noted for his scientific research into the electrical properties of acupoints, explains that when moxa is burned on the skin, some of the tissue dissolves and enters the bloodstream, triggering the immune response (1976/2000). This activation of the immune system by introducing a minute amount of foreign material into the body is much like vaccination, which involves inoculating the body with a minute amount of antigen to stimulate antibody production.

MOXA PRODUCTS

In preparing a moxa product, the leaves of the wild weed mugwort are dried and aged, and then crushed and sifted (Williams, 1996). Premium quality, finer grade moxa consists of the choicest part—the fluffy underside of the leaf—and is used for direct application to the skin, while medium or coarser grade moxa contains other parts of the leaf and is used for indirect application. One of the advantages of premium grade moxa is that it burns evenly, whereas the coarser grade burns erratically, sometimes breaking off in blazing chunks, sometimes expiring (Serizawa, 1976/2000).

DIRECT APPLICATION

Moxa comes in different forms for different applications. Loose moxa, also known as moxa punk (Figure 8-1), looks like speckled, yellow-brown moss and feels a bit like gritty lint. It can be rolled and compressed or pinched into a tiny cone shape; set directly on water-moistened skin, which keeps the moxa in place; and lit by rotating the tip of a burning incense stick in small circles. The rotation prevents the moxa from adhering to the incense stick (Serizawa, 1976/2000). The cone

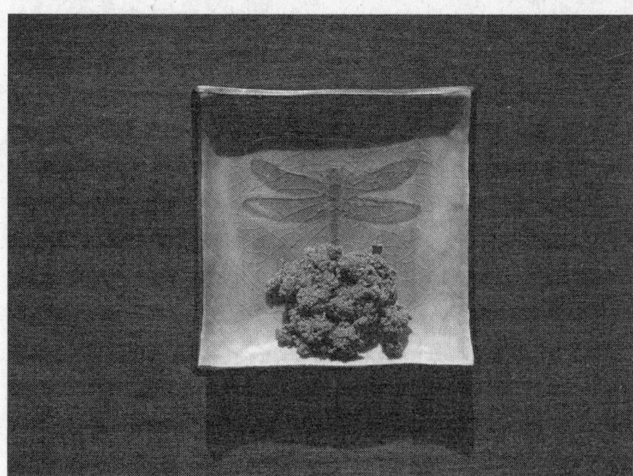

FIGURE 8-1 Loose moxa punk. Moxa punk has the texture of gritty lint. It can be placed directly on the skin or on top of a barrier, such as a thin slice of onion, garlic, or ginger.

smolders and burns down, and heat penetrates the point, stimulating Qi and blood flow. Although ancient texts advise burning the cone down to the skin, Western practitioners remove the cone with tweezers or a brush before blistering and scarring occur (Figure 8-2), usually when the client alerts the practitioner to a hot, stinging sensation. This treatment is repeated several times—usually three but up to seven times—and may be performed daily for up to three weeks.

INDIRECT APPLICATION

Loose moxa can also be placed on top of a base, such as a perforated slice of ginger, garlic, or onion; a flat piece of chive; a piece of gauze soaked in saltwater; a dab of miso or soybean paste (Serizawa, 1976/2000); a layer of salt poured into the navel; or a dollop of an herbal salve. Acupuncturists combine acupuncture and moxabustion by skewering a small cube of moxa on or wrapping it around the coiled end of an acupuncture needle so that the heat is transferred from the needle into the body (Williams, 1996).

Moxa also comes in rolls and sticks of various sizes for indirect application. Perhaps the most popular form is a long, cylindrical roll that looks like a cigar (Figure 8-3). The paper lining is peeled back, and the end is lit. The glowing tip is held half an inch to an inch above the acupoint and rotated in circles or pecked toward and away from the skin for a few minutes or intermittently for up to 15 minutes (Williams, 1996).

One way a practitioner can anticipate client discomfort is to place the index and middle fingers of the idle hand on either side of the acupoint as a heat gauge (Esher, 2001b). When the temperature begins to approach uncomfortable for the practitioner, she knows it will soon be uncomfortable for the client. The practitioner can

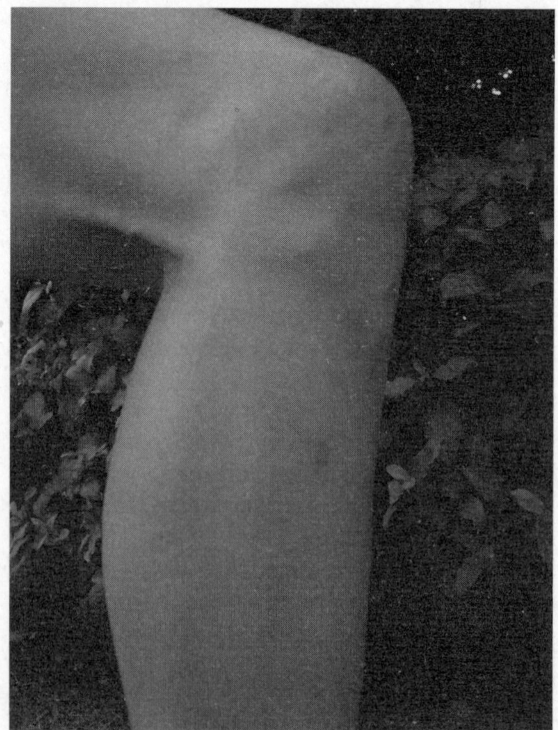

FIGURE 8-2 Moxa scar at St 36. This circular scar was created by holding a moxa roll or "cigar" above the point long enough to blister the tissues.

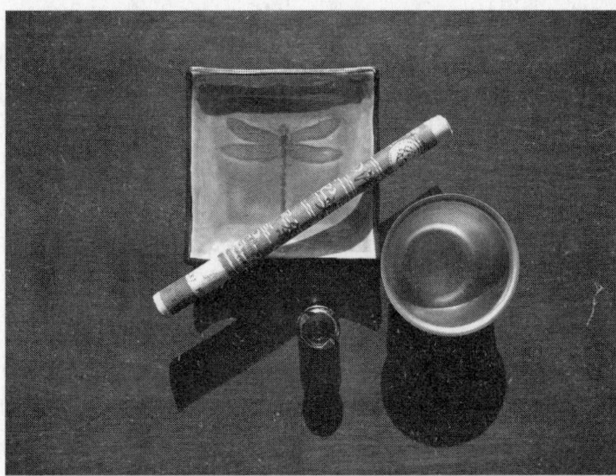

FIGURE 8-3 The popular moxa roll or "cigar" with snuffer and ash basin.

then withdraw the roll or move to another point even before the client alerts her. The accumulated ashes of the roll must be periodically tapped into a basin. The roll is extinguished by inserting it into a specially designed, snug-fitting snuffer or by plunging it into a bowl of sand or dirt (Beresford-Cooke, 2000). Alternatively, the smoldering end can be snipped off with scissors and dropped into water to eliminate any fire hazard.

Moxa sticks are much slimmer than moxa rolls; they look like incense sticks of varying thickness. The burning end can be held above the skin and rotated or pecked in the same manner as a moxa roll. Some moxa sticks are held inside a special applicator called a Tiger or Lion Warmer. The Tiger and Lion Warmers are chrome-plated, brass plungers with ventilation grates near the burning end that allow smoke to escape and a small hole in the convex end of the applicator that conducts the heat and moxa (see Figure 8-4). By pushing down on a coiled spring plunger, the practitioner can control within a certain range how near or far the moxa stick comes to the convex end, which can be applied directly to the skin until it becomes too hot.

VENTILATION

Burning moxa discharges a copious volume of smoke, which has a distinct, musky odor that can be mistaken for marijuana. Barbra Esher, a licensed acupuncturist and Asian healing arts columnist for *Massage Today*, bemusedly noted in one of her articles

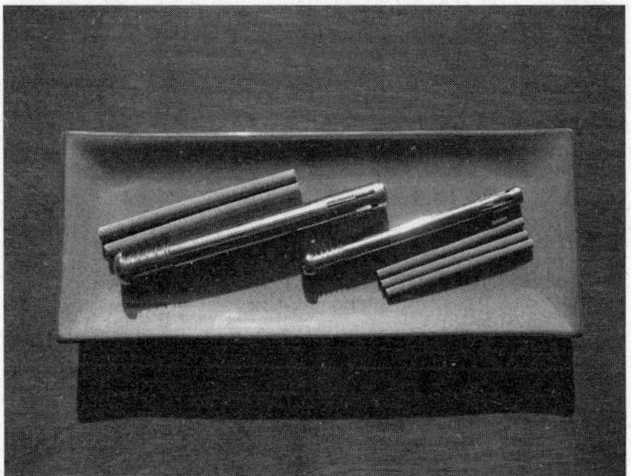

FIGURE 8-4 Moxa sticks beside Lion and Tiger Warmers.

that the police once appeared at her clinic, inquiring about the odor (2003, "Yin and Yang deficiency, part VI"). As with many TCM modalities that seem strange and mysterious to Westerners, educating the general public is part of the healing arts calling. Since moxa smoke can be fairly thick and the odor can cling long after a treatment session, good ventilation is important, or in good weather, moxa can be performed outdoors if feasible. Smokeless moxa is available, but it is not completely smokeless and odorless (Williams, 1996). It is also harder to ignite and is not preferred.

PRACTITIONER ADMINISTRATION VERSUS CLIENT SELF-ADMINISTRATION

As a therapy entailing some risk of accidental burning, moxa unfortunately raises concerns about malpractice liability. For example, when using the popular indirect method of a moxa roll, sometimes a glowing chunk of moxa will unexpectedly fall on the skin and must be briskly swept away and stamped out. Also, after the moxa roll has been burning awhile, the tip becomes sharper and hotter, and the likelihood of blistering increases. Because ordinary precautions cannot obviate mishaps and inadvertent overexposure is a possibility, those practitioners who prefer a conservative approach can instruct clients on self-administration rather than administering moxa to clients. (see Exhibit 8-1). As another precaution, a practitioner should not supply clients with moxa rolls but instead should direct clients to purchase moxa at an Asian market or through a mail-order supplier (see Appendix 4). This precaution further reduces liability for the practitioner (Esher, 2001a).

From a practical standpoint, teaching clients to self-administer moxa is wise because it affirms their responsibility and gives them power and control over their own health. Except for points on the back and hips, moxa is quite easily self-administered, especially on the hands, forearms, shoulders, chest, abdomen, lower legs, and feet, assuming the client is reasonably flexible. In fact, moxa requires a level of patience in holding the roll and a degree of sensitivity in monitoring the heat sensation that arguably are best performed by the recipient. Moreover, in a given Shiatsu session with limited time, most clients, if required to choose, prefer to receive hands-on therapy instead of moxa. But moxa is an extremely effective way to banish joint ailments aggravated by Cold and/or Dampness, and clients who could benefit should be taught how to supplement Shiatsu with moxa. Also, practitioners should moxa themselves, and especially those parts of the body, such as the hands, forearms, and shoulders, that are subject to fatigue and overuse strains that feel worse in cold damp weather.

From a professional standpoint, reserving moxa for self-administration is a double-edged sword. While a policy of abstention may be legally prudent, it is also professionally restrictive, limiting the scope of the healing modalities at the practitioner's disposal. A practitioner who has strong convictions about the benefits of moxa, having personally experienced them, should not balk at introducing moxa to clients. Ultimately, however, each practitioner must exercise his or her own best judgment, yet fear of being sued should not be the sole or dominant factor in the decision. The fact is that from a legal standpoint all treatments are risky to some extent. A practitioner can never control untoward circumstances, such as a client tripping over a futon, or account for idiosyncrasies in clients, such as a severe healing crisis, but that should not deter him or her from engaging in the healing arts.

MAGNETS

SEEDS AND PELLETS

Aside from moxabustion, acupoints can be stimulated with seeds, pellets, and magnets, which can be purchased through mail-order supplier (see Appendix 4). A **seed** or **pellet** can be taped over an acupoint to provide sustained acupressure

INSTRUCTIONS FOR SELF-ADMINISTERED MOXABUSTION

[Practitioner Name]
[Practitioner Contact Information]

ITEMS NEEDED:

Moxa cigar
Lighter
Bowl or basin to catch ash
Moxa cigar snuffer or a bowl of sand or scissors and water

INDICATIONS:

Coldness, dampness, weakness, stiffness, rigidity, especially when aggravated by cold, damp weather

CONTRAINDICATIONS:

As a heat therapy, moxabustion is contraindicated for Heat conditions, such as fever and inflammation, since radiant heat energy would exacerbate the symptoms. Moxa is also contraindicated for skin disorders or breaches in skin like pimples, rashes, burns, bruises, scrapes, cuts, scabs, and open wounds.

INSTRUCTIONS:

1. Ventilate by opening windows and turning on fans to direct smoke outside. Even better, perform outdoors whenever possible, as moxa smoke is thick and pungent, lingering long after treatment, and may cling to fabrics in clothing or upholstery.
2. Peel back the paper lining of the moxa cigar and light the end. Blow on the end until it looks like a glowing, red-hot poker.
3. Hold the glowing end half an inch or an inch above the acupressure point and rotate in circles or peck toward and away from the skin for a few minutes before a stinging sensation is felt, and then quickly withdraw.
4. Repeat up to 15 minutes on the same point or alternate treatment of several points.
5. Monitor the glowing end and beware of dropping ashes or glowing moxa chunks. To avoid the risk of burning, periodically tap the ash into a basin before it accumulates.
6. To extinguish, insert the moxa cigar into a specially designed plunger or a bowl of sand, or snip the smoldering end off with a pair of scissors and let the end drop into water.

WHERE TO OBTAIN MOXA CIGARS:

Most Asian markets or Asian medical suppliers such as:
Lhasa-OMS
230 Libbey Parkway
Weymouth MA 02189
1-800-722-8775
1-781-340-1071
www.LhasaOMS.com

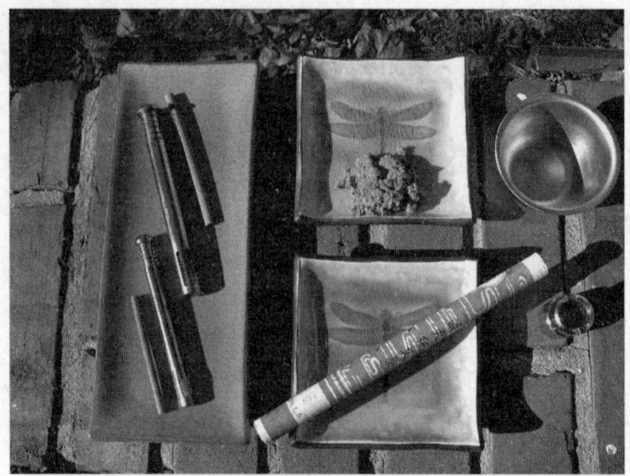

FIGURE 8-5 **Moxa supplies.**

lasting one to three days or longer. They are made of silver- or gold-plated aluminum or stainless steel and come mounted on a hypoallergenic adhesive plaster, such as surgical tape or Band-Aid tape. There may be one seed or pellet on the plaster or two or a cluster to stimulate a wider treatment area. Seed or pellet plasters can be applied after a Shiatsu session to prolong the effects of the treatment. They are also good self-help options when a particular ailment requires stimulation for a length of time or at a location that makes Shiatsu impracticable—for example, holding seeds or pellets in place on PC 6 to avert morning sickness during pregnancy or motion sickness during a car or boat ride. Most pharmacies now carry antinausea wristbands using seeds, pellets, magnets, or a combination thereof.

A Brief History of Magnet Therapy

Historically, many cultures have used magnets as a medical or experimental treatment regimen. Perhaps the earliest reference to magnet therapy occurs in the *Nei Jing*, which prescribes the application of lodestones, or natural magnets, to acupuncture points (Payne, 1997). Modern Eastern Europe, Russia, China, Korea, and Japan have all conducted extensive research on the therapeutic value of magnets (Null, 1998) and have incorporated magnet therapy into clinical practice and/or pursued it as a viable business enterprise. For example, in Japan the Ministry of Health officially recognizes the therapeutic value of magnets, which are routinely used by millions of Japanese in consumer products ranging from foot insoles to knee and wrist wraps to jewelry (Payne, 1997). Indeed, magnet therapy is Japan's twentieth largest industry.

Western Europe has followed suit with clinical research, but the United States still lags behind, primarily for ideological and economic reasons. Ever since the discovery of antibiotics to control infectious diseases, the study of medicine in the United States has been oriented toward biochemistry rather than biophysics, and drug therapies have been privileged over other interventions (Owen, 2000). As a practical result, pharmaceutical companies have dominated medical research and development through their funding imperatives. Naturally, their vested interest and economic incentive lie in promoting drug therapies, not alternative medical therapies like magnets (Owen, 2000). Nevertheless, public concern over the detrimental side effects of drug therapies and the clinical and economic success of certain patented electromagnetic inventions for the healing of bone fractures may indicate an eventual turn in medicine toward biophysics, or at least the mutual development of both medical disciplines.

MAGNETISM AND MAGNET THERAPY

No one completely understands what magnetism is. Suffice to say that it is a force that pulls or pushes, attracts or repels, and even twists materials susceptible to it (Payne, 1997). Magnetism occurs naturally during volcanic eruptions, when the electrons in molten metals, such as iron, cobalt, and nickel, are organized and aligned in the same direction as the earth's magnetic poles (Owen, 2000). Yet magnets can also be manufactured for consumer use. Commercial magnets are made of metals that support magnetism, such as iron, alloys of these metals, or compositions of these metals blended with other substances, such as iron and ceramic or iron and plastic.

Currently, there are two main forms of magnet therapy: permanent and intermittent. Permanent magnets are the previously mentioned synthetic version of lodestones found in nature, and intermittent electromagnetic devices are patented inventions. A **permanent magnet** emits a static magnetic field that provides constant magnetic stimulation, whereas a pulsing electromagnetic device emits a magnetic field whose direction alternates and whose concentration fluctuates, providing intermittent, varying electromagnetic stimulation (Null, 1998; Owen, 2000). The two therapies are similar, though not identical. At this point, **pulsing electromagnetic fields (PEMFs)** are the treatment of choice for healing acute injuries in which the integrity of the tissues is disrupted, such as bone fractures, while permanent magnets are suitable for mitigating chronic conditions in which the tissues are still intact but dysfunctional, such as joint pain and debility.

In a Shiatsu practice, permanent magnets can be incorporated into the session to enhance the treatment or applied after the session to prolong the life of the treatment. One way to incorporate magnet therapy into a session is to place a magnetic mattress pad on top of a futon and under a sheet for the client to rest on while receiving Shiatsu. The magnetic mattress pad will treat a large surface area—potentially the client's whole body if the client rotates during the session. This will augment the effects of Shiatsu.

To treat a smaller surface area, a magnetic pillow pad can be placed between a pillow and pillowcase or between a bolster and bolster cover or over the client's clothing—for example, on the lower back or abdomen while another area of the body is worked. No doubt some experimentally minded practitioners will want to apply Shiatsu through a magnetic pad; however, this is inadvisable for several reasons. The shape and mass of the magnets can make compression techniques uncomfortable, and the thickness and bulkiness of the pad can obscure navigation of the body's landmarks and sensitivity to De Qi.

Magnet therapy can be used after a session by giving the client a few magnets mounted on adhesive plasters to apply to key acupressure points for continued stimulation. Some permanent magnets feature a tiny protrusion in the center of the magnet that combines acupressure with magnetism. The client can wear these magnets for several days following the session. Once the adhesive plaster becomes worn or soiled, the magnet can be removed and remounted on a new plaster, which the client can purchase or the practitioner can provide at a future session. The client should be advised to discontinue use if any irritation or discomfort occurs.

MAGNET STRENGTH

Permanent magnets vary in strength, depending on several variables, especially their gauss rating and size: The higher the gauss rating and the larger the size, the stronger the magnet (Owen, 2000). The **gauss** rating is a measure of the strength of the magnet's attraction. Additionally, the distance between the magnet and the person affects its potency, since a magnet's power decreases with distance (Payne, 1997). Therapeutic magnets typically range in strength from 800 to 9,000 gauss, while the outer limit of therapeutic magnetic exposure is 20,000 gauss (Owen, 2000).

To put this in perspective, the magnetic field at the earth's surface ranges from 0.5 to 2 to 3 gauss (Owen, 2000); the average refrigerator magnet is about 50 to 100 gauss; a magnet of 500 gauss can lift a 2-pound iron weight; a magnet of 2,500 gauss can lift a 25-pound iron weight (Whitaker & Adderly, 1998); and a magnetic resonance imaging (MRI) diagnostic instrument, approved by the U.S. Food and Drug Administration (FDA), applies magnetic forces in the range of 650 to 15,000 gauss to the body (Payne, 1997).

Stronger magnets (2,500 gauss or more) should be used for shorter durations, such as the length of a Shiatsu session, while weaker magnets (800 gauss) may be held in place for several days and relocated as the pain shifts (Owen, 2000). Most research scientists, medical practitioners, and the World Health Organization agree that magnets in the therapeutic range of up to 20,000 gauss are safe (Owen, 2000; Whitaker & Adderly, 1998). This conclusion is drawn on the basis of research exploring the effects of short-term use of magnets. To date, no research has been conducted on the effects of long-term use of magnets, though many experts believe that the body adapts to magnetic input, rendering it ineffective after awhile, or that the body simply ignores magnetic input it does not need (Owen, 2000).

MAGNET SIDES

While most physicists believe there is little difference between the bionorth and biosouth sides of a magnet, most practitioners, especially acupuncturists, agree that the **bionorth** side (–) of the magnet calms and relaxes, retarding and inhibiting biological activity, whereas the **biosouth** side (+) stimulates and energizes, accelerating and promoting biological activity (Payne, 1997). In general, the bionorth side (–) is used to sedate Jitsu excess conditions, whereas the biosouth side (+) is used to tonify Kyo deficiency conditions. Both sides can be used alternately for balance, but in practice, the bionorth side (–) is more commonly applied, since it eases symptoms and reduces pain and inflammation. Some magnets are bipolar, containing alternating bionorth (–) and biosouth (+) polarities on the same side, but they do not penetrate as deeply and are therefore less effective than single-pole magnets for deep tissue pain, as in cases of lumbago or piriformis syndrome (Owen, 2000).

RESEARCH STUDIES ON PERMANENT MAGNETS

While abundant scientific research has been conducted in the United States on the efficacy of PEMFs, only a limited number of valid pilot studies—studies using less than 50 subjects—have been conducted on the benefits of permanent magnets. Nevertheless, these pilot studies were well designed and well executed by medical doctors, satisfying criteria of reliability including experiment replicability, placebo control, randomized sampling, double-blind participation of researchers and subjects, measurable results, and publication in a professional, peer-reviewed journal (Owen, 2000).

Though the research subjects in the pilot studies were seeking relief for specific disorders, such as diabetes, fibromyalgia, and postpolio symptoms, the study results may be applicable to those with similar problems arising from other causes. The Weintraub study (1991) demonstrated that magnets alleviate or eliminate numbness, burning, tingling, prickling, and sharp jolting sensations associated with nerve damage. The Baylor study (Vallbona, Hazelwood, & Jurida, 1997) demonstrated that magnets reduce pain in trigger points due to myofascial tension and degenerative arthritis, as well as in other parts of the body not directly stimulated by magnets. The Colbert study (Colbert, Markor, Benerji, & Pilla, 1999) demonstrated that magnets reduce site-specific pain, insomnia, and fatigue, leading to improved daily functioning, better sleep, and higher energy levels. And the Man study (Man, D., Man, B., & Plosker, 1999) demonstrated that magnets accelerate postsurgical recovery time, reduce postoperative ecchymosis (bruising) and edema, and diminish the need for postoperative analgesics. Additionally, none of the medical researchers reported any adverse side effects associated with magnet therapy.

These studies suggest that magnet therapy has a broad range of applications, including nerve pathology, chronic and acute muscle and joint pain, chronic fatigue and sleep disturbances, and recovery from injury and trauma. Despite the promising results of preliminary research, magnet therapy has yet to be approved by the FDA and embraced by the medical community; however, PEMFs have become the treatment of choice for healing bone fractures and for other osteopathic and orthopedic conditions (Owen, 2000).

MAGNET THEORIES

Although various theories have been advanced, currently no one can conclusively explain why magnet therapy works. Since a comprehensive survey of magnet theories is beyond the scope of this book, the interested reader is referred to *Pain-Free with Magnet Therapy* (2000) by Lara Owen, who has written a balanced overview on the subject. Those further interested in electromagnetic therapy may want to read *The Body Electric: Electromagnetism and the Foundation of Life* (1985) and *Cross Currents: The Perils of Electropollution, The Promise of Electromedicine* (1990), seminal works by Robert Becker, a medical doctor and pioneer in the field of energy medicine. More books may be found by contacting various distributors (see Appendix 4) or by using a search engine like Google (www.google.com) to search the World Wide Web.

MAGNET CONTRAINDICATIONS AND CAUTIONS

There are a few contraindications and cautions regarding magnets. As always, common sense should guide usage. If both sides of the magnet irritate or do nothing to improve the condition, discontinue its use. Magnets should not be applied near the heart of a person with a cardiac pacemaker or any other implanted electronic device, such as an insulin pump, as the magnets could interfere with its functioning (Null, 1998; Owen, 2000; Payne, 1997). Likewise, magnets should not be applied near the uterus of a pregnant woman, since the effects on the fetus are unknown as yet (Null, 1998; Owen, 2000; Payne, 1997). Magnets should not be applied to bleeding wounds, as magnets may interfere with the blood-clotting mechanism; nor should they be applied to infections or malignancies, since the biosouth pole could stimulate the growth of microbial pathogens and cancer cells (Null, 1998). There is some uncertainty about whether magnets are appropriate for persons prone to epileptic seizures. Some sources recommend exercising caution, since such persons can be sensitive, while others recommend magnet therapy, since low-level PEMFs have proven helpful in reducing seizures (Owen, 2000). Finally, as a practical precaution, magnets should not be placed near credit cards, magnetic recording tapes, compact discs, watches, or any other sensitive magnetic device that could be damaged by such exposure.

GUA SHA

Gua Sha, also spelled *guasha* or *gwasha*, is a skin-scraping technique used extensively in China in both clinical and nonclinical settings. Although formerly part of the erudite medical tradition, Gua Sha has subsequently filtered down into every stratum of society through a mainstreaming process called medical sedimentation and is now practiced in the home (McCollum, 2003). Its popularity as a folk remedy, however, does not negate its efficacy as a treatment. The mainstreaming of Gua Sha in China suggests that it is economical, practical, and beneficial to many.

Gua means to scrape, rub, scratch, or apply friction at the surface (McCollum, 2003; Nielsen, 2002). Sha refers to the pathogenic agent and its manifestation on the body's surface when expelled (McCollum, 2003). According to TCM, Sha is both the pernicious evil trapped in the body and the petechiae—the raspberry rash-like blotches—that surface during scraping. Gua, or scraping, draws up and releases Sha, the deleterious agent that is embedded in the tissues, resulting in Sha, what appears like a reddish skin abrasion that lingers for a few days.

GUA SHA LUBRICANTS AND INSTRUMENTS

As a healing modality, Gua Sha is simple, relatively easy to perform, and effective—hence, its popularity. The skin is first lubricated with saltwater, oil, or a liniment, lotion, or salve. In China, peanut oil is preferred, but in the West, Tiger Balm and Vicks® VapoRub® or their generic versions are preferred. Vicks is particularly good for Heat conditions, since the active ingredients in it—camphor, menthol, and eucalyptus—are cooling, whereas extra-strength Tiger Balm is good for Cold conditions, since the clove in it is warming (Esher, 2001b, Unraveling the lower back pain puzzle). In practice, any liniment, balm, or lotion, and especially one that treats the presenting condition—whether respiratory congestion, muscular soreness, or aches and pains in the joint—can be applied topically. Quality liniments and balms usually contain essential oils with antiseptic, analgesic, and rubefacient properties that promote the circulation of blood, lymph, and Qi; promote tissue regeneration; reduce pain; improve mobility; and disinfect.

After the skin is lubricated, it is held taut and pressed and scraped with a tool. Any tool that has a smooth, rounded lip-like edge that does not grate or gouge the recipient can be used for scraping. In China, popular tools include a slice of polished water buffalo horn, a plastic soup spoon resembling a miniature ladle, and the edge of a coin or jar lid (Nielsen, 2002). In the West, a Tiger Balm jar lid is commonly used, though some practitioners prefer a Chinese soup spoon, available at any Asian market. The lid of a Vicks VapoRub jar is unsuitable, though, because the edge is too sharp and rough. (see Figure 8-6.)

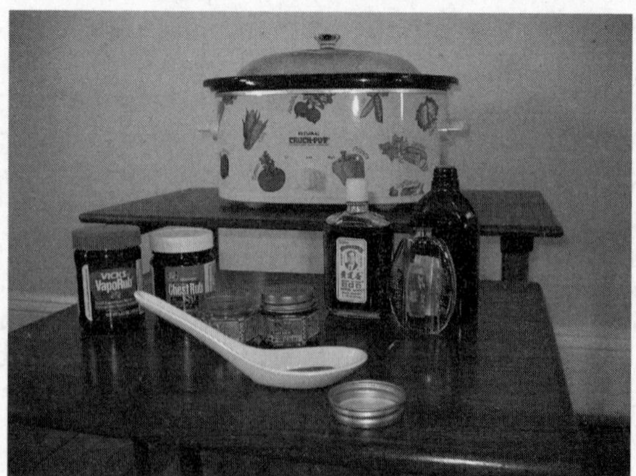

FIGURE 8-6 Gua Sha supplies and tools. Supplies include Vicks VapoRub (or a generic version) or Tiger, Eagle, or some other brand-name balm. Scraping tools include a Chinese soup spoon and Tiger Balm lid. The crock pot is soaking a hot towel to conclude treatment.

In addition to scraping, the skin can be pinched between the fingers (Tsien Sha) or slapped (Pak Sha), but these techniques are less common (McCollum, 2003). Areas that are commonly scraped include the sides and back of the neck, the back, the hips, and the upper chest. In general, the technique is performed in overlapping swaths, moving in a downward and outward direction to expel pathogenic agents.

GUA SHA USES AND INDICATIONS

Gua Sha is a versatile therapy that treats a number of disorders, including seasonal illnesses. It is useful around the turn of a season when people typically get ill or any time a cold or influenza epidemic occurs. Gua Sha expels Pernicious Influences—deleterious environmental agents like Wind, Cold, Heat, and Damp that block Qi flow and manifest in the body as chilliness, fever, systemic malaise, distension, achiness, and stiffness of the limbs. Traditionally, scraping is applied at the onset of an illness like a cold to prevent the illness from settling in the body or to prevent it from transmogrifying into something far worse, like a flu, bronchitis, or pneumonia. If the illness has already taken hold and embedded itself, Gua Sha can be applied to purge pathogens and expedite recovery time. Applying Gua Sha at the first sign or inkling of illness can ward off the illness, leaving the client feeling normal the next day, while applying it during an illness can reduce the length and severity of the illness (McCollum, 2003).

Because the Asian tradition of working on sick clients contravenes a Western contraindication against infectious illness, the practitioner should exercise caution and good judgment. To avoid contracting the illness, the practitioner should feel healthy and abstain from working on the client during the acute, contagious phase of the illness, when the client first begins to manifest dramatic symptoms such as sneezing and coughing. Other precautions can be taken, if desired—ventilating the room; spraying the room with an airborne mister that contains eucalyptus; wearing a facial mask; and disinfecting the hands, doorknobs, light switches, and any other contact surfaces after treatment.

With respect to thermal imbalances, Gua Sha is an adaptogenic therapy: The treatment conforms to the client's particular need (Nielsen, 2002). Hence, Gua Sha can cool a client who feels hot and warm a client who feels cold. As an exterior releasing technique, Gua Sha is especially effective in dispelling excess Heat and dissipating fullness. Heat usually manifests as flushed red skin, a palpable emanation of radiant heat from the body, and an uncomfortable sensation of heat within the body. Sometimes a client may not present obvious signs of Heat, but when Gua Sha is applied, the petechiae will appear very red, indicating the release of Heat. Fullness manifests as an uncomfortable internal pressure and surface distension, usually from a buildup and stasis of fluid. An example is premenstrual bloating.

Gua Sha can also be applied to sore, aching muscles after strenuous or unaccustomed physical exercise or manual labor. Gua Sha disperses the congestion of stagnant fluids in the tissues and dislodges and discharges waste products—metabolic acids and the debris of microtrauma—that are encapsulated in muscles. Gua Sha raises these agents—stagnant fluids, acids, and bio-debris—to the surface membrane, where they are released through the pores or where the extensive network of capillaries flushes them away (Belko, 1993). This relieves soreness, achiness, stiffness, and debility.

To review, those who can benefit from Gua Sha are clients who feel as if they are on the verge of an illness or who have had trouble overcoming a lingering illness, those who present signs of Heat or fullness, and those who feel sore, stiff, and fatigued from exertion. In fact, any client who shows signs of Sha during diagnostic palpation is a good candidate for Gua Sha. The diagnostic procedure for Sha is fairly straightforward. To determine the presence of Sha, the practitioner palpates the general area of complaint and locates any specific constriction and tenderness.

The practitioner then presses the client's flesh with the fingertips and removes them quickly. If the fingertip pressure leaves pale, almond-shaped after-images of the fingertips that are slow to fade, there is Sha and blood stagnation, and Gua Sha is indicated. This assessment procedure is called **press and blanch** (Nielson, Guetersloh, & Verlag fuer Ganzheitliche Medizin, 2002).

GUA SHA THEORIES

Two main theories explain the effectiveness of Gua Sha. TCM theory recognizes that the interior and exterior of the body are interrelated and that the fluid movement of vital substances is necessary for health. According to TCM, Gua Sha is a dynamic, exterior releasing technique that propels Qi, blood, and fluids, especially where they are sluggish or stuck, thereby positively influencing internal organ function (Nielsen, Guetersloh, & Verlag fuer Ganzheitliche Medizin, 2002). Gua Sha also expels pathogens hovering in the surface layer, preventing them from descending into and embedding in the deeper tissues of the body.

Western theory also recognizes that the interior and exterior of the body are connected, albeit through the contiguous system of connective tissue in the body rather than through Qi or vital substances (Nielsen, Guetersloh, & Verlag fuer Ganzheitliche Medizin, 2002). By pressing into the subcutaneous fascia, the practitioner irrigates the tissues with blood, promoting normal cell respiration—nutrient delivery and waste removal—at both superficial and deeper levels of the body.

OBTAINING INFORMED CONSENT

The only unpleasant side effect of Gua Sha is cosmetic in nature, albeit superficial and transient. Scraping leaves painless but conspicuous **petechiae**—raised, reddish speckles of encapsulated acids on the skin—which look a bit like road rash or a constellation of hickeys (Nielsen, Guetersloh, & Verlag fuer Ganzheitliche Medizin, 2002). The discoloration usually disappears within two to four days, but if vigorous scraping is done or the recipient has sluggish circulation, it could take longer to resolve. Consequently, the Shiatsu practitioner should always obtain the client's informed consent before performing Gua Sha, especially if the client is concerned about appearance. However, it is best to emphasize the benefits and not dramatize the temporary blemishing that occurs.

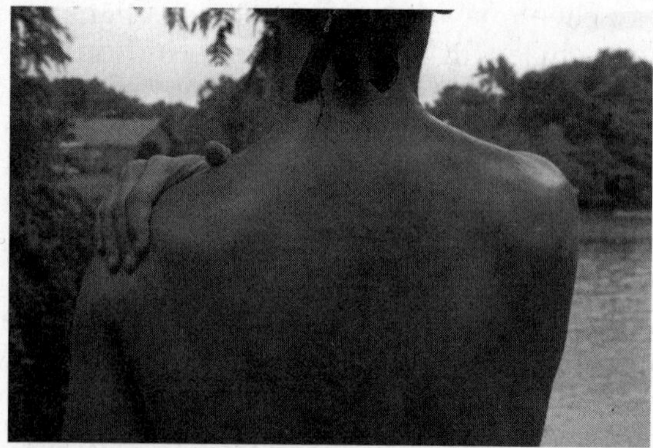

FIGURE 8-7 Petechiae.
Scraping extravasates blood, leaving painless patches of red speckles that look a bit like road rash. The marring is temporary and fades in a few days, but it is one reason to obtain informed consent prior to commencing treatment. (See Color Plate 4.)

GUA SHA PROTOCOL AND TECHNIQUES

To perform Gua Sha, the practitioner positions the client so that the area to be treated is exposed and easily accessible and the muscles are in a relatively neutral position conducive to relaxation—neither taut from stretching nor tense from contracting (Nielsen, Guetersloh, & Verlag fuer Ganzheitliche Medizin, 2002). If, for example, the client is seated, the head should be tilted slightly forward in flexion to expose the neck area, but not too far forward, since holding the weight of the head against gravity could pull and strain the posterior muscles of the neck. To work the area between the shoulder blades while the client is seated, the practitioner should direct the client to cross the arm over the chest, and hold the opposite shoulder; this position opens the interscapular border. Gua Sha can, of course, be done in any recumbent position as well.

The practitioner begins above the site of complaint and ends below it, working downward toward the feet and outward toward the extremities in overlapping longitudinal swaths; the downward and outward direction facilitates the expulsion of pathogens trapped in the body (McCollum, 2003). For example, to scrape the upper back the practitioner starts at the base of the neck on the midline of the body on the Governing Vessel, moves laterally 1.5 cun to the inner Bladder Meridian, moves laterally another 1.5 cun (3 cun total) to the outer Bladder Meridian, and then moves over the shoulder and down the arms as necessary. A good releasing point for the shoulder is Bl 43. To scrape the lower back and hips, the practitioner starts at the midback and scrapes downward over the lower back and sacrum, outward over the hips, and down, the legs as necessary. A good releasing point for the lower back is Bl 23; for the hips, the point is GB 30.

To ward off an impending illness like a cold or flu, the practitioner should include points that boost the immune function and resistance, such as Bl 12, Bl 13 (the Lung Shu point), Bl 14 (the Pericardium Shu point), Bl 15 (the Heart Shu point), Lu 1 (the Lung Mu point), Ki 27, and CV 17 (the Pericardium Mu point).

The scraping tool should be angled close to the flesh, raised only 10 to 15 degrees above the surface, with just enough space to permit the practitioner's fingers to wrap underneath the tool to hold it (Figure 8-8) (Nielsen, Guetersloh, & Verlag fuer Ganzheitliche Medizin, 2002). The practitioner's fingers or thumb should be in constant contact with the client's skin during the stroke so that the client feels the practitioner's hand initiating and leading the stroke, while the tool follows. Pressure should be applied firmly into the fascia rather than superficially on the skin.

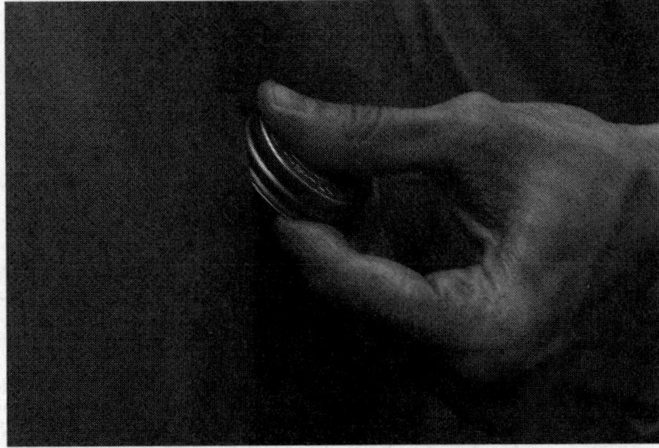

FIGURE 8-8 **Angle of scraping tool.** The scraping tool is angled close to the flesh—at about 15 degrees—allowing enough space to permit the fingers to wrap underneath the tool to guide the stroke.

A single stroke is applied only in a unilateral direction and never as a return stroke or backstroke; rather, the tool is lifted and reset. Strokes should be 4 to 6 inches in length and repeated 7 to 11 times in overlapping swaths until the Sha surfaces or the area begins to sting (Nielsen, Guetersloh, & Verlag fuer Ganzheitliche Medizin, 2002). Only then should the practitioner move to the next parallel swath.

CHASING THE DRAGON

Although the client's complaint and the press and blanch assessment will suggest a general treatment plan, the practitioner should strive to tailor the Gua Sha session, using the client's ongoing feedback about the shifting path of the pain. This means following the pain where it migrates. For example, what initially begins as lumbago may turn into hip pain after the low back has been scraped and the pain in the low back has diminished or disappeared. Custom-designing the Gua Sha treatment to pursue the path of the pain is called **chasing the dragon** in China (Nielson, Guetersloh, & Verlag fuer Ganzheitliche Medizin, 2002). After scraping an area, the practitioner should palpate it again to verify and confirm a change in the tissues. After Gua Sha, palpation should feel pleasant, not irritating or painful, to the client. In other words, any previous tenderness or sensitivity in the tissues should be reduced or resolved.

GUA SHA CONTRAINDICATIONS

Contraindications to Gua Sha are any abnormal skin condition, including contusions, abrasions, lacerations, scabs, open wounds or sores, burns, rashes, pimples, moles, and skin tags (McCollum, 2003; Nielsen, Guetersloh, & Verlag fuer Ganzheitliche Medizin, 2002). The practitioner should work around any pimples, moles, or skin tags, covering them with a finger to avoid inadvertently severing them with the scraping tool. If the entire back or other prospective scraping area is covered with pimples, moles, or skin tags, Gua Sha is contraindicated. If the client is on blood-thinning medication, caution should be exercised; the practitioner should treat a limited area and assess the client's reaction before proceeding further (Nielsen, Guetersloh, & Verlag fuer Ganzheitliche Medizin, 2002). Gua Sha should not be performed on the abdomen of a pregnant woman; however, it may be performed on the woman's lower back, sacrum, and hips, even during delivery. Finally, Gua Sha should not be performed more than once every two weeks.

SIGNIFICANCE OF SHA APPEARANCE

The color and form of the Sha, as well as the speed with which it surfaces, are diagnostic signs (Nielsen, Guetersloh, & Verlag fuer Ganzheitliche Medizin, 2002). Sha that is difficult to raise, requiring a high number of strokes, indicates deep or longstanding blood stagnation. Red Sha, especially very red Sha, indicates excess Heat (Figure 8-9). Quite likely, the client's skin will turn lobster red from palpation during assessment, even before Gua Sha is performed. Very dark or brown Sha indicates Heat and a deficiency of Yin in the blood. This kind of Sha may be found in athletes who regularly engage in prolonged, strenuous Yang activities and who have to maintain a low body weight, such as marathon runners and cyclists. Blue or purple Sha indicates long-term blood stagnation. Small or pale Sha indicates a blood deficiency. Such Sha may be found in thin or vegan clients whose diets may render them slightly malnourished.

ENDING A GUA SHA SESSION

A pleasant, optional way to end a Gua Sha session is to soak a towel in hot water with or without ground ginger root and apply it as a hot compress on the area that has been scraped (Figures 8-10 through 8-12) (McCollum, 2003). As soon as the towel

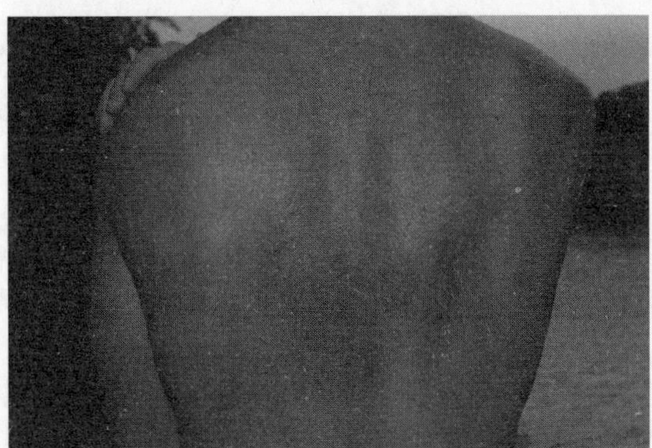

FIGURE 8-9 Color of Sha as a diagnostic sign. This model's Sha is quite red, indicating Heat. (See Color Plate 4.)

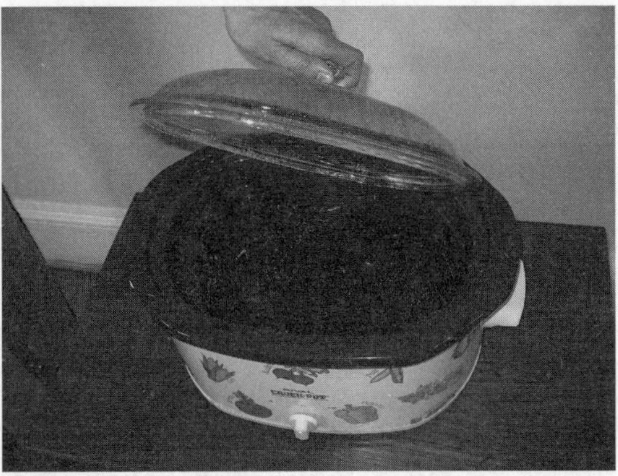

FIGURE 8-10 Towel soaking in hot water inside a crock pot.

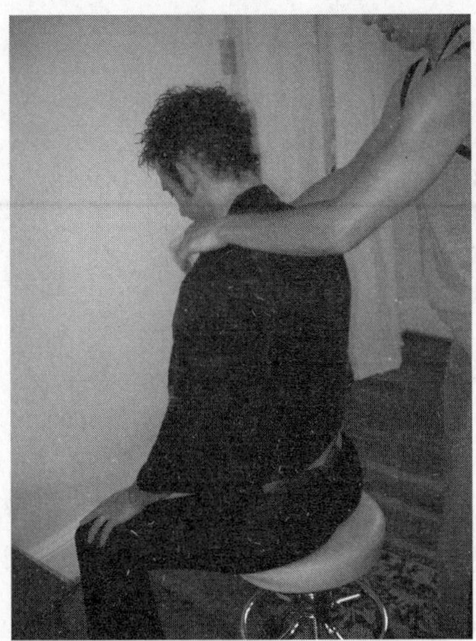

FIGURE 8-11 Drape steaming towel. A pleasant but optional way to conclude Gua Sha is to soak and heat a towel in a crock pot, wring it out, and drape it over the client while it is still billowing steam.

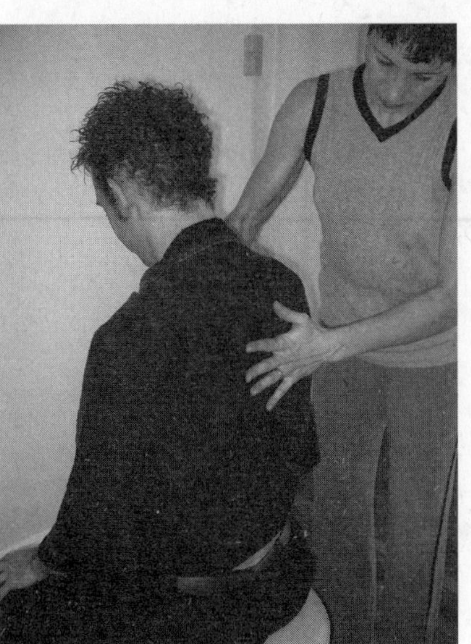

FIGURE 8-12 Pat down. The moist, hot towel can also be used to wipe off any residual balm. Once the towel begins to cool, remove it promptly and direct the client to dress immediately.

begins to cool, it should be removed, and any residual moisture or salve should be wiped off with a dry towel to prevent the client's clothes from being stained. The client should immediately dress and cover the scraped area, especially in cold weather, taking care not to expose the area to Cold, since the pores are still open.

In the days following Gua Sha, the client should practice moderation in all things: "no drugs, booze, sex, fasting or feasting, and no hard labor" (Nielson, Guetersloh, & Verlag fuer Ganzheitliche Medizin, 2002). The client should wear a shirt to bed at night until the Sha fades. As a courtesy and professional service, the practitioner may want to prepare an information sheet on Gua Sha for the client to share with family members, friends, or other health practitioners (see Exhibit 8-2).

GUA SHA HANDOUT FOR CLIENTS

[Practitioner Name]
[Practitioner Contact Information]
Gua Sha is a therapeutic technique widely practiced in China. The word *Gua* means to scratch, scrape, rub, or apply friction at the surface. *Sha* refers to any deleterious agent, such as heat, metabolic wastes or irritants, or pathogens that are embedded and entrapped in the tissues and that are raised to the surface and released by scraping. Thus, Gua Sha is a form of therapeutic abrasion or extraction that draws deleterious agents to the superficial skin layer, where they can be released through the pores or where the rich capillary bed can flush them away.

Gua Sha, or scraping, is painless but results in temporary petechiae, clusters of tiny reddish bumps that resemble a patch of hickeys or road rash. With normal circulation, the petechiae fade in two to three days.

Gua Sha has many benefits. It promotes blood and fluid flow in areas of stagnation, enhancing cell respiration—the uptake of oxygen and nutrients and the discharge of wastes. It relieves soreness, reduces pain, and increases mobility. It cools overheated tissues and warms cold tissues. It can even ward off the onset of a cold or expedite recovery.

On the day of Gua Sha, you should not engage in strenuous exercise; however, light exercise and stretching are fine.

Following Gua Sha, while the pores are still open, you are advised to immediately and thoroughly cover the area, avoiding exposure to any inclement or extreme weather, especially cold wind, cold dampness, or heat. Wearing a T-shirt to bed for a few days is recommended. In the days following Gua Sha, you should practice moderation in all things, avoiding overindulgence or deficiency in food, drink, and physical exertion.

This will educate the client and others about the benefits of Gua Sha and hopefully obviate concern about the temporary appearance of petechiae.

Usually, the client's condition will improve immediately, but sometimes it will worsen slightly before getting better. If the press and blanch assessment technique reveals evidence of Sha again after a week, most likely the client is engaging in behaviors that compromise the Wei Qi or defensive armor (Nielsen, Guetersloh, & Verlag fuer Ganzheitliche Medizin, 2002), and lasting change will come only through lifestyle reform.

REFERENCES

Academic American Encyclopedia (vol. 12). (1981). "Kinetic Theory of Matter." Princeton, NJ: Arete.

Belko, K. R. (1993, October). Sports acupuncture. *Muscle & Fitness*, 87–89, 200–203.

Beresford-Cooke, C. (2000). *Shiatsu theory and practice: A comprehensive text for the student and professional*. Edinburgh: Churchile Livingstone.

Colbert, A. P., Markov, M. S., Benerji, M., & Pilla, A. A. (1999). Magnetic mattress pad use in patients with fibromyalgia: A randomized double-blind pilot study. *Journal of Back & Musculoskeletal Rehabilitation, 13*, 19–31.

Cooney, J. (2000, December). Magnets as health care: Some observations and pointers. *Bloomingnews*.

Esher, B. (2001a). Asian healing arts: Depression and the Five Elements, part 2. *Massage Today, 1*(5), 15, 21.

Esher, B. (2001b). Asian healing arts: Unraveling the lower back pain puzzle. *Massage Today, 1*(10), 14, 20.

Esher, B. (2003). Asian healing arts: Yin and Yang deficiency, part VI. *Massage Today, 3*(3), 18–19, 22.

Man, D., Man, B., & Plosker, H. (1999). The influence of permanent magnetic field therapy on wound healing in suction lipectomy patients: A double-blind study. *Journal of Plastic & Reconstructive Surgery,* 104(7):2261–8.

McCollum, H. (2003, May 31). Lecture. Gua Sha workshop conducted at the Cayce/Reilly School of Massotherapy in Virginia Beach, Virginia.

Nielsen, A. (Director), Guetersloh, M. (Producer), & Verlag fuer Ganzheitliche Medizin (Producer). (2002). *Gua Sha—Step by step—A visual guide to a traditional technique for modern practice.* [Videocassette].

Null, G. (1998). *Healing with magnets*. New York: Carroll & Graf.

Owen, L. (2000). *Pain-free with magnet therapy*. Roseville, CA: Prima Health.

Payne, B. (1997). *Magnetic healing: Advanced techniques for the application of magnetic forces*. Twin Lakes, WI: Lotus Press.

Serizawa, K. (2000). *Tsubo: Vital points for oriental therapy*. Tokyo: Japan Publications. (Original work published 1976.)

Vallbona, C., Hazelwood, C. F., & Jurida, G. (1997). Response of pain to static magnetic fields in post-polio patients: A double blind pilot study. *Archives of Physical Medicine & Rehabilitation, 78*, 1200–1203.

Weintraub, M. (1991). Magnetic bio-stimulation in painful diabetic peripheral neuropathy: A novel intervention—A randomized, double-placebo crossover study. *American Journal of Pain Management, 9*, 8–17.

Whitaker, J., & Adderly, B. (1998). *The pain relief breakthrough: The power of magnets*. Boston: Little, Brown.

Williams, T. (1996). *The complete illustrated guide to Chinese medicine: A comprehensive system for health and fitness*. Shaftesbury, England: Element Books.

Yamamoto, S., & McCarty, P. (1993). *Whole health Shiatsu: Health and vitality for everyone*. Tokyo: Japan Publications.

STUDY QUESTIONS

1. What is moxabustion?
2. For what general conditions is moxa indicated?
3. For what general conditions is moxa contraindicated?
4. What physical effects does moxa stimulate?
5. In what way is moxa more than just a heat therapy?
6. Describe the direct or scarring method of applying moxa.
7. Is blistering or scarring done in the West?

8. Give a few examples of bases that are placed between the client and the moxa.

9. Describe the indirect method of applying moxa.

10. Aside from verbal feedback, how else can a practitioner gauge when the moxa gets too hot for the client?

11. Why is ventilation important when using moxa?

12. What risk does moxa entail?

13. Is there an alternative to performing moxa on a client?

14. Why is moxa suitable for self-administration?

15. What areas of the body are especially accessible to self-administration?

16. What do seeds and pellets do?

17. How can seeds and pellets be incorporated into a Shiatsu practice?

18. How can magnets be incorporated into a Shiatsu practice?

19. How long should one apply stronger magnets (those in excess of 2,500 gauss)?

20. How long should one apply weaker magnets?

21. What effect does the bionorth side (–) of a magnet have, and for what conditions is bionorth indicated?

22. What effect does the biosouth side (+) of a magnet have, and for what conditions is biosouth indicated?

23. What is Gua Sha?

24. The word *Sha* has two meanings. Define *Sha*.

25. Identify a few lubricants that can be topically applied for Gua Sha.

26. For what condition is Vicks® VapoRub® suitable?

27. For what condition is Tiger Balm suitable?

28. In the West, what instruments are used to scrape?

29. For what purpose is Gua Sha traditionally used?

30. What other conditions are indicated for Gua Sha?

31. What does the term *adaptogenic* mean with respect to Gua Sha?

32. Explain how Gua Sha works from a TCM perspective.

33. Explain how Gua Sha works from a Western perspective.

34. Why is it important to get the client's informed consent before performing Gua Sha?

35. How long do the petechiae typically last?

36. Describe the diagnostic procedure for determining the presence of Sha.

37. Give instructions on scraping technique (angle of instrument, depth of pressure, direction of stroke, length of stroke, repetitions of stroke).

38. What areas of the body should one Gua Sha for frozen shoulder?

39. What areas of the body should one Gua Sha for hip pain?

40. What is the significance of the treatment approach called chasing the dragon?

41. Identify some contraindications to Gua Sha.

42. How should one proceed with pimples, moles, and skin tags?

43. How often can Gua Sha be done?

44. What is the diagnostic significance of the color of Sha (red, brown/dark, blue/purple, light)?

45. Why should the client immediately cover up after Gua Sha?

46. What post-treatment advice should one give the client?

47. If the client's Sha returns soon after treatment, what does that suggest about the client's lifestyle?

48. What special properties do liniments have?

49. For what conditions are liniments beneficial?

COMPLEMENTARY HEALING MODALITIES TEST (45 POINTS)

MATCHING. FOR SOME QUESTIONS, MORE THAN ONE ANSWER IS CORRECT.

A. Moxabustion
B. Seeds and pellets
C. Magnets
D. Gua Sha
E. Liniments and balms

____**1.** Topical essential oil therapy.

____**2.** Herbal heat therapy.

____**3.** Acupressure therapy.

____4. Abrasion therapy.

____5. Therapeutic force that attracts or repels.

____6. Folk remedy.

____7. Antiseptic and analgesic properties.

____8. Active ingredients include menthol and camphor.

____9. Wards off seasonal illnesses.

____10. Prolongs acupressure at home and work.

____11. Dissipates Heat and fullness.

____12. Warms Cold and evaporates Dampness.

____13. Discharges metabolic waste products.

____14. Mobilizes sluggish blood, lymph, and Qi.

____15. Stimulates Qi flow at home and work (prolonged administration).

____16. Boosts immune response and alkalizes blood.

____17. Soothes aches, pains, strains, and sprains.

____18. Contraindicated for Heat conditions.

____19. Contraindicated by pimples, moles, and abnormal skin conditions.

____20. Contraindicated near cardiac pacemakers, insulin pumps, and other similar implants.

TRUE OR FALSE. CIRCLE THE CORRECT ANSWER.

True False 21. Moxabustion is one of the four classical healing modalities of TCM.

True False 22. The herb used for moxa is a member of the hemp family.

True False 23. Moxa is good for weakness and tiredness.

True False 24. When using moxa punk, follow the ancient texts with regard to blistering and scarring.

True False 25. When using a moxa cylinder, hold it steadily over the point until the client says, "Ouch."

True False 26. In practice, the bionorth side (–) of a magnet is used more than the biosouth side (+) because it eases symptoms and reduces pain.

True False 27. Place the biosouth side (+) on an area that is tense and spastic.

True False **28.** Place the bionorth side (–) on a malignant tumor to retard its growth.

True False **29.** Place the biosouth side (+) on the abdomen of a pregnant woman to stimulate the growth of the fetus.

True False **30.** Weaker magnets can be left on for days, whereas stronger magnets (in the range of 2,500 to 9,000 gauss) should be applied only for a short period of time.

True False **31.** A magnet of sufficient polarity can induce heart muscle contraction and can therefore be used to reinforce a cardiac pacemaker.

True False **32.** In TCM, Sha refers to pathogenic agents embedded in the body.

True False **33.** To determine the presence of Sha, press the flesh and quickly remove your fingers; a red after-image of your fingers that is slow to fade indicates the presence of Sha.

True False **34.** Gua Sha strokes are performed inward toward the midline and upward toward the head.

True False **35.** To raise the Sha more thoroughly and quickly, apply pressure on the backstroke as you return the instrument to its starting position.

True False **36.** Chasing the dragon, means repeating the strokes a few more times on an area once it begins to sting.

True False **37.** Gua Sha lightly over a bruise to expedite tissue regeneration.

True False **38.** After Gua Sha, the client can engage in strenuous exercise or relax with a few beers if he wants.

True False **39.** To release stubborn Sha that is difficult to raise, repeat the treatment three days in a row, if necessary.

SHORT ANSWER/CASE STUDIES

40. Your client has sore muscles from weightlifting. She mentioned that she is going to attend a cocktail party tonight and is planning to wear a low-cut evening dress; tomorrow she is going to the beach and plans to wear a bikini. Would you Gua Sha? Why or why not? (1 point)

____

____

41. Your client's arthritis has gotten worse recently because of the cold, damp weather. The massage therapy room is an enclosed space without windows. Would you moxa? Why or why not? (1 point)

____

____

42. Your client is going on a boat ride but is concerned about getting seasick. What complementary healing modality would you recommend that could prevent or mitigate her seasickness? (1 point)

____

____

43. Your client recently ordered a 9,000 gauss magnet. He has pain in his right hip from tense gluteal muscles, so he plans to wear the adhesive magnet with the biosouth side (+) facing his buttocks for about a week. What advice would you give him? (3 points)

____

____

9

PRACTICE PRELIMINARIES

OBJECTIVES

- To observe contraindications and cautions for Shiatsu
- To modify Shiatsu for special populations, such as cancer patients, the elderly, and pregnant women
- To advise clients how to maximize their Shiatsu experience and how to ameliorate a healing crisis
- To use proper body mechanics and principles of compression
- To position and prop the client with pillows and bolsters to maximize comfort

KEY TERMS

Contraindications	Seiza	Prone
Local	Hara	Supine
Systemic	Two-Hand Connectedness	
Healing Response/Healing Crisis	Mother/Son Hand Technique	

Before launching into Shiatsu practice, some preliminaries must be covered, including contraindications and cautions, modifications for the elderly and pregnant women, helpful information to give first-time clients, principles of proper body mechanics and the application of pressure, tips on specific techniques, and client positions.

CONTRAINDICATIONS

A **contraindication** is any condition for which Shiatsu is inappropriate, usually because manual manipulation could aggravate the condition or because the condition poses a health hazard. If the condition is **local**, or isolated to a limited area of the body, the contraindication may be partial, and Shiatsu is restricted only as to that specific site. However, if the condition is **systemic**, or widespread, and affects the whole body, the contraindication may be total, and Shiatsu is avoided altogether. Most contraindications follow commonsense guidelines and public health policies. Abiding by contraindications not only protects the practitioner's health and the public health, but also reduces the likelihood of malpractice liability lawsuits.

In general, Shiatsu should not be given in cases of acute, infectious or contagious illness, whether the client's or the practitioner's. This includes colds, flus, bronchitis, strep throat, and all communicable illnesses, especially in their contagious stage, which is usually at the onset of the illness.

One exception to this general rule is the application of Gua Sha for the specific purpose of preventing a cold or flu or expediting recovery from a lingering cold or flu (see Chapter 8: Gua Sha Uses and Indications). If the practitioner owns a private massage practice or works on friends and family in a home setting, this specific application is the prerogative of the practitioner, who assumes the risk of exposure. On the other hand, if the practitioner works at a business belonging to another person, such as a spa, salon, clinic, or gym, the business owner has discretion on assumption of risk. In such case, the practitioner and business owner should agree in advance on the use of Gua Sha for prevention or recovery, and necessary precautions should be taken to reduce the chance of spreading an illness. The best time to administer Gua Sha to prevent an illness from lodging in the body is when the client starts to feel worn down, but before overt symptoms like coughing, sneezing, sore throat, nasal congestion or drainage, headache, fever and chills manifest.

SKIN DISORDERS

Non-contagious skin disorders and minor skin injuries are usually a partial rather than a total contraindication. In most cases, the practitioner can work around the isolated site of the skin problem, as for example, a laceration, abrasion, burn, scab, or other wound, or a patch of acne, eczema, or psoriasis.

Because the client customarily wears clothing during a Shiatsu session, Shiatsu can be administered without direct skin-to-skin contact. The lack of direct skin contact gives the Shiatsu practitioner greater latitude than a massage practitioner in choosing whether or not to work on a client who has certain contagious skin conditions. For instance, the practitioner can still administer Shiatsu to a client who has a case of poison ivy, poison oak, or athlete's foot, as long as treatment is given through clean clothing and socks and direct skin-to-skin contact is avoided (Chow, 2002). Poison ivy and poison oak are types of contact dermatitis (skin inflammation) caused by an allergic reaction following exposure to the offending substance, while athlete's foot is caused by a fungus.

Other conditions that are more widespread or suspicious-looking may require medical guidance. In the absence of medical guidance, the practitioner should exercise his or her own best judgment, and in doubtful cases, err on the side of caution. Skin infections, such as impetigo, are absolutely contraindicated. Skin infections can be identified by symptoms such as blisters, eruptions, discharges, ulcerations, and encrustations.

Gua Sha has broader contraindications for skin conditions than Shiatsu because it requires direct contact on non-breached, non-problematic skin (see Chapter 8: Gua Sha Contraindications). Obviously, the practitioner should not apply Gua Sha on rashes or wounds. Further, certain skin conditions such as widespread pimples or moles, which are not contraindicated for Shiatsu, are contraindicated for Gua Sha because of the potential for rupturing or severing the skin.

SOFT TISSUE AND BONE INJURIES AND OTHER ANOMALIES

Soft tissue injuries are usually a local contraindication. The practitioner should not give Shiatsu on the site of a soft tissue injury, such as a muscle strain or joint (ligament) sprain, especially during the acute inflammatory phase of the injury, but may work around the area to facilitate blood, lymph, and energy flow and to promote the body's own regenerative power. The inflammatory response, which lasts between 24 and 72 hours, can be identified by the presence of redness, heat, swelling, pain, and debility of the affected tissues. Other soft tissue contraindications include contusions (bruises), sensitive scars, and abnormal lumps of any kind, including cysts, lipomas, and tumors. Additionally, in cases of hernia—the bulging protrusion of an organ through its containing wall—the hernia should not be pressed, and stretches that flex or extend the spine should be avoided (Chow, 2002).

Bone injuries, such as fractures and dislocations, are another local contraindication. A fracture occurs when a bone cracks, breaks, or shatters, and a dislocation occurs when two or more contiguous bones that constitute a joint are misaligned or disconnected. The practitioner should not perform Shiatsu on bone injuries, although he or she may work on the uninjured opposite side of the body to stimulate a reflexive healing response.

CARDIOVASCULAR DISORDERS AND DISEASES

Cardiovascular disorders and diseases require partial or total abstention, depending on the nature and scope of the problem. Although Shiatsu does not stimulate circulation as much as modalities like Swedish and deep tissue massage, it still enhances blood flow and could therefore be hazardous to a client with a circulatory disorder. Consequently, Shiatsu should not be given to a client who has a serious cardiovascular disease, such as hemophilia. Hemophilia is a rather rare disease, usually affecting only men, in which the blood coagulating mechanism is impaired (Chow, 2002). On a hemophiliac, Shiatsu could induce hemorrhaging.

Other systemic cardiovascular diseases are more common, and the presence of certain predisposing factors requires a conservative approach to Shiatsu. Predisposing factors include stress, a sedentary lifestyle, a diet high in cholesterol, an overweight or obese body type, smoker status, male gender, and age over 40, especially when conditions that are precursors to heart attacks—such as arteriosclerosis, hardening of the arteries, and angina pectoris, heart disease—have been diagnosed. In such case, the practitioner should generally avoid ischemic compression—deep, static pressure—and specifically avoid pressing on the main arteries of the body: the carotid artery of the neck, the brachial arteries of the armpits, the aorta of the abdomen, and the femoral arteries of the legs (Chow, 2002). A complication that may accompany arteriosclerosis is an abdominal aortic aneurysm, a blood-filled bulge in the wall of the main artery. Ampuku (abdominal massage) is contraindicated, and especially pressure on the midline of the abdomen above and below the navel, an area that overlies the route of the aorta.

Local cardiovascular disorders may also require local abstention. For example, if a client is diagnosed with phlebitis—inflammation of the deep veins—in the legs, the practitioner should avoid the legs but can give Shiatsu to the rest of the body. Phlebitis is associated with the presence of thrombi or blood clots. Should a thrombus exist, it could be dislodged by manual manipulation and enter the bloodstream, where it could eventually block an artery to a vital organ and precipitate a vascular accident, such as a stroke—the interruption of blood flow to the brain (Chow, 2002).

Another condition that requires local abstention is varicose veins of the legs. Varicose veins are abnormally dilated and have damaged nonreturn valves, causing blood flow to back up and pool in the extremities (Chow, 2002). They can be identified by their gnarled, engorged, blue/green noodle-like appearance. Because the structural integrity of varicose veins is impaired, pressure can cause them to rupture, which is why manual manipulation should be avoided. However, the practitioner can work elsewhere on the legs and the rest of the body.

A final example of a cardiovascular condition that requires modifying Shiatsu is an episode of hypertension, or blood pressure that is higher than 120 systolic/80 diastolic (Chow, 2002). During an episode of hypertension, vigorous and dynamic techniques that are deep, fast, and traveling should be avoided, since they could increase blood flow and elevate blood pressure even further. However, calming techniques that are moderate to light and slow or stationary may be done. Holding certain acupressure points, namely Bl 10, GB 20, and LI 11, which are all noted for their tonic effects on hypertension, may provide relief (Junying & Zhihong, 1997).

When delivering Shiatsu to persons with cardiovascular diseases:

- Avoid Shiatsu on a person diagnosed with hemophilia.
- Screen for risks of cardiovascular disease (overweight or obese, sedentary, stressed, smoker, male, 40+); avoid ischemic compression, especially near major arteries; avoid ampuku.

- Avoid the region of phlebitis and the specific site of varicose veins.
- Avoid deep, vigorous, dynamic techniques during an episode of hypertension.

OTHER CONTRAINDICATIONS

Thermal disorders constitute another set of contraindications. These include fever and chills; hyperthermia or abnormally high body temperature, a result of dehydration and exposure to high ambient air temperature and/or humidity; and hypothermia or abnormally low body temperature, a result of exposure to low ambient air temperature, rain, and wind. Still other contraindications include extreme debility or exhaustion, intoxication, and untreated or untreatable mental disorders, like schizophrenia or Alzheimer's disease, that make a person emotionally volatile and unstable. Giving Shiatsu to clients with mental disorders like schizophrenia or Alzheimer's requires caution or a doctor's release.

CANCER

Cancer is a broad category of diseases characterized by the uncontrolled growth of abnormal cells (Chamness, 1993). For nearly two decades, a protracted controversy over whether bodywork is appropriate for cancer patients has deterred many massage therapists, including Shiatsu practitioners, from working on cancer patients. Curiously, the absolute contraindication against bodywork has been perpetuated, in the main, by massage therapy educators whose default mode is conservative (McConnellogue, 2000). This contraindication is premised on the as yet unfounded assumption that manual manipulation could facilitate or expedite the spread of cancer by enhancing circulatory and lymph flow or could metastasize a malignant tumor by breaking off a fragment, which could migrate into the distribution channels of the blood or lymph system. Although researchers still do not fully understand how cancer spreads, the very same factors that cause cancer—heredity and environment—are implicated, not bodywork. Moreover, an increase in blood and lymph flow is beneficial; otherwise, many oncologists would never encourage their patients to exercise, which they do.

The growing consensus in favor of bodywork is premised on research about the general benefits of massage, as well as specific benefits for cancer patients. Bodywork stimulates blood and lymph flow, which augments nutrient distribution, waste elimination, immune function, and tissue regeneration (McConnellogue, 2000). It also relaxes muscle tension, improves mobility, ameliorates pain, and reduces stress, as evidenced by lowered heart rate, respiratory rate, blood pressure, and cortisol or stress hormone levels (MacDonald, 1995). It diminishes the tissue swelling of lymphedema caused by chemotherapy, radiation, or surgical procedures, such as a mastectomy (Bunce, Mirolo, Hennessy et al., 1994; Brennan & Weitz, 1992; Badger, 1986; Zanolla, Monzeglio, Balzarini et al., 1984) and mitigates fatigue (McConnellogue, 2000). Equally important to the cancer patient is relief from anxiety and depression (Ferrell-Torry & Glick, 1993; Wilkinson, 1995) and from a sense of social alienation and dissociation from the body (Chamness, 1993). Although bodywork cannot treat or cure cancer, it does reduce suffering, provide comfort, and improve morale, which, in turn, can improve patient outcome (McConnellogue, 2000).

The quest for ways to improve patient experiences and outcomes has led to reliance on teams of medical experts and the use of complementary modalities as adjuncts to allopathic medicine. This trend, along with increased funding for massage research and the growing use of massage in hospitals, outpatient centers, and rehabilitation clinics, indicates medical approval of bodywork as a means to improve the quality of a cancer patient's life during treatment and remission (McConnellogue, 2000), not just hospice care. For a comprehensive treatment of the subject of bodywork on cancer patients, the interested reader is referred to Gayle MacDonald's *Medicine Hands: Massage Therapy for People with Cancer.*

A Shiatsu practitioner who is motivated to work on a cancer patient should first obtain the oncologist's and the patient's written consent and should consult the oncologist on an ongoing basis about the nature and location of the cancer and any modifications that may be necessary (McConnellogue, 2000). Additionally, obtaining the patient's written authorization for the release of medical information and records is highly advisable (Chamness, 1993).

When giving Shiatsu to cancer patients, several precautions are necessary. Because radiation and chemotherapy compromise a cancer patient's immune system, reducing the white blood cell count and increasing the risk of illness and infection, the practitioner should be ultrathorough in personal hygiene (Chamness, 1993), washing up to the elbows in antibacterial soap before touching the patient. Moreover, if the practitioner feels unwell or if a member of the practitioner's household is ill, he or she should abstain from giving Shiatsu until the episode is passed.

A patient undergoing radiation to annihilate cancer cells or prevent them from proliferating will have areas of the body that are off-limits to Shiatsu due to the presence of a tumor and/or tissue irritation or damage from radiation (Chamness, 1993). Areas targeted for radiation may be identified by a radiologist's ink markings, and the skin is likely to be dry or burned (McConnellogue, 2000). Such areas should be avoided.

A patient undergoing radiation or chemotherapy could experience suppressed bone marrow functioning with abnormally low blood platelet counts. Such a patient will have a compromised blood clotting function and will be susceptible to bruising or bleeding. In mild cases of compromised blood clotting, Shiatsu must be gentle to prevent bruising or bleeding; in extreme cases, as when the patient is hospitalized for impaired blood clotting, Shiatsu is contraindicated (Chamness, 1993). Additionally, cancer affecting the bones may render the patient susceptible to fractures (McConnellogue, 2000). Again, Shiatsu must be light to prevent bone breakage.

A patient undergoing chemotherapy through intravenous infusion will be confined to a hospital bed and will have either a port, a small chamber inserted subcutaneously near the shoulder, or a catheter tube in place that affects how Shiatsu is administered. Not only should the practitioner avoid Shiatsu near and around the device, where the tissues are often inflamed, but also the practitioner must take care to avoid disrupting or dislodging the device during treatment and must adapt the treatment, including patient positioning, to accommodate the device and to promote patient comfort (Chamness, 1993; McConnellogue, 2000).

Various surgical procedures will also affect the timing, nature, and scope of Shiatsu. The practitioner should always obtain the oncologist's written permission for treatment following surgery. In general, a practitioner should refrain from giving Shiatsu within 24 hours of a needle biopsy that aspirates a tumor site; after that, general Shiatsu that avoids the site may be acceptable (Chamness, 1993). A longer moratorium follows more radical procedures, such as a lumpectomy, the surgical removal of a mass from breast tissue. Light Shiatsu to remote areas, such as the hands and feet, may be acceptable 48 hours after surgery.

When delivering Shiatsu to cancer patients:

- Consult the oncologist about the cancer.
- Obtain the oncologist's and the patient's written consent.
- Obtain the patient's authorization for the release of medical records.
- Wash with antibacterial soap up to the elbows before touching the patient.
- Postpone treatment if feeling unwell or if a household member is ill.
- Avoid tumors.
- Avoid radiation-treated areas.
- Avoid disrupting or dislodging a catheter or port.

- Avoid surgical sites.
- In general, use lighter pressure and gentler techniques.
- Focus on patient comfort.

SPECIAL POPULATIONS

THE ELDERLY

Because the elderly may have reduced immune function, the same precautions regarding personal hygiene apply as with cancer patients: The practitioner should wash with antibacterial soap up to the elbows before working and should avoid working if he or she is feeling unwell or has been around someone who feels unwell. Except in the case of robust clients, a practitioner should give lighter and gentler Shiatsu to the elderly. Also, certain positions, especially the prone position, may be uncomfortable due to the stiffness and rigidity of the cervical and lumbar spine and the musculoskeletal distortions of age. Place a pillow under the chest and/or abdomen, and a bolster under the ankles, or avoid the prone position altogether.

Osteoporosis, a degenerative bone disease, is of particular concern for the elderly, especially elderly white women, who have the greatest risk of developing it. Physical signs that may indicate the presence of osteoporosis include a delicate bone structure; general frailty or infirmity; the use of a cane or walker; thoracic kyphosis, a stooped posture characterized by a dowager's hump or hunch back; and cervical flexion, a drooping or forward-jutting head. If a client is diagnosed with or is suspected of having osteoporosis, the practitioner should exercise caution and avoid deep or dynamic pressure, since the bones are porous and brittle and the risk of breaking them is great. Only light pressure should be applied. Heavy instruments like knuckles, fists, forearms, elbows, and knees should be eliminated altogether, as should any jostling and pummeling techniques.

If an elderly client has an artificial joint, such as a hip replacement, the practitioner should avoid traction, body mobilization techniques (BMTs), and passive stretches on the artificial joint, though he or she may work on the opposite side of the body to stimulate a reflexive healing response.

Osteoarthritis and rheumatoid arthritis may afflict the elderly. Osteoarthritis is a degenerative joint disease caused by the deterioration of cartilage and bones due to attrition, or wear and tear (Rados, 2005). It usually affects weight-bearing joints, such as the knees and hips, more than other joints, though a genetically inherited form can affect the spine and hands as well. Shiatsu, and especially BMTs and passive stretches that mimic exercise, may provide some relief. By contrast, rheumatoid arthritis is an autoimmune disease that damages and destroys the synovial lining that lubricates the joint, as well as the cartilage that cushions the joint, leading to loss of joint integrity and bone attrition. In early stages, rheumatoid arthritis is characterized by inflammation, stiffness, and pain in the joints and, in later stages, by instability, severe deformity, and decrepitude of the joints. Techniques that are safe to administer to the average person could dislocate the joints and damage the associated neurovascular structures of a person with rheumatoid arthritis (Chow, 2002). Because of the risk of injury, Shiatsu should be given only with a doctor's prescription and great caution.

When delivering Shiatsu to elderly clients:

- Wash with antibacterial soap up to the elbows.
- Postpone treatment if feeling unwell or if a household member is ill.
- Avoid the prone position if uncomfortable, or use props.
- In general, use lighter pressure and gentler techniques.
- Screen for risk of osteoporosis: frailty, thoracic kyphosis, and cervical flexion; if present, avoid deep, dynamic pressure and industrial-strength body tools.

- Avoid traction, BMTs, and stretches on an artificial joint.
- Obtain a doctor's consent to work on a client with rheumatoid arthritis and proceed with caution.

PREGNANT WOMEN

During pregnancy, several modifications to Shiatsu are necessary, including changes in the level of pressure and the positioning of the client, as well as the restriction against working on certain areas or acupressure points. Most Shiatsu authorities agree that the practitioner should avoid deep pressure or vigorous techniques below knee level. However, at least one authority on prenatal massage advises against anything but very light pressure—5 grams or the weight of a nickel—on the legs, due to the increase in fibrogenic or blood coagulating activity during pregnancy and as long as 10 weeks postpartum (Stillerman, 1996, 2004). Fibrogenesis prevents hemorrhaging during labor but also increases the risk of thrombi or blood clots in the legs. These blood clots could be dislodged by manual manipulation, enter the bloodstream, and precipitate a vascular accident, such as a stroke—hence, the ultraconservative approach of applying very light pressure to the legs. To determine the presence of a blood clot, the practitioner applies the homen test by dorsiflexing the client's relaxed foot. If the client feels a radiating sensation anywhere in the leg, Shiatsu is contraindicated, and the client should be referred to a physician for further testing.

The secretion of the hormone relaxin at weeks 10–14, while limbering the mother and widening her pelvis for the passage of the child through the birth canal, contributes to joint laxity and instability (Stillerman, 1996, 2004). Consequently, the Shiatsu practitioner should exercise caution when applying stretches or BMTs, as the soft tissues are limber and could be strained and the joints are hypermobile and could be displaced.

Shiatsu should not be administered while a client is suffering from morning sickness. However, acupressure to PC 6 (Figure 9-1) can mitigate nausea. Additionally, the

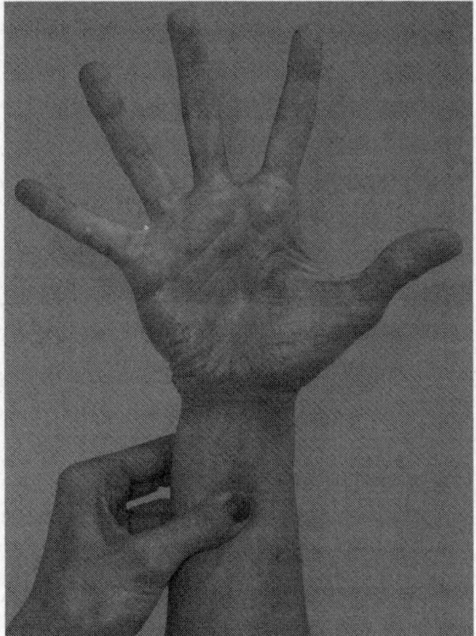

FIGURE 9-1 PC 6.
2 cun (2 thumb widths) above the inner wrist between the two wrist flexor tendons. This anti-emetic point is good for countering nausea experienced during pregnancy. The client may obtain a magnetic and/or seed/pellet (acupressure) wristband from most pharmacies to wear to avert morning sickness.

client can obtain an anti-emetic wristband at most pharmacies that she can wear during the first trimester to control morning sickness and vomiting.

Other contraindications to Shiatsu include bleeding, premature labor, pre-eclampsia, eclampsia, and placenta previa (Stillerman, 1996, 2004). Pre-eclampsia is a toxic condition marked by high blood pressure, severe headaches, and pitted edema, and eclampsia is the potentially fatal version of it. To test for pitted edema and pre-eclampsia, the practitioner presses the flesh near the outer ankle and releases it. If the indentation and blanching of the practitioner's fingerprint do not resolve by a count of five, Shiatsu is contraindicated, and the client should be referred to a physician. Placenta previa is the attachment of the placenta to the lower rather than the upper portion of the uterus; Shiatsu is contraindicated.

Some techniques or areas of the body are contraindicated during pregnancy but later become useful during labor or postpartum. For example, ampuku or abdominal massage is best avoided during pregnancy, though it is quite helpful postpartum to induce uterine involution—the shrinking of the uterus to its former size and the return of the uterus to its subumbilical location (Stillerman, 1996, 2004). Moxabustion, a type of heat therapy, is usually not applied during gestation, especially not below the knees, but can be applied to Bl 67 (Figure 9-2) around the thirtyeighth week to rotate a breech presentation, if necessary.

Certain acupressure points are strictly prohibited during pregnancy because they draw energy downward and could induce a miscarriage. These are LI 4, named The Great Eliminator for its expulsion function; Sp 6, Three Yin Crossing, the quintessential female energy point in the body; and GB 21, Shoulder's Well. (see Figures 9-3 to 9-5.) However, these same points—LI 4, Sp 6, and GB 21—can be vigorously and repeatedly stimulated just before the due date to induce labor and during labor to expedite delivery.

Additionally, Sp 10, Ocean of Blood, can be stimulated after birth to discharge the contents of the uterus, including the placenta and lochia (Stillerman, 2004). Sp 3 can be stimulated postpartum to ease the severity of the hormonal drop that contributes to postpartum blues (Stillerman, 1996, 2004). Finally, the following points can be stimulated to encourage lactation or milk letdown in nursing

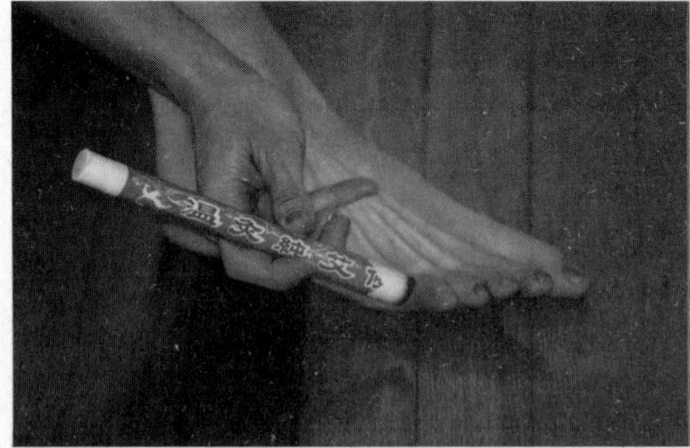

FIGURE 9-2 Bl 67.
At the outer corner of the nailbed of the little toe. If the fetus is not in the head-down position by the thirtyeighth week, moxabustion—an herbal heat therapy—can be applied to this point to rotate a breech presentation (see Chapter 8 on complementary modalities). Moxa cigars can be purchased at some health food stores, at most Asian markets, or through an Asian medical supplier (see Appendix 4).

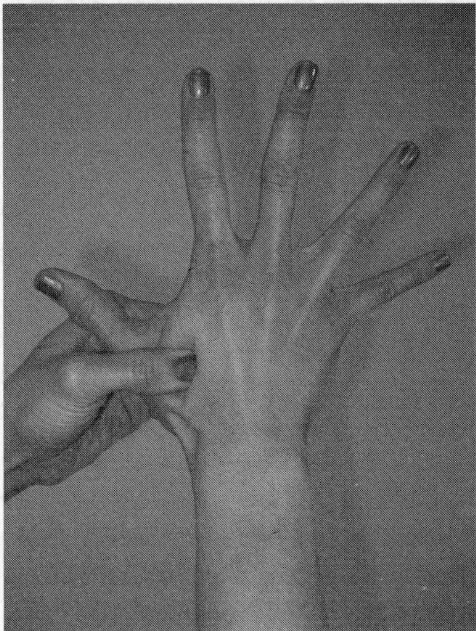

FIGURE 9-3 LI 4.
In the web of flesh between the index finger and thumb; press toward the first metacarpal. This point is contraindicated during pregnancy because it draws energy downward and facilitates expulsion from the body, possibly inducing miscarriage, but it is useful in labor to expedite delivery of the child.

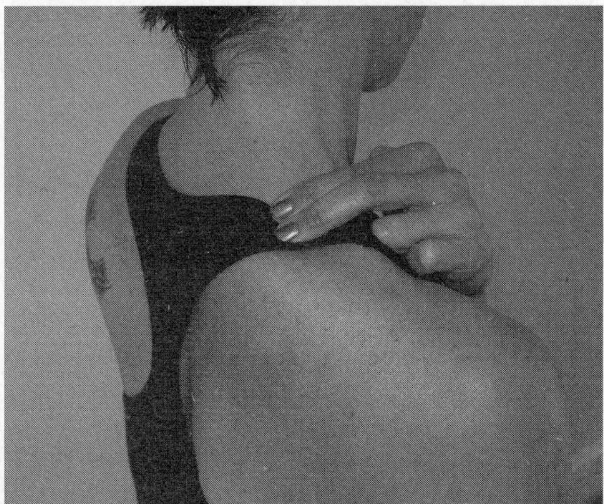

FIGURE 9-4 GB 21.
On the belly of the upper trapezius. This point is contraindicated during pregnancy but useful in labor.

mothers: GB 21, Lu 1 (Letting Go), St 13, St 16 (Breast Window), and CV 17 (Stillerman, 1996, 2004; Gach, 1990). The interested reader is referred to Appendix 1, the glossary of acupoints for the locations of these points.

In addition to the caveat against stimulating certain points during pregnancy, certain positions are contraindicated, either because they are uncomfortable or because they are dangerous. Although the prone position does not pose any danger to the fetus, which is cushioned in a sac of amniotic fluid, the prone position may

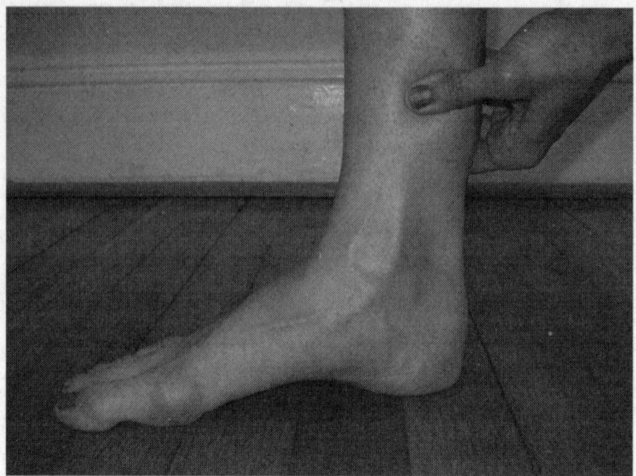

FIGURE 9-5 Sp 6.
Three cun (4 finger widths) above the medial malleolus (inner ankle); press toward the tibia. This point is contraindicated during pregnancy but useful in labor.

become uncomfortable for the mother during the second trimester due to her protruding abdomen. If this is the case, the prone position should be avoided. In advanced stages of pregnancy, the supine position is contraindicated because the weight of the fetus can compress the mother's inferior vena cava, restricting or blocking blood flow back to the heart and causing dizziness or lightheadedness. When the prone position becomes uncomfortable or the supine position is contraindicated, the sidelying position should be used instead.

When delivering Shiatsu to pregnant women:

- Use the sidelying position during the second and third trimesters.
- Avoid deep or vigorous techniques below knee level.
- Exercise caution when applying stretches or BMTs.
- Avoid contraindicating conditions: morning sickness, pre-eclampsia, eclampsia, and placenta previa.
- Avoid contraindicated points: LI 4, GB 21, and Sp 6.

PRE- AND POST-SHIATSU-SESSION ADVICE FOR CLIENTS

Before the Shiatsu session, the practitioner should advise a new or first-time client how to maximize the experience. The client should avoid eating a heavy meal or drinking alcohol before the session. By the same token, the client should not arrive hungry but may eat a light snack to ward off hunger pangs. The client should wear loose, comfortable, natural-fiber clothing such as cotton sweatpants and a T-shirt during the session and should refrain from wearing perfume, cologne, or a fragrant deodorant, since all these can mask the client's natural odor, which is helpful for assessment. Ideally, the client should reserve the day of the Shiatsu treatment as a day of rest or moderate activity, not undertaking stressful or demanding tasks before or after the session and not rushing into or out of the appointment.

After the session, the client might experience a **healing response** or **healing crisis**, especially if the client has not had much bodywork and/or is toxic. Signs of toxicity that increase the likelihood of a healing response include the smell of smoke, indicating that the client is a smoker or exposed to secondhand smoke; dry skin and dry hair; skin that adheres to the tissues underneath it rather than being easy to pluck up and scrunch; soft tissues that feel hard and resistant rather than supple and pliable; and joints that are stiff and rigid rather than mobile.

A healing response indicates that the body is processing toxins and may include the following symptoms: general fatigue or malaise, muscle aches or stiffness, headache, frequent urination, stomach upset or diarrhea, and irritability or mild depression. These symptoms usually pass within 24 hours, leaving the client feeling much better than before the session. However, the client can do a few things to facilitate the cleansing process: drink plenty of water to flush metabolic wastes from his system and prevent the tissues from reabsorbing toxins; soak in a hot, Epsom salt bath to relieve any soreness; rest and get a good night's sleep; and exercise lightly or stretch the following day, if desired.

PRINCIPLES OF PROPER BODY MECHANICS

Because Shiatsu is a healing art, practitioners tend to focus exclusively on the client's welfare and comfort and forget or neglect their own. While doing Shiatsu, the practitioner should periodically check posture and body mechanics and make adjustments to prevent strain and injury. Consistently observing proper form increases the effectiveness of any given technique, the practitioner's enjoyment, and the quality and longevity of the practitioner's career. The main principles of good body mechanics are maintaining a low center of gravity, facing the client with the hara, and using leverage to apply pressure.

Maintaining a low center of gravity means having a broad and heavy base of support. This principle is used in engineering to ensure structural stability. For example, ships are loaded with heavy cargo at the bottom to give them ballast; otherwise, they could capsize. Buildings are built with a solid concrete and steel foundation. For the Shiatsu practitioner, stability is gained by working from a position that is low to the ground, spread wide, and bottom heavy. A number of positions provide such stability: crawling on all fours, sitting in **seiza**—the kneeling, Japanese meditation position in which the sit bones rest on the heels, spreading the knees farther apart in a triangle like a samurai sitting in council, spreading the legs wide in a kneeling lunge, and squatting low to the ground like a Sumo wrestler. (See Figures 9-6 to 9-10.) Of course, many of these positions require flexibility in the hips, knees, and ankles and may take practice.

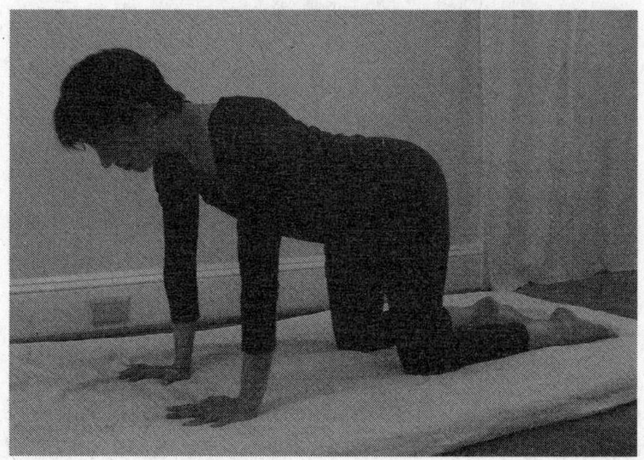

FIGURE 9-6 **Crawl.**
The weight of the torso is transferred in a straight line through the shoulders to the hands.

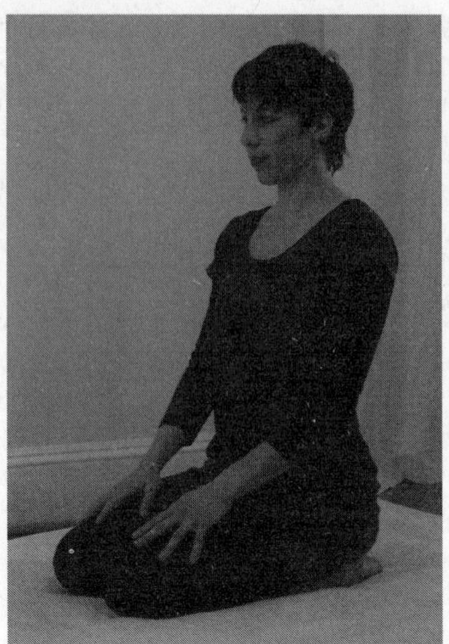

FIGURE 9-7 Seiza.
The Japanese meditation position. A pillow can be placed between the thighs and calves for comfort.

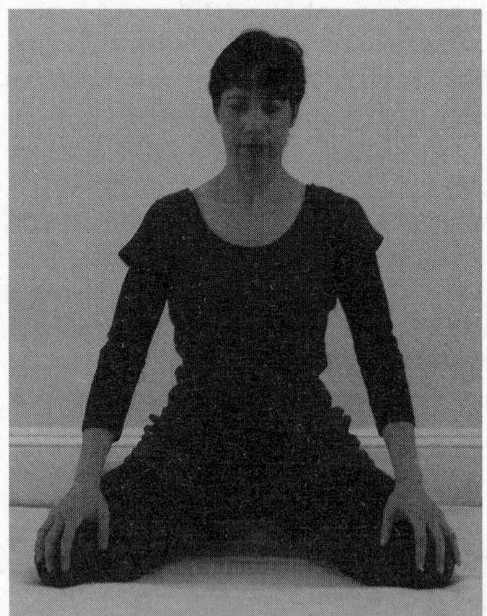

FIGURE 9-8 Samurai seat.
Spreading the knees apart to form a triangular base confers greater stability.

Facing the client with the **hara**, or abdomen and hips, increases power and reduces strain. In general, the practitioner's hips should point directly toward the target area on the client. In this position, the practitioner's center of power and gravity is directly behind the hands and arms so that the technique can be delivered with maximum power and minimum effort. The practitioner should never work from any awkward position that entails twisting. If the practitioner experiences discomfort or strain while exerting pressure, the practitioner should check hara alignment in relation to the client to see whether he or she is incorrectly

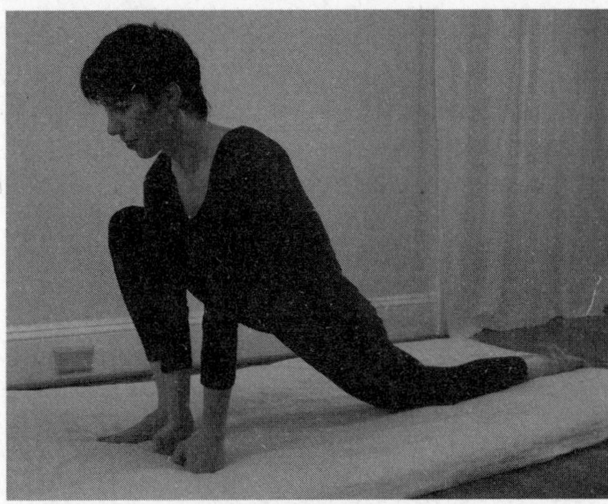

FIGURE 9-9 **Kneeling lunge.** This position requires flexibility in the iliopsoas and rectus femoris (hip flexors). There is also a side variation of the kneeling lunge (not pictured) that requires flexibility in the adductors (inner thighs).

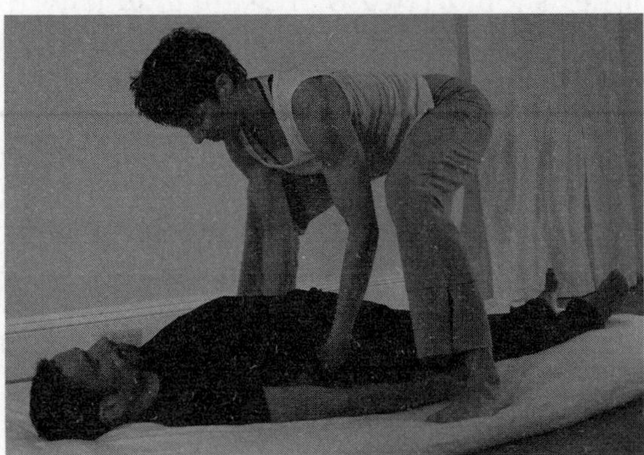

FIGURE 9-10 **Sumo wrestler squat.** This straddling squat is optimal for working the client's center or midline. In contrast to kneeling beside the client, this position does not require you to twist your torso, an important mechanical advantage.

torqueing the body. If the target area is beside, rather than directly in front of, the navel, the practitioner should reposition immediately.

Using leverage to apply pressure means harnessing the power of gravity. The practitioner should harness the power gravity by leaning the body weight into the client rather than marshalling strength to push, which can lead to strain or exhaustion. Logistically, the practitioner must rise above the client and sink weight into the client. Additionally, the practitioner should initiate all movements from the hara or core rather than the extremities—hands, arms, and shoulders. For example, when applying a compression technique, such as acupressure, the practitioner should shift and transfer the weight of the hips forward and downward into the client rather than thrusting with the hands and arms. When jostling the client, the practitioner should oscillate the hips, not the shoulders or arms: The hips, not the shoulders or elbows, should rock and sway back and forth. Moving from the hara not only preserves the practitioner's hands and arms, but also feels more powerful and stable to the client.

To use proper body mechanics:

- Maintain a low center of gravity.
- Face the target area with the hara.
- Use leverage: Lean into the client.
- Move from the hara, not the extremities.

PRINCIPLES OF APPLYING PRESSURE

The angle at which pressure is applied and the quality of entry into and exit from the target area are important. In general, the practitioner should apply pressure at a right angle or perpendicular to the target area to ensure contact with the client's vital energy. Applying pressure at an oblique angle, such as 45 degrees, diminishes the accuracy and effectiveness of the technique. Pressure should be applied gradually until the practitioner feels resistance or has "hit bottom." Easing into the technique smoothly gives the tissues time to adapt to the load and feels less intrusive or invasive to the client than an abrupt, bolting entry. Once pressure has been applied, the practitioner should hold the pressure for a few seconds—ideally for a count of three—or longer if necessary. Stationary, sustained pressure gives the muscles a chance to relax and melt under the load and attracts vital energy to the area. Finally, the practitioner should release pressure gradually to avoid jarring the client.

The effectiveness of any compression technique can be further enhanced if the practitioner images that he or she is penetrating through the target area to the opposite side of the body. Martial artists use this principle of intention to increase the power of their strikes: They concentrate on punching through rather than at the opponent. Likewise, the practitioner should apply pressure through rather than on a client.

Another important principle is coordinating movement with breathing. Bodybuilders coordinate weightlifting with exhalation to increase their power and core stability. During exhalation, the muscles of the hara, and especially the transverse abdominus that wraps around the waist like a corset or back brace, are engaged, providing support for the spine and power for movement. The abdominal muscles and the intercostals (ribcage muscles) contract to decrease space in the abdominal and thoracic cavities in order to expel air from the lungs. For the practitioner and the client, exhalation is the optimal time to give or receive pressure. Hence, the practitioner should try to breathe and move with the client's natural rhythm. As the client exhales, the practitioner exhales and applies pressure, and as the client inhales, the practitioner inhales and releases pressure. Coordinating movement with breathing is particularly important when working on the client's back or abdomen, as unsynchronized pressure interferes with the client's respiration and feels uncomfortable. The practitioner should never press down while the client is attempting to inhale and the ribcage and abdomen are expanding.

Compression techniques should be applied in a progressive fashion from general to specific or from broad to sharp, beginning with padded techniques and graduating to more focused and intense techniques, as appropriate. Initially, compressions should be applied with broad, flat surfaces like the palms and heels of the hands, all four fingerpads, and the fleshy belly of the forearms, as when crawling on the client. The pressure level should be gentle to moderate at first. After the tissues are sufficiently warmed and loosened by the preliminary work, more intense techniques may be applied. Sharp, pointed surfaces like the thumbs, knuckles, and elbows may be used, and deeper levels of pressure may be delivered. If this principle of working from general to specific is disregarded, the client will most likely find the treatment invasive or hurtful, even if the client likes deep, focused pressure.

When applying pressure:

- Apply pressure at an angle perpendicular to the surface area.
- Penetrate through the surface area to the opposite side.
- Apply pressure gradually on exhaling.
- Sustain stationary pressure for three seconds or more.
- Release pressure gradually on inhaling.
- Progress from general to specific and light/moderate to deep compression.

SPECIAL HAND TECHNIQUES

Zen Shiatsu, a style developed by Shizuto Masunaga, uses two special hand techniques—two-hand connectedness and the Mother/Son hand technique—that enrich the Shiatsu repertoire. **Two-hand connectedness**, or "two as one," is a subtle energetic technique that takes some practice to experience but occurs naturally when the practitioner is deeply absorbed and relaxed in the work. As with standard two-handed techniques, the practitioner places both palms or thumbs on the client's body but concentrates on feeling an energy loop from one hand to the other hand to the client, like a closed circuit of bioelectricity (Masunaga & Ohashi, 1997; Beresford-Cooke, 2000; Jarmey & Mojay, 1999). Initially, the practitioner may have to imagine or envision the circuit of energy before experiencing it. However, if the practitioner feels particularly engrossed in the bodywork and attuned to or "in synch" with the client during a Shiatsu session, the experience of energetic connection may emerge naturally, along with the feeling of immersion in the bodywork or fusion with the client. The purpose of two-hand connectedness is to experience practitioner-client harmony and unity, a goal of all good personal and professional relationships. An additional benefit is that two-hand connectedness develops mental concentration and focus, reducing the mediocrity in service that comes with distraction.

The **Mother/Son hand technique** differs from the standard two-handed compression, in which both hands do the same thing at the same time. With the Mother/Son hand technique, the two hands are doing different tasks and performing different functions. (See Figures 9-11 to 9-21.) The Mother hand applies static,

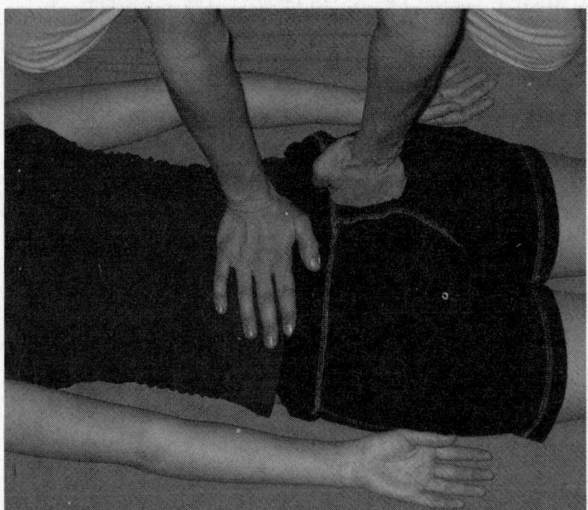

FIGURE 9-11 Mother/Son: Bl 23 & Bl 53. The Mother hand rests bilaterally on both Bl 23 points while the Son fist presses all around the hip and pauses at Bl 53.

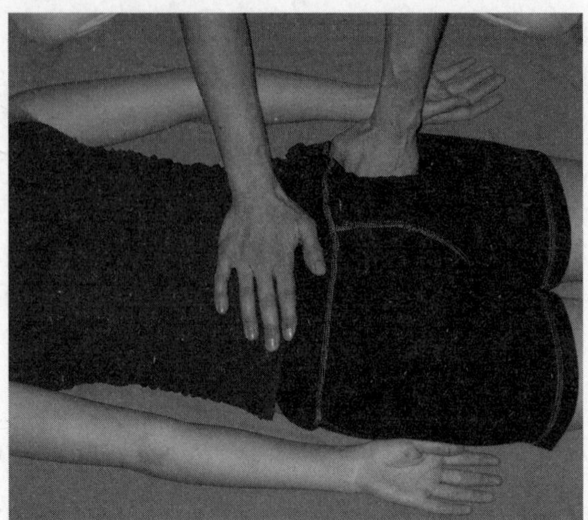

FIGURE 9-12 **Mother/Son: Bl 23 & GB 30.** The Mother hand rests bilaterally on both Bl 23 points while the Son fist presses all around the hip and pauses at the GB 30.

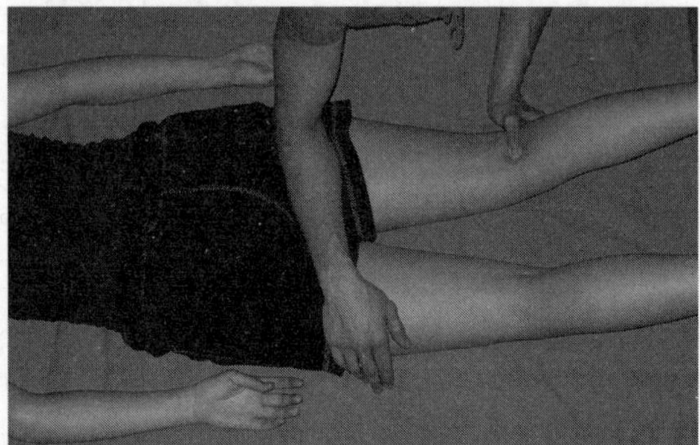

FIGURE 9-13 **Mother/Son: Bl 36 & Bl 40.** The Mother forearm rests on Bl 36 while the Son hand presses down the Bladder Meridian of the thigh and pauses at Bl 40.

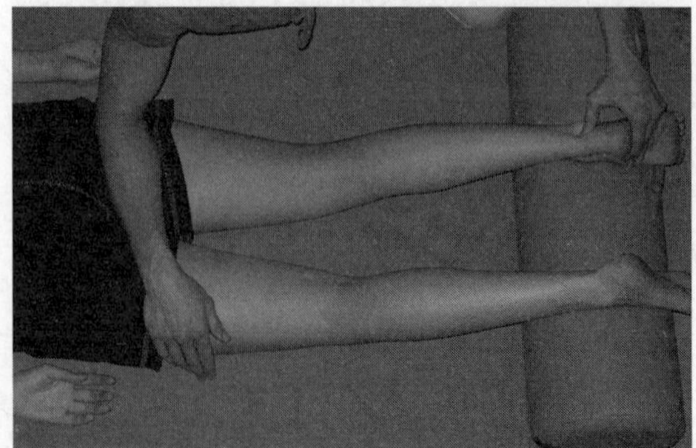

FIGURE 9-14 **Mother/Son: Bl 36 & Bl 60.** The Mother forearm rests on Bl 36 while the Son thumb presses down the Bladder Meridian of the calf and stops at Bl 60.

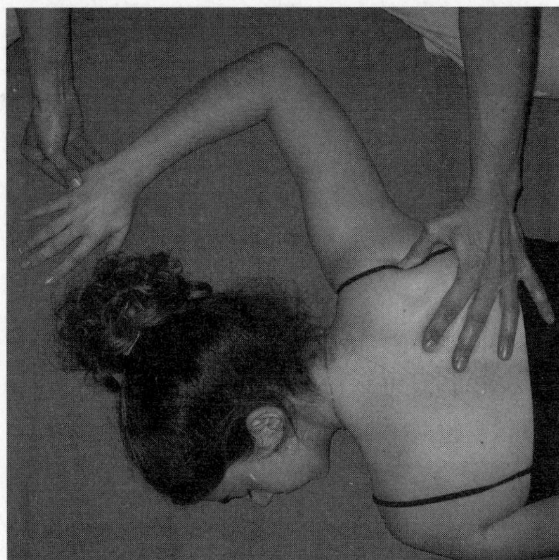

FIGURE 9-15 **Mother/Son: SI 11 & SI 3.** The Mother thumb holds SI 11 while the Son thumb presses down the Small Intestine Meridian of the arm and stops at SI 3.

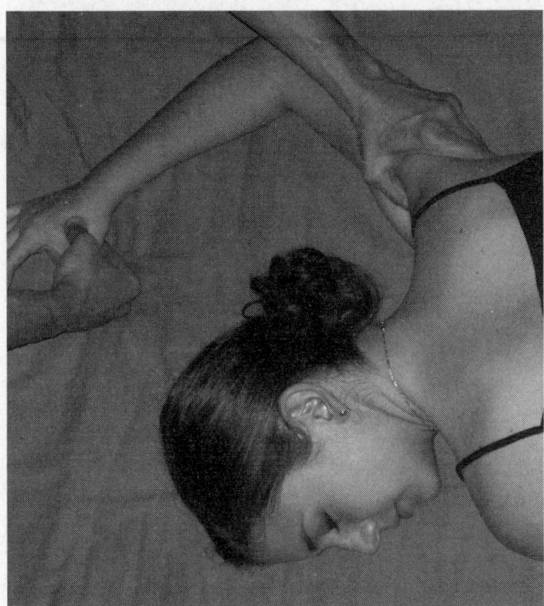

FIGURE 9-16 **Mother/Son: LI 15 & LI 4.** The Mother thumb holds LI 15 while the Son thumb presses down the Large Intestine Meridian of the arm and stops at LI 4.

stationary pressure, usually on or near the torso, generating warmth by drawing and attracting vital energy to the area, while the Son hand applies active, dynamic pressure along the length of a limb and directs vital energy through it (Masunaga & Ohashi, 1997). For example, to work the arm, the Mother hand stays planted on the shoulder while the Son hand compresses the arm from the shoulder to the wrist. To work the front of the leg, the Mother hand stays planted on the abdomen

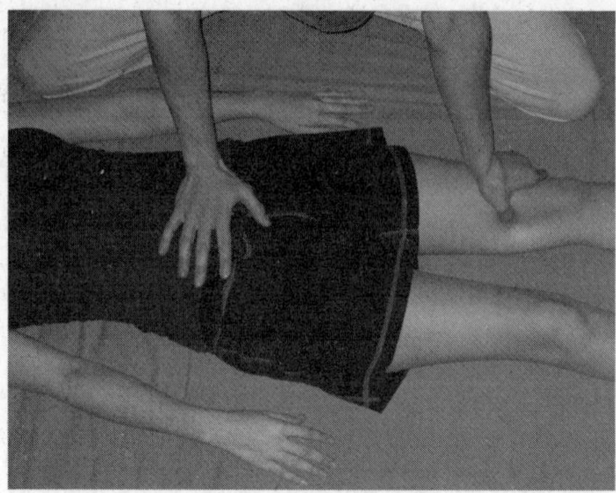

FIGURE 9-17 Mother/Son: CV 4 & Sp 10. The Mother hand rests on CV 4 while the Son thumb presses down the Spleen Meridian of the thigh to Sp 10.

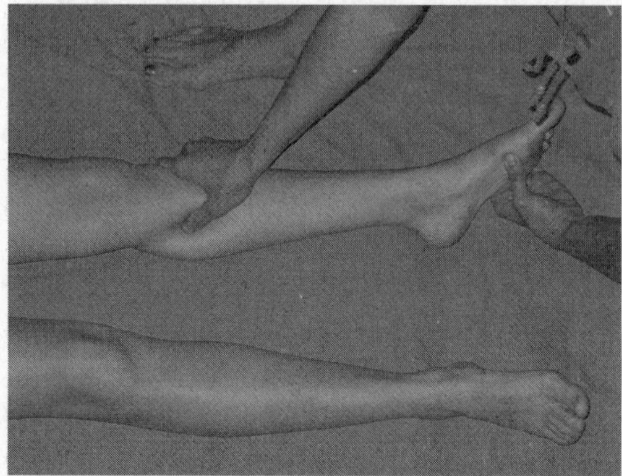

FIGURE 9-18 Mother/Son: Sp 9 & Sp 3. The Mother hand relocates to Sp 9 while the Son thumb presses down the Spleen Meridian of the leg to Sp 3.

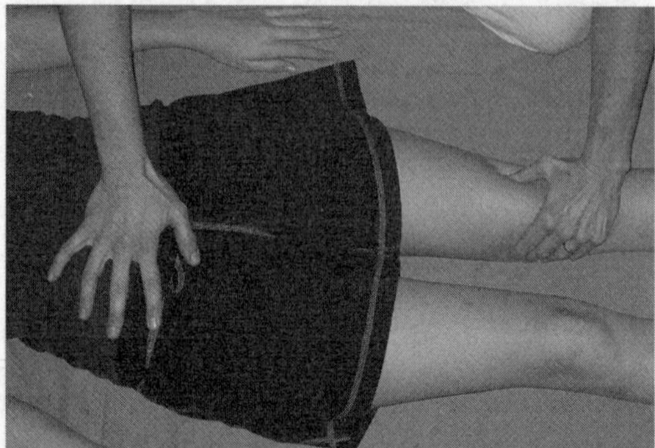

FIGURE 9-19 Mother/Son CV 4 & St 34. The Mother hand rests on CV 4 while the Son thumb presses down the Stomach Meridian of the thigh and pauses at St 34.

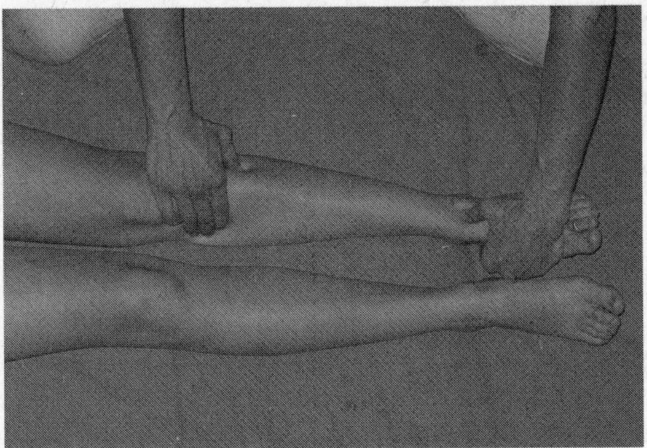

FIGURE 9-20 Mother/Son St 36 & St 41. The Mother hand relocates to St 36 while the Son thumb presses down the Stomach Meridian of the leg to St 41.

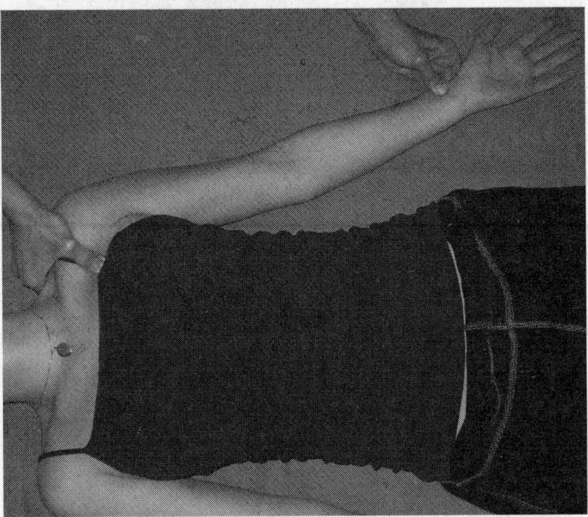

FIGURE 9-21 Mother/Son Lu 1 & Lu 7. The Mother thumb holds Lu 1 while the Son thumb presses down the Lung Meridian of the arm and stops at Lu 7.

or hip while the Son hand compresses the leg from the hip to the ankle. To work the hip, the Mother hand rests on the sacrum or lower back while the Son hand compresses the hip. If the client's limbs are too long for the practitioner to reach the distal extremities, the practitioner can relocate the Mother hand near the knee while the Son hand works the lower leg and foot.

The Mother/Son hand technique has several client-specific purposes. It is preferred if the client has difficulty relaxing because the limbs are tense, tender, or even painful to touch. Planting one hand near the core of the body is comforting and reassuring, and using only one hand to apply dynamic pressure is less intense than using both hands. The Mother/Son hand technique is also preferred if the client has a weak or cold lower back or abdomen, as the sustained presence of the Mother hand will warm it. It is also preferred if the client's energy reserves are low, as when the client is fatigued, exhausted, or otherwise infirm or ill, as this technique is gentler than two-handed compression.

On the other hand, two-handed compression—in which both hands actively apply the same pressure technique along a limb—is preferable if the client likes deep pressure or a vigorous treatment, if a stronger effect is desired, or if the client needs to discharge or release pent-up energy. Most of the protocols in this book demonstrate two-handed compression, but the practitioner should use the Mother/Son hand technique if, as noted above, the client is experiencing hypersensitivity, weakness, coldness, or tiredness.

POINTERS ON SPECIFIC TECHNIQUES

In addition to the general principles of applying pressure, there are specific pointers for using various body tools. The nails should be trimmed very short to avoid gouging the client when applying finger or thumb techniques, and any rings should be removed to avoid poking or grating the client when applying fist techniques. When using the palms, the palms should mold to the contour of the body,

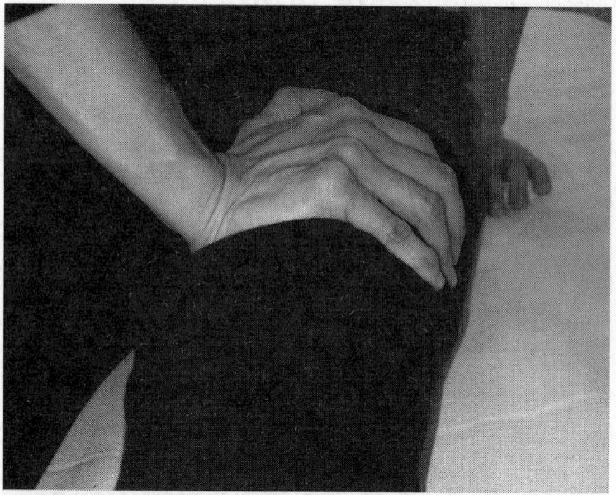

FIGURE 9-22 Palm, correct. Your hand should mold to the contours of the client's body to maximize contact and stability.

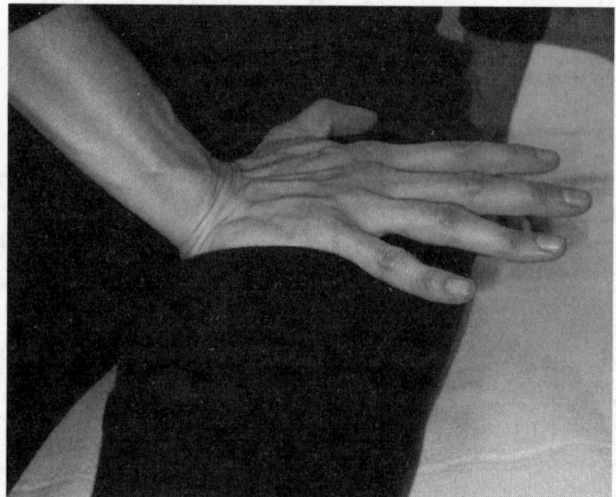

FIGURE 9-23 Palm, incorrect. Extending your fingers creates unnecessary tension in your forearm, wrist, and hand and is not as comforting to the client as full hand contact.

maximizing contact and minimizing strain on the forearm extensors. (See Figures 9-22 and 9-23.) When using the fingers pads, all the fingers should be used together unless specific acupressure points are being stimulated on the face. In general, the index and middle fingers apply most of the pressure, while the others brace or reinforce these two.

When using the thumb, pressure should be applied with the pad of the thumb, as this surface feels best to the client and preserves the structural integrity of the thumb (Figure 9-24). Occasionally, the tip of the thumb may be used for acupressure points located in relatively inaccessible bony hollows around the wrist (TH 4; LI 4, 5; SI 3; Ht 7; Lu 9) or ankles (GB 40; St 41) or in other locations that require more precision than the pad of the thumb (Figure 9-25). However, the tip of the thumb should be used sparingly and reserved for small entry points, as the tip often produces a sensation that is too sharp and the thumbnail may inadvertently gouge the client. Pressure should never be applied with the interphalangeal joint—the joint between the distal and proximal phalanges of the thumb—because this entails hyperextending the shaft of the thumb, which may strain or injure it. Likewise, the metacarpal joint or base of the thumb should never be fully extended and abducted—drawn backward and away from the index finger in the side splits—while applying pressure, as this could strain several thumb tendons, the extensor pollicis longus and brevis and abductor pollicis longus. Lastly, the thumb should never be used in isolation. It should always be stabilized, supported, and reinforced by bracing the other fingers against the body. (See Figures 9-26 to 9-28).

When using fists, the surface of the fist that makes contact when a punch is thrown is the same surface that contacts the client during fist compression: technically, the proximal phalanges, or base segment of the fingers (Figure 9-29). The practitioner's weight is distributed evenly on this surface. When using the knuckles, the fingertips are tucked under, and pressure is applied with the interphalangeal joints, the joints between the base and middle segments of the fingers. To increase strength and stability, the base segments of the fingers should be extended and aligned with the metacarpals (bones of the palm) so that the practitioner's weight is transferred in a straight line through the wrist to the interphalangeal joints during knuckle compression. (See Figure 9-30.)

The elbow should be used only on firm, fleshy muscles, such as the upper and middle trapezius (shoulders) and gluteals (hips). The elbow should never be used on bone or on an area where the flesh is thin. Pressure can be focused or diffused by

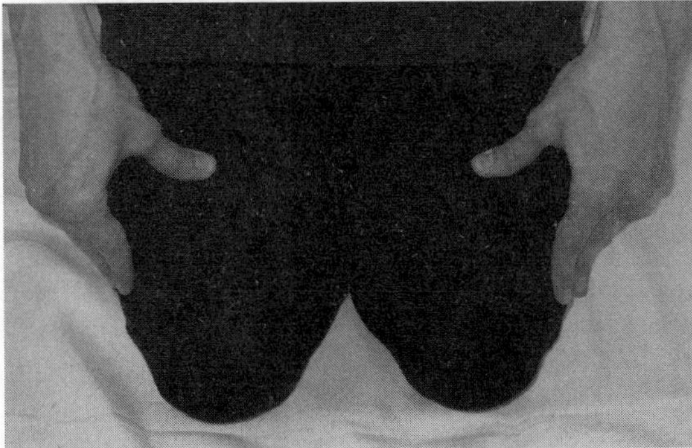

FIGURE 9-24 Thumb pads, correct. The thumb pads offer the best sensation for the client and are the safest for you to use.

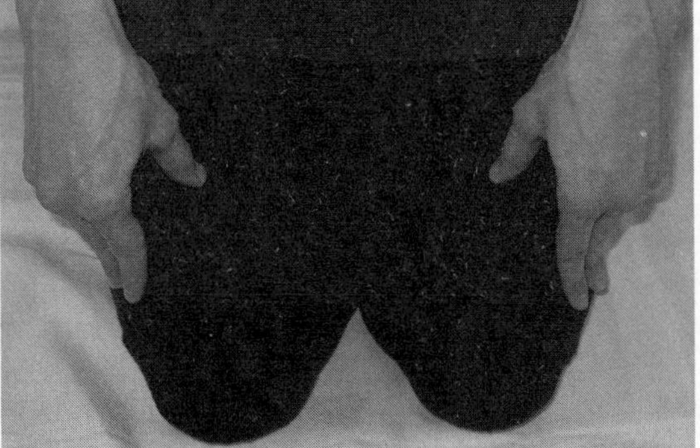

FIGURE 9-25 Thumb tips, incorrect. Because the thumb tips produce a sharp sensation and because the thumbnail may gouge, the tips should be reserved for certain points, such as LI 5, whose access or entry is too small for the thumb pad.

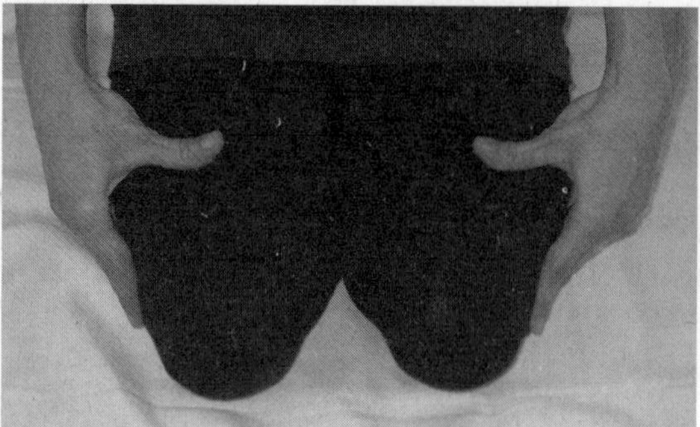

FIGURE 9-26 **Thumb joints, incorrect.**
Hyperextending the thumb should be avoided because it offers no mechanical advantage and risks straining the interphalangeal joint (the joint between the distal and proximal phalanges of the thumb).

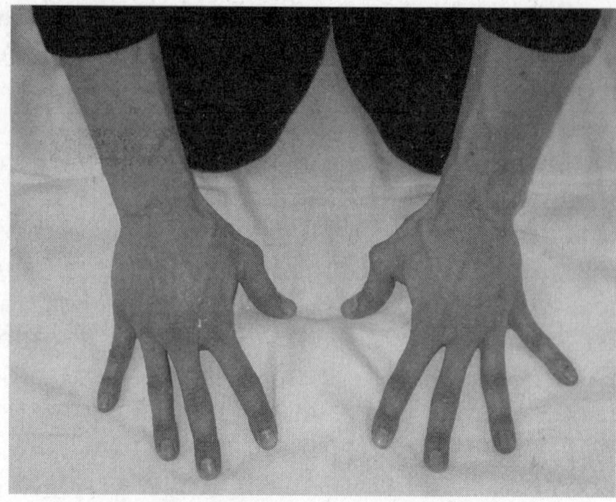

FIGURE 9-27 **Thumbs reinforced by fingers, correct.**
Whenever possible, the thumbs should be braced and reinforced with full finger contact on the client. Additionally, the thumbs should be as close to the index fingers as possible.

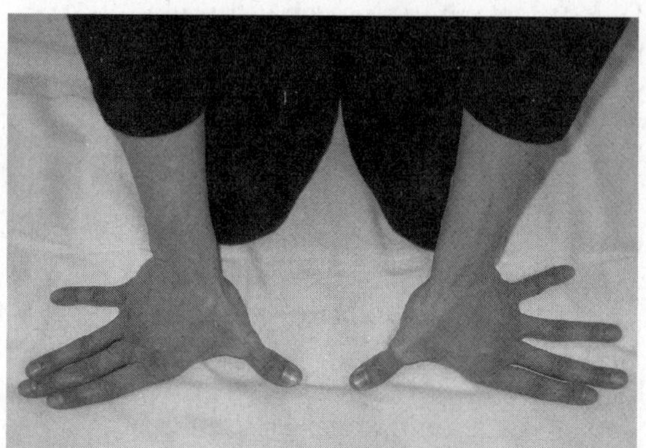

FIGURE 9-28 **Thumbs splayed, incorrect.**
Splaying the thumbs should be avoided because it offers no mechanical advantage and abducts the thumbs too far, increasing the risk of strain or injury.

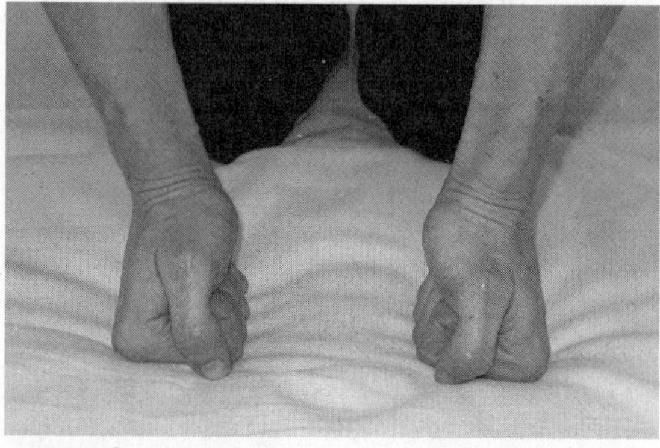

FIGURE 9-29 **Fists.**
The fingers are curled and tucked into the palm, and pressure is applied with the proximal phalanges—the base segments of the fingers.

decreasing or increasing the angle of the elbow. To soften and blunt the sharpness of the elbow tip for more diffused pressure, the practitioner extends the elbow, partially straightening the arm so that the elbow angle increases to greater than 90 degrees (Figure 9-31). To sharpen and intensify the elbow tip for more focused pressure, the practitioner flexes the elbow, bending the arm so that the elbow angle decreases to less than 90 degrees (Figure 9-32).

The knees should also be reserved for firm, fleshy muscles, such as the gluteals and hamstrings (back of the thighs). Like the elbows, the knees should never be used on bone or on an area where the flesh is thin. When using both knees, the practitioner should stabilize his or her own body by placing the hands and the balls of the feet on the floor beside the client. This prevents wobbling or slipping and controls the application of body weight. (See Figure 9-33.)

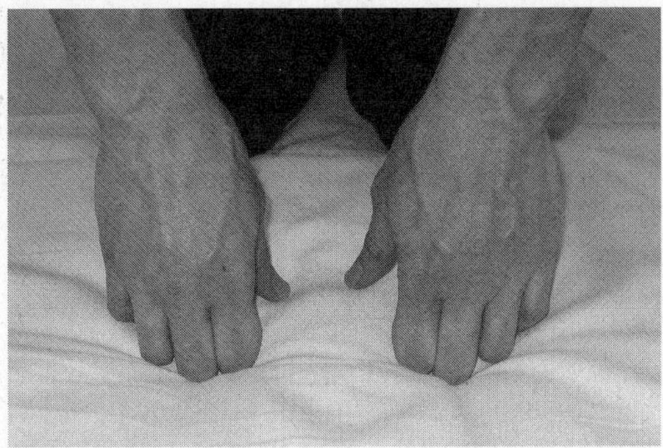

FIGURE 9-30 Knuckles.
The fingertips are curled under and pressure is applied with the interphalangeal joints between the base and middle finger segments. To increase strength and stability, the base segments of the fingers should be flush or level with the back of the hand so that weight is transferred in a straight line through the wrist to the interphalangeal joints.

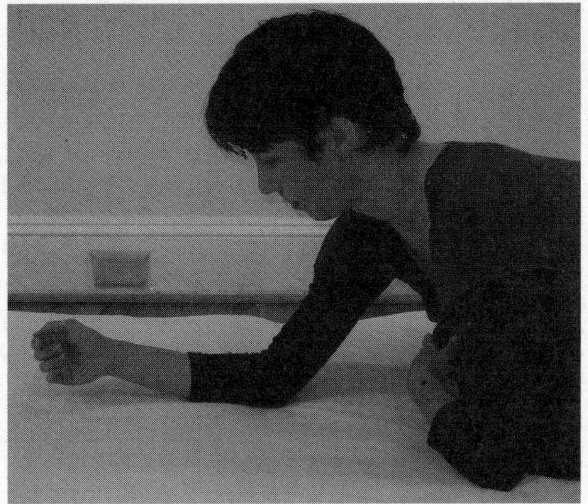

FIGURE 9-31 Elbow, blunt angle.
Extend the elbow joint and straighten the arm to reduce the intensity of elbow pressure. The elbow should be used only on thick, muscular surfaces, never on bony surfaces such as the sacrum or soft surfaces such as the abdomen.

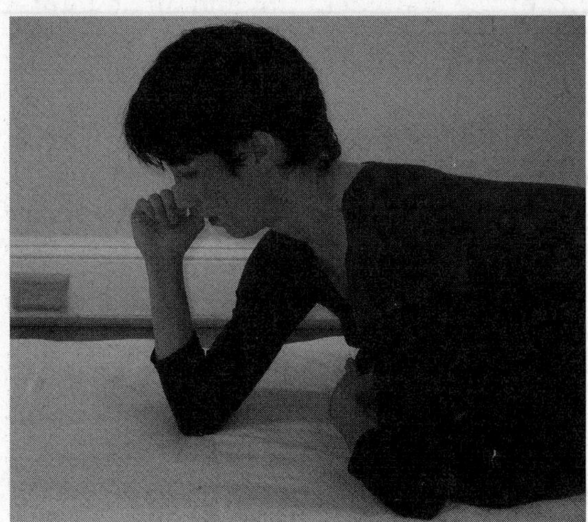

FIGURE 9-32 Elbow, sharp angle.
Flex the elbow joint and bend the arm to increase the intensity of elbow pressure. The elbow is typically used to disperse stagnation, often associated with excess muscle tension.

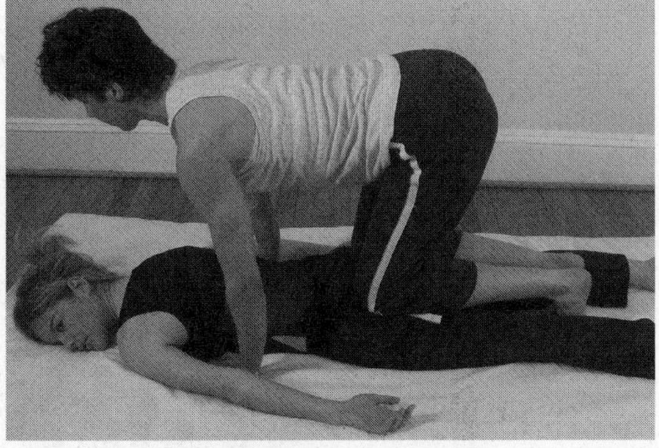

FIGURE 9-33 Knees.
When compressing the gluteals or hamstrings, you should stabilize yourself by placing your hands on the ground beside the client's torso and the balls of your feet between the client's legs. The knees should be used only on thick, muscular surfaces, never on bony or soft surfaces.

The feet should be reserved for the arches of the client's feet, upper shoulders, hips, and backs of legs. If the practitioner is standing while administering foot pressure, one foot or part of both feet should stay in touch with the ground for stability. The practitioner should never walk on the client unless he or she receives special training to do so. Different parts of the foot deliver varying intensities of pressure. The ball of the foot delivers the gentlest pressure; the side of the foot, firmer pressure; and the heel of the foot, the strongest pressure.

CLIENT POSITIONS

Practitioners must consider whether and for how long to place a client in the prone, supine, or sidelying position. Each position has advantages and disadvantages as to the accessibility of certain body parts and the comfort level of special populations. The **prone** or face down position is preferable for working the back, hips, and backs of the legs, which primarily correspond to the Bladder Meridian. However, the prone position may be uncomfortable and difficult to sustain for clients with neck or lower back problems, since the client must lie with the neck rotated for an extended period of time and the lordotic curve of the lower back is usually accentuated, increasing compressive strain. Additionally, the prone position may be uncomfortable for clients with large breasts, large bellies, or feet that flex but do not point. Ways to accommodate these clients include periodically rotating the head from side to side to prevent stiffness; placing a pillow under the abdomen to reduce lumbar lordosis, or swayback; placing a pillow or bolster under the ankles to reduce plantarflexion, or pointing of the feet; and spending less time in the position (Figure 9-34). The prone position is generally contraindicated for pregnant women during the second trimester because of maternal discomfort, but this caveat depends on how much the abdomen is protruding and the mother's subjective experience.

The **supine** or face up position is preferable for working the abdomen, chest, arms, and their corresponding Meridians—Lung, Pericardium, and Heart—and the front and inside of the legs and their corresponding Meridians—Stomach, Spleen, Liver, and Kidney. It is also the best position for facilitated stretches and body mobilization techniques, especially rotations of the shoulder, hip, and ankle joints. However, the supine position may become uncomfortable after awhile, especially for the sacrum, lower back, and knees. Ways to alleviate discomfort include using a thicker, more cushioned mat and placing a pillow or bolster under the knees to reduce sacral pressure, lumbar lordosis, hyperextension of the knees, and lateral rotation of the legs (Figure 9-35). The supine position is contraindicated for women in advanced stages of pregnancy because the weight of the fetus compresses the mother's inferior vena cava, restricting or blocking venous return to the heart.

The **sidelying** position is good for working the sides of the body, especially the outside of the torso and legs, which correspond to the Gallbladder Meridian, and the inside of the legs and the associated Spleen, Liver, and Kidney Meridians. However, the sidelying position can be quite demanding for the practitioner,

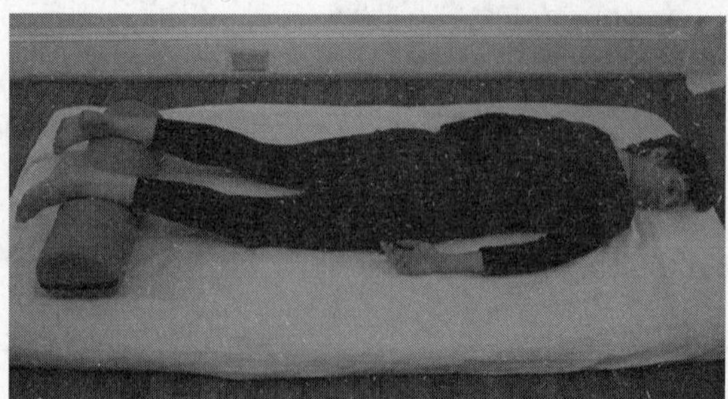

FIGURE 9-34 Prone position. Placing a bolster under the client's ankles reduces pressure on the dorsal surface of the feet and strain on the lower back. Additionally, a pillow may be placed under the abdomen to reduce lumbar lordosis/swayback (not shown).

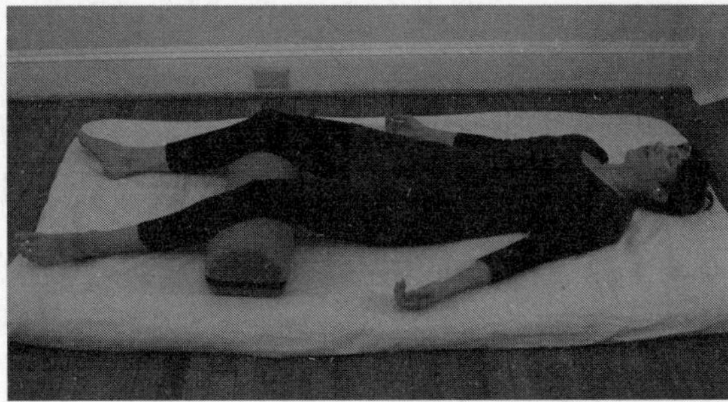

FIGURE 9-35 Supine position. Placing a bolster under the client's knees reduces pressure on the lower back and the backs of the knees and prevents the legs from rotating laterally (outward) too far.

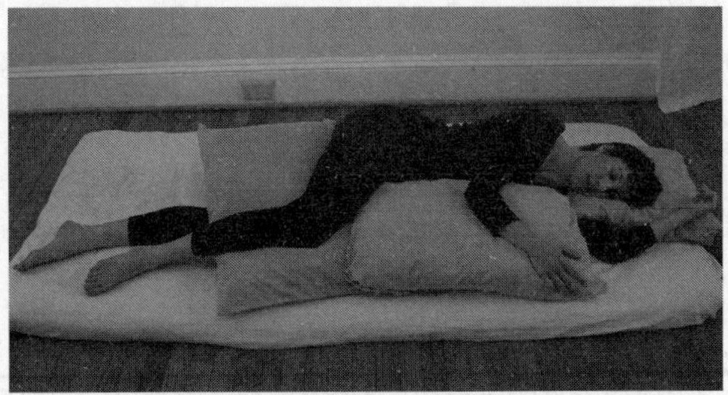

FIGURE 9-36 Sidelying position. Placing a pillow between the head and shoulder aligns the cervical vertebrae, and placing a pillow between the legs aligns the pelvis, stacking the hips. A pillow may also be placed under the uppermost arm for comfort and support.

requiring continual maneuvering and angling of position to treat body parts located in different planes. For example, in treating the back, the practitioner must apply pressure sideways without the assistance of gravity. Additionally, the sidelying position often requires the practitioner to support or stabilize the client with counterpressure. For example, since the client is stacked one shoulder on top of the other and one hip on top of the other—a somewhat precarious position—the practitioner must brace the client when applying pressure on the hips and back; otherwise, the client will collapse forward into a semiprone position. Finally, more props are needed in the sidelying position than any other. A pillow is placed under the client's head to maintain alignment of the cervical spine; another is placed under the uppermost leg to maintain alignment of the hips and pelvis, and another is placed under the uppermost arm for additional support and comfort, if desired (Figure 9-36). Sidelying is the primary position used for pregnant women and clients who find the other positions uncomfortable. It is also a pleasant variation on the standard prone and supine positions.

The seated position on the floor is a good option for a short session focusing on the upper shoulders and neck. However, it is not preferred for a number of reasons. First, the practitioner must actively support the client's body weight, which can be awkward and difficult if there is a disparity in size and shape between the practitioner and client and if the practitioner lacks agility. Second, in spite of this support, the client usually cannot relax as completely as he or she could in a recumbent position, since postural muscles must be engaged to maintain verticality. Third, sitting is a position that is overemphasized in modern living, in deskwork, transportation, and entertainment. Too much sitting can impair the function of the Stomach and Spleen Meridians, which are related to digestion and cognition (Gach, 1990). Nevertheless, the seated position may be an excellent alternative for someone who wants an abbreviated session to release shoulder and neck tension, clear the mind, energize, and uplift the emotions.

MERIDIAN STRETCHES, TRACTION, BMTS, AND FACILITATED STRETCHES

Meridian stretch positions are limb positions that raise a Meridian to the surface, stretch its associated muscles, and stimulate energy flow. The Bladder and Stomach Meridians require the practitioner to actively support and transport the leg into a passive stretch that must be held in midair with effort (a facilitated stretch). All other Meridians can be stretched more easily by placing the limb in the desired stretch position on the floor or across the body or by propping the limb so that it is relaxed but suspended. Shiatsu may then be given to the limb in the Meridian stretch position with no extra effort but with extra effect. (See Figures 9-37 to 9-55.)

Facilitated stretches are most effective and least painful or injurious if they are administered after compression techniques, which prepare the tissues for elastic tension by warming and loosening them and boosting blood, lymph, and Qi flow. The best progression for movement therapy in order of increasing complexity is traction, then joint mobilization, and finally facilitated stretch. Traction entails pulling on an extremity to decompress a joint that may have become compacted by the inexorable drag of gravity or poor posture. Joint mobilization entails gently swinging or rocking a joint or moving it through a partial or full range of motion, such as circumduction; this loosens the joint and promotes mobility. Facilitated stretching entails supporting a limb or body part and transporting it to its outermost

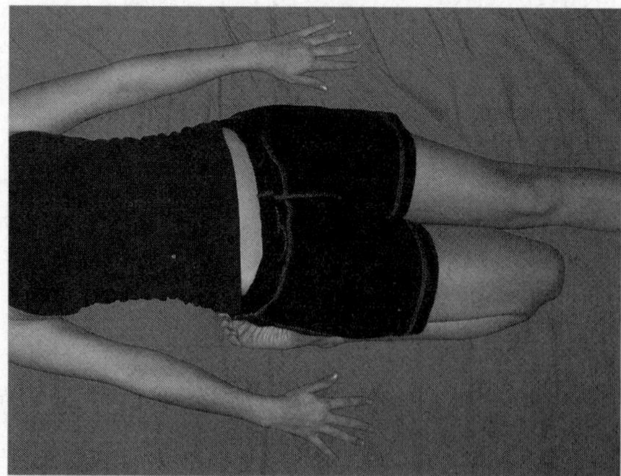

FIGURE 9-37 Stomach and Spleen Meridian stretch, supine.
This is the traditional passive Stomach and Spleen Meridian stretch position. Since few Westerners can rest comfortably in this position or receive Shiatsu while doing so, active stretches are used instead.

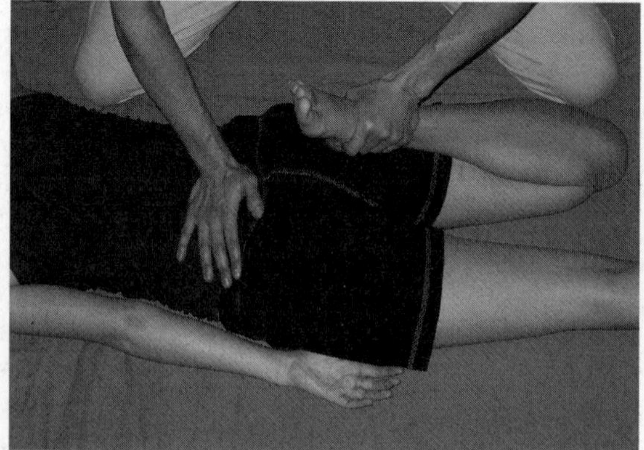

FIGURE 9-38 Stomach and Spleen Meridian stretch, prone.
Stabilize the low back and sacrum, and press client's heel toward the ischial tuberosity (sit bone). The Stomach and Spleen Meridians correspond to the quadriceps (front thigh). This is an active, facilitated stretch rather than a passive one.

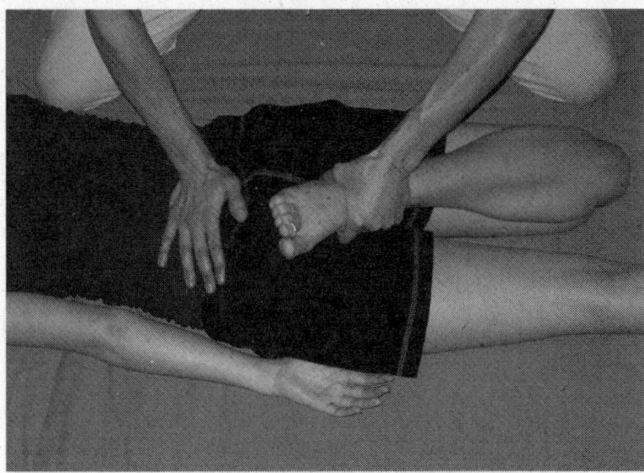

FIGURE 9-39 **Stomach Meridian stretch, prone.**
To emphasize the Stomach Meridian, draw the heel medially toward the coccyx. The Stomach Meridian roughly corresponds to the vastus lateralis or outer quadriceps.

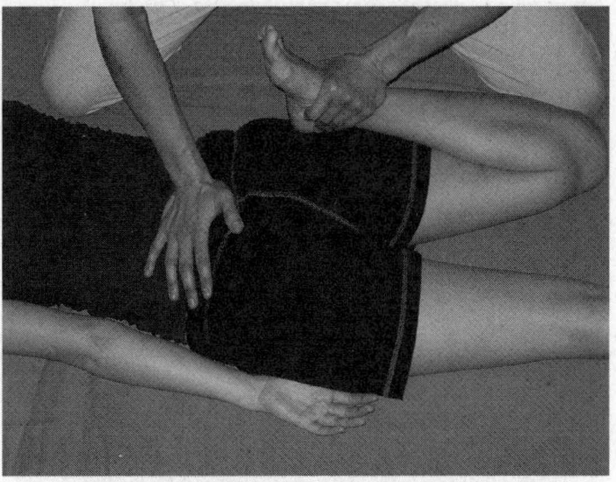

FIGURE 9-40 **Spleen Meridian stretch, prone.**
To emphasize the Spleen Meridian, draw the heel laterally toward the hipbone. The Spleen Meridian roughly corresponds to the vastus medialis or inner quadriceps.

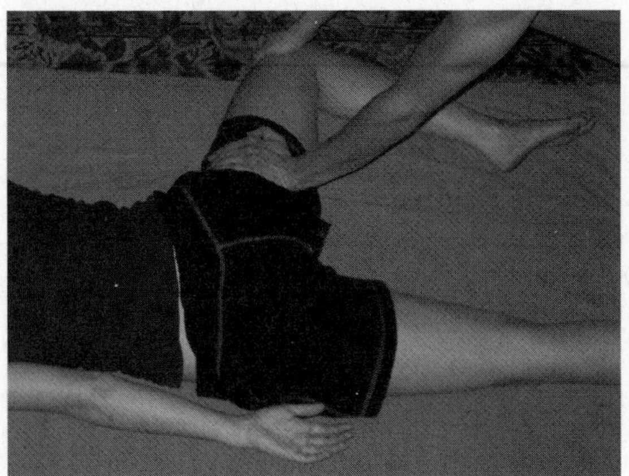

FIGURE 9-41 **Gallbladder Meridian stretch, prone.**
Bend the client's knee and rotate the leg outward. The Gallbladder Meridian roughly corresponds to the border between the iliotibial band and the biceps femoris (outer hamstring).

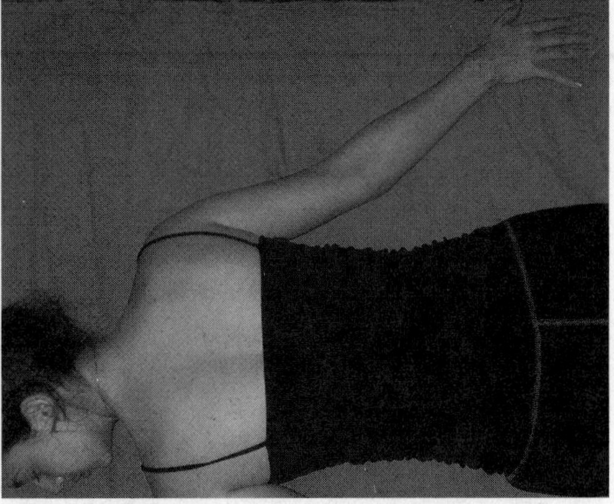

FIGURE 9-42 **Large Intestine Meridian stretch, prone.**
Set the arm, palm downward, about 45 degrees away from the body. The Large Intestine Meridian roughly corresponds to the division between the anterior and medial deltoids of the shoulder and the brachioradialis or radial surface of the posterior forearm.

range of motion so that the associated muscles are extended to their maximum length. Facilitated stretches are held for at least 10 seconds and may be repeated several times, as desired. These stretches release tension and energy stagnation or blockage (Lundberg, 1992).

Traction, BMTs, and facilitated stretches should be administered slowly, smoothly, and carefully. A conscientious, gingerly approach to stretching is advisable for several reasons. First, it enables the practitioner to gauge the condition

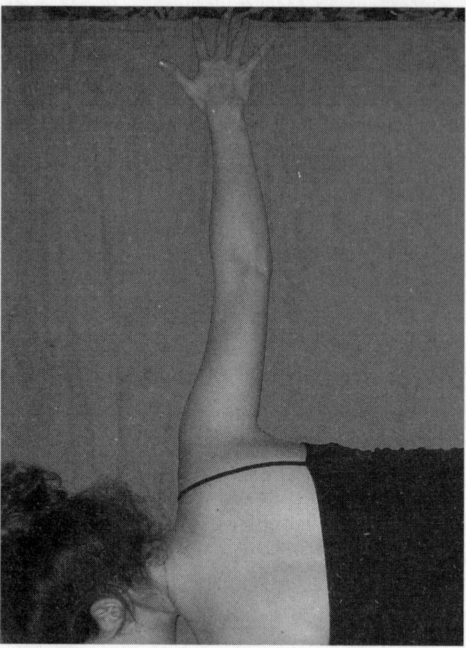

FIGURE 9-43 Triple Heater Meridian stretch, prone.
Set the arm, palm downward, 90 degrees away from the body. The Triple Heater Meridian roughly corresponds to the division between the medial and posterior deltoids of the shoulder, the lateral head of the triceps, and extensor digitorum or interosseus surface of the posterior forearm (between the radius and the ulna).

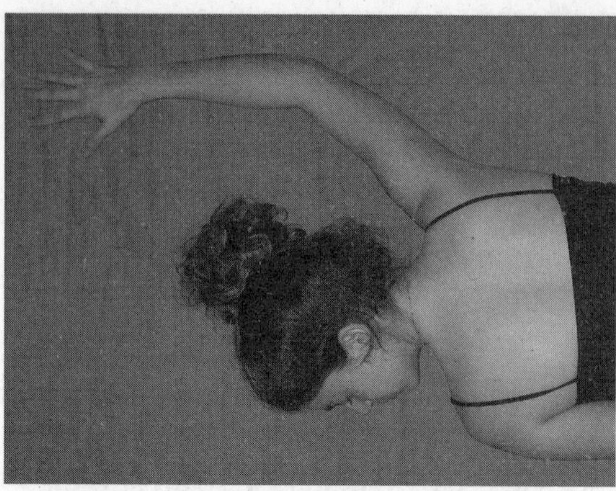

FIGURE 9-44 Small Intestine Meridian stretch, prone.
Set the arm, palm downward about 120 degrees away from the body. The Small Intestine Meridian roughly corresponds to the long head of the triceps and the extensor carpi ulnaris or ulnar surface of the posterior forearm.

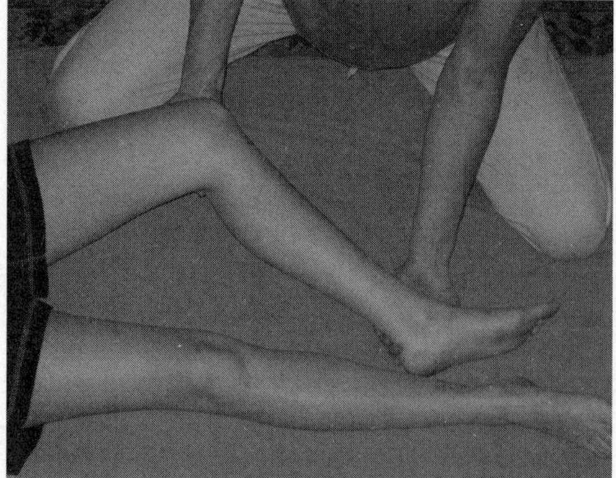

FIGURE 9-45 Spleen Meridian stretch, supine.
Bend the client's knee and laterally rotate the leg, placing the heel just above ankle level. The Spleen Meridian roughly corresponds to the vastus medialis or inner quadriceps. If the client's leg does not comfortably rest on the ground, support it under the knee with your hand or a pillow.

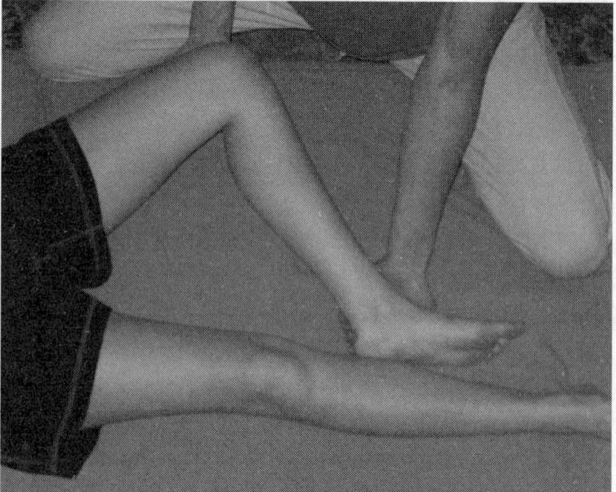

FIGURE 9-46 Liver Meridian stretch, supine.
Place the heel at calf level to expose more of the inner thigh. In the legs, the Liver Meridian roughly corresponds to the sartorius attachment at the inner knee and the adductor longus of the inner thigh.

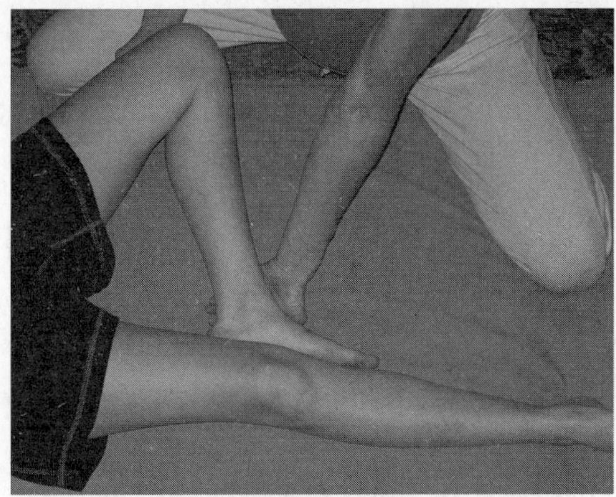

FIGURE 9-47 **Kidney Meridian stretch, supine.**
Place the heel at knee level to expose even more of the inner thigh. The Kidney Meridian roughly corresponds to the border between the gracilis and adductor magnus (deep adductors) and semimembranosus (inner hamstring). When working the Kidney Meridian near the groin, take care to avoid the genitals.

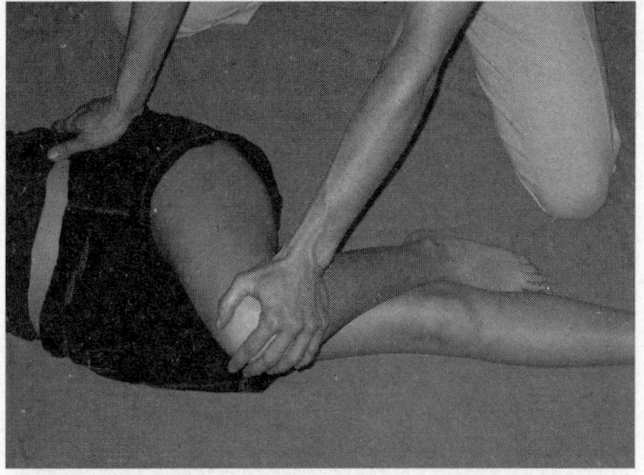

FIGURE 9-48 **Gallbladder Meridian stretch, supine.**
Rotate the leg medially. The Gallbladder Meridian roughly corresponds to the border between the iliotibial band and the biceps femoris (outer hamstring).

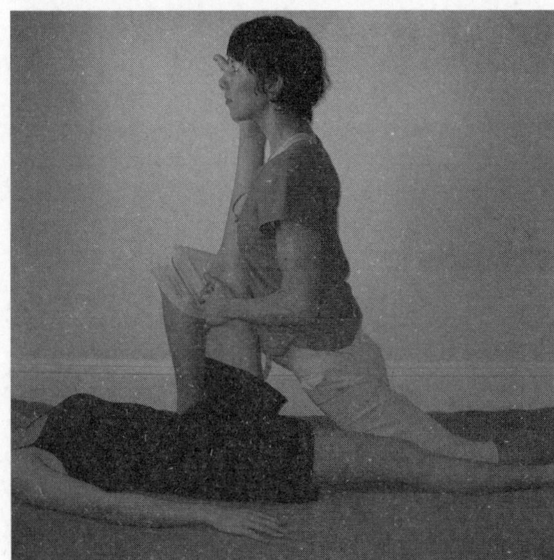

FIGURE 9-49 **Bladder Meridian stretch, supine.**
Like the Stomach and Spleen Meridians, the Bladder Meridian must be actively rather than passively stretched. The Bladder Meridian corresponds to the hamstring group (back of the thigh). Prop the ankle on the shoulder and brace the thigh above the knee.

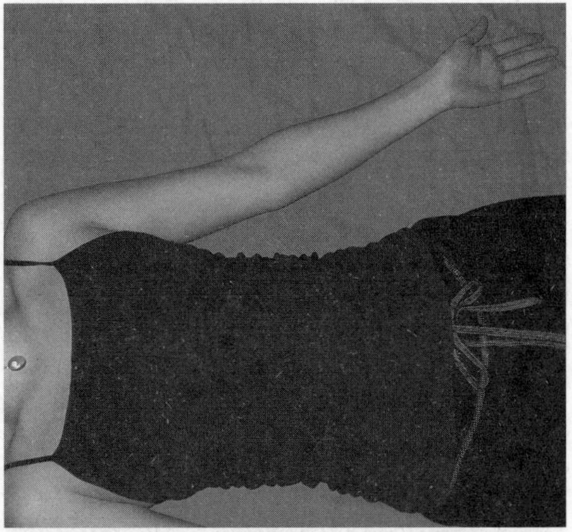

FIGURE 9-50 **Lung Meridian stretch, supine.**
Set the arm, palm upward, about 45 degrees away from the body. The Lung Meridian roughly corresponds to the long head of the biceps brachii and the flexor pollicis longus or radial surface of the anterior forearm.

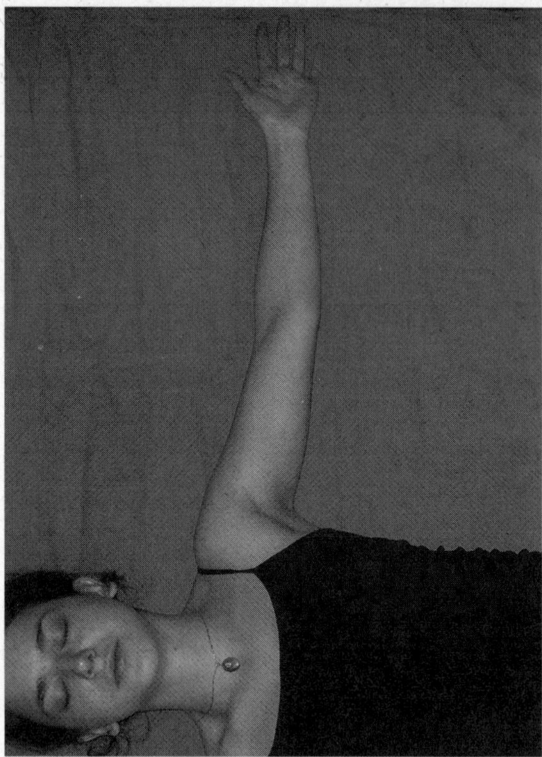

FIGURE 9-51 **Pericardium Meridian stretch, supine**
Set the arm, palm upward, 90 degrees away from the body. The Pericardium Meridian roughly corresponds to the division between the two heads of the biceps brachii and the flexor carpi radialis or the interosseus surface of the anterior forearm (between the radius and the ulna).

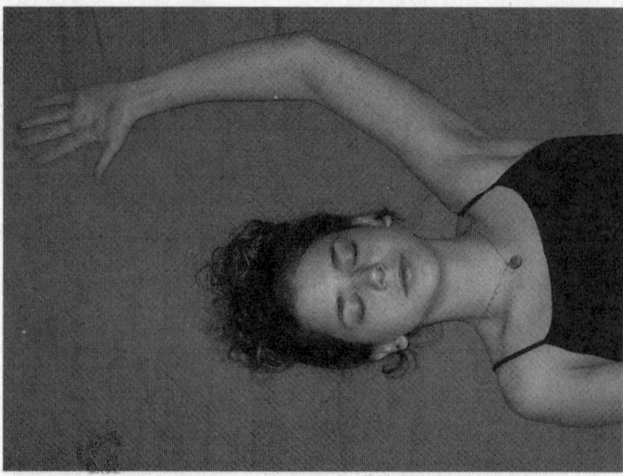

FIGURE 9-52 **Heart Meridian stretch, supine.**
Set the arm, palm upward, about 120 degrees away from the body. The Heart Meridian roughly corresponds to the short head of the biceps brachii and the flexor carpi ulnaris or the ulnar surface of the anterior forearm.

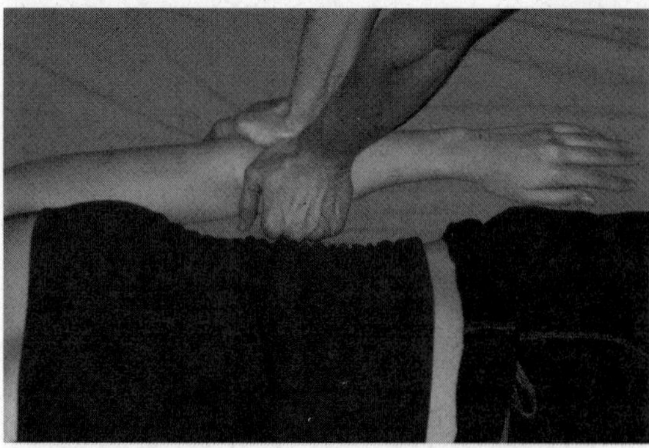

FIGURE 9-53 **Large Intestine Meridian stretch, supine.**
Set the arm, palm downward about 45 degrees away from the body. The Large Intestine Meridian roughly corresponds to the division between the anterior and medial deltoids and the brachioradialis or radial surface of the posterior forearm.

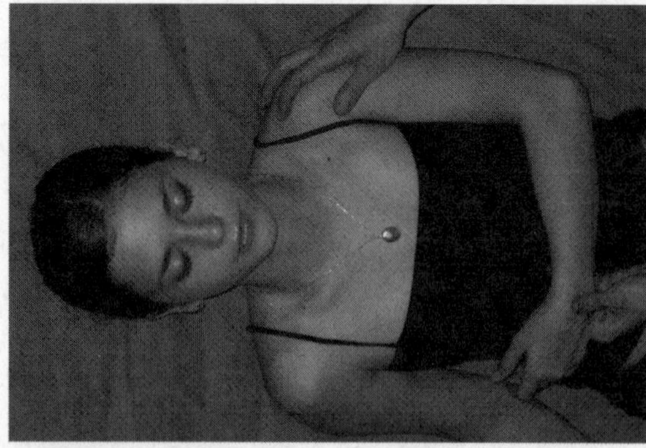

FIGURE 9-54 **Triple Heater Meridian stretch, supine.**
Place the arm, palm downward, across the torso. The Triple Heater Meridian roughly corresponds to the division between the medial and posterior deltoids of the shoulder, the lateral head of the triceps, and the extensor digitorum or interosseus surface of the posterior forearm (between the radius and the ulna).

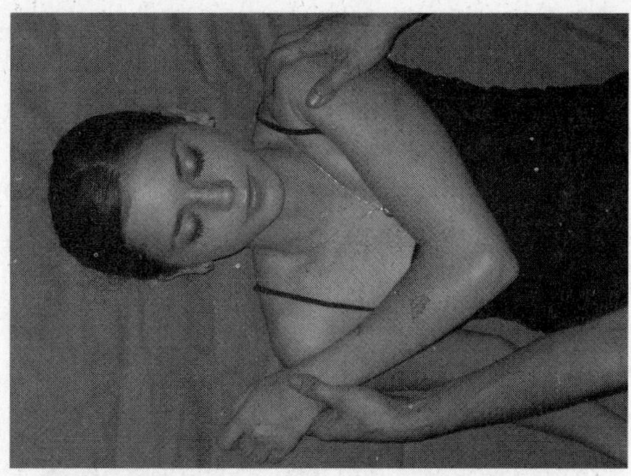

FIGURE 9-55 **Small Intestine Meridian stretch, supine.**
Place the arm palm downward, across the chest. The Small Intestine Meridian roughly corresponds to the long head of the triceps and the extensor carpi ulnaris or ulnar surface of the posterior forearm.

of the tissues and the quality of energy. For example, limpness, slackness, or laxity indicates a lack of muscle tone or deficient vital energy, while tension, tightness, stiffness, or rigidity indicates excess muscle tone or blocked energy (Lundberg, 1992). Second, it gives the tissues time to adapt to a new length, and third, it prevents pain or strain. The practitioner should never force, jerk, or bounce a stretch, as these maneuvers may result in injury.

REFERENCES

Badger, C. (1986). The swollen limb. *Nursing Times* (England), *82*(31), 40–41.

Beresford-Cooke, C. (2000). *Shiatsu theory and practice: A comprehensive text for the student and professional.* Edinburgh, Churchill Livingstone.

Brennan, M., & Weitz, J. (1992). Lymphedema 30 years after radical mastectomy. *American Journal of Physical Medical Rehabilitation, 71*, 12–14.

Bunce, I., Mirolo, B., Hennessy, J., et al. (1994). Post-mastectomy lymphedema treatment and measurement. *Medical Journal of Australia, 161*, 125–128.

Chamness, A. (1993). Massage therapy and persons living with cancer: Some basic information for the massage therapist. *Massage Therapy Journal, 32*(3), 53–54, 56–65.

Chow, K. T. (2002). *Thai Yoga massage: A dynamic therapy for physical well-being and spiritual energy*. Rochester, VT: Healing Arts Press.

Ferrell-Torry, A., & Glick, O. (1993). The use of therapeutic massage as a nursing intervention to modify anxiety and the perception of cancer pain. *Cancer Nursing, 16*(2), 93–101.

Gach, M. (1990). *Acupressure's potent points: A guide to self-care for common ailments.* New York: Bantam.

Jarmey, C., & Mojay, G. (1999). *Shiatsu: The complete guide* (Rev. ed.). London: Thorsons.

Junying, G., & Zhihong, S. (1997). *Practical Traditional Chinese Medicine & pharmacology: Acupuncture and moxibustion*. Beijing, New World Press.

Lundberg, P. (1992). *The book of Shiatsu: A complete guide to using hand pressure and gentle manipulation to improve your health, vitality, and stamina*. New York: Fireside.

MacDonald, G. (1995). Massage for cancer patients: A review of nursing research. *Massage Therapy Journal, 34*(3), 53–54, 56.

Masunaga, S., & Ohashi, W. (1997). *Zen Shiatsu: How to harmonize Yin and Yang for better health*. Tokyo: Japan Publications. (Original work published 1977).

McConnellogue, K. (2000). The courage of touch: Massage and cancer story. *Massage & Bodywork, 15*(6),12–16, 18–20.

Rados, C. (2005, March–April). Helpful treatments keep people with arthritis moving. *FDA Consumer Magazine*, Retrieved June 5, 2005, from http://www.fda.gov/fdac/features/2005/205_pain.html.

Stillerman, E. (1996). *MotherMassage: Massage during pregnancy*. Unpublished reference manual.

Stillerman, E. (2004, July 23–25). Lecture presented at a MotherMassage® workshop at the Cayce Reilly School of Massotherapy, Virginia Beach, Virginia.

Wilkinson, S. (1995). Aromatherapy and massage in palliative care. *International Journal of Palliative Nursing, 1*(1), 21–30.

Zanolla, R., Monzeglio, C., Balzarini, A., et al. (1984). Evaluation of the results of three different methods of postmastectomy lymphedema treatment. *Journal of Surgical Oncology, 26*, 210–213.

STUDY QUESTIONS

1. What is a contraindication?
2. To whom does the contraindication apply—the client or the practitioner or both?
3. Why is it important to avoid Shiatsu when there are contraindications?
4. Give a few examples of infectious or contagious illnesses that are contraindications.
5. Why might a practitioner still work on a client who has a skin disorder?
6. Give a few examples of skin disorders that are contraindications.
7. Apart from avoiding the site of a soft tissue injury or anomaly, what can a practitioner do to promote healing at the site?
8. Give a few examples of soft tissue maladies that are contraindications.
9. Apart from avoiding the site of a bone injury, what can a practitioner do to promote healing at the site?
10. What are the risk factors for cardiovascular disease?
11. How should one modify Shiatsu for a client who presents these risk factors?

12. Why is it dangerous to work on the site of phlebitis?
13. Can one still give Shiatsu to a client who has varicose veins?
14. Why should one avoid Shiatsu on an inflamed site?
15. Identify a few other conditions that are contraindications.
16. Is Shiatsu indicated or contraindicated for cancer patients?
17. Whose permission should one obtain before administering Shiatsu to a person diagnosed with cancer?
18. How should one modify Shiatsu for a cancer patient?
19. How should one modify Shiatsu for an elderly client?
20. What precaution should a practitioner take for a client who has osteoporosis?
21. What specific techniques should one avoid on an artificial joint?
22. What conditions of pregnancy are absolute contraindications for Shiatsu?
23. Which acupressure points are contraindicated during pregnancy and why?
24. On what areas of the body should one avoid deep pressure during pregnancy?
25. Which position usually becomes uncomfortable during the second trimester of pregnancy?
26. What kinds of clothes should a client wear for Shiatsu?
27. What is a healing response?
28. Identify a few signs of client toxicity that indicate the possibility of a healing response.
29. How long does a healing response typically last?
30. Identify a few symptoms of a healing response.
31. What can a client do to mitigate the effects of a healing response?
32. What features characterize a low center of gravity?
33. Why should a practitioner maintain a low center of gravity?
34. Which working positions have a low center of gravity?
35. What is the hara?
36. Which part of the practitioner's body should face the target area of work?
37. Why should one face one's work (what are the advantages)?

38. How can a practitioner gain leverage over a client?

39. Which part of the body should initiate movement and power—the hara or the extremities?

40. Why should one move from the hara (what are the advantages)?

41. At what angle should one apply pressure?

42. Why should one apply and release pressure gradually?

43. How long should one hold an acupressure point?

44. What principle of intention from the martial arts should one use to increase the effectiveness of pressure?

45. What principle of breath control from bodybuilding should one use to increase the effectiveness of pressure?

46. Why should one progress from general to specific or broad to sharp compression techniques?

47. Give a few examples of general versus specific compression techniques.

48. What is two-hand connectedness?

49. Describe the Mother/Son hand technique used in Zen Shiatsu.

50. The Mother/Son hand technique is particularly appropriate for what client conditions?

51. When is the two-handed compression preferable?

52. What part of the palm should contact the client?

53. What part of the thumb applies pressure?

54. How can one prevent strain to the thumb tendon?

55. How can one blunt the sharpness of the elbow tip?

56. How can one accentuate the sharpness of the elbow tip?

57. What parts of the body are suitable for elbow techniques?

58. What parts of the body are unsuitable for elbow techniques?

59. How should one stabilize oneself when using the knees?

60. What parts of the body are suitable for knee work?

61. What parts of the body are unsuitable for knee work?

62. What parts of the body are suitable for foot techniques?

63. Which Meridian is especially accessible in the prone position?

64. What client conditions make the prone position uncomfortable?

65. How can one improve client comfort in the prone position?

66. Which position is superior for facilitated stretches and BMTs?

67. Which Meridians are accessible in the supine position?

68. How can one improve client comfort in the supine position?

69. Why is the supine position contraindicated for women in advanced stages of pregnancy?

70. Which position is ideal for women at any stage of pregnancy?

71. Which Meridian is especially accessible in the sidelying position?

72. How can one improve client alignment and comfort in the sidelying position?

73. Should facilitated stretches be administered before or after compressions?

74. Describe how a facilitated stretch should be performed and what maneuvers should be avoided.

PRACTICE PRELIMINARIES TEST (35 POINTS)

SHORT ANSWER

1. What is a contraindication?____________

2. How can a practitioner promote healing at a site that cannot be worked because of a contraindication? ____________

3. Give an example of a cardiovascular contraindication that is local, not systemic. ____________

4. How should one modify a session for a cancer patient? ____________

5. How should one modify a session for an elderly client? ____________

6. On what area of a pregnant client's body should one abstain from applying heavy pressure? ____________

7. Identify one acupressure point that is contraindicated during pregnancy. ____________

MATCHING. LETTER MAY BE USED MORE THAN ONCE.

A. Low center of gravity
B. Hara
C. Leverage
D. General to specific

____**8.** Sink your body weight into the client rather than using muscle strength.

____**9.** Begin by applying broad, flat surfaces at medium pressure; end by applying focused, sharp surfaces at deeper pressure.

____**10.** Harness the power of gravity to minimize your effort.

____**11.** A solid, stable foundation; a bottom-heavy, broad base of support.

____**12.** Used to initiate movements.

____**13.** Examples include kneeling, kneeling lunge, and squat.

____**14.** Faces the target area of work.

MATCHING. LETTERS MAY BE USED MORE THAN ONCE.

A. Two-hand connectedness
B. Mother/Son hand technique
C. Two-handed compression

____**15.** The static hand holds the torso while the dynamic hand works the limb.

____**16.** Forms a closed circuit of vital energy between practitioner and client.

____**17.** Both hands are active, performing the same technique.

____**18.** Preferable when a stronger effect is desired.

____**19.** Preferable when the client is hypersensitive to touch.

TRUE OR FALSE. CIRCLE THE CORRECT ANSWER.

True False **20.** Apply pressure at a 45 degree (oblique) angle.

True False **21.** Apply and release pressure quickly with a pumping action as if performing CPR.

True False **22.** Inhale when applying pressure, and exhale when releasing pressure.

True False **23.** Use the pad, not the tip, of the thumb on easily accessible acupressure points.

True False **24.** Reserve the use of elbows and knees for firm, fleshy areas of the body.

True False **25.** Facilitated stretches are best applied before compression techniques.

True False **26.** To promote flexibility, swift thrusting stretches and rhythmically bouncing stretches are most effective.

MATCHING. LETTERS MAY BE USED MORE THAN ONCE.

A. Prone
B. Supine
C. Sidelying

____27. Best position for passive stretches and BMTs.

____28. May be uncomfortable after the first trimester of pregnancy or once the abdomen protrudes.

____29. Contraindicated in advanced stages of pregnancy.

____30. Suitable for any stage of pregnancy.

____31. Uncomfortable for clients with neck or lower back problems, large breasts, large abdomens, or tight ankles.

____32. Place a pillow under the head to keep the cervical spine (neck) in alignment with the rest of the spine.

____33. Improve client comfort by propping pillows under the uppermost arm and leg.

____34. Improve client comfort by periodically rotating the head from one side to the other and by propping a pillow under the abdomen and a bolster under the ankles.

____35. Improve client comfort by propping a bolster under the knees.

10

PRONE UPPER BODY PROTOCOL

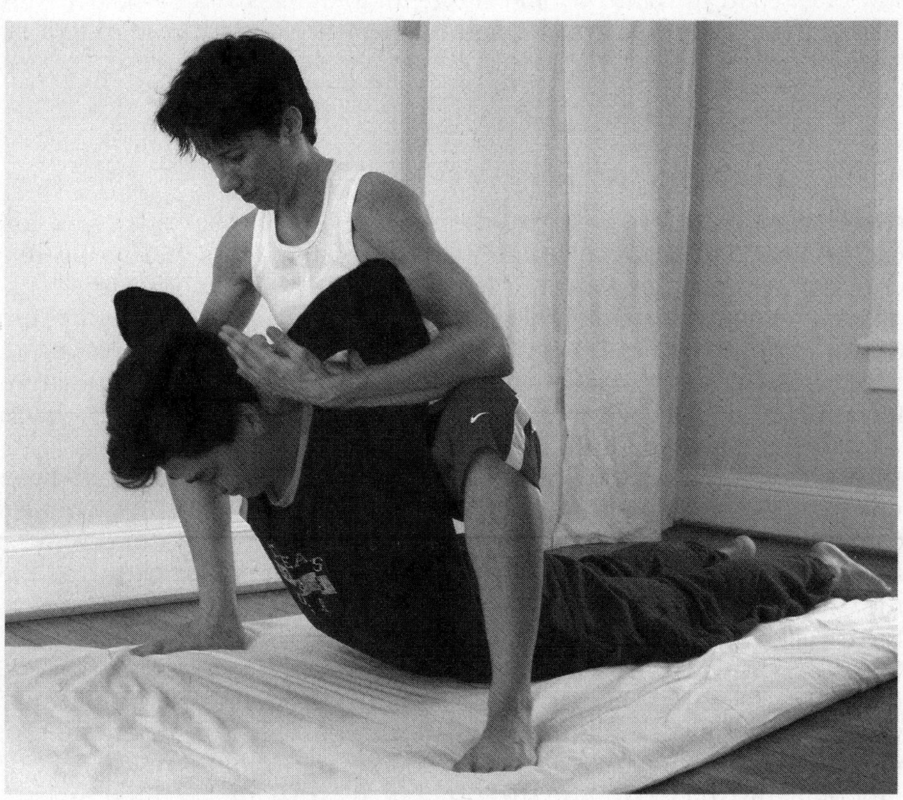

THERAPEUTIC EMPHASIS

The prone upper body protocol emphasizes the Yang Meridians of the arm—the Large Intestine (LI), Triple Heater (TH), and Small Intestine (SI) Meridians—as well as the inner and outer Bladder (Bl) Meridian of the back. Focused work on these Meridians and key acupressure points can benefit clients who have painful obstruction syndrome—localized muscular soreness and joint aches—in the back, shoulder, elbow, forearm, wrist, and hand; clients whose Meridians assess as Kyo or Jitsu or are otherwise symptomatic; and clients who present physical disorders or psychological disharmonies associated with the corresponding elements.

CAUSES OF DISCOMFORT AND TREATMENT STRATEGIES

A client can develop painful obstruction syndrome from hard manual labor, vigorous exercise, participation in sports events or performing arts, or any unaccustomed activity that subjects the body to a stress load to which it has not adapted. Even customary but prolonged low-load activities or repetitive low-load activities such as those required by most occupations can cause painful obstruction syndrome. To disperse blood and fluid stagnation, sore and fatigued muscles should be squeezed and rubbed. To clear blockages in energy flow, key acupressure points in the associated muscles should be pressed and held or pressed and subjected to friction. If soreness extends along the pathway of a Meridian, the entire Meridian should be given Shiatsu. The listed examples in the section below target isolated areas of the posterior upper body that can become sore and fatigued from exertion. For photos of point locations on a human model, see Appendix 1. For illustrated charts of Meridian locations, see the Flow of Qi chart in Figure 2-1 and "Posterior Meridians and Associated Musculature" on p. 205. For an illustrated chart of the Shu/Yu Bladder Meridian points, see Figure 7-6.

KEY ACUPRESSURE POINTS FOR THE POSTERIOR UPPER BODY

- **Outer Forearms:** The wrist extensor muscles on the back side of the forearm can become sore from wrist extension exercises, any activity that requires dexterity of the fingers—such as keyboarding, playing an instrument like the piano or guitar, and signing for the deaf—or any activity that requires moving or controlling a load with the wrist hyperextended—such as delivering a backhand stroke in tennis or racquetball. Give Shiatsu to the Yang Meridians of the forearm and acupressure to forearm points LI 11 and LI 10 and to hand and wrist points LI 4, LI 5, TH 4, TH 5, SI 5, and SI 3.
- **Outer Upper Arms:** The triceps can become sore from doing elbow extension exercises like dumbbell "kickbacks," barbell "nose bashers," cable pulls, dips, and push-ups; mowing a lawn; depressing an air pump; or pushing a disabled car. Give Shiatsu to the TH and SI Meridians, whose pathways traverse the tricep group, and acupressure to TH 13, TH 12, TH 11, and TH 10 to relieve the triceps.
- **Shoulder Stabilizers:** The rotator cuff is a group of small accessory muscles that assist in shoulder movements, stabilize the shoulder, and are easily strained, especially from lifting heavy weights or using a lot of force in shoulder movements. Give Shiatsu to the SI Meridian and acupressure to SI 12 on the supraspinatus and to SI 11 on the infraspinatus, two rotator cuff muscles.
- **Upper Shoulders:** The upper trapezius, levator scapulae, and supraspinatus (upper shoulder muscles) can become sore from doing exercises that elevate the shoulders and slightly abduct the arms like shoulder shrugs or from carrying hand luggage or suitcases through long airport terminals. Give acupressure to the upper trapezius (Bl 10, GB 20, and 21) and supraspinatus (SI 12).
- **Upper Shoulders and Side of Shoulders:** The upper trapezius, levator scapulae, supraspinatus, and deltoid (upper and outer shoulder muscles) can become sore from doing exercises that elevate the shoulders and fully abduct the arms like military presses or from engaging in manual labor like painting walls and ceilings, cleaning overhead light fixtures, and trimming high tree branches. Additionally, these muscles can become sore from service industry occupations that require lifting and holding the arms up—such as hairstyling, dental hygiene, stocking shelves, and scanning and bagging consumer products—and from office work—such as keyboarding and operating a mouse, especially on the dominant right side. Give Shiatsu to the LI and TH Meridians that traverse the deltoid and press acupressure points in the upper trapezius (Bl 10, GB 20, and GB 21), supraspinatus (SI 12), and deltoid (LI 14, LI 15, and TH 14) to relieve these muscles.
- **Back of Shoulders and Upper Back:** The posterior deltoid (outer rear shoulder muscle), middle trapezius, and rhomboids (between the shoulder blades) can become sore from shoulder retraction and arm extension exercises

like rowing, as well as from raking, and uprooting unwanted vegetation. Give acupressure to the posterior deltoid (SI 10), middle trapezius, and rhomboids (Bl 11–14 and Bl 41–43) to relieve these muscles.

- **Middle and Lower Back:** The lower trapezius, latissimus dorsi (middle to lower back muscles) and teres major (posterior armpit muscle) can become sore from doing shoulder depression exercises like pull-ups or cable pull-downs, from rock or pole climbing, swimming, and chopping with an ax. Give acupressure to points in the teres major (SI 9), lower trapezius (Bl 15–20 and Bl 44–49), and latissimus dorsi (Bl 16–25 and Bl 45–52) to relieve these muscles.
- **Lower Back:** The erector spinae (a group of postural muscles that support the spinal column) and quadratus lumborum (a lower back muscle) can become sore from doing spinal extension exercises like leg, arm, and torso raises in the prone or crawl position and from working in a bent or stooped posture to clean floors, garden, or wash a vehicle. The lower back can also feel strained from excessive sitting. Give Shiatsu to the inner and outer Bladder Meridians and acupressure to key points on the erector spinae and quadratus lumborum (Bl 21–25 and Bl 51, 52) to relieve these muscles.
- **Here are the key acupressure points in various locations:**
  Hand: LI 4, SI 3
  Wrist: LI 5, SI 5, TH 4, TH 5
  Forearm: LI 10, LI 11
  Elbow: TH 10, SI 8
  Shoulder: GB 21, LI 14, LI 15, TH 14, SI 9, SI 10, SI 11, SI 12
  Neck: Bl 10, GB 20
  Upper back: Bl 11–14 and Bl 41–43
  Middle back: Bl 15–20 and Bl 44–49
  Lower back: Bl 21–25 and Bl 51, 52

Kyo Jitsu Imbalances

A client with a Meridian that is demonstrably Kyo (empty and deficient) or Jitsu (full and excessive) should be given Shiatsu to the Meridian. To assess the Yang Meridians of the arm in the prone position, place the arm, palm down, at a 45 degree angle from the body for the Large Intestine Meridian, at a 90 degree angle for the Triple Heater Meridian, and at a 120 degree angle for the Small Intestine Meridian (see the discussion of Meridian stretches in Chapter 9). Unlike the Yang Meridians of the arm, the Bladder Meridian of the back does not have a stretch position. Facilitated spinal flexion or forward bending is necessary to stretch the Bladder Meridian of the back.

Palpate along the Meridian, feeling the quality of the tissues and the quality of energy (see “Qualities of Kyo and Jitsu” and “Meridian Diagnosis” in Chapter 6). Tissues in a Jitsu Meridian feel firm and toned or even hypertonic (tense), whereas tissues in a Kyo Meridian feel limp and flaccid (soft and flabby) or, conversely, hard and tough. Additionally, Jitsu tissues may feel warm or hot to the touch and may look red, in contrast with Kyo tissues, which may feel cool or cold and may look pale. A Jitsu Meridian feels firm, lively, and buoyant to the touch, but a Kyo Meridian feels recessive, void, or shut. Kyo in the Bladder Meridian can make the back unnaturally rigid and impenetrable like a wooden board or coat of armor. When the back is hard from Kyo, the tissues do not yield when pressed and the torso does not sway when rocked.

Pressure on Jitsu tends to elicit a sharp or painful sensation that subsides with continued therapy. Pressure on Jitsu may also elicit a jump response like a muscle twitch or a startle response like a jerk. However, because Jitsu is reactive and volatile, it also relaxes quickly. By contrast, Kyo is relatively impassive (nonresponsive). Pressure on Kyo tends to elicit a soothing, dull sensation that satisfies a deep ache or no sensation at all. Unlike Jitsu, pressure on Kyo does not initiate immediate change. Kyo tissues tend to feel inert, requiring prolonged holding, like a block of ice that needs to thaw.

To sedate a Jitsu Meridian, apply stimulating techniques to disperse stagnation and congestion and to release blocked Qi (see "Application of Techniques" and Table 6-1 in Chapter 6). Two-handed compression can be used to cover more surface area and to intensify the effect. Compression along the Meridian should be moderate to deep, fairly brisk, and rhythmic, following a downward and outward direction or countercurrent to the flow of the Meridian (see "Direction of Movement" in Chapter 6). Additionally, kenbiki (jostling, torsion wringing, and cross-fiber friction) and tapotement (pummeling) can be applied. Specific Jitsu dispersal techniques include the traveling fist twist, S-move with wriggling thumbs, prayer elbows, and side of the hand squeeze down the Bladder Meridian.

To tonify a Kyo Meridian, apply nurturing techniques to draw and gather Qi to the area of deficiency (see "Application of Techniques" and Table 6–1 in Chapter 6). The Mother/Son hand technique may be used when the arms present signs of deficiency—lack of tone, emaciation, weakness, coldness, or edema (fluid retention)—or are too hyperirritable for Jitsu dispersal techniques. Place the Mother hand like a warm compress on a deficient area like Bl 13 (Lung Shu/Yu point), Bl 15 (Heart Shu/Yu point), Bl 20 (Spleen Shu/Yu point), Bl 23 (Kidney Shu/Yu point), or GV 4 (Source Qi point), or use the Mother hand to hold a key acupressure point, such as LI 4, TH 4, or SI 3, while the Son hand presses the length of the Meridian (see Practice Exercise 6-1). Pressure should be light to moderate and fairly slow and steady, following an upward and inward direction or concurrent with the flow of the Meridian (see "Direction of Movement" in Chapter 6).

Certain activities, if done habitually on a long-term basis or to excess on a short-term basis, such as standing, sitting, or lying down, can tax a Meridian, leading to an energetic imbalance in the Meridian (Gach, 1990). Prolonged standing, required by some occupations, strains the Bladder and Kidney Meridians, leading to lumbago and weariness, while prolonged lying down, as when convalescing from an injury or illness, strains the Large Intestine and Lung Meridians, adversely affecting breathing and bowel movements. Give Shiatsu to these Meridians.

ELEMENT TYPE IMBALANCES

Clients who present a constellation of physical disorders or psychological disharmonies associated with a particular element should be given Shiatsu to the Yang and Yin Meridians of that element. The Large Intestine Meridian is associated with the Metal element type and the Lung and Large Intestine organ functions. The Triple Heater and Small Intestine Meridians are associated with the Fire element type and the Heart, Pericardium, Triple Heater, and Small Intestine organ functions. The Bladder Meridian is associated with the Water element type and the Kidney and Bladder organ functions.

For a profile on the element types, see Chapter 4, and for a description of element imbalances, see Chapter 5. Additionally, Table 4-1 summarizes correspondences for each of the Five Elements, Table 7-4 summarizes physical disorders associated with each element's organ pair; and Table 7-5 summarizes psychological disharmonies associated with each element.

SHU/YU POINTS

The prone upper body protocol is unique among protocols in that the whole body and psyche can be positively influenced by pressing the points along the inner and outer Bladder Meridians of the back (for further explanation, see "Nerve Reflex Arc Theory", "Relaxation Response Theory", and "Posterior/Anterior Point Combinations" in Chapter 7). Points along the inner Bladder Meridian correspond to various organ functions, while points along the outer Bladder Meridian correspond to the psychological capacities of the organs (for a list of inner Bladder Meridian Shu/Yu points associated with organ ailments, see Table 7-4; for a list of outer Bladder Meridian points associated with psychological imbalances, see Table 7-5; for an illustrated chart of Shu/Yu points, see Figure 7-6). Shiatsu to the inner Bladder Meridian stimulates, soothes, and harmonizes organ function, while Shiatsu to the outer Bladder Meridian calms, clarifies, and uplifts the mind and emotions. Aside from giving Shiatsu to

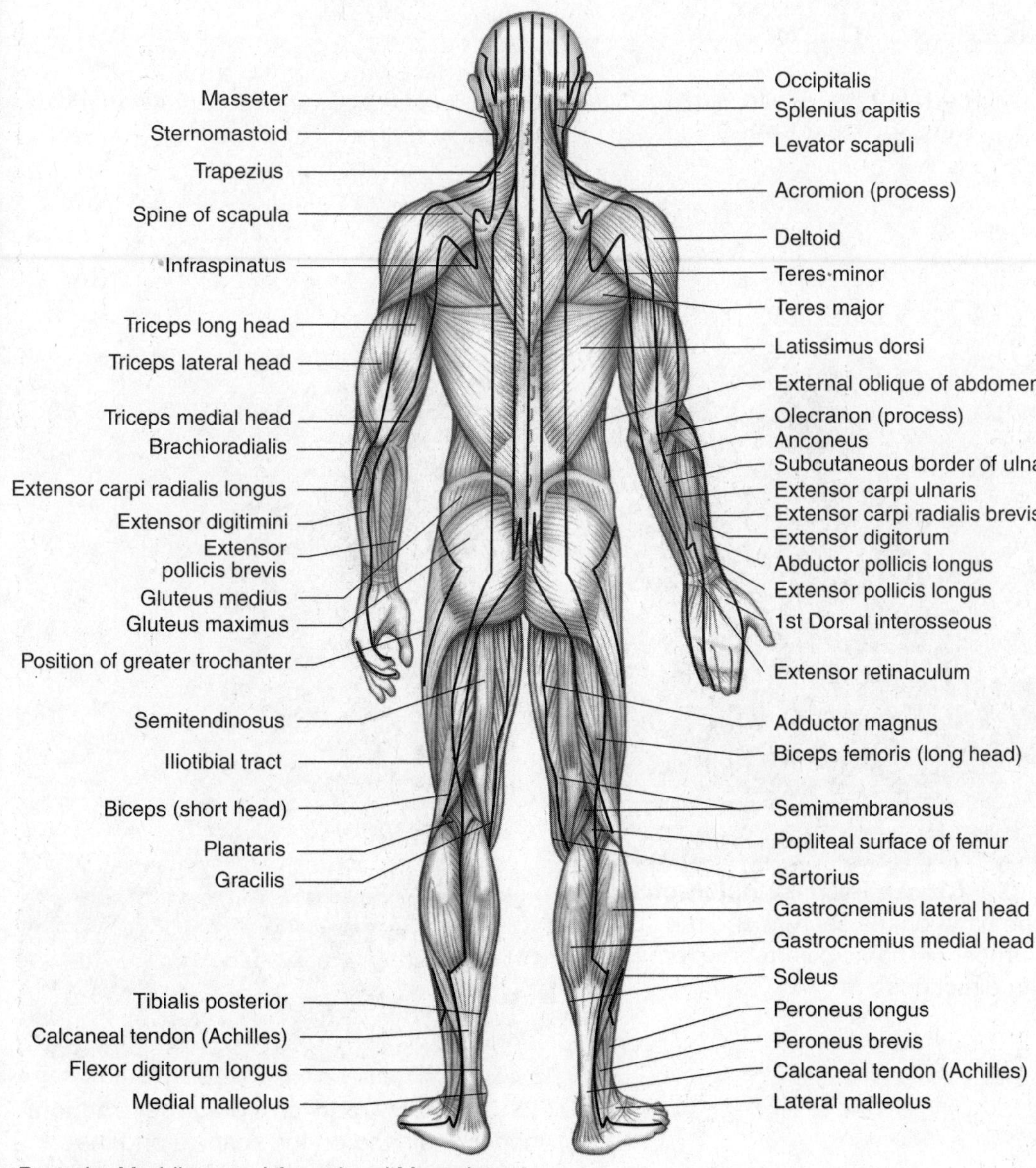

Posterior Meridians and Associated Musculature. (See Color Plate 5.)

all the Bladder Meridian points to revitalize the client, certain points on the inner Bladder Meridian can be emphasized if the client presents a physical disorder associated with an organ imbalance. Similarly, certain points on the outer Bladder Meridian can be emphasized if the client presents psychological distress associated with an organ disharmony. Because of its salubrious effect on the body-mind, Shiatsu to the back is included in every session and should be considered central to the practice.

CLIENT COMFORT

To increase client comfort, place a pillow under the abdomen and a bolster under the ankles, and remind the client to rotate the neck periodically to avoid stiffness. When working only one shoulder, direct the client to rotate the head in the opposite direction to open the shoulder and to avoid inadvertent contact with the face while working the shoulder.

REFERENCE

Gach, M. (1990). *Acupressure's potent points: A guide to self-care for common ailments.* New York: Bantam.

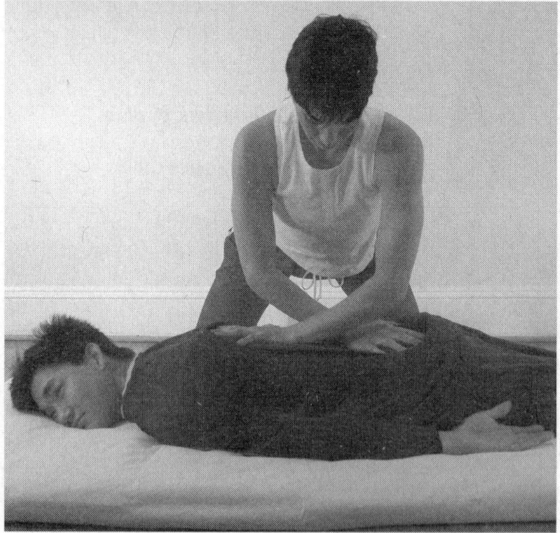

FIGURE 10-1 **Crossed-arm spinal traction.** Anchor one hand on the sacrum and the other on lumbar or thoracic vertebrae; press in opposite directions.

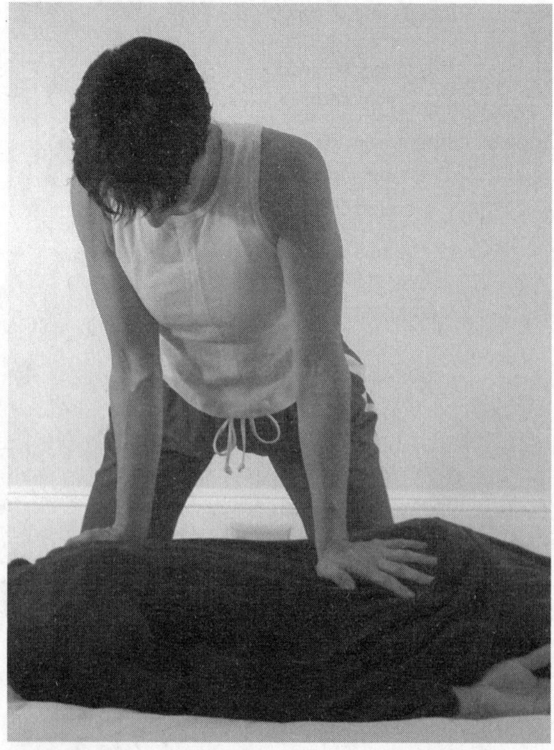

FIGURE 10-2 **Open-arm diagonal traction.** Anchor one hand on the scapula and the other on the pelvic crest; press in opposite directions.

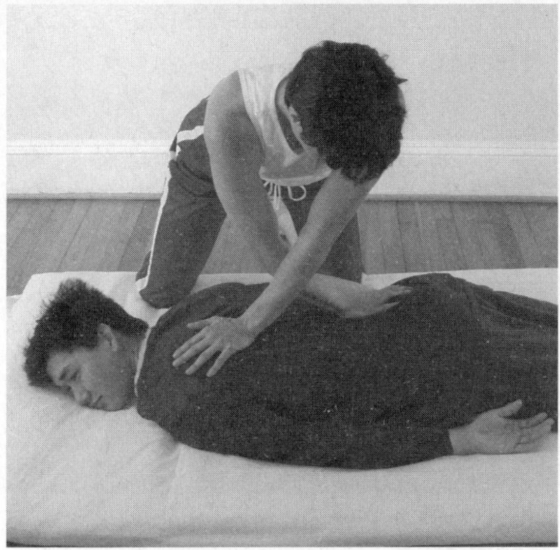

FIGURE 10-3 **Crossed-arm diagonal traction (variation).**
Anchor one hand on the scapula and the other on the pelvic crest; press in opposite directions.

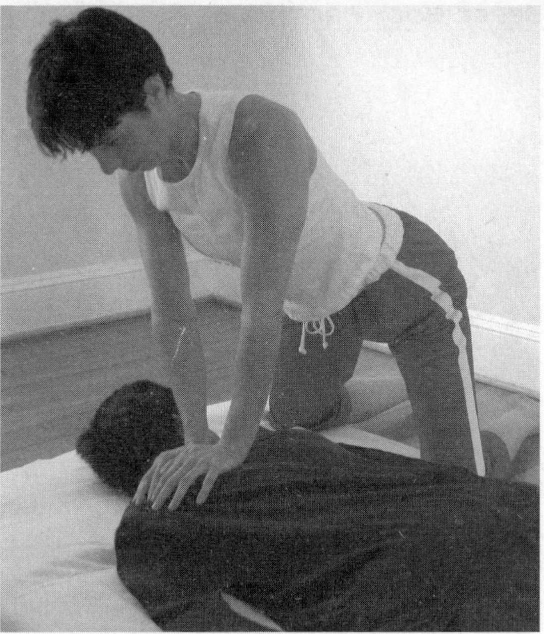

FIGURE 10-4 **Kenbiki with the heels of the hands.**
Plant the heels of your hands on the opposite side of the spine, covering the inner Bladder Meridian and possibly the outer Bladder Meridian (coverage depends on how wide the client's back is and how large your hands are). Press and rock down the Bladder Meridian. The client's body should undulate from the jostling.

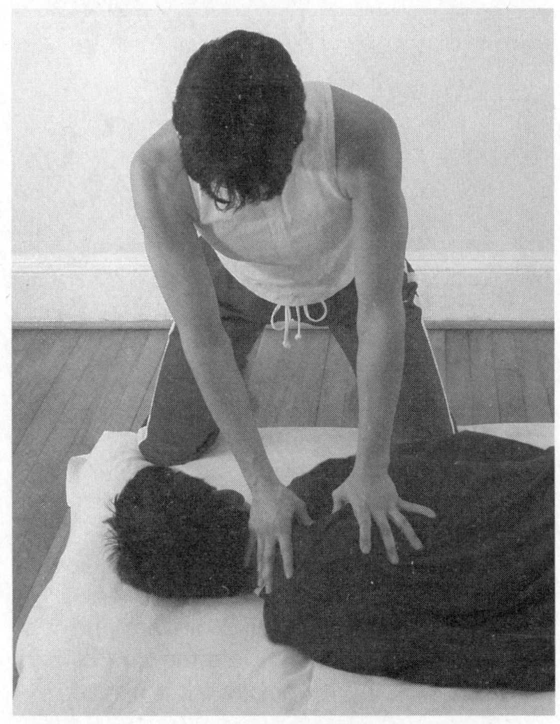

FIGURE 10-5 **Kenbiki with the thumbs.**
Plant your thumbs on the opposite side of the spine on the inner Bladder Meridian; press and rock, scooting down the Bladder Meridian. The client's body should undulate from the jostling.

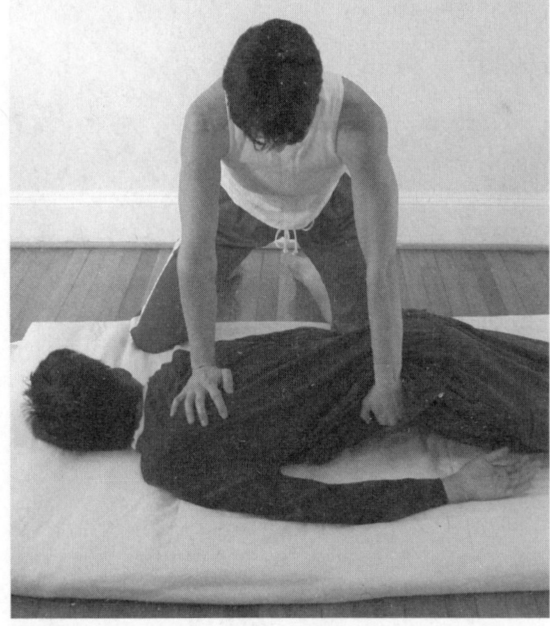

FIGURE 10-6 **Torso torsion.**
Plant one hand on the upper Bladder Meridian and scoop the other under the hip. Press down on the Bladder Meridian with the upper hand and pull up on the hip with the lower hand. Repeat several times, moving down the Bladder Meridian with the upper hand. Repeat Figures 10–4 through 10–6 on the other side.

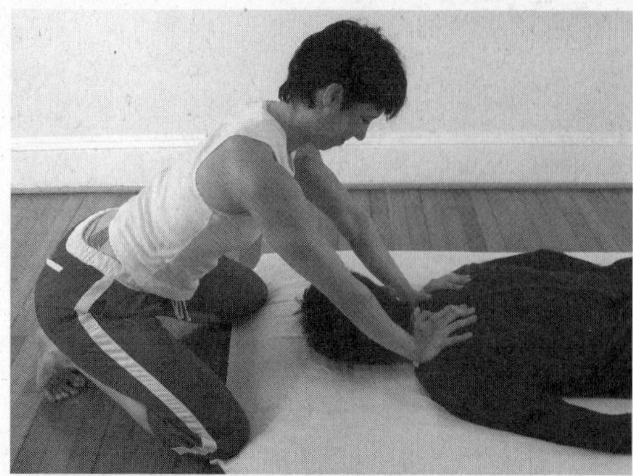

FIGURE 10-7 Palm press on the shoulders.
Variation: Alternate pressing with the left and right hands to create a seesaw motion of the upper shoulders.

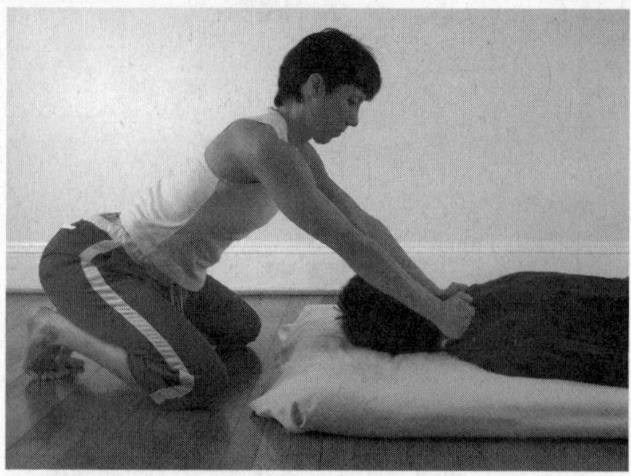

FIGURE 10-8 Fist press on the shoulders.
Variation 1: Alternate pressing with the left and right hands.
Variation 2: Simultaneously press and torque (fist twist).

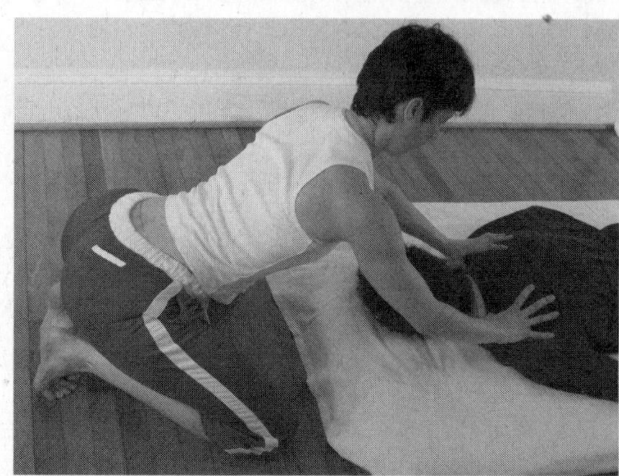

FIGURE 10-9 Thumb press on the shoulders.
Variation: Press and rock; hold GB 21.

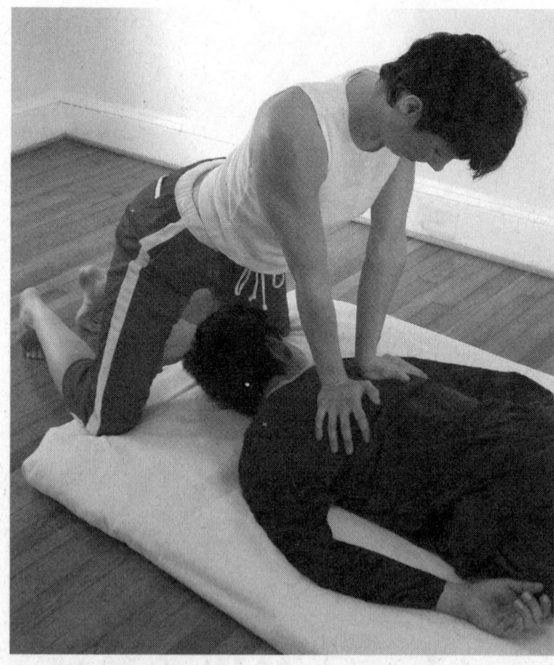

FIGURE 10-10 Palm press down the Bladder Meridian.
Shift the weight of your hips forward and press straight down; straddle the client's head to reach the lower back, if possible.

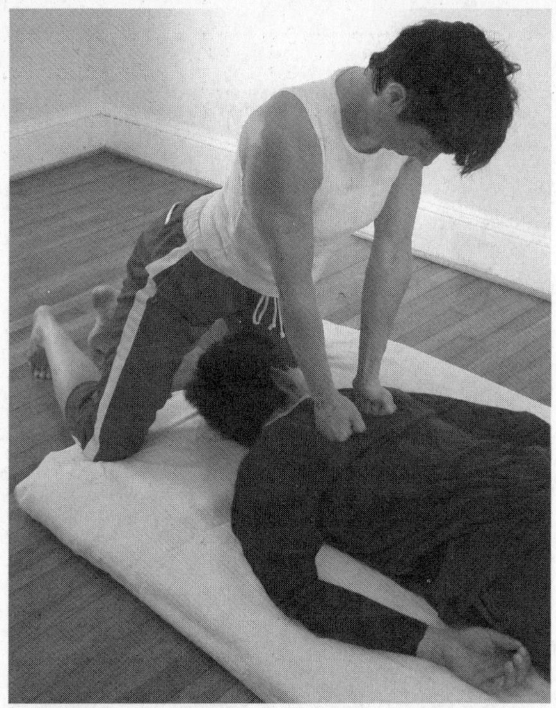

FIGURE 10-11 Fist press down the Bladder Meridian.
Wrists should face one another; shift the weight of your hips forward and press straight down; straddle the client's head to reach the lower back, if possible.

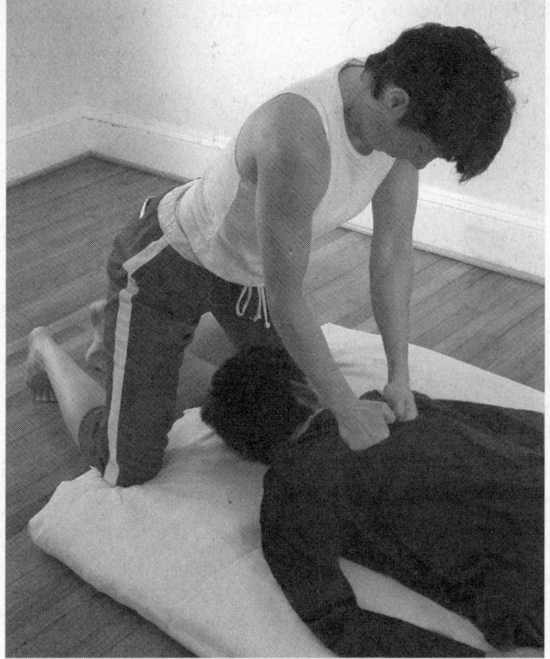

FIGURE 10-12 Fist twist down the Bladder Meridian.
With pronated forearms, sink and hook your fists into the muscle belly; then torque outward (supinate the forearms).

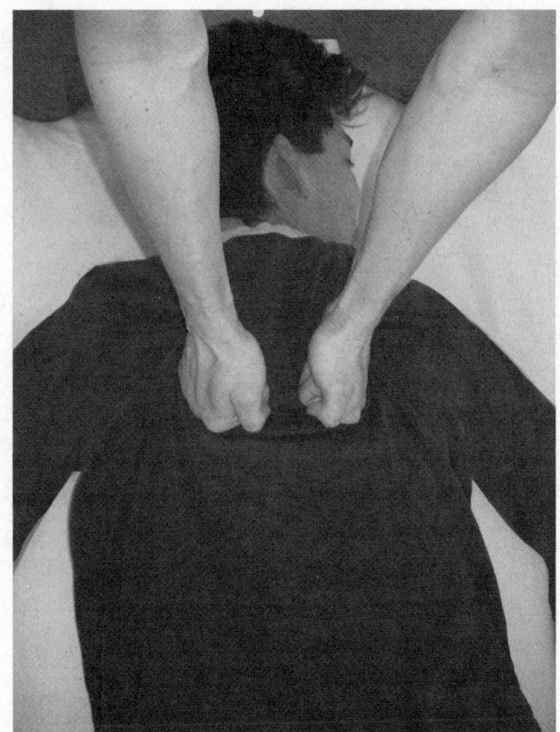

FIGURE 10-13 Close-up of fist twist.
You should feel your fists wringing the muscle, and the client's clothing should spiral. This friction technique disperses stagnation.

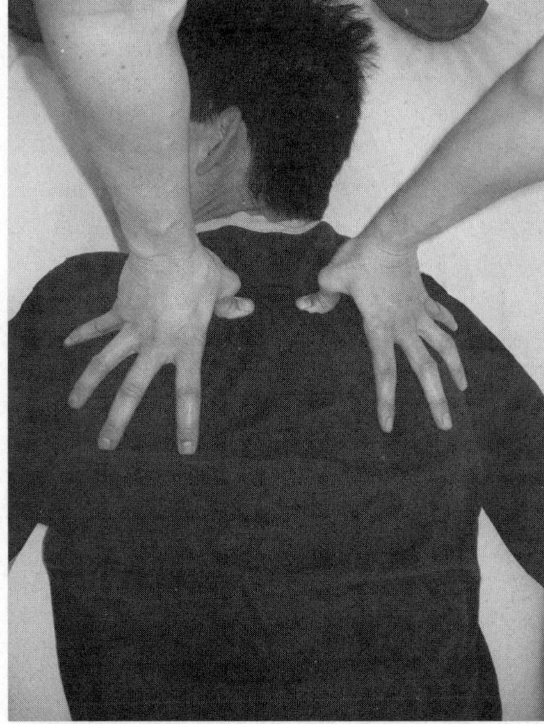

FIGURE 10-14 Thumb press down the inner Bladder Meridian.
This technique benefits the organs via associated acupoints (Shu/Yu points).

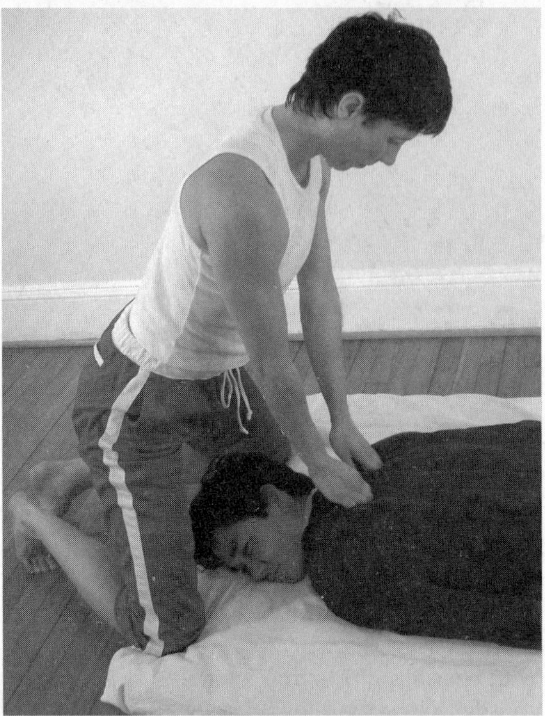

FIGURE 10-15 Knuckle press down the inner Bladder Meridian.
This can be done in addition to, or instead of, the thumb press (to spare the thumbs).

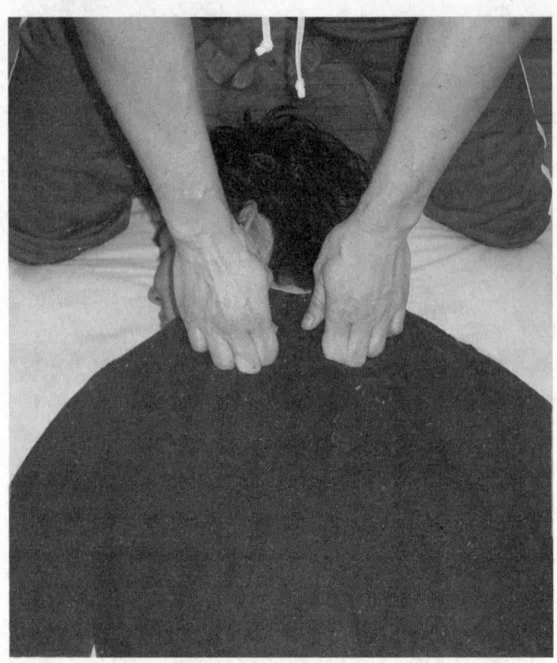

FIGURE 10-16 Close-up of knuckle press down the Bladder Meridian.

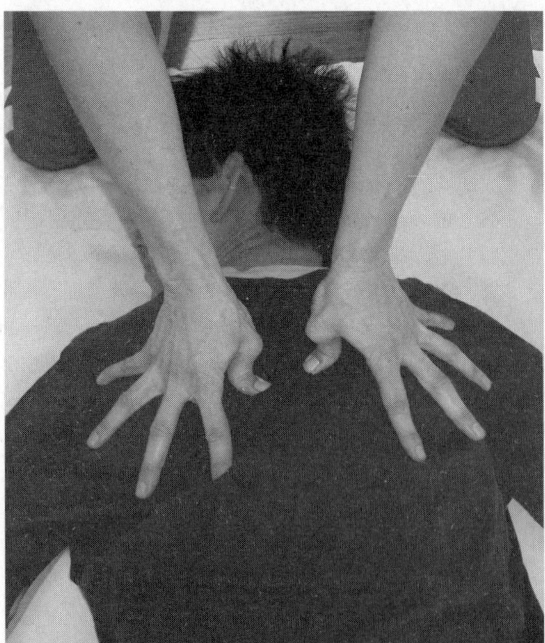

FIGURE 10-17 S-move down the Bladder Meridian.
With your thumbs side by side, press straight down, hooking into the muscles; next, arc one thumb forward and the other backward; then reverse, wriggling several times in place; relocate and repeat.

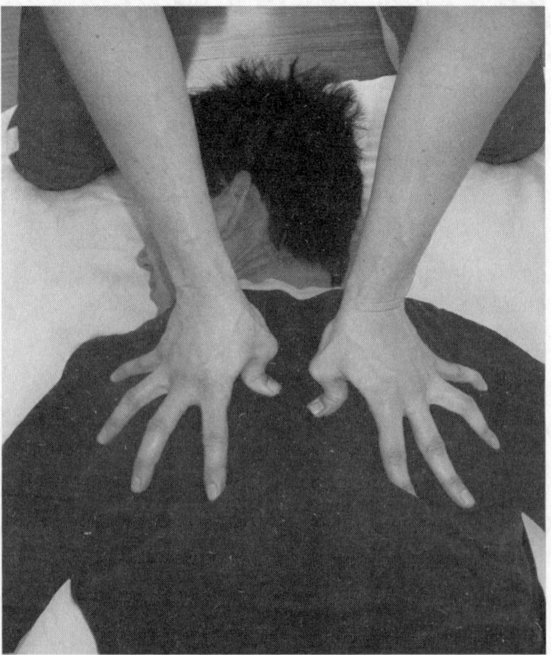

FIGURE 10-18 S-move down the Bladder Meridian.
The wriggling of your thumbs traces an invisible letter "S." This friction technique disperses stagnation. To avoid thumb strain, you may use your knuckles instead.

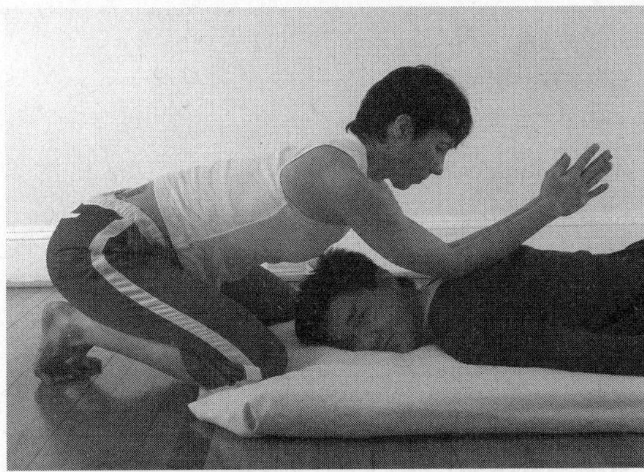

FIGURE 10-19 Prayer elbows, open position.
Plant your elbows on the Bladder Meridian with your arms partially extended (an obtuse angle of the arm blunts the point of the elbow and softens the sensation).

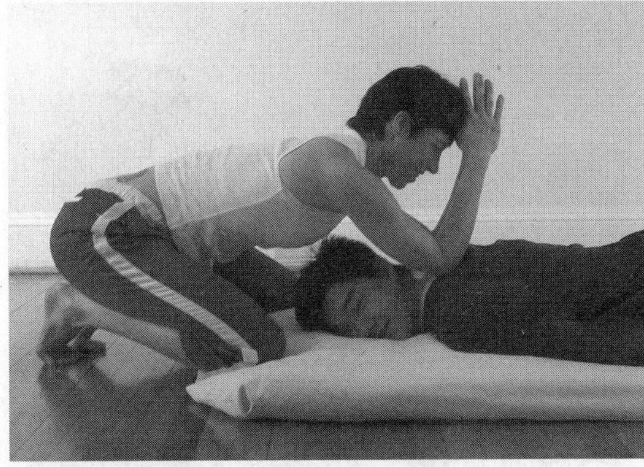

FIGURE 10-20 Prayer elbows, closed position.
Draw your hands to your forehead (an acute angle of the arm sharpens the point of the elbow and intensifies the sensation). Inch down and repeat, traversing the length of the Bladder Meridian.

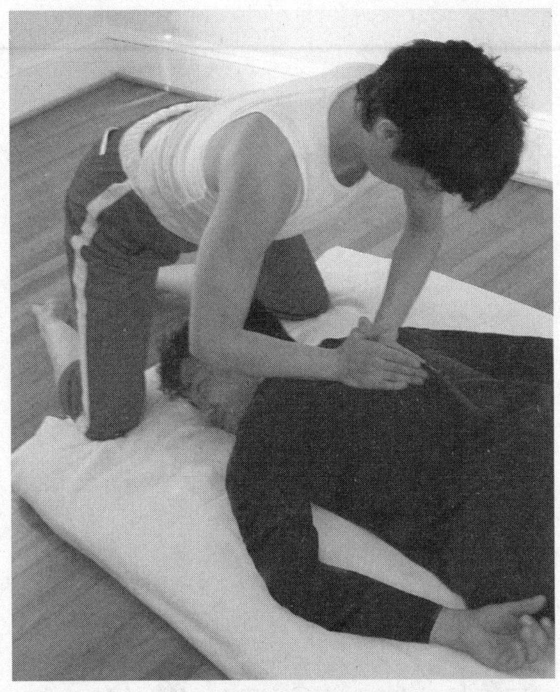

FIGURE 10-21 Sides of the hands squeeze the outer Bladder Meridian.
Hook and scoop the muscles, squeezing them toward the midline.

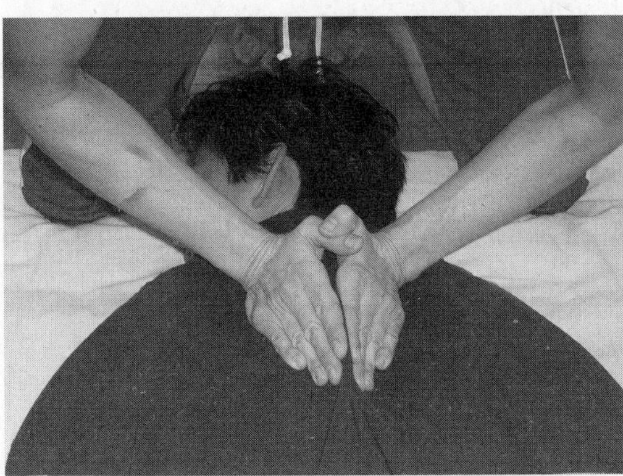

FIGURE 10-22 Close-up of sides of the hands squeeze.
You should feel the client's tissues bunch up and see the client's clothes wrinkle.

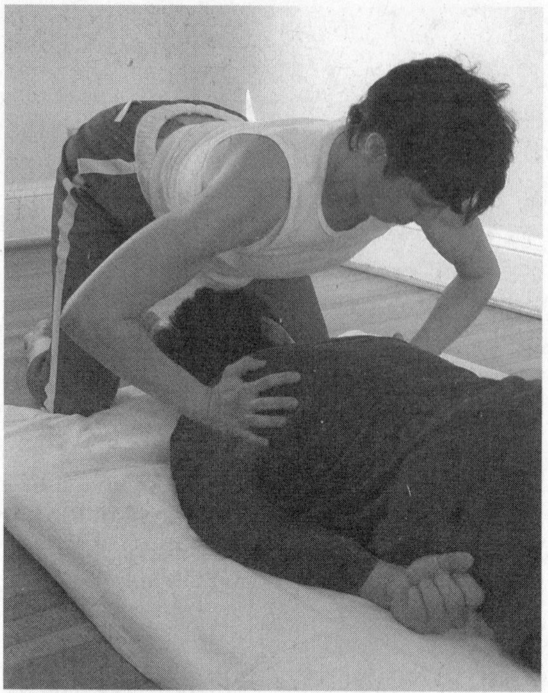

FIGURE 10-23 **Sides of the hands compress the shoulders.**
Press your palms in toward the midline. Relocate your hands farther down the sides of the body and repeat, traversing the Gallbladder Meridian along the ribcage and waist.

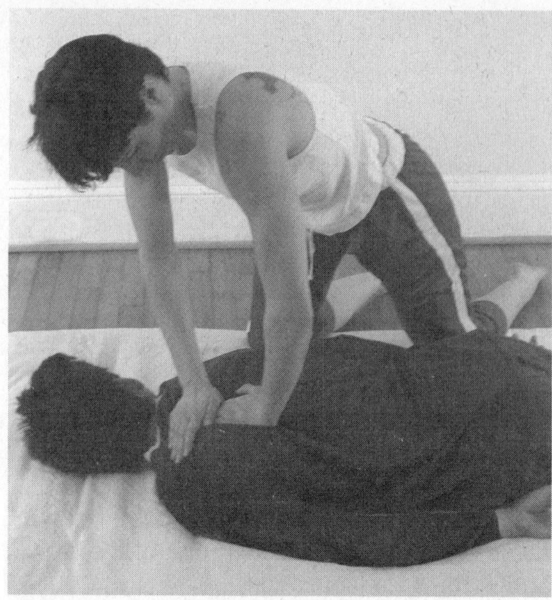

FIGURE 10-24 **Side of the hand under the scapula.**
Press the side of your hand along the vertebral border of the scapula. On some clients, your hand will slide underneath the scapula.

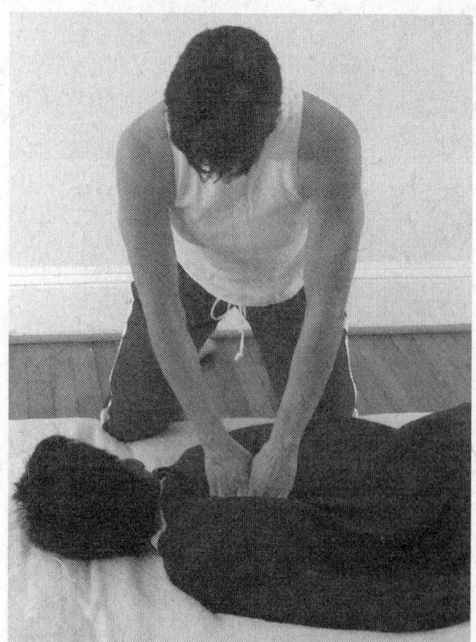

FIGURE 10-25 **Knuckles under the scapula.**
Press your knuckles along the vertebral border of the scapula.

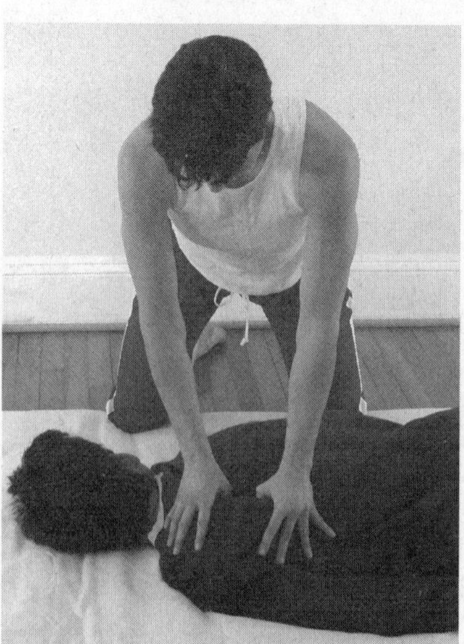

FIGURE 10-26 **Thumbs under the scapula.**
Press your thumbs along the vertebral border of the scapula.

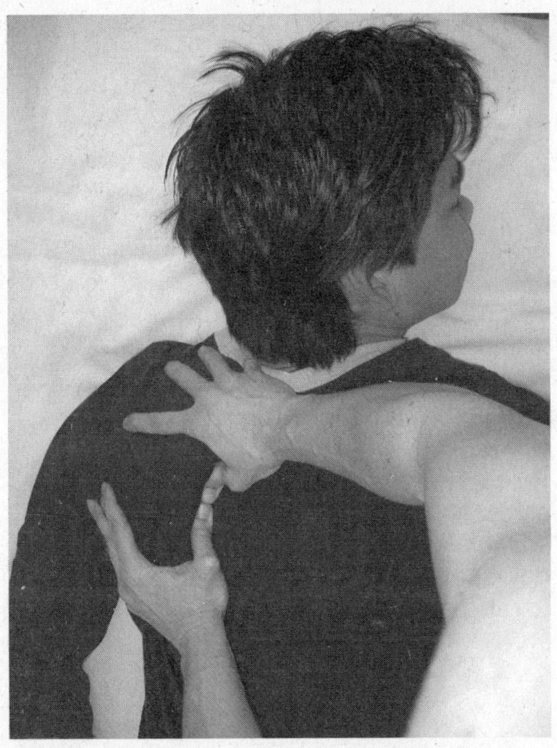

FIGURE 10-27 Close-up of thumbs under the scapula.

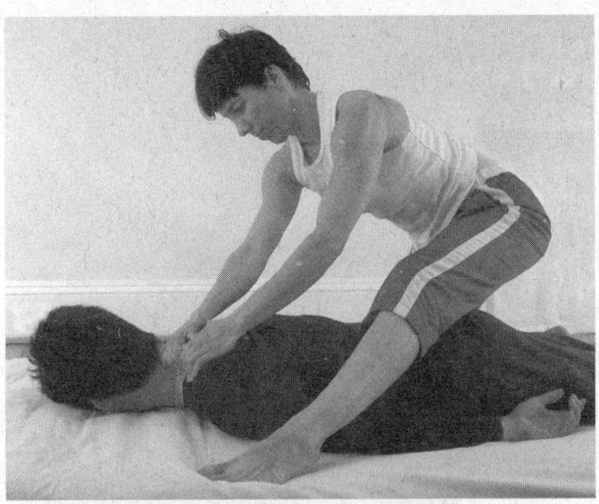

FIGURE 10-28 Shoulder squeeze.
Straddle the client in a kneeling lunge. Grab and squeeze the upper shoulder and lean back.

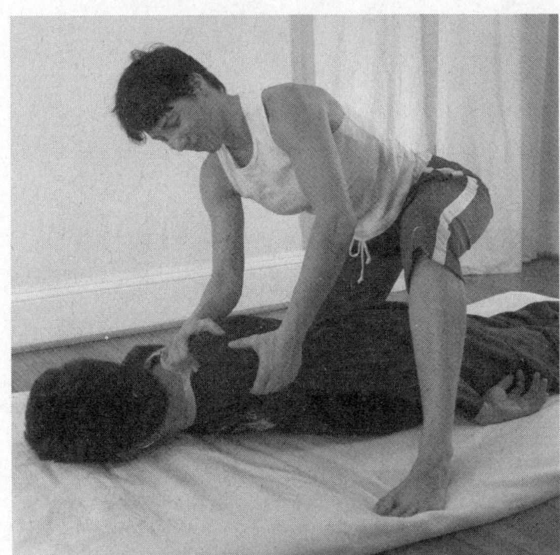

FIGURE 10-29 Shoulder rotation.
Grab the upper shoulder with your inner hand; scoop under the front of the shoulder with your outer hand. Rotate.

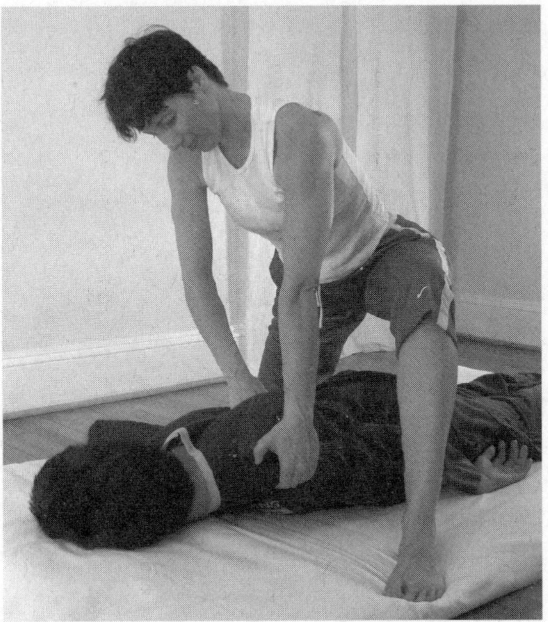

FIGURE 10-30 Shoulder traction, knuckle compression.
Scoop your outer hand under the front of the shoulder; plant your knuckles at the scapular border; pull up with your outer hand and press down with your inner hand; repeat along the border of the scapula.

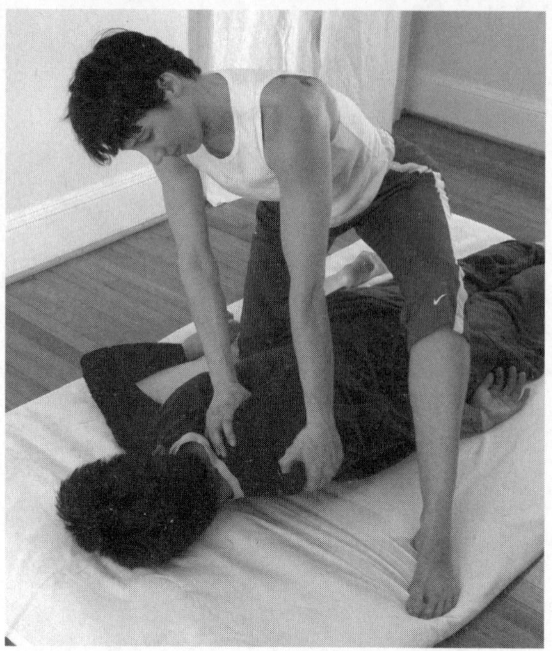

FIGURE 10-31 **Shoulder traction, thumb compression.**
Follow the steps from Figure 10-30 using your thumbs.

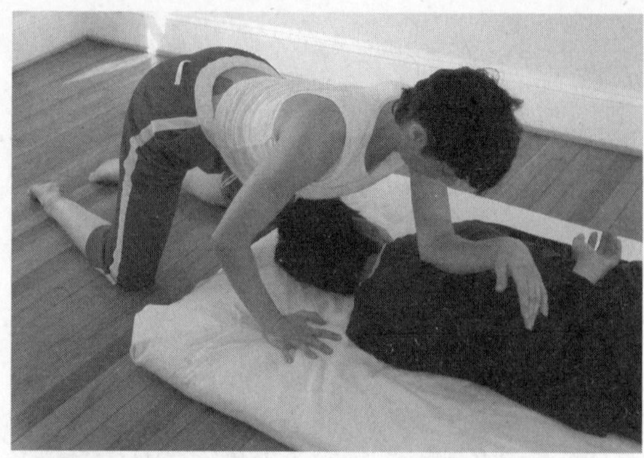

FIGURE 10-32 **Elbow press, scapular border.**
Relocate at the client's head and press your elbow along the vertebral border of the scapula. Option: If the client has good shoulder mobility, hook one arm behind the back to raise and define the scapular border.

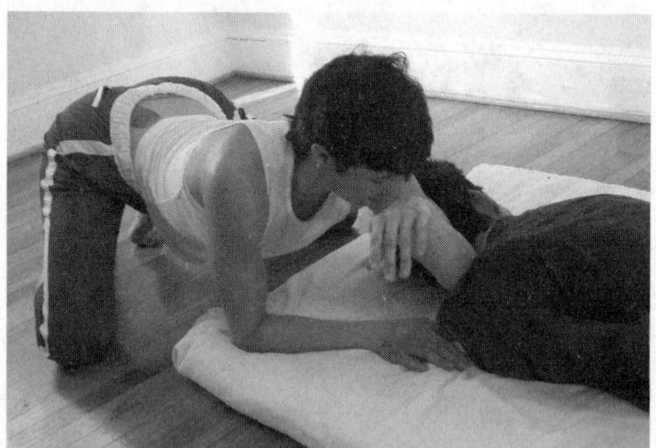

FIGURE 10-33 **Elbow press, upper shoulder.**
Crouch down to press GB 21 on top of the shoulder. Repeat Figures 10–24 through 10–33 on the other side.

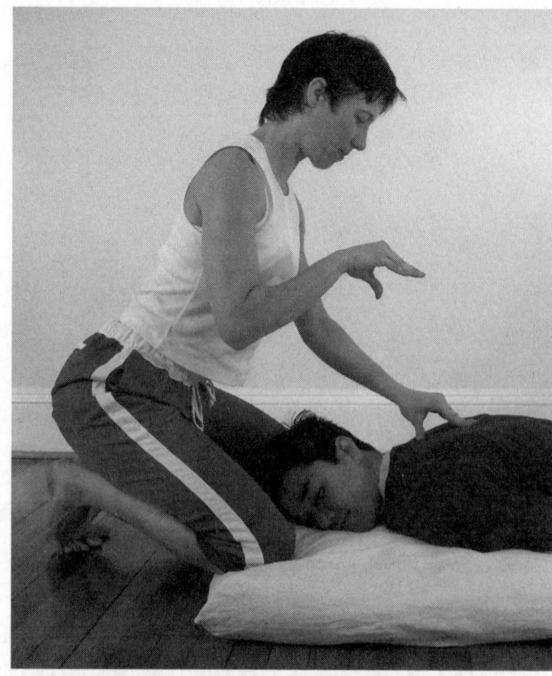

FIGURE 10-34 **Pecking/Tapping.**
Pelt the client with firm fingertips, alternating right and left sides. This and the following pummeling techniques are stimulating and disperse stagnation.

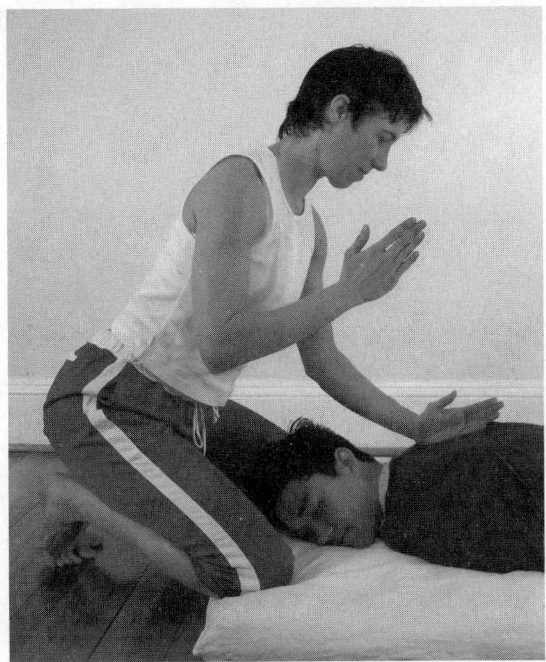

FIGURE 10-35 **Single-handed hacking/chopping.**
Hack the client with the sides of your hands, alternating right and left. Avoid strong percussion near the kidneys.

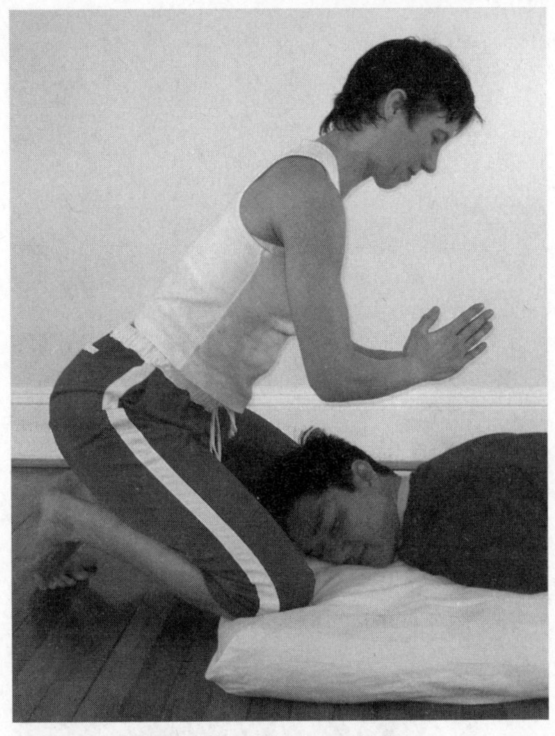

FIGURE 10-36 **Double-handed hacking/chopping.**
Hold your hands in a loose prayer position and hack. Avoid strong percussion near the kidneys.

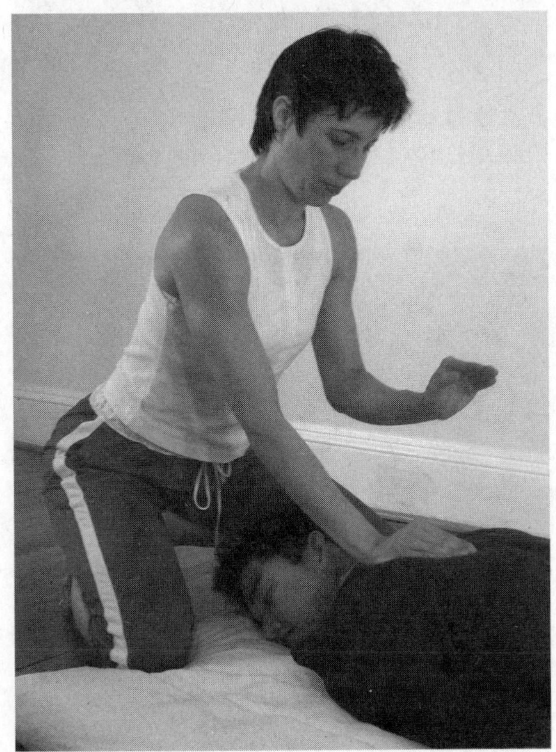

FIGURE 10-37 **Cupping.**
Mold your hands into an arc and pummel.

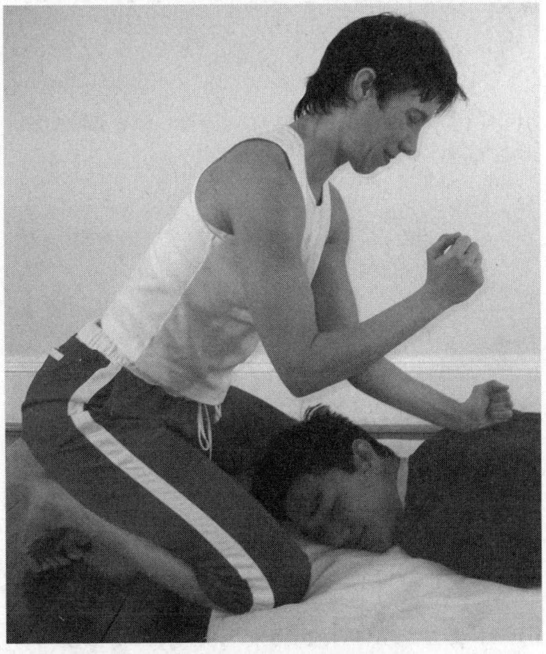

FIGURE 10-38 **Pounding/beating.**
Hold your hands in loose fists and pummel. Avoid strong percussion near the kidneys.

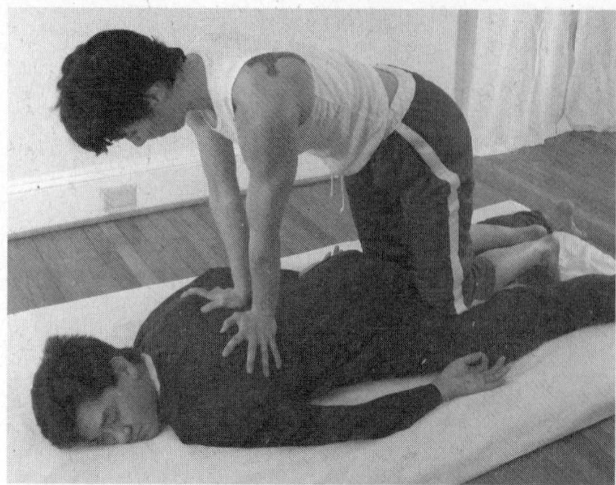

FIGURE 10-39 **Palm press down the Bladder Meridian.**
Place the balls of your feet between the client's legs and lightly kneel on the backs of the thighs below the ischial tuberosities (sit bones). Palm press down the back.

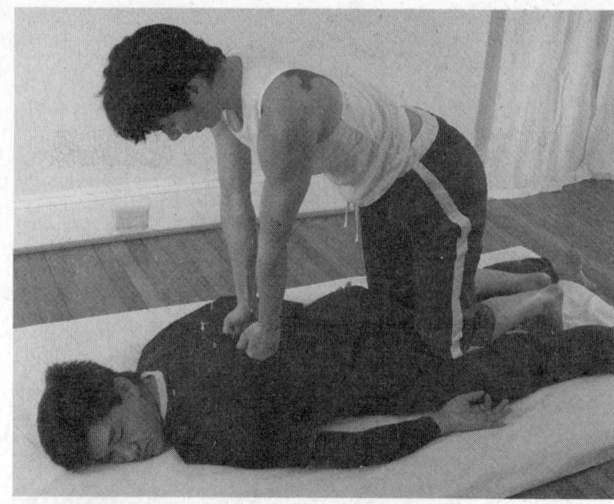

FIGURE 10-40 **Fist press down the Bladder Meridian.**
Repeat with fists.

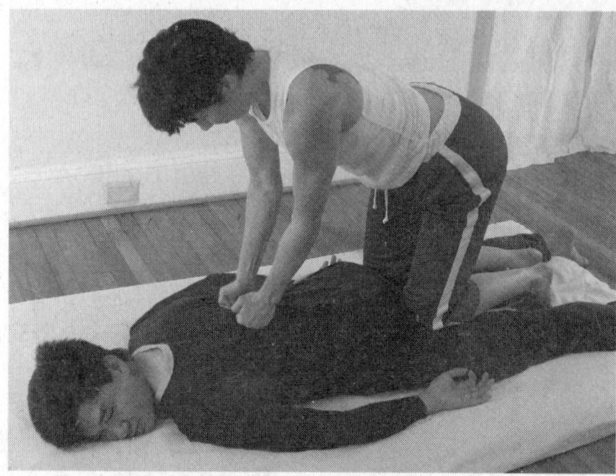

FIGURE 10-41 **Fist twist down the Bladder Meridian.**

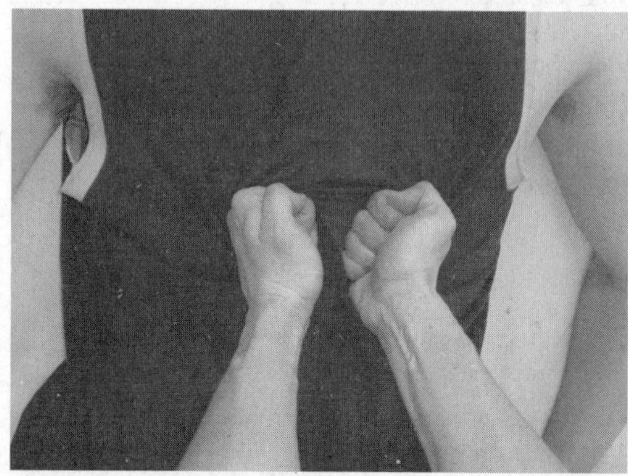

FIGURE 10-42 **Close-up of fist twist.**

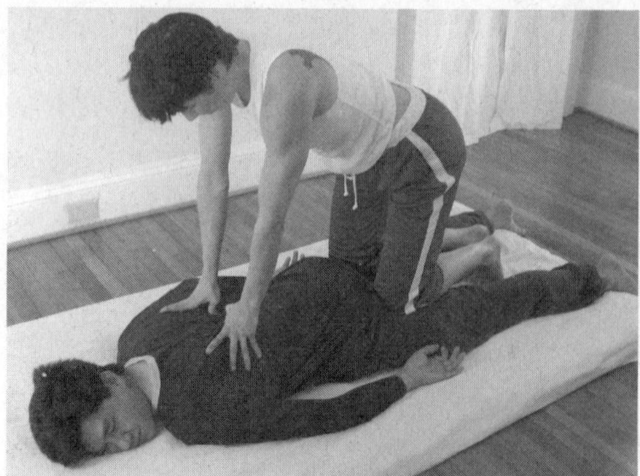

FIGURE 10-43 **Thumb press down the Bladder Meridian.**
Working from this angle enables you to reach the lower lumbar and sacral points on clients with long torsos.

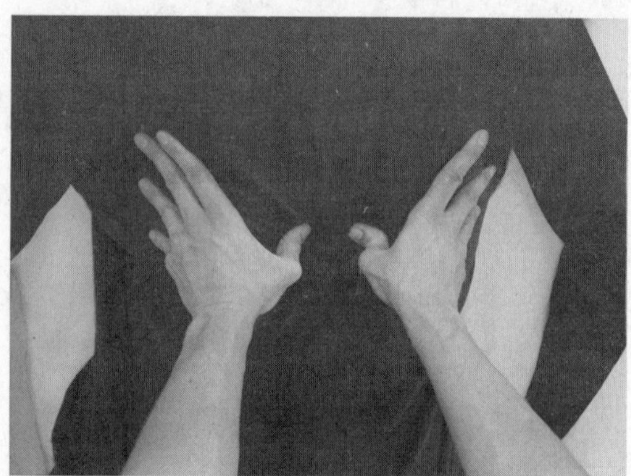

FIGURE 10-44 **Close-up of thumb press.**

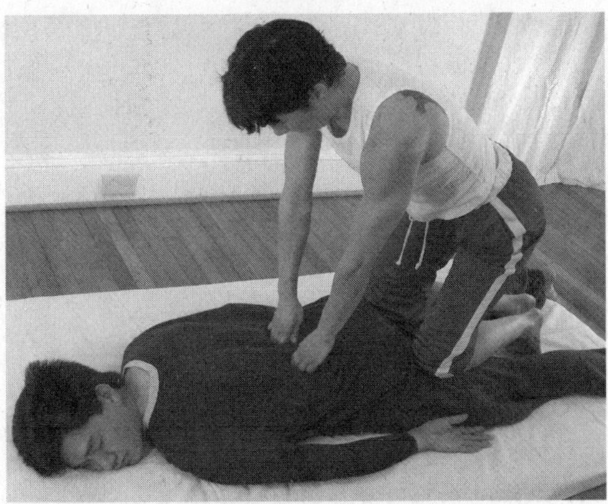

FIGURE 10-45 **Knuckle press down the Bladder Meridian.**
Keep the metacarpals (of your palm) in line with your proximal phalanges (first set of finger joints); do not buckle your metacarpophalangeal joints and collapse into a fist position.

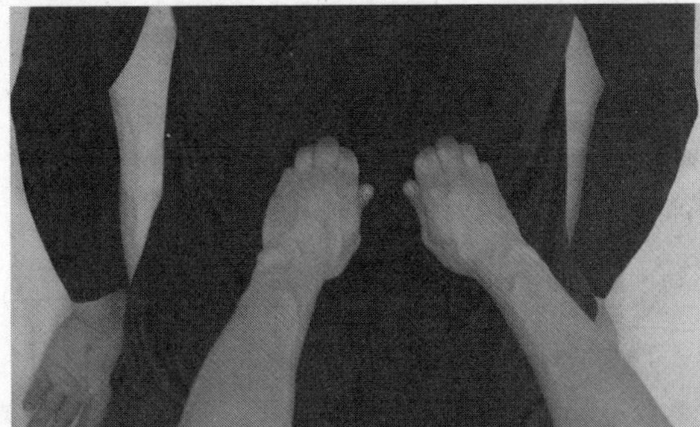

FIGURE 10-46 **Close-up of knuckle press.**

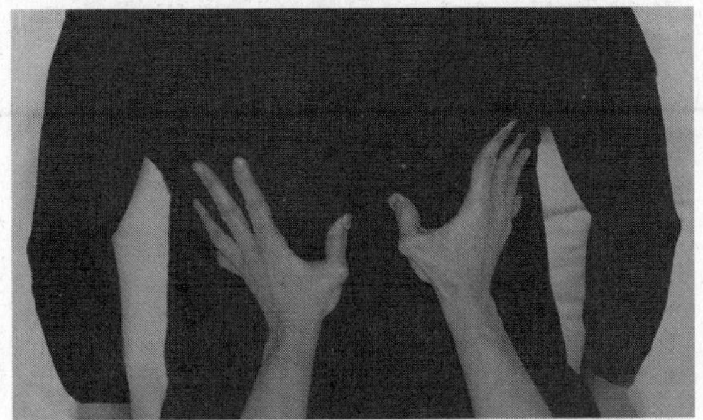

FIGURE 10-47 **S-move down the Bladder Meridian.**
As you wriggle the thumbs, the client should jiggle slightly.

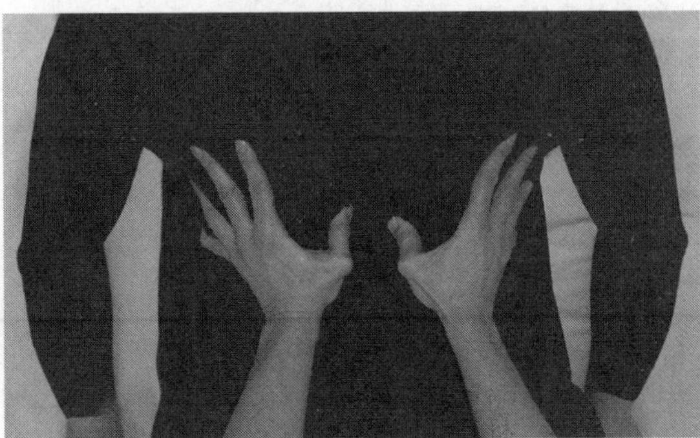

FIGURE 10-48 **S-move down the Bladder Meridian.**

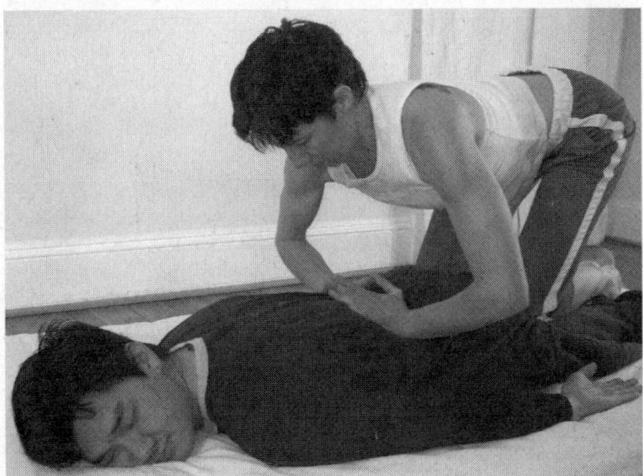

FIGURE 10-49 **Side of the hand squeeze.**
Scoop and bunch the muscles toward the midline, stimulating the outer Bladder Meridian. Alternative: Use clasped hands.

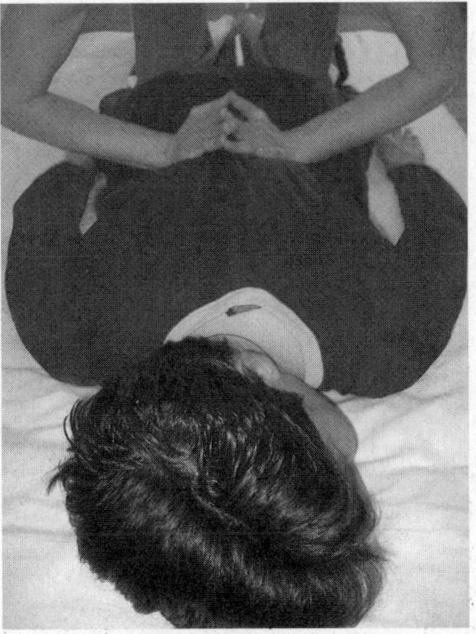

FIGURE 10-50 **Front view of side of the hand squeeze.**

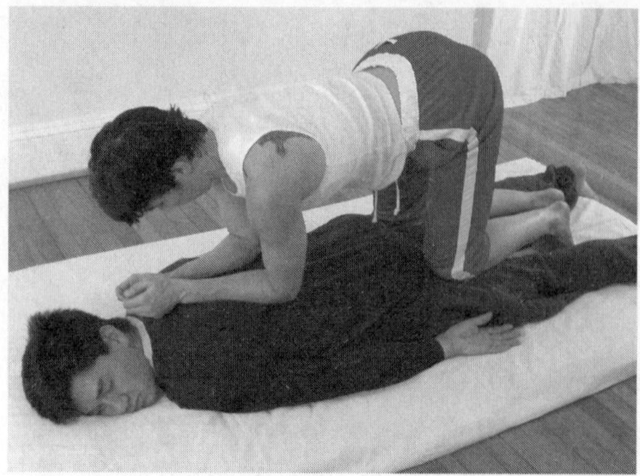

FIGURE 10-51 **Crawl.**
Crawl on the client's back with your forearms. "Iron" the erector spinae muscles by compressing and rolling sideways over them. Avoid the spine.

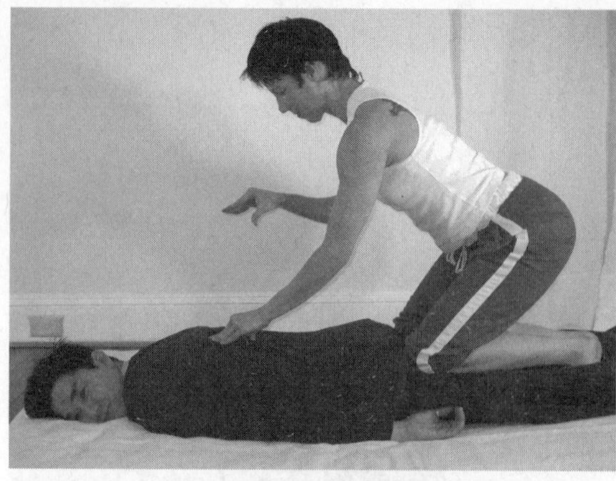

FIGURE 10-52 **Pecking/tapping.**
Pummeling techniques are for Jitsu excess conditions (tension), not Kyo deficiency conditions (chronic fatigue).

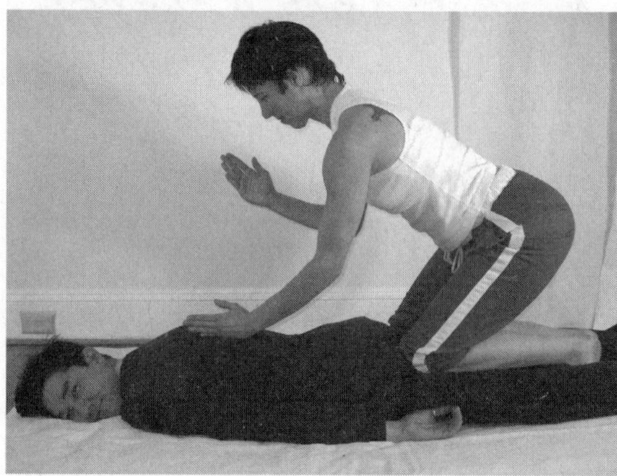

FIGURE 10-53 **Single-handed hacking/chopping.**
Pummeling should never jar the client. Avoid excessive force.

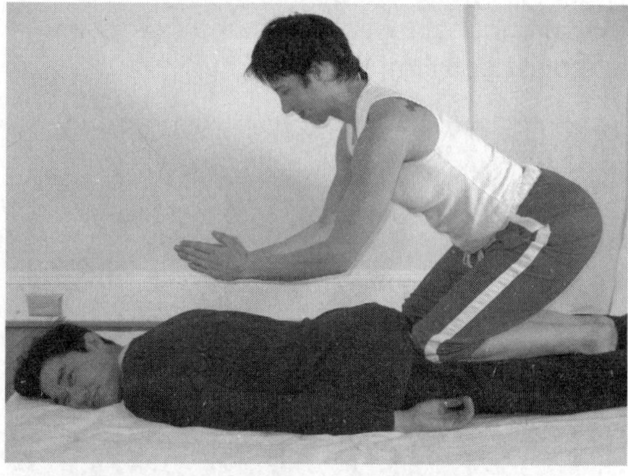

FIGURE 10-54 **Double-handed hacking/chopping.**
Hacking is particularly suitable for large, dense muscles such as the hamstrings, calves, and quadriceps (not shown here).

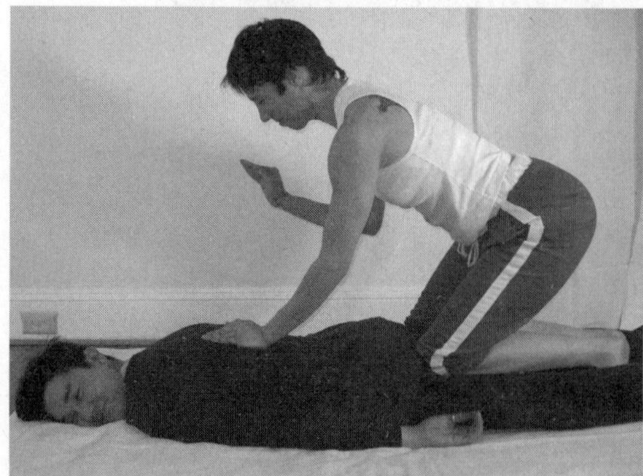

FIGURE 10-55 **Cupping.**
Cupping is the mildest pummeling technique.

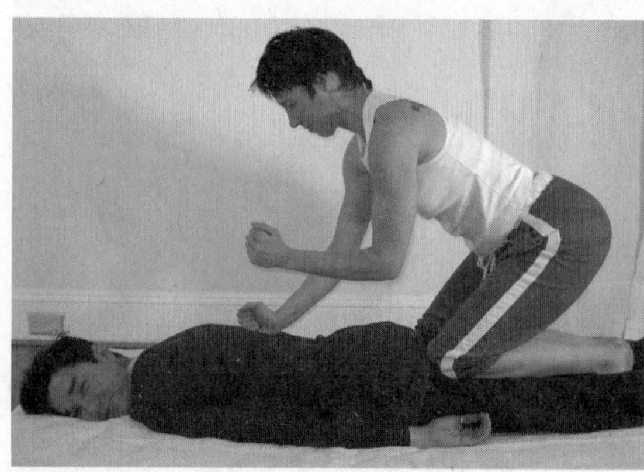

FIGURE 10-56 **Pounding/beating.**
Pounding is particularly suitable for large, dense muscle groups such as the gluteals (not shown here).

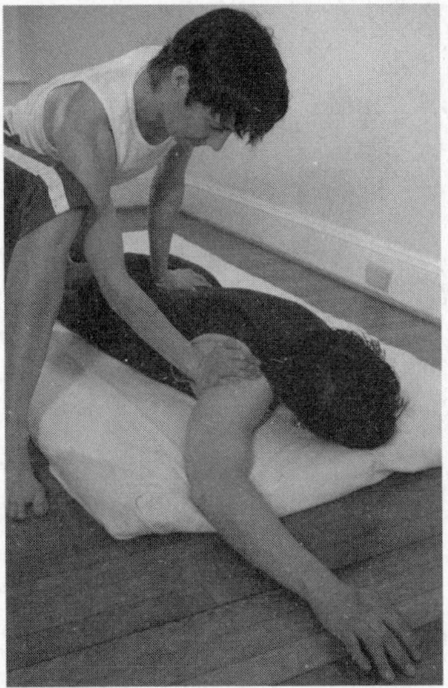

FIGURE 10-57 **Palm press on the rotator cuff.**
Extend the client's arm overhead to open the rotator cuff and stretch the Small Intestine Meridian. Prop your arm against your thigh for leverage, or kneel, directly facing client (not shown here). Palm press the posterior scapula and axilla.

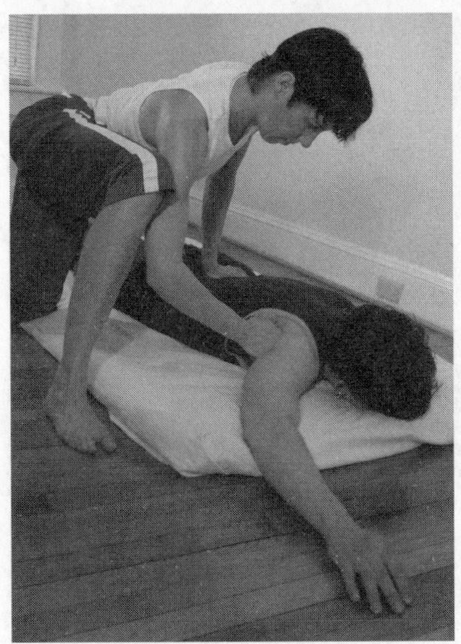

FIGURE 10-58 **Fist press and twist on the rotator cuff.**
Apply static and dynamic (twisting) fist pressure to the posterior scapula and axilla.

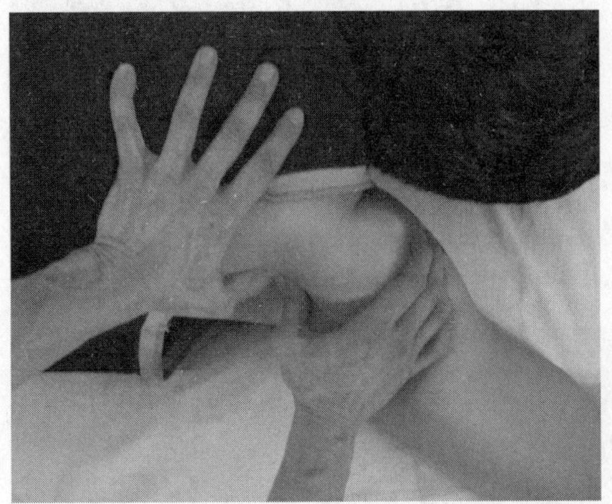

FIGURE 10-59 **SI 9.**
On the teres major at the axillary border (armpit crease) when the arm hangs down.

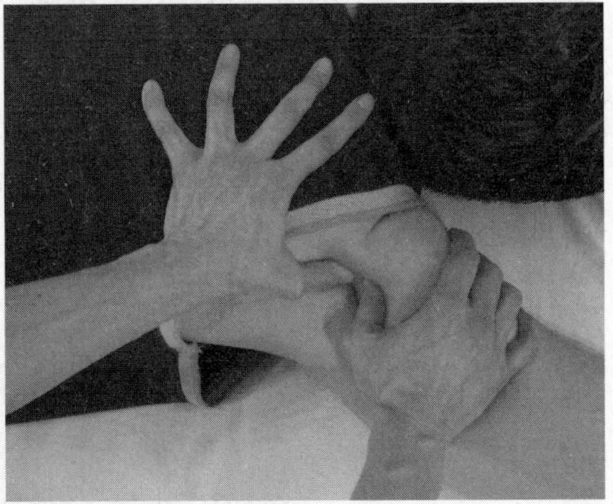

FIGURE 10-60 **SI 10.**
On the posterior deltoid.

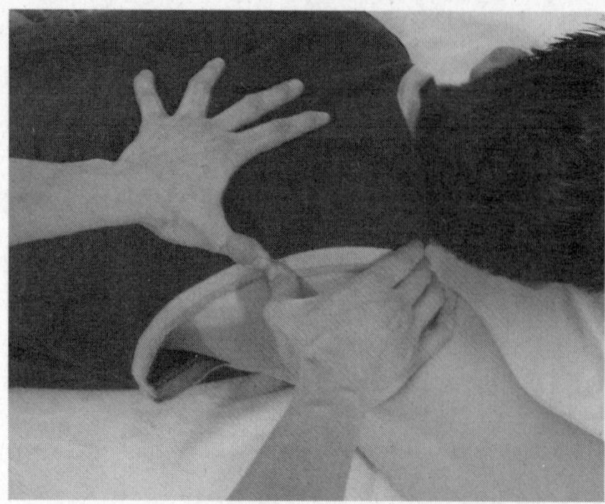

FIGURE 10-61 SI 11.
On the infraspinatus in the center of the scapula.

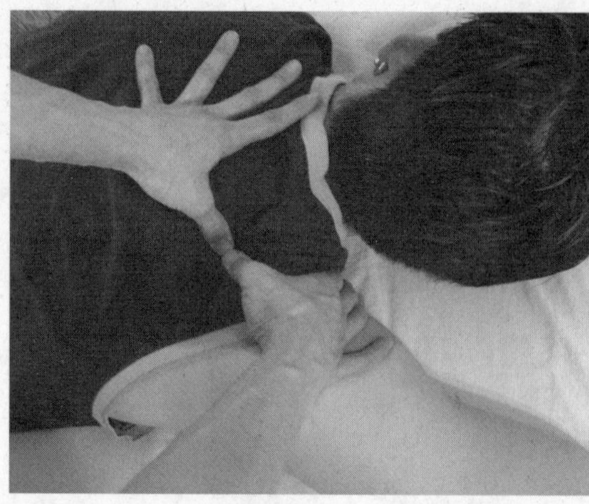

FIGURE 10-62 SI 12.
On the supraspinatus above the spine (bony ridge) of the scapula.

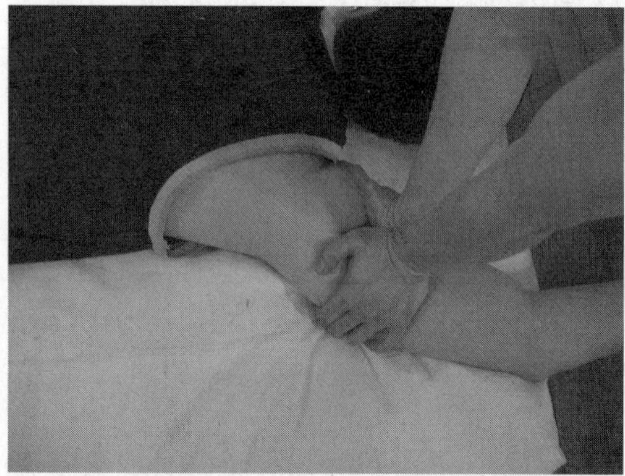

FIGURE 10-63 Butterfly, upper arm.
Wrap your fingers around the arm, press with the heels of your hands, and squeeze with your fingers like a tourniquet, moving down the Yang Meridians of the arm.

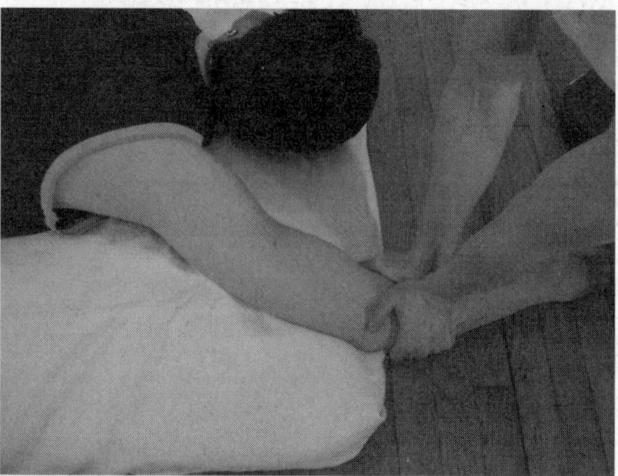

FIGURE 10-64 Butterfly, forearm.
Traditionally, three passes of compressions are applied along the length of a limb or Meridian, but the number can be modified to meet the client's needs.

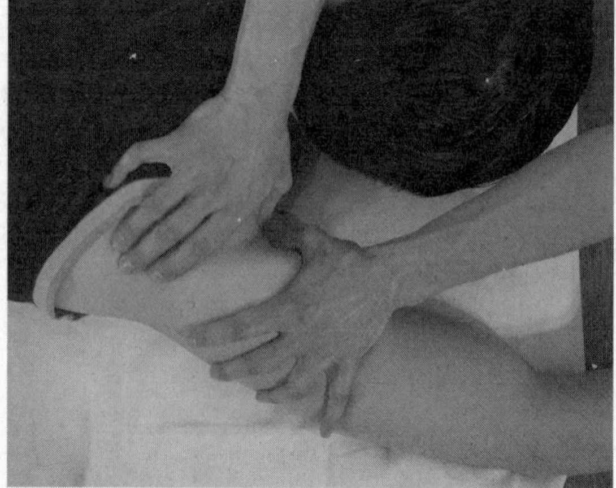

FIGURE 10-65 LI 15.
In the anterior (front) of the two dimpled notches when the arm is abducted (raised overhead).

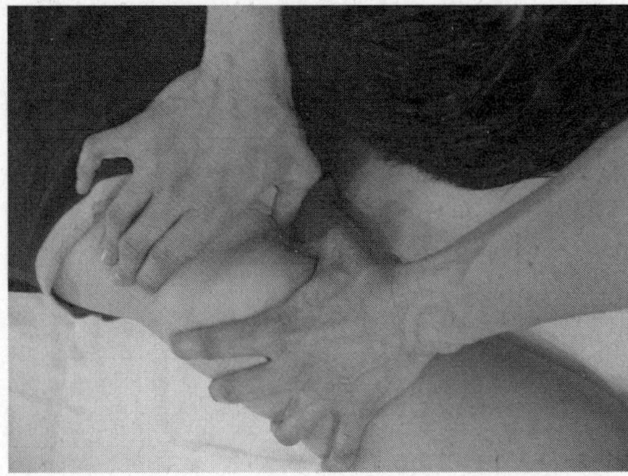

FIGURE 10-66 **Close-up of LI 15, arm at 120 degrees.**
Note: Traditionally, the 120 degree arm angle is reserved for the Small Intestine Meridian and the 45 degree arm angle for the Large Intestine Meridian. However, the upper Large Intestine Meridian points are easier to locate and treat with the arm raised because abduction defines the deltoid, making it bulge and dimple, and also slackens the muscle, making the Large Intestine Meridian points easier to penetrate.

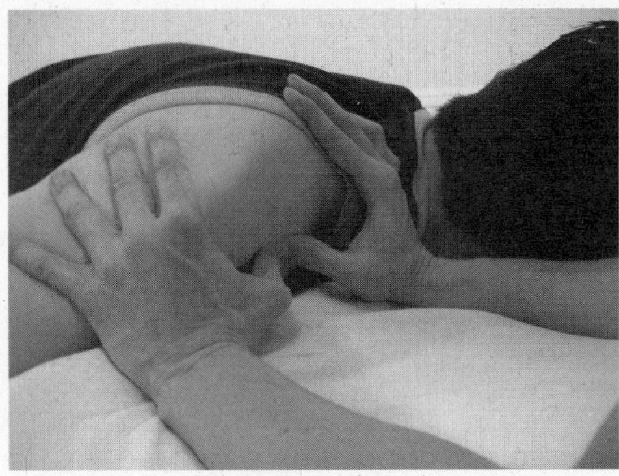

FIGURE 10-67 **LI 15, arm at 45 degrees.** Compare this traditional arm position for the Large Intestine Meridian (45 degree angle) with Figure 10–66 (120 degrees). At 45 degrees, the deltoid does not bulge and dimple, the muscle is taut from being in a relatively stretched position, and you must crouch lower to apply thumb pressure when the client is in the prone position.

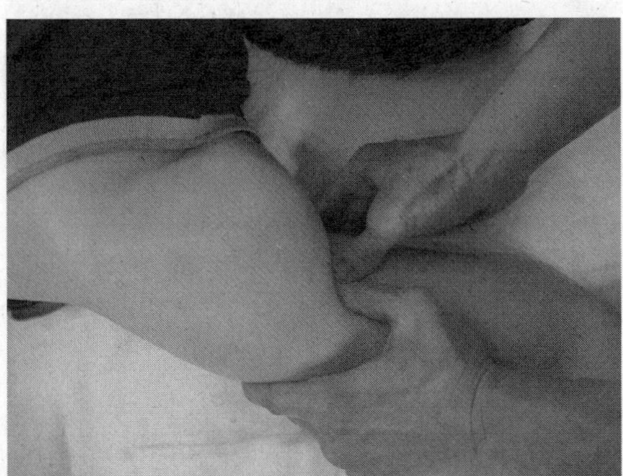

FIGURE 10-68 **LI 14, arm at 120 degrees.** Just in front of and above the deltoid insertion on the humerus.

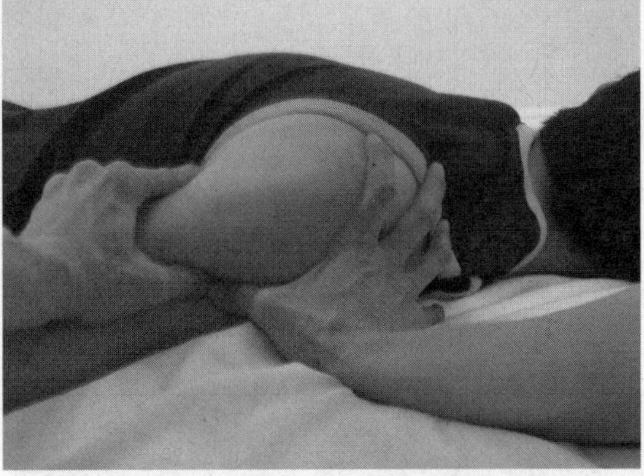

FIGURE 10-69 **LI 14, arm at 45 degrees.** Compare this traditional arm position (45 degrees) with Figure 10–68 (120 degrees). Again, the deltoid is flattened, so that its attachment to the humerus is not as pronounced, and you must crouch lower to apply thumb pressure.

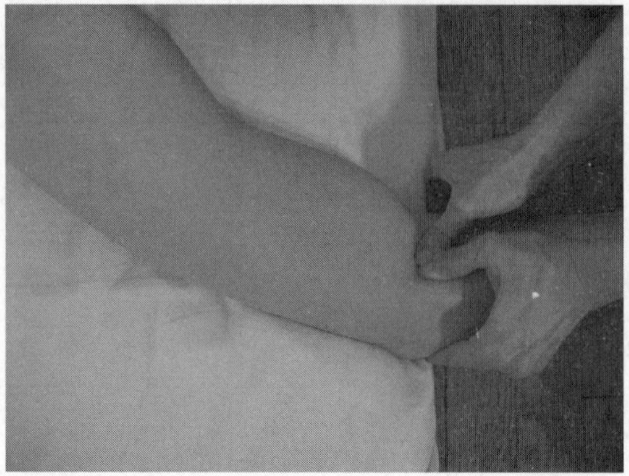

FIGURE 10-70 **LI 11.**
On the posterior forearm at the elbow joint toward the radial (thumb) side.

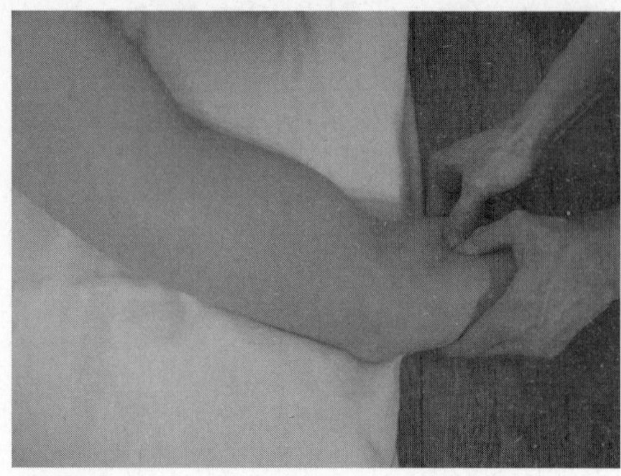

FIGURE 10-71 **LI 10.**
On the posterior forearm 2 cun below the elbow joint.

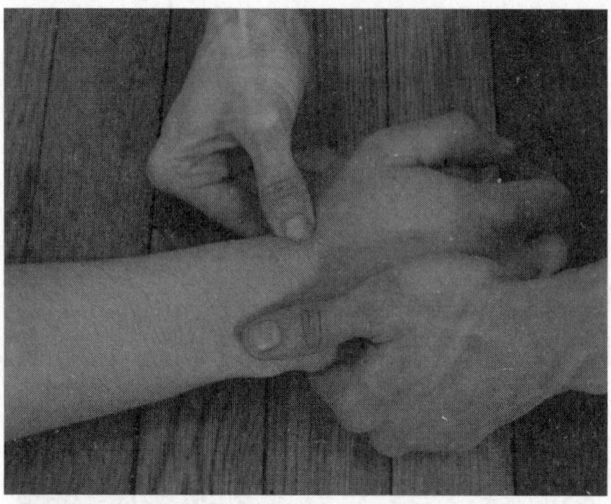

FIGURE 10-72 **LI 5.**
In the hollow between the two tendons at the base of the thumb.

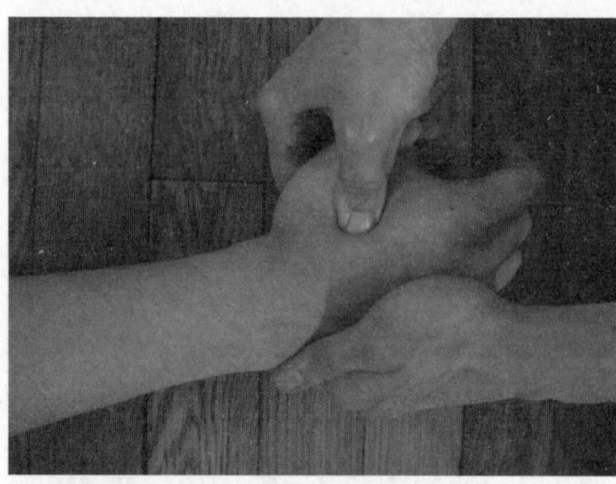

FIGURE 10-73 **LI 4.**
In the fleshy web between the thumb and forefinger; press toward the forefinger.

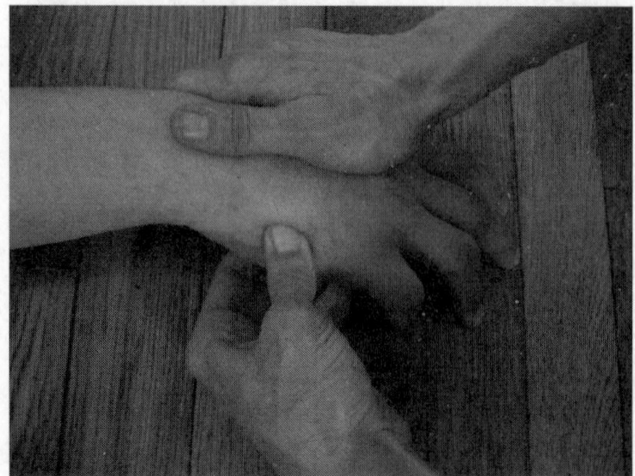

FIGURE 10-74 **SI 3.**
On the side of the hand above the fifth metacarpal joint (the knuckle of the little finger).

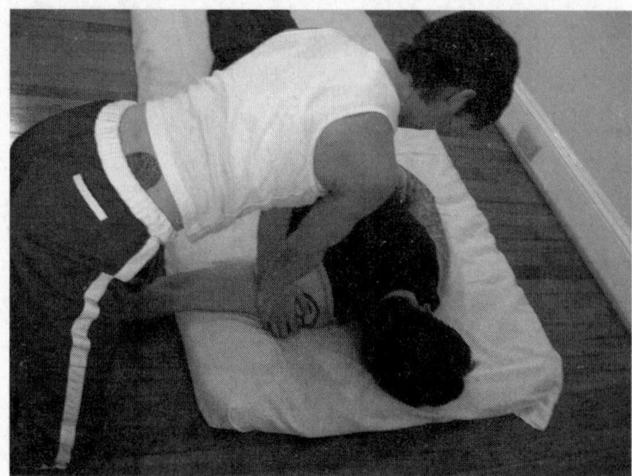

FIGURE 10-75 **Butterfly.**
Hand squeeze down the Yang Meridians of the arm, second pass. The arm is in the Triple Heater Meridian position (90 degree angle).

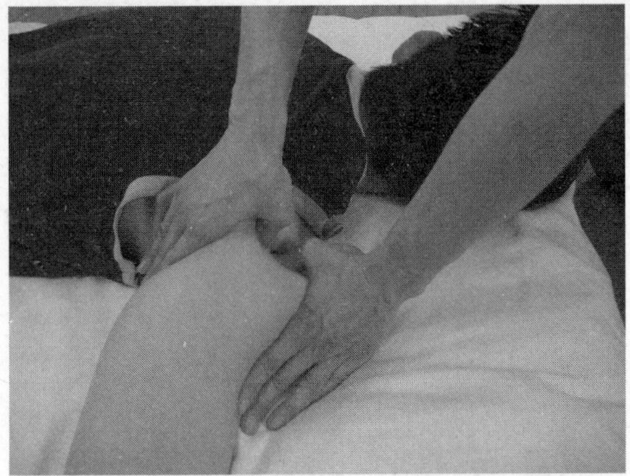

FIGURE 10-76 **TH 14.**
In the posterior (back) of the two dimpled notches when the arm is abducted (raised).

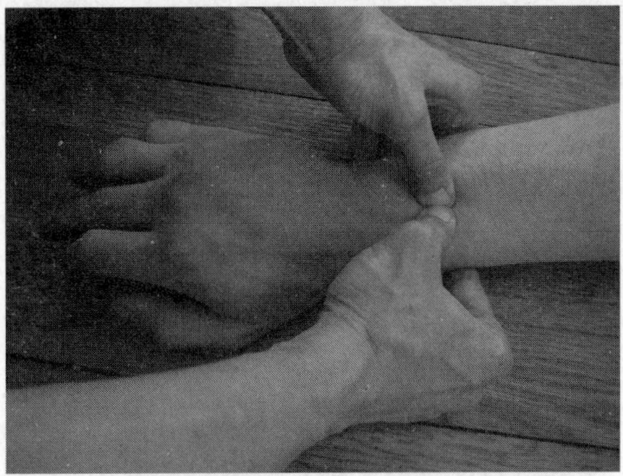

FIGURE 10-77 **TH 5.**
Two cun above the posterior wrist between the radius and the ulna.

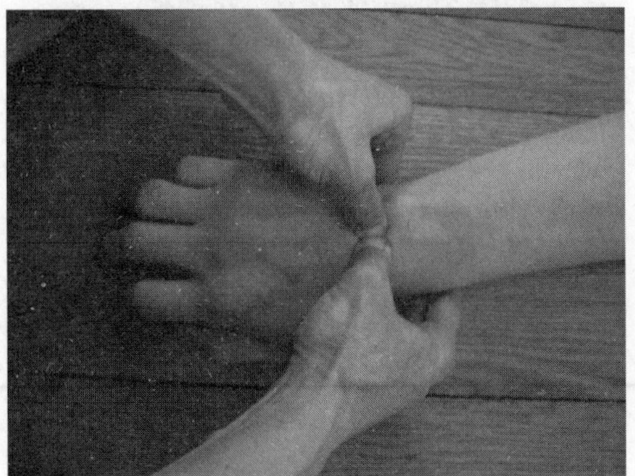

FIGURE 10-78 **TH 4.**
Near the middle of the posterior wrist but closer to the little finger side.

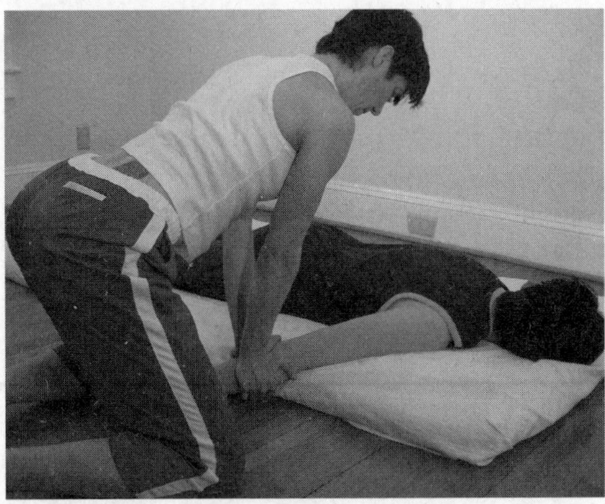

FIGURE 10-79 **Butterfly.**
Hand squeeze down the Yang Meridians of the arm, third pass. The arm is in the Large Intestine Meridian position at a 45 degree angle.

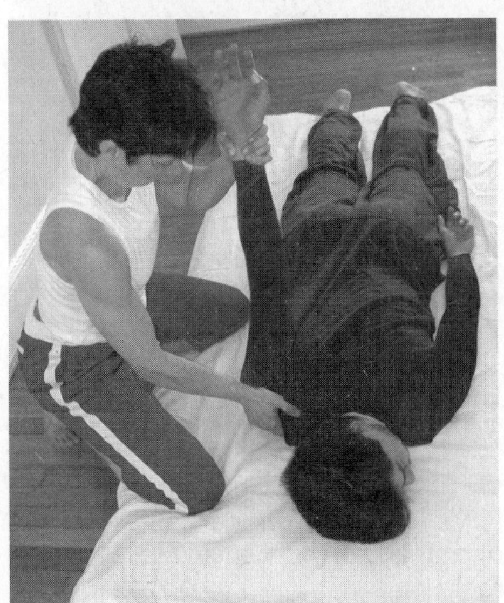

FIGURE 10-80 **Arm extension: anterior deltoid and bicep stretch.**
The client's arm faces palm up. Grab the wrist; stabilize the shoulder, and raise the arm until resistance is felt. The client's elbow should be straight.

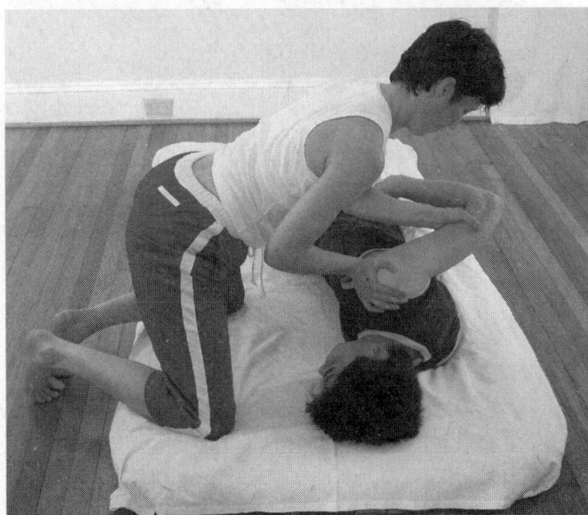

FIGURE 10-81 **Bent-arm pectoralis and bicep stretch.**
Grab the client's arm above the elbow and support the front of the shoulder; push the bent arm and shoulder toward the opposite side of the body.

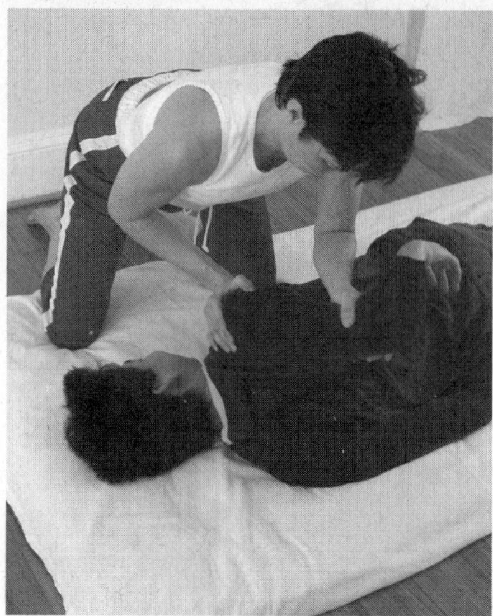

FIGURE 10-82 **Back view of bent-arm pectoralis and bicep stretch.**
Repeat Figures 10–57 through 10–82 on the other side.

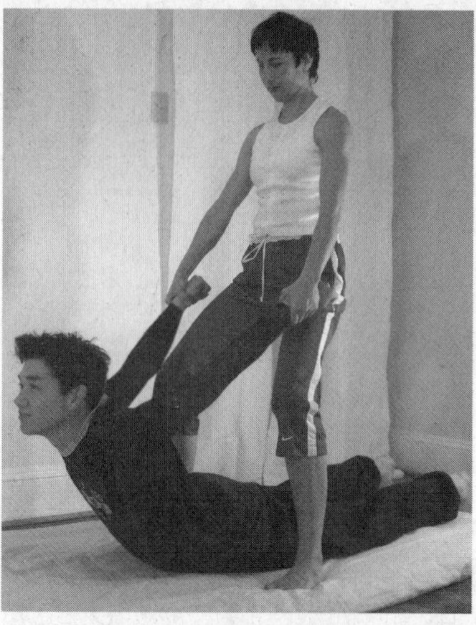

FIGURE 10-83 **Standing chest stretch.**
Straddle the client at hip level and grab the wrists. Stand up and lean back. Repeat this pectoral and bicep stretch several times as desired. Omit on clients larger and heavier than you or clients with lower back problems.

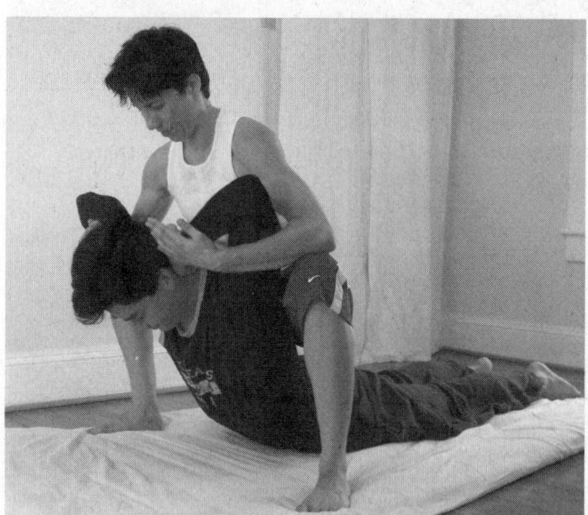

FIGURE 10-84 **Squatting chest stretch, center.**
Straddle the client and instruct the client to clasp the hands behind the head. Squat down and scoop your forearms under the client's arms. Lift the client's torso and set your elbows on your thighs for support.

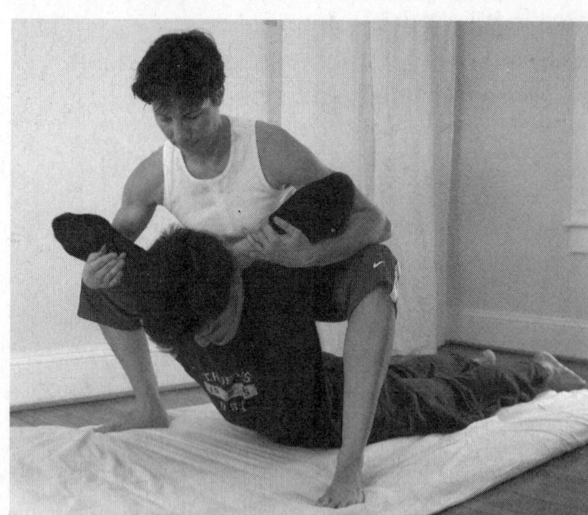

FIGURE 10-85 **Squatting chest stretch, left.**
Twist left. This technique should not be applied on clients who are substantially larger and heavier than you or clients with lower back problems.

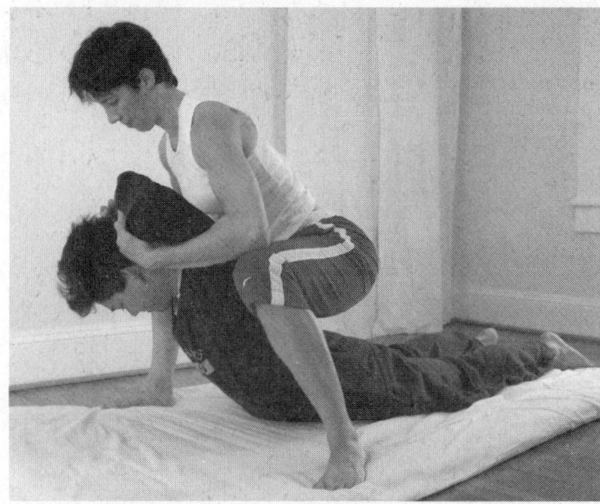

FIGURE 10-86 Squatting chest stretch, right.
Twist right. This technique should also not be performed if you cannot squat comfortably and stably.

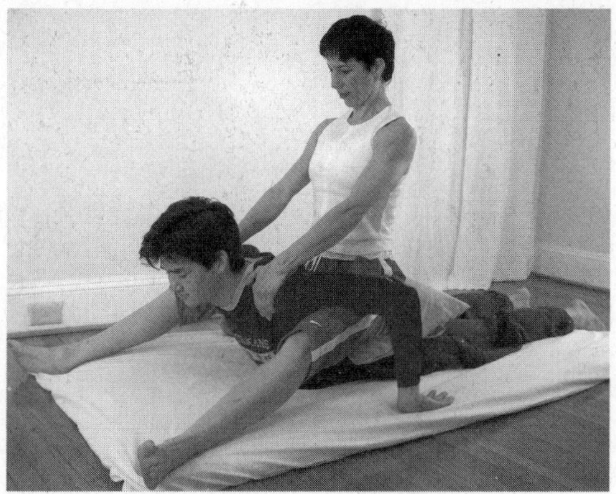

FIGURE 10-87 Seated chest stretch.
Sit on the client's sacrum (a pillow adds a comfort and privacy barrier, if desired). Drape the client's arms over your legs. Scoop your hands under the front of the client's shoulders and lean back. Repeat several times as desired.

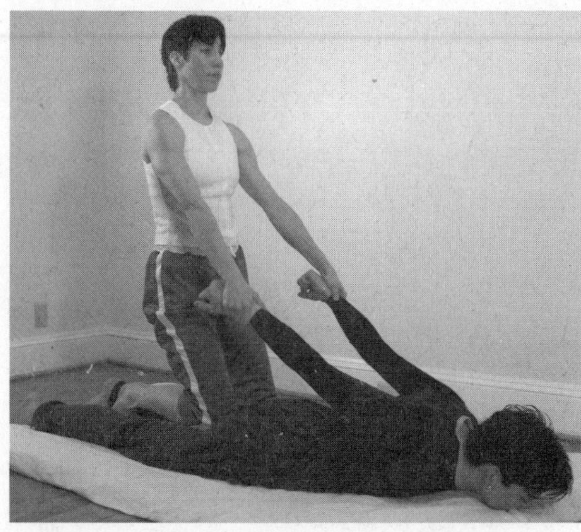

FIGURE 10-88 Kneeling chest stretch, phase 1.
Set the balls of your feet between the client's legs and kneel on the client's ischial tuberosities (sit bones). Grab the client's wrists; rise to an upright kneeling position.

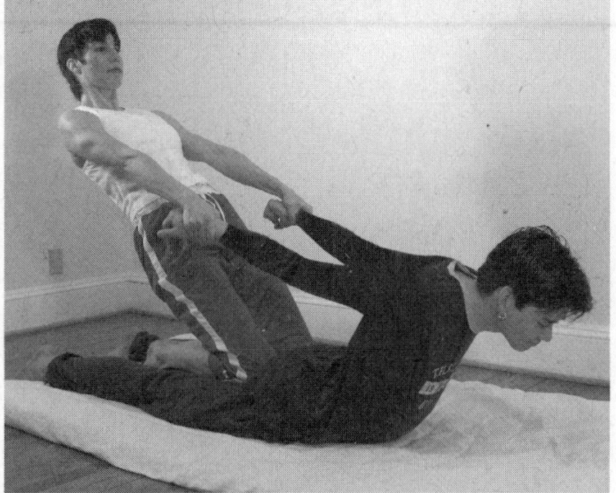

FIGURE 10-89 Kneeling chest stretch, phase 2.
Lean back. Repeat several times as desired. Omit on clients who have lower back problems.

11

Prone Lower Body Protocol

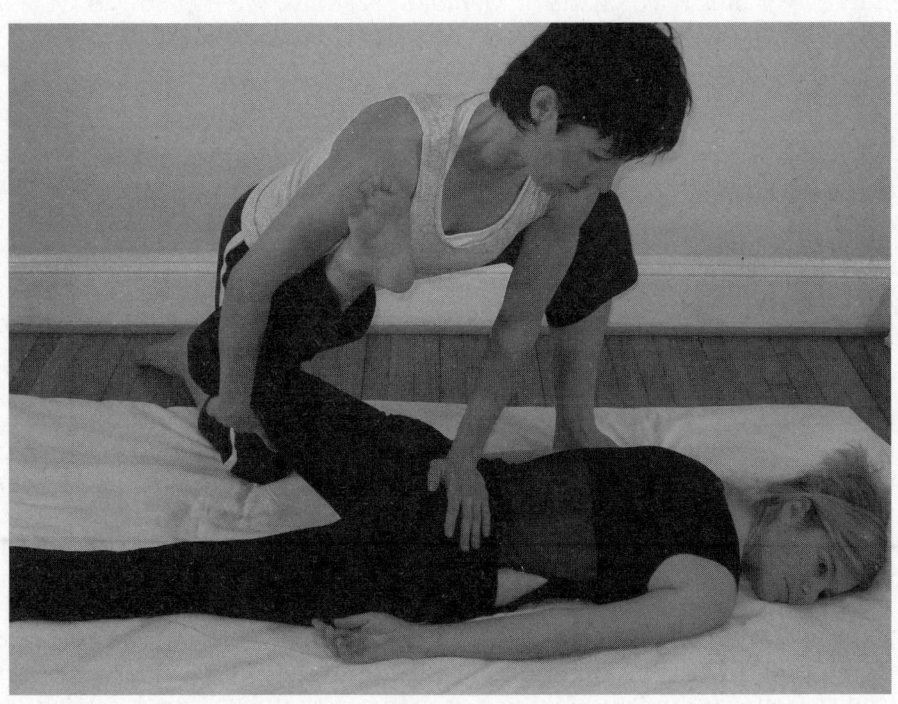

Therapeutic Emphasis

The prone lower body protocol emphasizes the Yang Meridians of the hip and leg: the Bladder (Bl), Gallbladder (GB), and Stomach (St) Meridians. Focused work on these Meridians and key acupressure points can benefit clients who have painful obstruction syndrome—localized muscular soreness and joint aches—in the hips, backs and sides of the thighs, calves, sides of the lower legs, and soles of the feet; clients whose Meridians assess as Kyo or Jitsu or are otherwise symptomatic; and clients who present physical disorders or psychological disharmonies associated with the corresponding elements.

Causes of Discomfort and Treatment Strategies

Because the muscles of the hips and legs are relatively large and powerful, a client is more likely to develop painful obstruction syndrome in the lower body from vigorous or unaccustomed exercise and participation in sports events, performing arts, and outdoor recreational activities than from ordinary manual labor or prolonged or repetitive low-load occupational activities. To disperse blood and fluid stagnation, sore and fatigued muscles should be pressed, squeezed, and rubbed. To clear blockages in energy flow, key acupressure points in the associated muscles should be pressed and held or pressed and subjected to friction. On the large muscles of the hips and posterior thighs, acupressure may be given with strong body tools like knuckles, elbows, and knees if appropriate for the client. If soreness extends along the pathway of a Meridian, the entire Meridian should be given Shiatsu. The listed examples in the section below target isolated areas of the posterior lower body that can become sore and fatigued from exertion. For photos of point locations on a human model, see Appendix 1. For illustrated charts of Meridian locations, see the Flow of Qi chart in Figure 2-1 and "Posterior Meridians and Associated Musculature" on p. 230.

KEY ACUPRESSURE POINTS FOR THE POSTERIOR LOWER BODY

- **Back of Hips:** The gluteus maximus (buttock muscle) can become sore from doing hip extension exercises like leg lifts in the prone or crawl positions, squats, lunges, and leg presses; running and climbing; and working out on a treadmill, stairmaster, recumbent bike, or elliptical cardio machine. Additionally, this muscle may become sore from prolonged sitting. Give Shiatsu to the hip and sacrum and acupressure to Bl 53 and Bl 54.
- **Side of Hips:** The hip abductors—the gluteus medius and minimus (buttock muscles on the side of the hip), tensor fascia latae (muscle on the side of the hip), and iliotibial band (band of connective tissue on the side of the thigh)—can become sore from leg abduction exercises; lateral traveling movements made in tennis, basketball, and racquetball; and hip stabilization, as when balancing on one leg or breaking the momentum of a swing in golf or baseball. Give Shiatsu to the hips, especially the outer edges of the hips, and lateral thigh, and acupressure to GB 30 and GB 31.
- **Back of Thighs:** The hamstrings (posterior thigh muscles) can become sore from doing hip extension and knee flexion exercises like hamstring curls, as well as from running and biking. Give Shiatsu to the Bladder Meridian on the posterior thigh and acupressure to Bl 36, Bl 37, and Bl 40.
- **Calves:** The gastrocnemius and soleus (calf muscles) can become sore from doing knee flexion and plantarflexion exercises like heel raises, jumping as in basketball and volleyball, leaping as in dance, and propelling oneself forward as in power walking, walking in sand, hiking uphill, and running. They can also become sore from wearing high heels, which places these muscles in a contracted position for a prolonged period of time. Give Shiatsu to the Bladder Meridian in the calves and acupressure to Bl 40, Bl 56, and Bl 57. Pinch Bl 60 and Ki 3 on either side of the Achilles tendon.
- **Outer Shins:** The anterior tibialis (shin muscle) can become sore from doing ankle flexion exercises like toe taps and toe raises, from hiking uphill in boots, from prolonged weight bearing in a lunge position, and from absorbing the shock of running and landing from aerial jumps. Those clients with tight ankles or lateral shin splints should have these muscles worked. The peroneals (outer lower leg muscles) can become sore from lateral movements as in ice skating and rollerblading and ankle stabilization as when walking, hiking, or running on uneven surfaces. Give Shiatsu to the Stomach and Gallbladder Meridians in the lower leg and acupressure to St 36, St 41, GB 34, and GB 40.
- **Soles of Feet:** The foot flexors and plantar fascia (connective tissue) on the soles of the feet can become sore from pointing the feet as in ballet and gymnastics from doing heel raises, from absorbing the shock of running, and from walking in sand or walking uphill. They can also become sore from pronation (collapsed arches) and the condition of plantar fascitis. Give Shiatsu to the soles of the feet and acupressure to Ki 1 and Sp 3.

- **Here are the key acupressure points in various locations:**
  Hips: Bl 53, Bl 54, GB 30
  Posterior thighs: Bl 36, Bl 37, Bl 40
  Lateral thighs: GB 31
  Posterior calves: Bl 56, Bl 57
  Outer shin: St 36, GB 34
  Ankles: Bl 60, Ki 3, GB 40, St 41
  Feet: Ki 1, Sp 3

KYO JITSU IMBALANCES

A client with a Meridian that is demonstrably Kyo (empty and deficient) or Jitsu (full and excessive) should be given Shiatsu to the Meridian. To place the Gallbladder Meridian of the leg in the stretch position, bend the knee and rotate the leg outward to raise the surface. There is no Bladder Meridian stretch position for the leg in the prone position. Hip flexion and knee extension are necessary to stretch the Bladder Meridian of the leg, which is best done in the supine position as a facilitated stretch.

Palpate along the Meridian, feeling the quality of the tissues (see "Qualities of Kyo and Jitsu" and "Meridian Diagnosis" in Chapter 6). Jitsu tissues feel firm and toned, whereas Kyo tissues often feel mushy, flabby, and slack or, alternatively, very hard and tough. A Jitsu Meridian feels resistant but springy, whereas a Kyo Meridian feels bottomless or unyielding and inert. Initially, pressure on a Jitsu Meridian may elicit a lancinating (lightning bolt) sensation that abates with continued therapy. This may be accompanied by a groan or exclamation from the client, a startle response like a jerk, or a jump response like a muscle twitch. These reactions are more common when the side of the hips, lateral thighs, and calves, which tend toward hypersensitivity, are worked. Pressure on a Kyo Meridian tends to elicit a soothing, dull sensation or no sensation. When the sensation is agreeable, the client may sigh or request the practitioner to remain in the area or repeat the technique.

To sedate a Jitsu Meridian, apply stimulating techniques to disperse stagnation and congestion and to release blocked Qi (see "Application of Techniques" and Table 6-1 in Chapter 6). Two-handed compression can be used to cover more surface area and to intensify the effect. Compression along the Meridian should be moderate to deep, fairly brisk, and rhythmic, following a downward and outward direction or countercurrent to the flow of the Meridian (see "Direction of Movement" in Chapter 6). Additionally, kenbiki (jostling, torsion wringing, and cross-fiber friction) and tapotement (pummeling) can be applied. Specific Jitsu dispersal techniques include the fist twist, treading "cat paw" knuckles, elbow friction, and kneeling crawls on the hips; dynamic forearm techniques, such as "rolling pin" on the hamstrings and "sawing" on the calves; and pincer grip jostling of the calves.

To tonify a Kyo Meridian, apply nurturing techniques to draw and gather Qi to the area of deficiency (see "Application of Techniques" and Table 6-1 in Chapter 6). Specific two-handed Kyo tonification techniques include butterfly hands, double fists, and double forearms, which provide a broad, flat, noninvasive form of compression. The Mother/Son hand technique may be used when the legs present signs of deficiency—lack of tone, emaciation, weakness, coldness, edema (fluid retention), or varicose veins—or are too hyperirritable for Jitsu dispersal techniques. Place the Mother hand like a warm compress on a deficient area like Bl 23 and GV 4, or use the Mother hand to hold a key acupressure point like Ki 1 while the Son hand presses the length of the Meridian (see Practice Exercises 6-1). Pressure should be light to moderate and fairly slow and steady, following an upward and inward direction or concurrent with the flow of the Meridian (see "Direction of Movement" in Chapter 6).

Certain activities, if prolonged, such as standing, sitting, or lying down, can strain the function of a Meridian, leading to an energetic imbalance in the Meridian

(Gach, 1990). Excessive standing, required by some occupations, strains the Bladder and Kidney Meridians, leading to lumbago and weariness. Excessive physical activity or inactivity can strain the Gallbladder and Liver Meridians, inducing cramps and spasms. Give Shiatsu to these Meridians.

ELEMENT TYPE IMBALANCES

Clients who present a constellation of physical disorders or psychological disharmonies associated with a particular element should be given Shiatsu to the Yang and Yin Meridians of that element. The Gallbladder Meridian is associated with the Wood element type and the Liver and Gallbladder organ functions. The Bladder Meridian is associated with the Water element type and the Kidney and Bladder organ functions. The Stomach Meridian is associated with the Earth element type and the Spleen and Stomach organ functions. When Yang element types (Wood, Fire, and driven Water) manifest symptoms of stress-related disorders in the head,

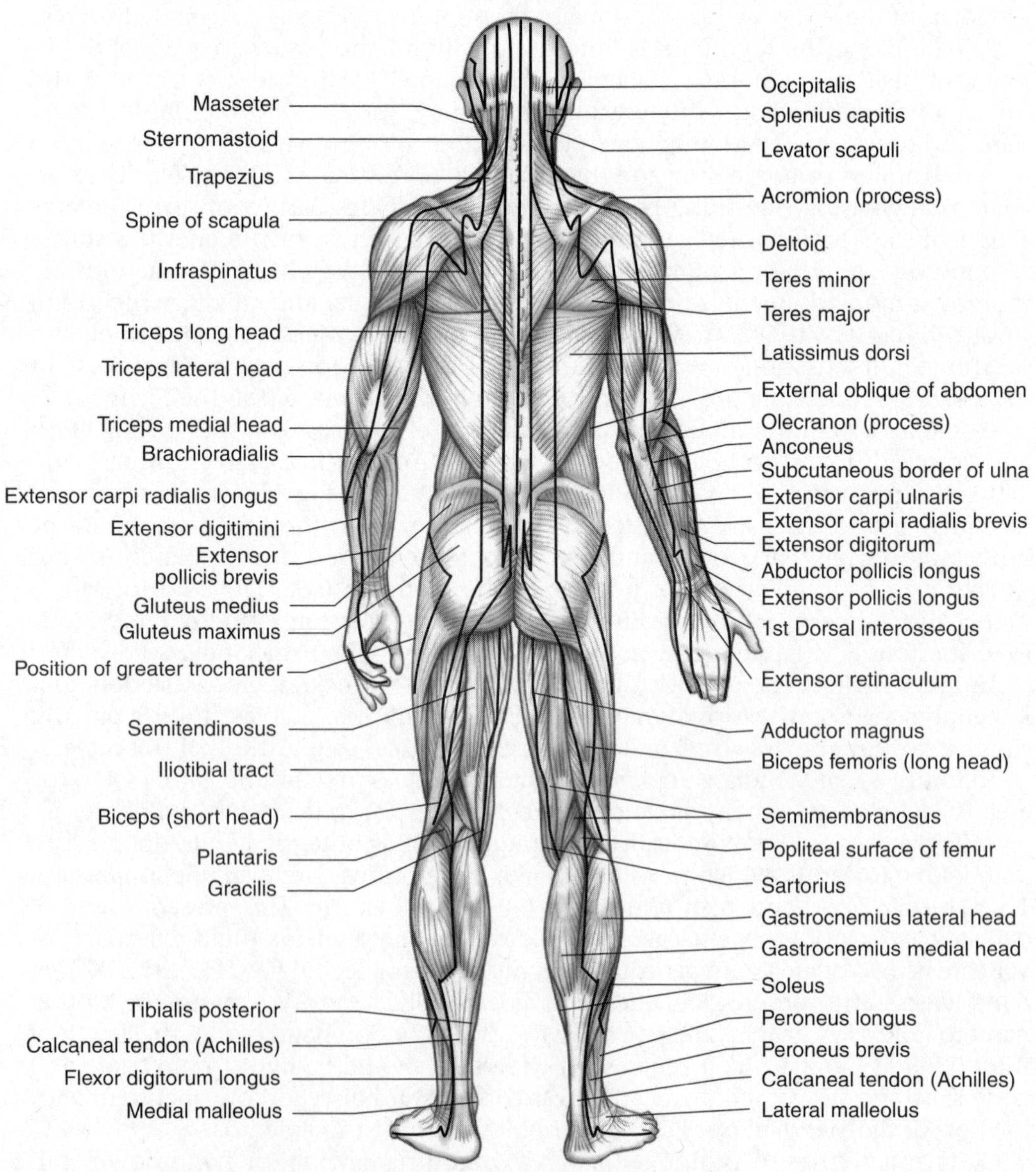

Posterior Meridians and Associated Musculature. (See Color Plate 5).

neck, and shoulders, acupressure to the lower body, especially the feet, is helpful to draw energy downward. Ki 1 lowers Qi that flares upward toward the head.

For a profile on the element types, see Chapter 4, and for a description of element imbalances, see Chapter 5. Additionally, Table 4-1 summarizes correspondences for each of the Five Elements; Table 7-4 summarizes physical disorders associated with each element's organ pair; and Table 7-5 summarizes psychological disharmonies associated with each element.

CLIENT COMFORT

Remind the client to rotate the neck periodically to prevent stiffness. If the client has lower back problems or tight ankles, place a pillow under the abdomen and a bolster under the ankles to increase client comfort, and minimize the time spent in this position, using the supine alternatives for working the Bladder and Gallbladder Meridians.

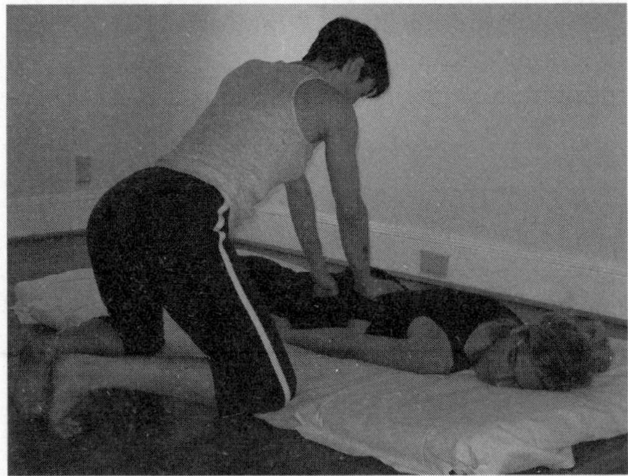

FIGURE 11-1 Fist rock.
Plant your stationary hand on the client's sacrum, and compress the gluteals with the dynamic hand, rocking the hips.

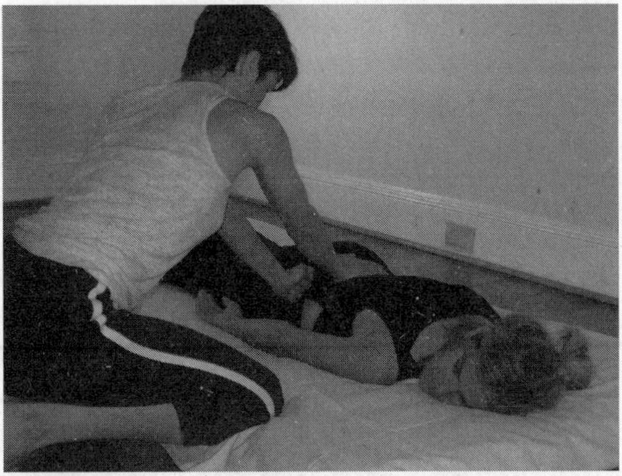

FIGURE 11-2 Fist rock.
Relocate your fist until you have worked the entire gluteal surface, including the abductors on the side of the hip.

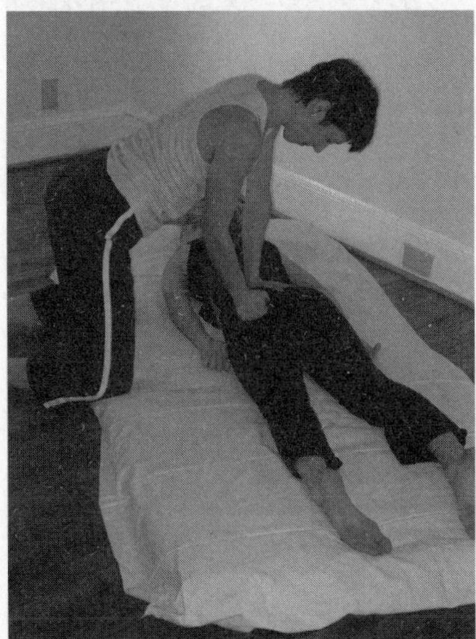

FIGURE 11-3 Fist twist.
Press down and twist. Do not slip over the client's clothes or superficial tissues; engage the deeper muscle layers and then twist.

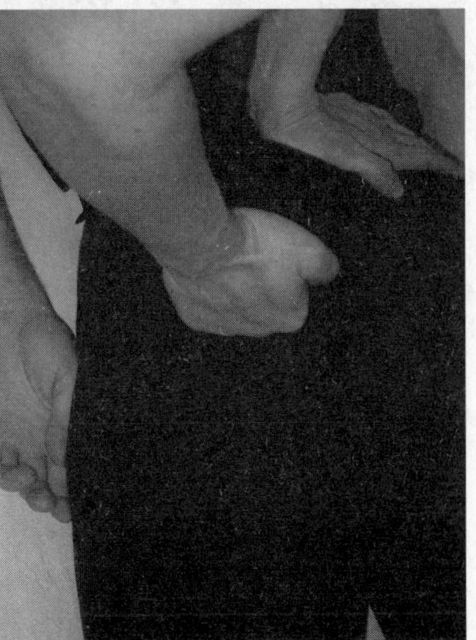

FIGURE 11-4 Close-up of fist twist.
Relocate your fist repeatedly, wringing the entire surface of the buttock, including the abductors on the side of the hip.

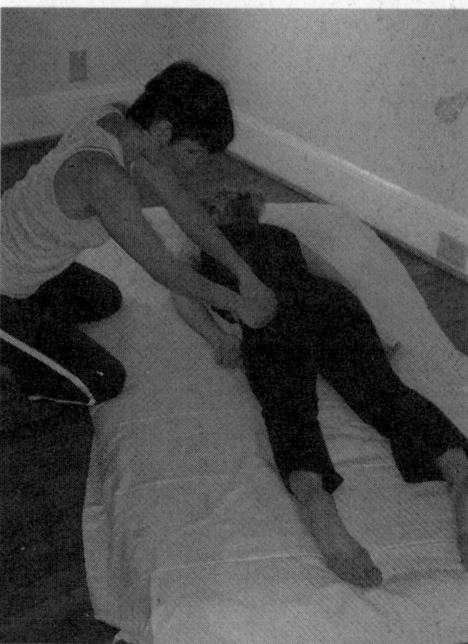

FIGURE 11-5 Knuckles, static pressure.
Sink your knuckles into the muscle attachments around the hip bone.

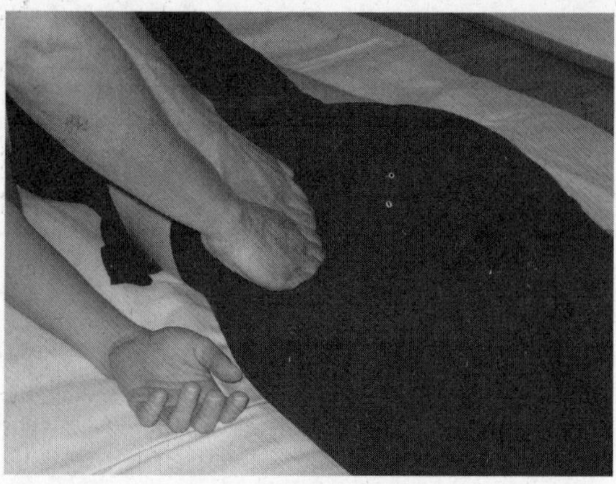

FIGURE 11-6 Knuckles, dynamic pressure.
Combine compression with transverse (side to side) friction or circular (rotary) friction for a more stimulating alternative.

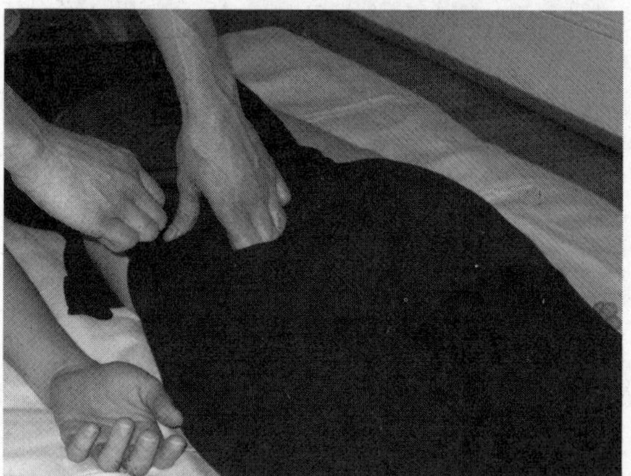

FIGURE 11-7 Knuckles, treading: "cat paws."
Press the knuckles of one hand and then those of the other hand into gluteals, alternating rhythmically.

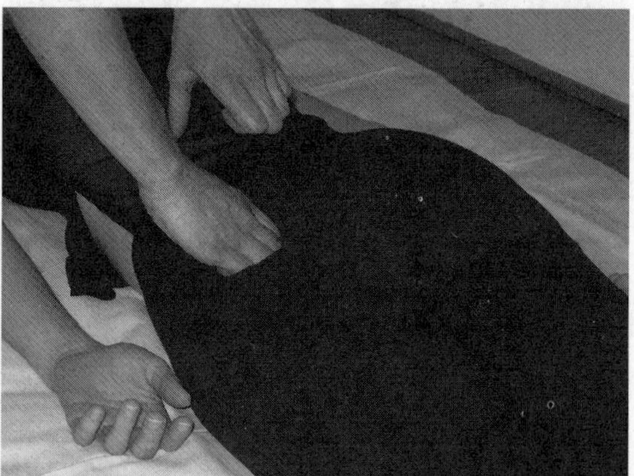

FIGURE 11-8 Knuckles, treading: "cat paws."
The client's hips should oscillate from the jostling.

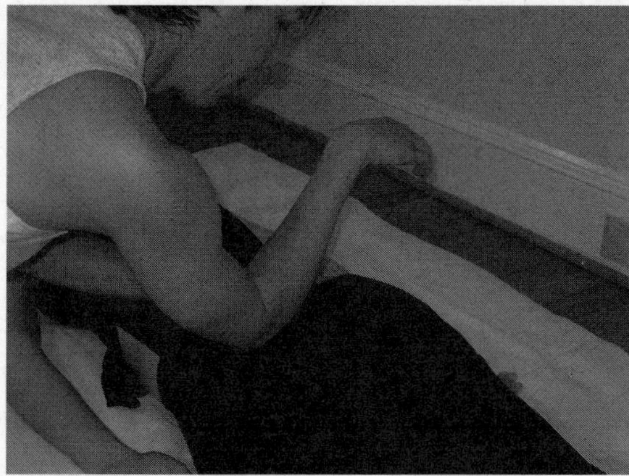

FIGURE 11-9 Elbow.
Sink your elbow into the client's gluteals, covering the entire surface of the hip. To decrease the sharpness of the sensation, extend the elbow; to increase the sharpness, flex the elbow.

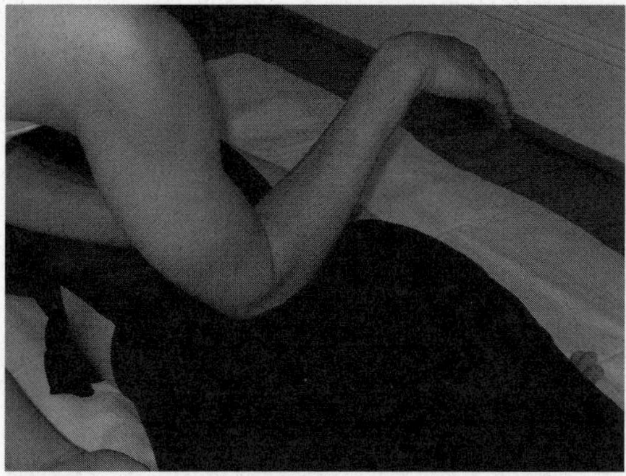

FIGURE 11-10 Bl 53.
Pause at Bl 53, on the buttock in line with the second sacral foramen.

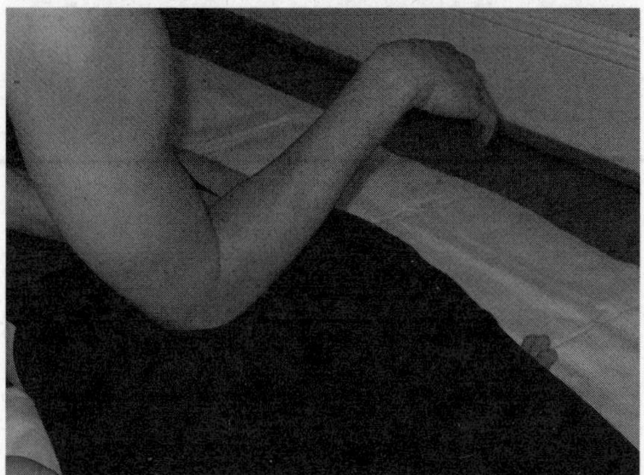

FIGURE 11-11 Bl 54.
Pause at Bl 54, on the buttock in line with the fourth sacral foramen.

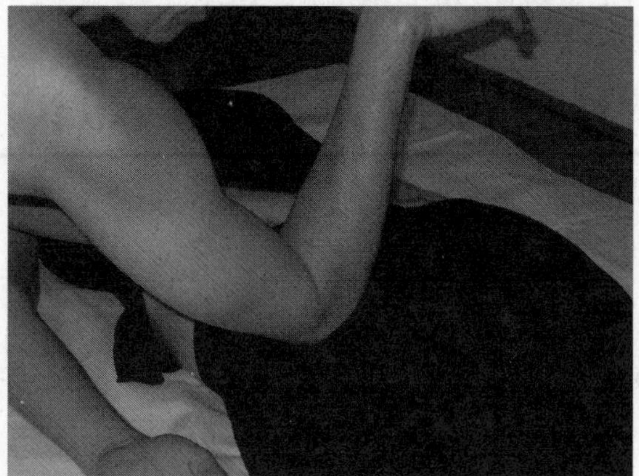

FIGURE 11-12 GB 30.
Pause at GB 30, on the buttock about two-thirds of the way between the sacrum and the greater trochanter of the femur (hipbone).

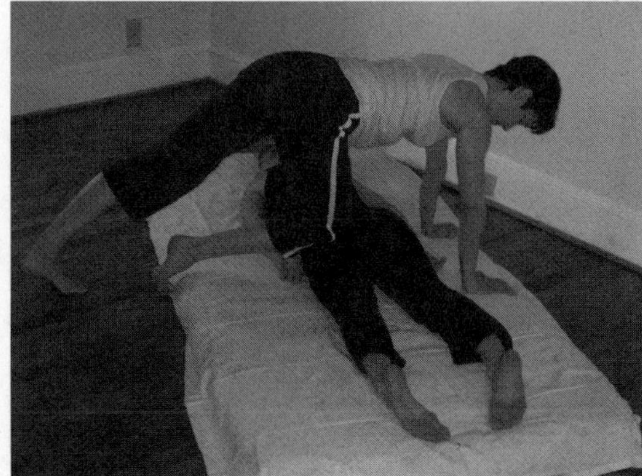

FIGURE 11-13 Knee.
Straddle the client in a push-up position. Sink your knee into the client's gluteals.

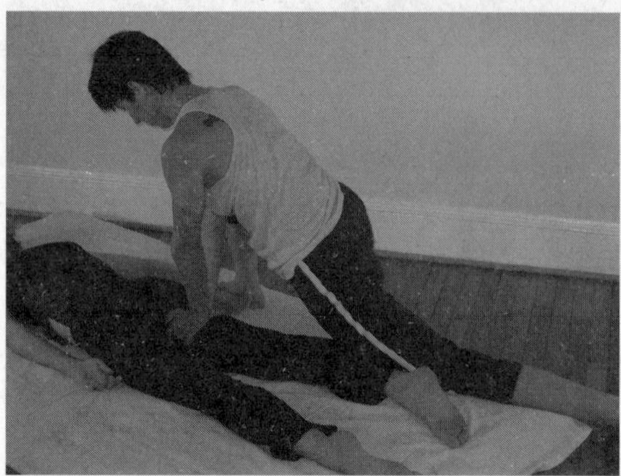

FIGURE 11-14 **Butterfly.**
In a kneeling lunge, palm press the hamstrings (Bladder Meridian) from hip to knee.

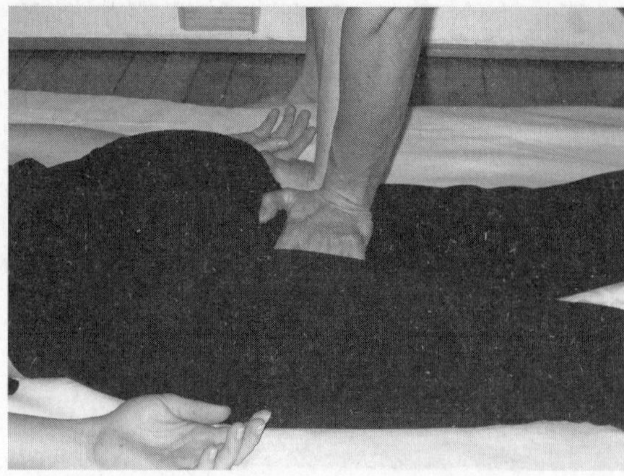

FIGURE 11-15 **Close-up of butterfly.**
Lighten the pressure when you reach the back of the knee.

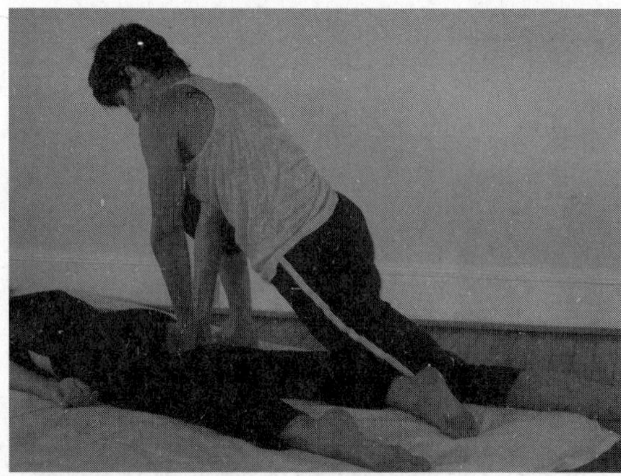

FIGURE 11-16 **Double fist press.**
In a kneeling lunge, fist press the hamstrings (Bladder Meridian) from hip to knee. The heels of the hands should be facing each other.

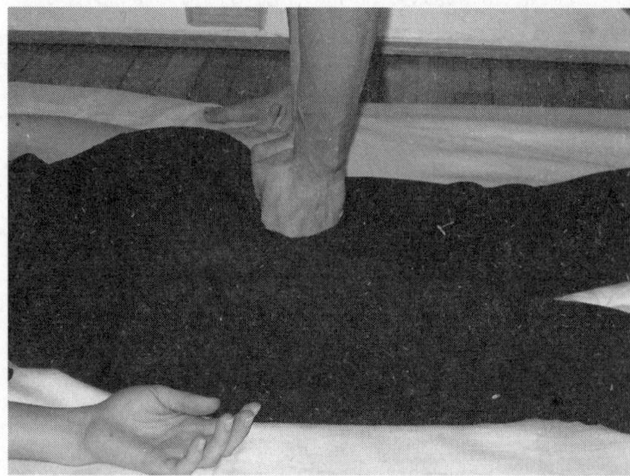

FIGURE 11-17 **Close-up of double fist press.**
Lighten the pressure when you reach the back of the knee.

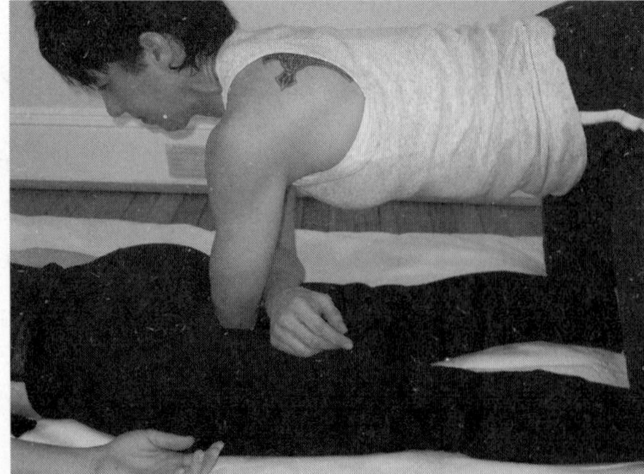

FIGURE 11-18 **Double forearms.**
In a kneeling straddle, press the hamstrings (Bladder Meridian) with both forearms from hip to knee. Lighten the pressure on the back of knee.

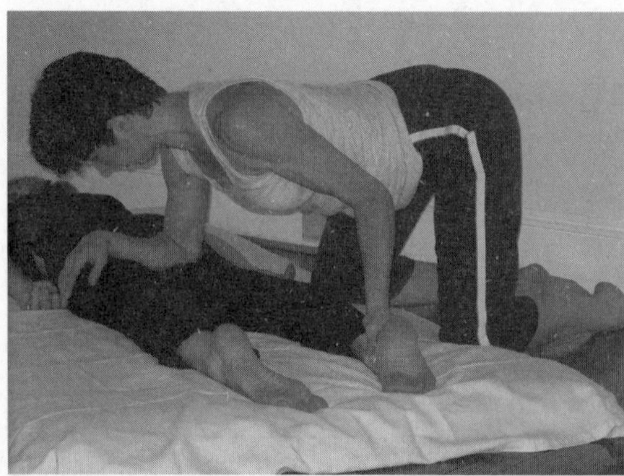

FIGURE 11-19 **Bl 36.**
Press your elbow into the hamstring attachment at the ischial tuberosity (sit bone) and traction the ankle with the opposite hand. Variation: Add transverse friction.

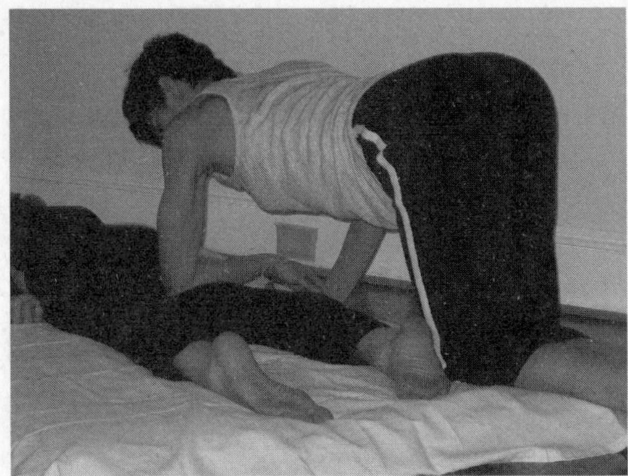

FIGURE 11-20 **Forearm: "rolling pin," palm down.**
Sink your forearm, palm down, into the hamstrings.

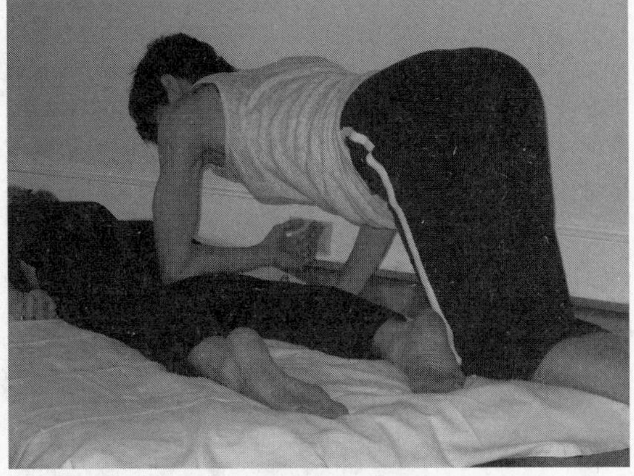

FIGURE 11-21 **Forearm: "rolling pin," palm up.**
Rotate your forearm, palm up, rolling and flattening the muscle. Repeat several times in place; then relocate lower on the leg and repeat.

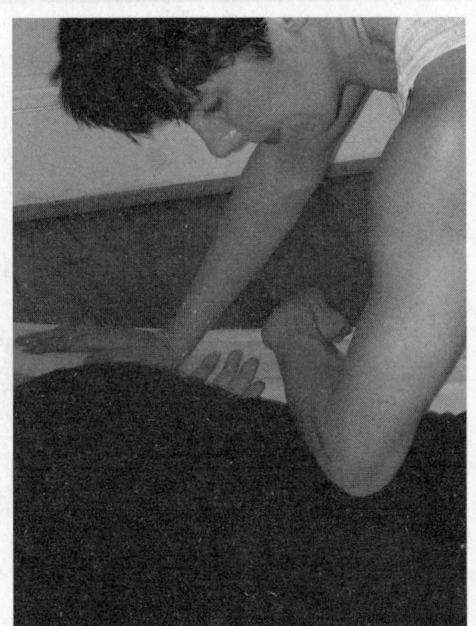

FIGURE 11-22 **Close-up of forearm: "rolling pin," palm down.**
Do not slip over the surface tissue, but engage the deeper muscle layers.

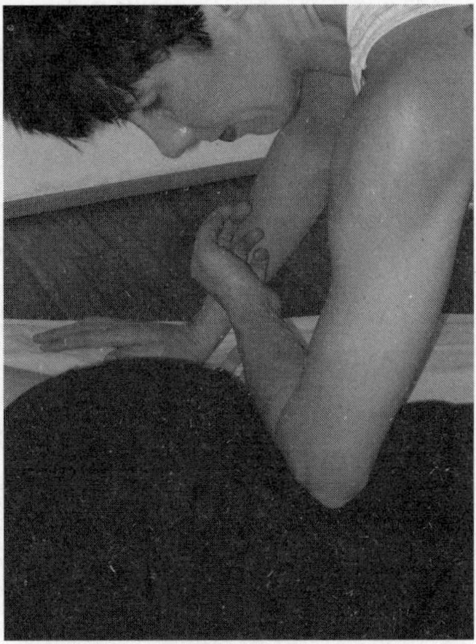

FIGURE 11-23 **Close-up of forearm: "rolling pin," palm up.**
This is a stimulating technique that can be used to disperse stagnation.

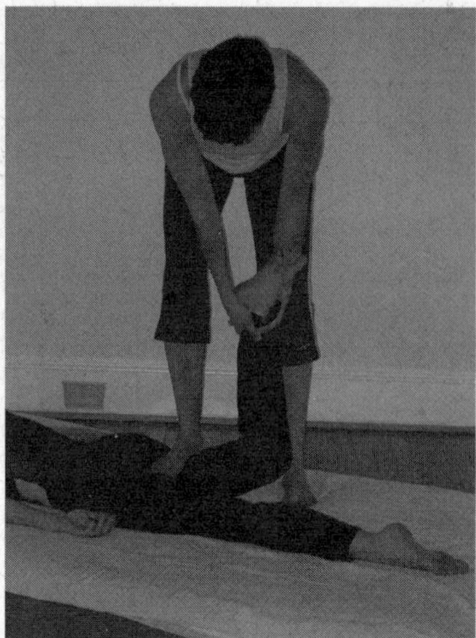

FIGURE 11-24 **Foot press with traction.** Grab the client's ankle with both hands. Plant your foot on the hamstrings. Push down with your foot and pull up on the ankle. Relocate your foot and repeat.

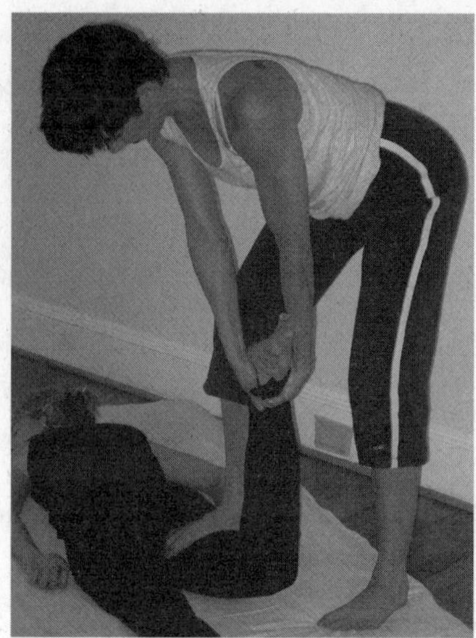

FIGURE 11-25 **Foot press with traction.** Omit this technique if you have lower back problems, or feel strain in your lower back or if your client's leg is heavier than you can comfortably lift. Repeat techniques in Figures 11–1 through 11–25 on the other side.

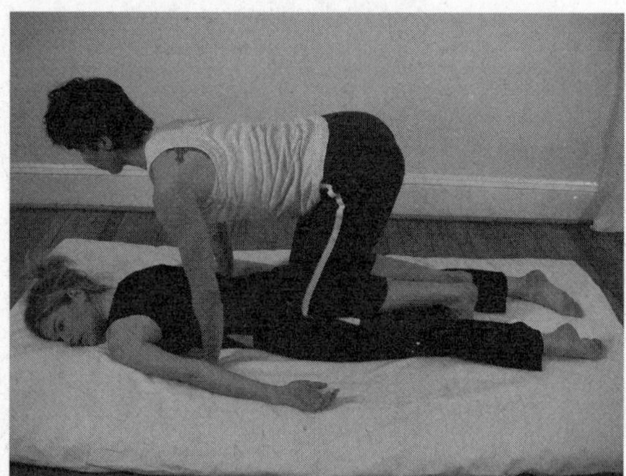

FIGURE 11-26 **Double knees.** The client's legs must be spread apart. Place your hands on either side of the client's torso and the balls of your feet between the client's legs. Kneel on the client's gluteals; transfer your weight back to your feet before relocating your knees.

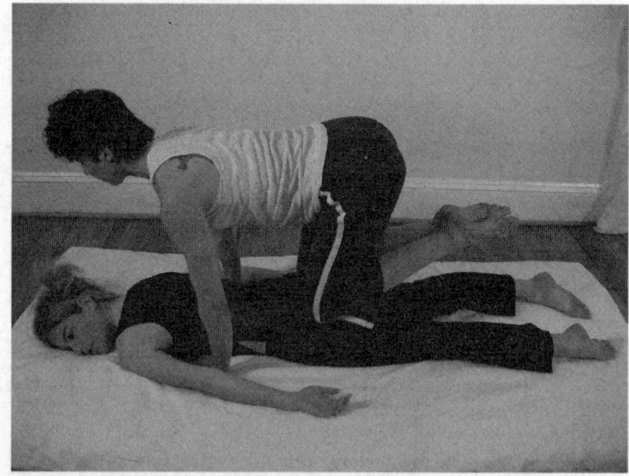

FIGURE 11-27 **Double knees, sharper angle.** To intensify the sensation, draw your feet up or create friction by alternately squeezing your knees together and drawing them apart or by sliding one knee forward and the other backward as in a crosscountry skiing motion.

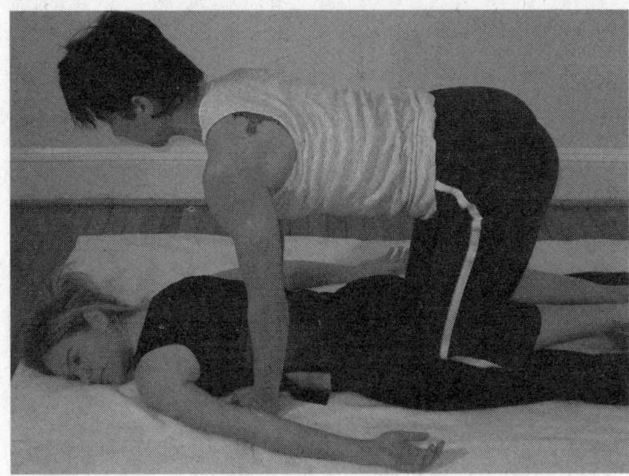

FIGURE 11-28 **Double knees, descending.** Kneel on the hamstrings at the Bladder Meridian. Lift and reset your knees farther down by transferring your weight to your feet between compressions. Stop just above knee level: Do not use this technique on the backs of the knees. This technique may be applied to the calves as well, providing the calves are warmed and prepared with preliminary techniques and providing the client enjoys deep pressure on the calves.

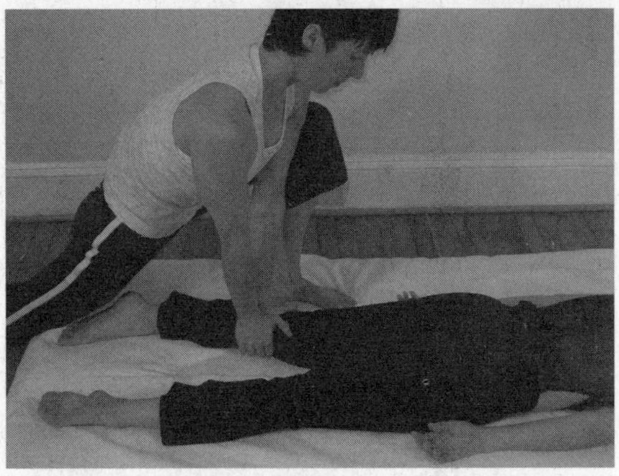

FIGURE 11-29 **Butterfly.** Palm press the calf (Bladder Meridian) from knee to ankle.

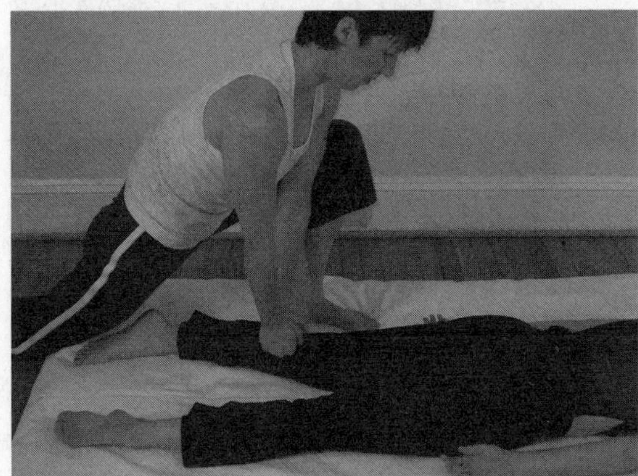

FIGURE 11-30 **Double fists.** Again, press the calf from knee to ankle. This technique can be oriented sideways, if preferred (you would then assume the kneeling samurai position).

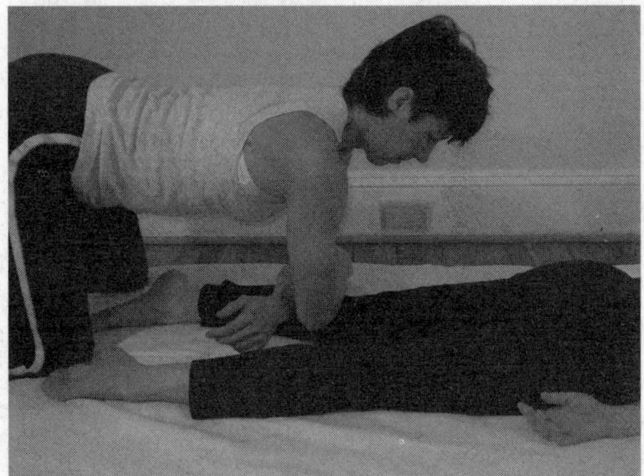

FIGURE 11-31 **Double forearms.** Leaning on both forearms, press the calf (Bladder Meridian) from knee to ankle.

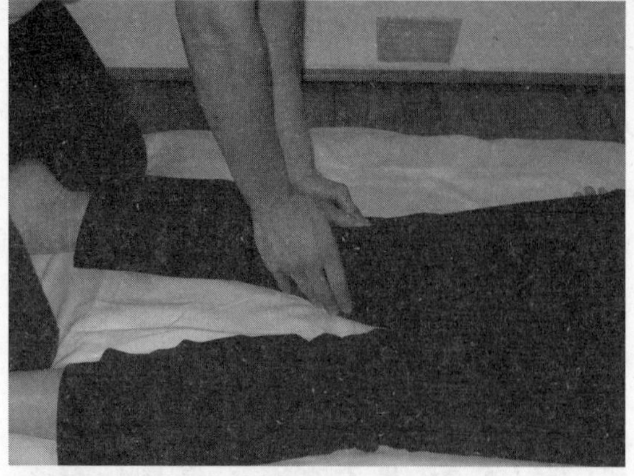

FIGURE 11-32 **Bl 40.**
Thumb press the calf, beginning at Bl 40, on the popliteal crease (back of the knee) between the two hamstring tendons. Apply light to moderate pressure on this point.

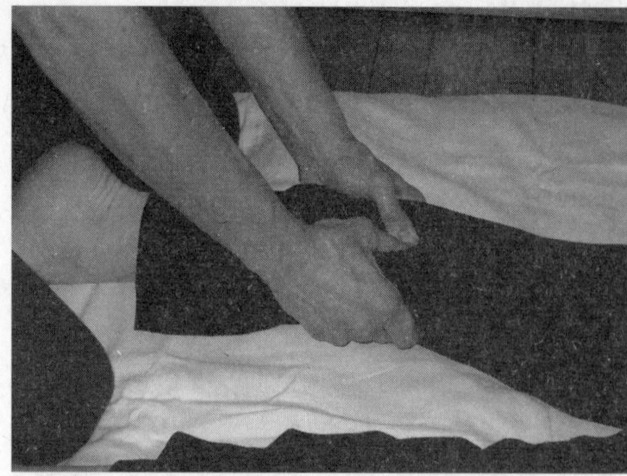

FIGURE 11-33 **Bl 56.**
Pause at Bl 56, on the high point of the belly of the gastrocnemius (superficial calf muscle).

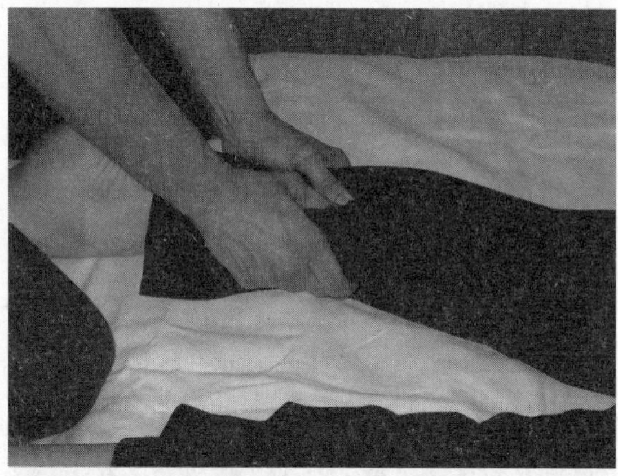

FIGURE 11-34 **Bl 57.**
Pause at Bl 57, where the belly of the calf tapers and the soleus (deeper calf muscle) is accessible.

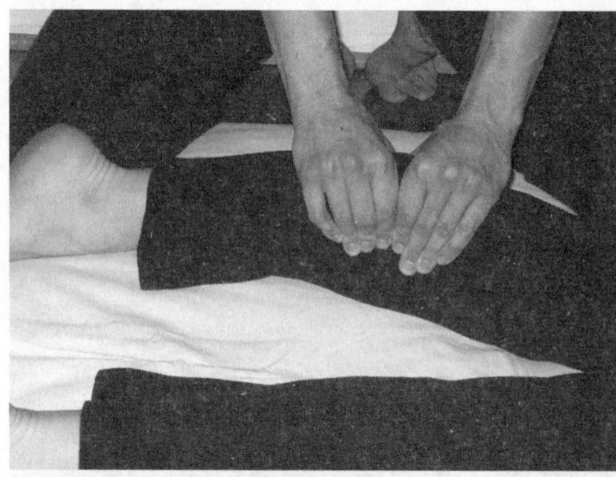

FIGURE 11-35 **Hand squeeze.**
Turn sideways to face the calf. Using a pincer grip, squeeze the calf between your fingertips and thumbs, moving from knee to ankle.

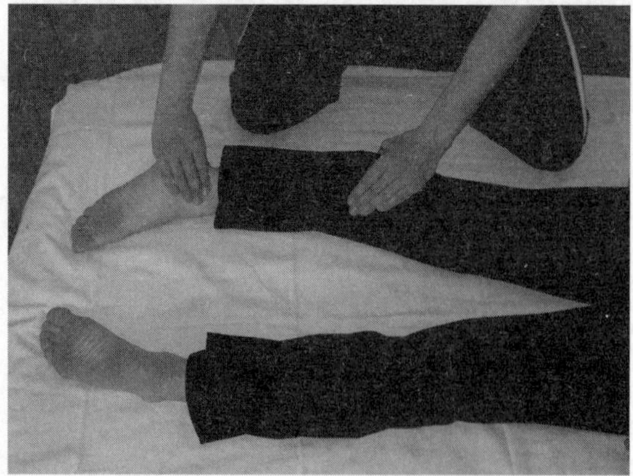

FIGURE 11-36 **Kenbiki, torquing calf outward.**
Stabilize the client's heel with one hand and grab the calf with the other. Using a firm pincer grip, jostle the calf vigorously, gradually scooting toward the ankle.

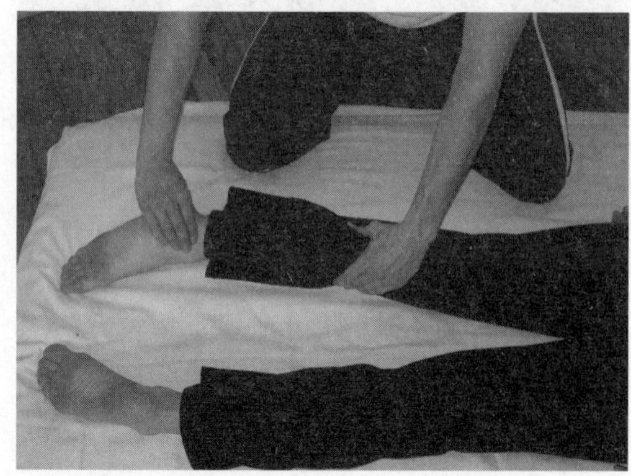

FIGURE 11-37 **Kenbiki, torquing calf inward.**
This stimulating technique is good for dispersing stagnation (calf tension and tightness).

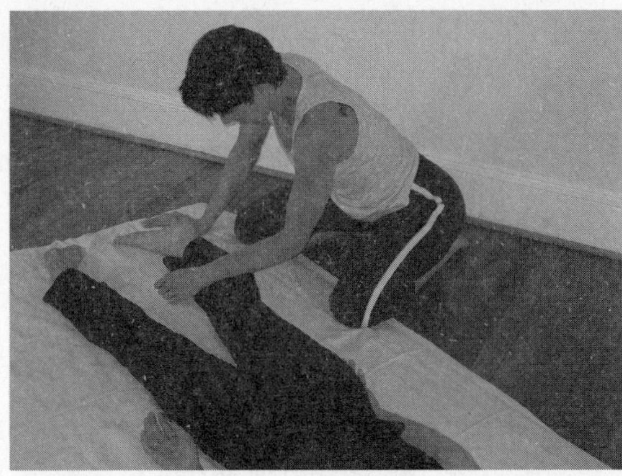

FIGURE 11-38 **Sawing forearm, lateral pull.** Using the fleshy part of your inner forearm (not the bony ulna), press into the calf and pull outward toward you. The client's leg should rotate medially (inward).

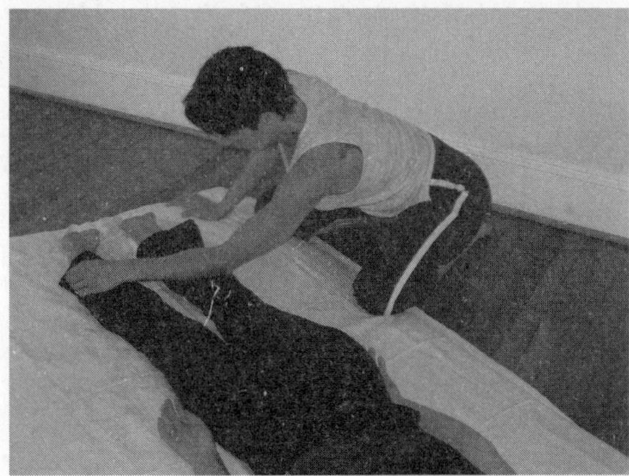

FIGURE 11-39 **Sawing forearm, medial push.** Still pressing the calf, push away. The client's leg should rotate laterally (outward). Alternate pushing and pulling, gradually scooting toward the ankle. This is another dispersal technique.

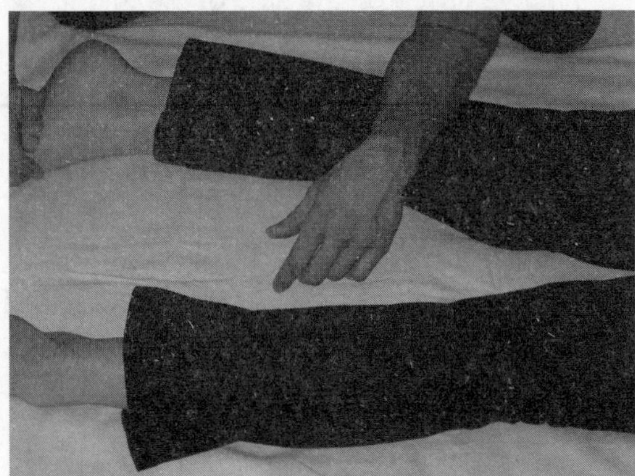

FIGURE 11-40 **Close-up of sawing forearm, pull.** The client's leg will rotate inward and outward as you pull and push.

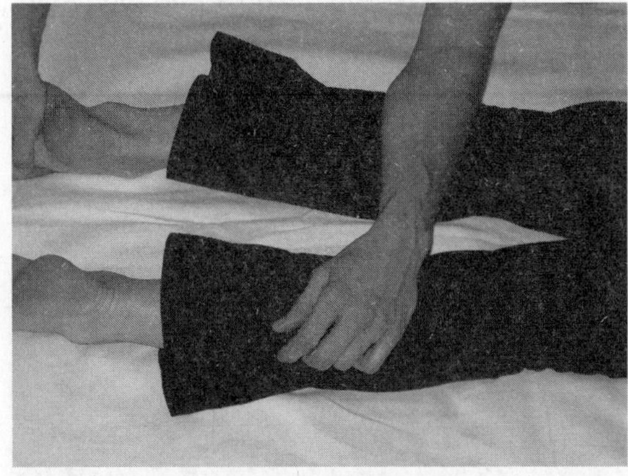

FIGURE 11-41 **Close-up of sawing forearm, push.**

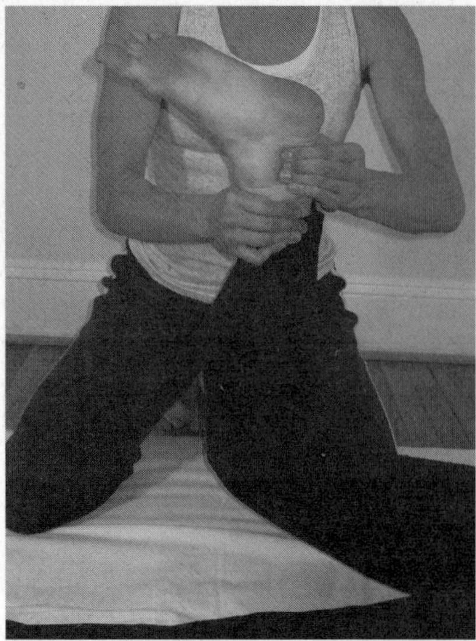

FIGURE 11-42 Press Ki 3 and Bl 60.
Lift and support the lower leg with one hand. With the other, squeeze the inner ankle (Ki 3) and outer ankle (Bl 60) on either side of the Achilles tendon, using a pincer grip. Variation: Raise the lower leg off the ground and wriggle back and forth on the pressure points, applying kenbiki.

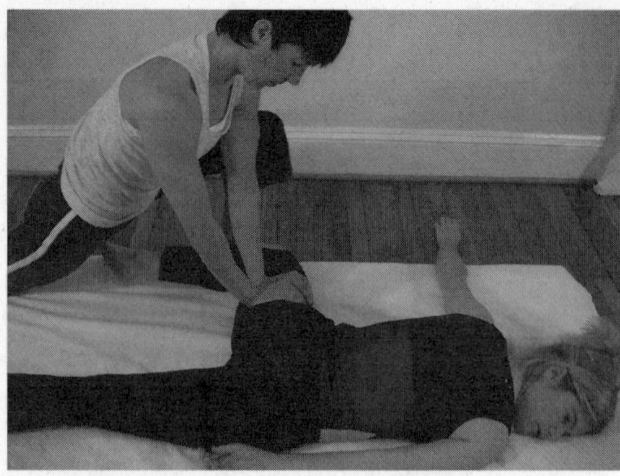

FIGURE 11-43 Heel of the hand compression on the Gallbladder Meridian.
Rotate the client's leg laterally to expose Gallbladder Meridian. Face the client's head in a kneeling lunge. Press the heels of your hands under the vastus lateralis and iliotibial tract (the broad band of muscle and connective tissue on the side of the thigh). Press from hip to knee.

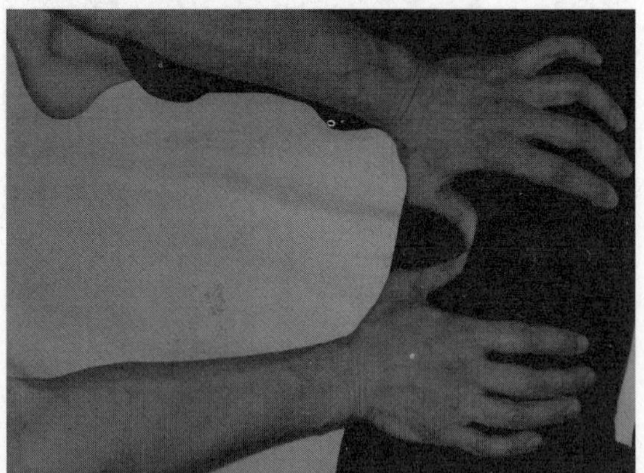

FIGURE 11-44 Double thumbs on GB 31.
Press your thumbs under the vastus lateralis and iliotibial tract. Work from hip to knee, pausing at GB 31, about halfway down the outer thigh.

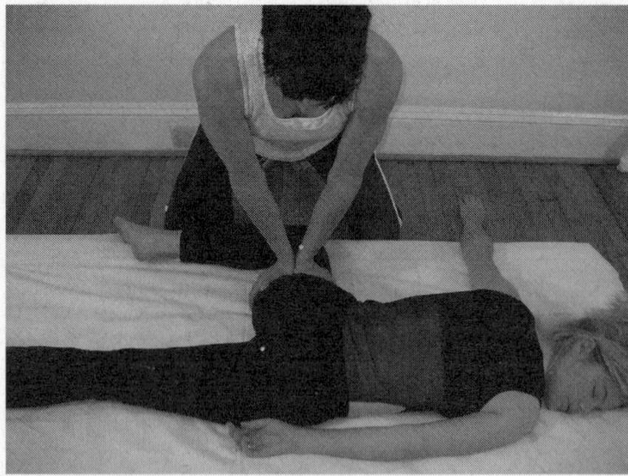

FIGURE 11-45 Butterfly on the Gallbladder Meridian.
Reposition yourself, facing the client's hip in a kneeling samurai stance. Compress muscle against bone, moving from hip to knee.

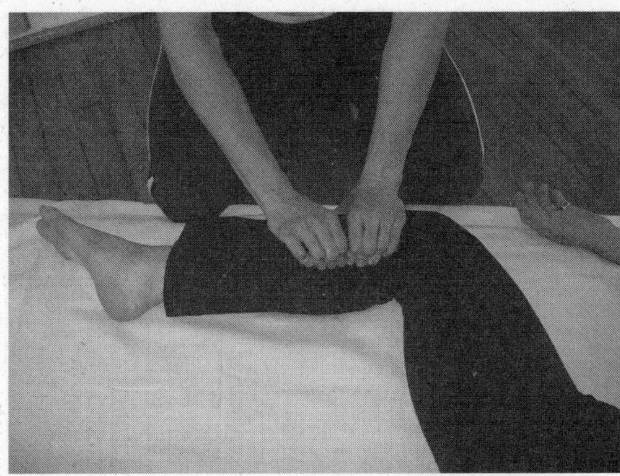

FIGURE 11-46 Fingertip squeeze.
Face the client's shin. Press your thumbs along the Stomach or Gallbladder Meridian from knee to ankle while your fingers squeeze the calf.

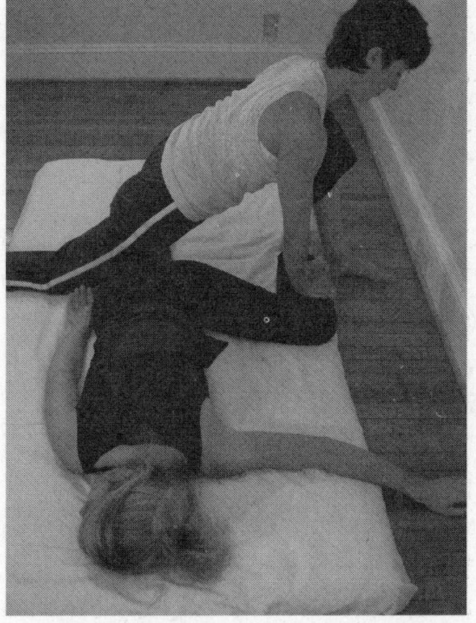

FIGURE 11-47 Heel of the hand press on the Stomach and Gallbladder Meridians.
Remain in the kneeling samurai stance (not shown), as in Figure 11–46, or relocate to face the calf in a kneeling lunge (shown) and press the heels of your hands along the lower leg.

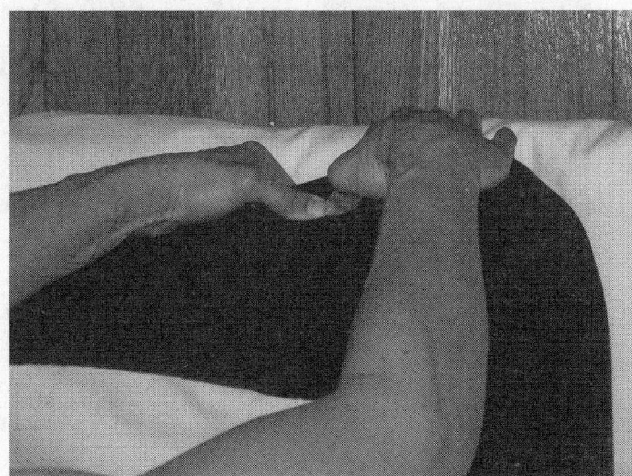

FIGURE 11-48 St 36.
Three cun (4 finger widths) below the patella (kneecap) slightly under the tibia (shinbone).

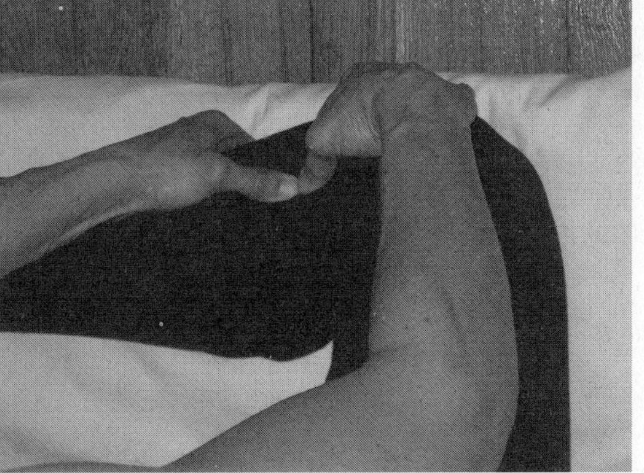

FIGURE 11-49 GB 34.
In front of and below the head of the fibula. To locate the head of the fibula, feel for a small, bony knob just lateral to the shin.

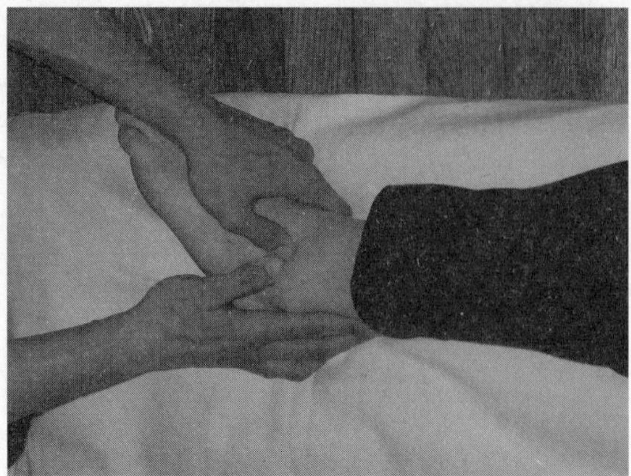

FIGURE 11-50 **GB 40.**
In the depression in front of the lateral malleolus (outer anklebone).

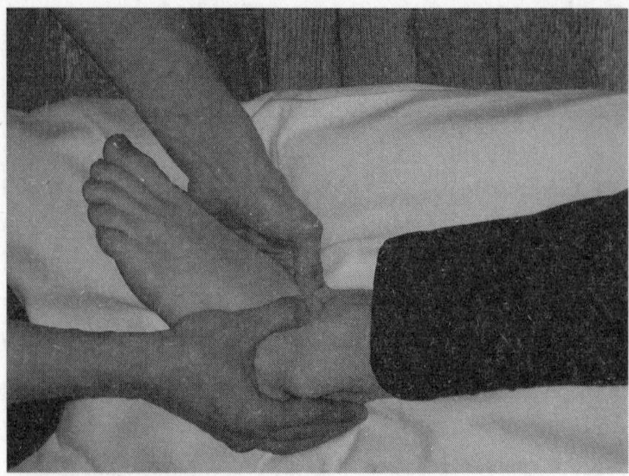

FIGURE 11-51 **St 41.**
At ankle level between the extensor hallicus longus tendon of the big toe and the extensor digitorum longus tendon of the other four toes. To define these tendons, ask the client to flex the foot.

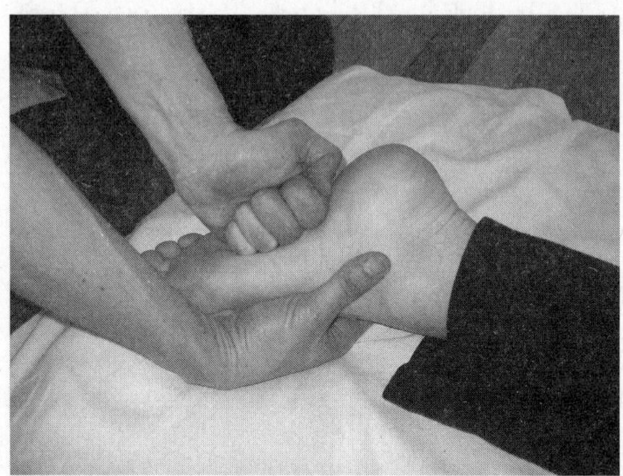

FIGURE 11-52 **Fist twist.**
Straighten the client's leg and apply the fist twist to the entire sole of the foot.

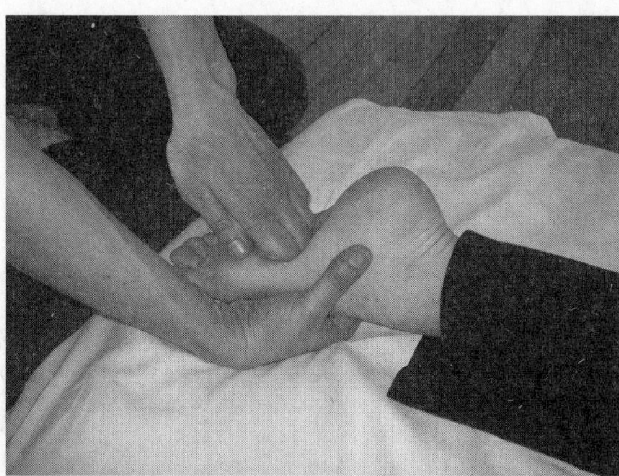

FIGURE 11-53 **Knuckles.**
Apply static pressure and transverse or circular friction with the knuckles to the entire sole of the foot.

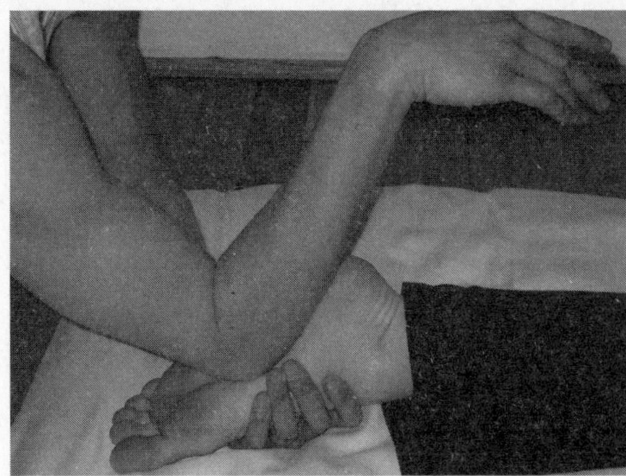

FIGURE 11-54 **Elbow.**
Apply elbow pressure to the entire sole of the foot.

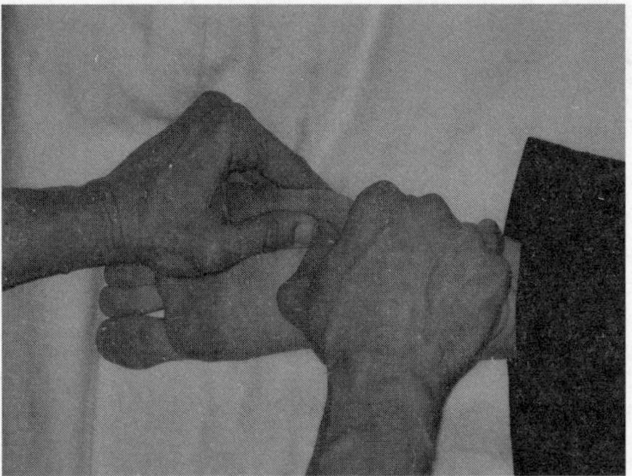

FIGURE 11-55 **Pincer grip.**
Pinch the side of the foot, pressing the thumbs along the lateral edge and the fingers along the fifth metatarsal. The latter corresponds to the Bladder Meridian, which terminates at the outer nailbed of the little toe.

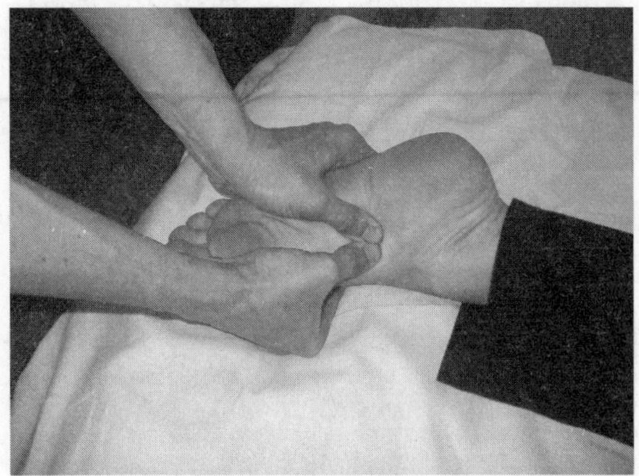

FIGURE 11-56 **Thumb press.**
Press the thumbs along the medial arch. This corresponds to the Spleen Meridian, which terminates at the inner nailbed of the big toe.

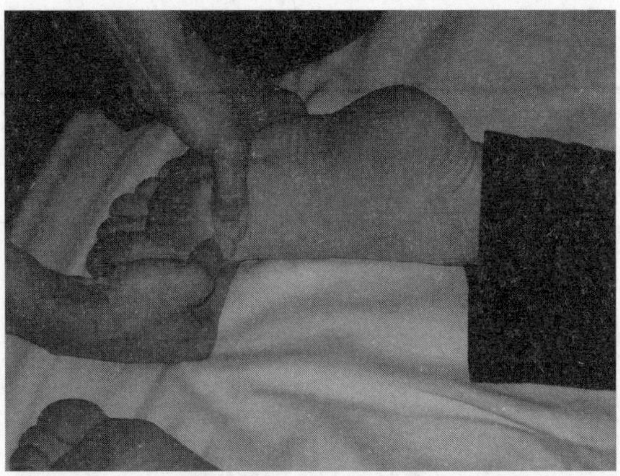

FIGURE 11-57 **Sp 3.**
On the medial arch of the foot, just above the first metatarsal.

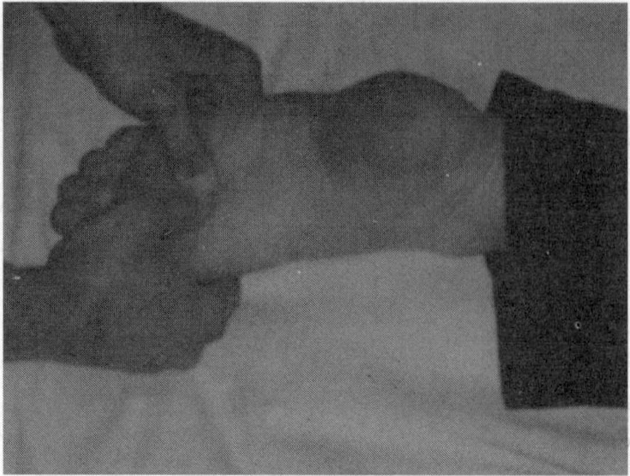

FIGURE 11-58 **Ki 1.**
On the sole of the foot just above the ball of the foot between the second and third metatarsals.

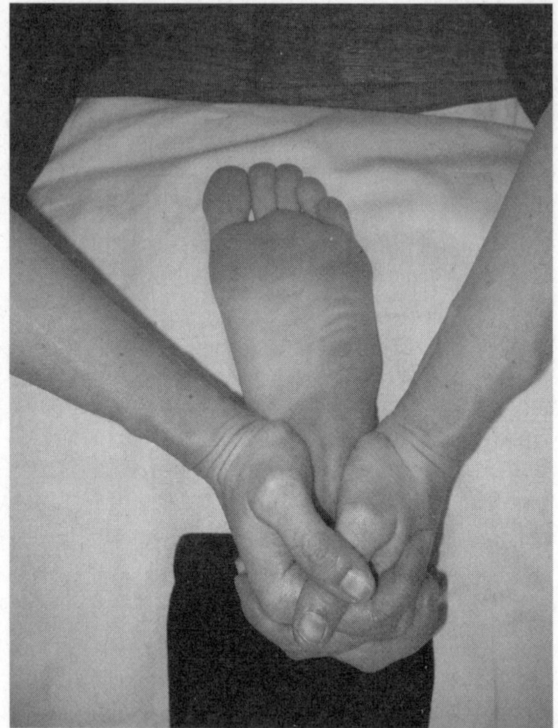

FIGURE 11-59 **Heel rub.**
Clasp your hands, squeeze, and rub the heels of your hands across the inner and outer heel.

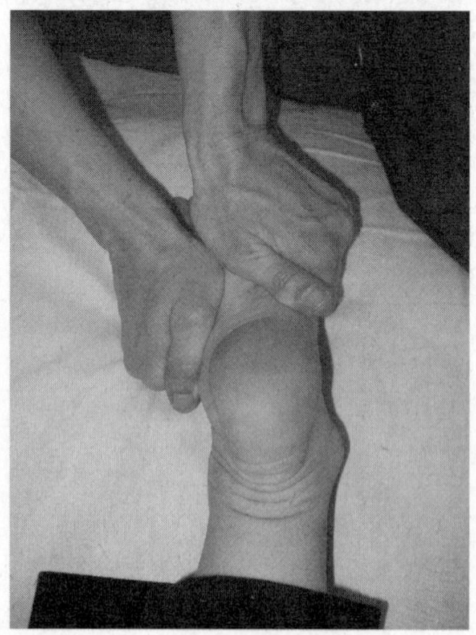

FIGURE 11-60 **Inversion.**
Hold the sides of the foot and rotate medially (inward).

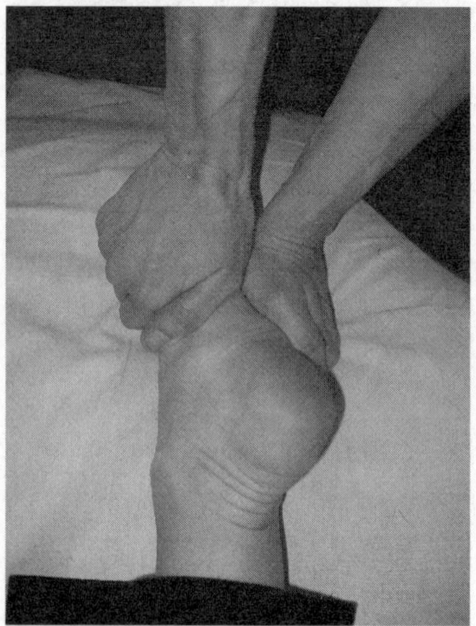

FIGURE 11-61 **Eversion.**
Rotate laterally (outward). Alternate inversion and eversion rapidly to mobilize the foot.

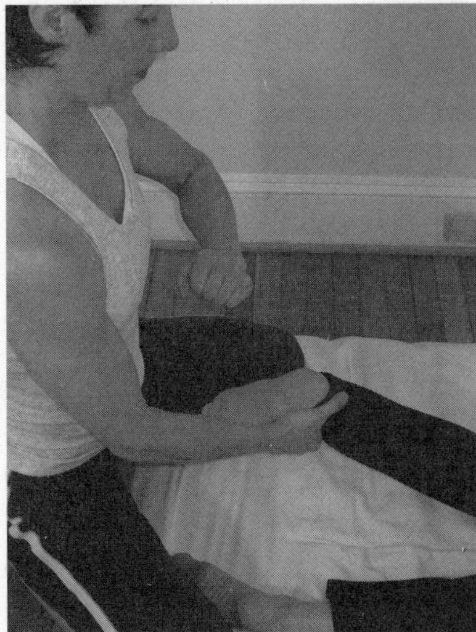

FIGURE 11-62 Pounding.
Support the dorsal surface of the foot. Pound the heel firmly with your fist. This is a stimulating technique.

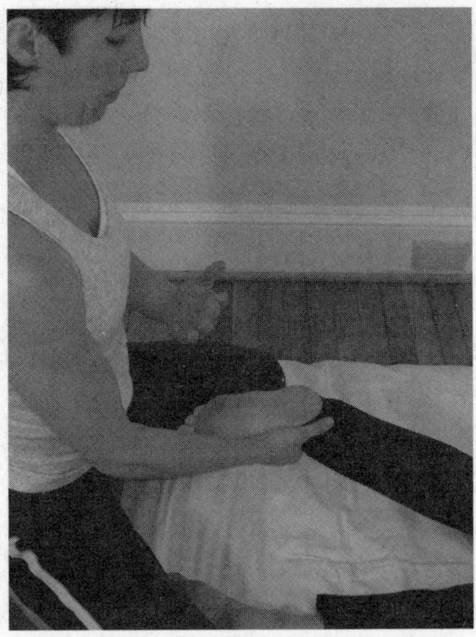

FIGURE 11-63 Slapping.
Slap the sole of the foot with the back of your hand. This is a stimulating technique.

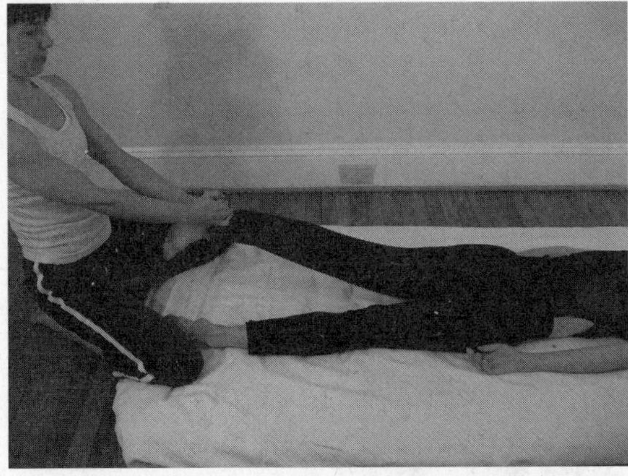

FIGURE 11-64 Leg traction.
Cup one hand under the dorsal surface of the client's foot and the other over the heel. Pull and hold, or pull and jostle.
Repeat techniques in Figures 11–29 through 11–64 on the other side.

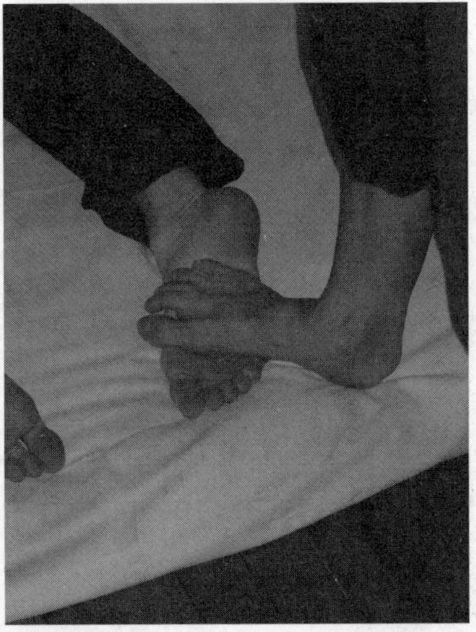

FIGURE 11-65 Foot treading, ball of the foot.
The ball of the foot provides the lightest pressure. Tread on one foot at a time. Shift your weight back and forth between your supporting leg and your working leg.
Repeat on the other foot.

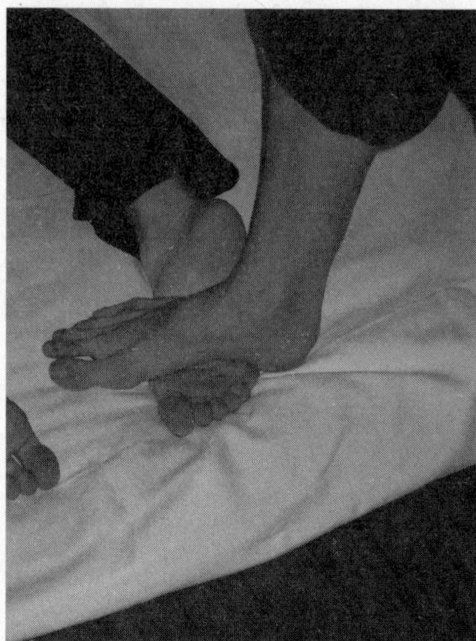

FIGURE 11-66 Foot treading, side of the foot.
The side and sole of the foot provide moderate pressure. Shift your weight back and forth. Repeat on the other foot.

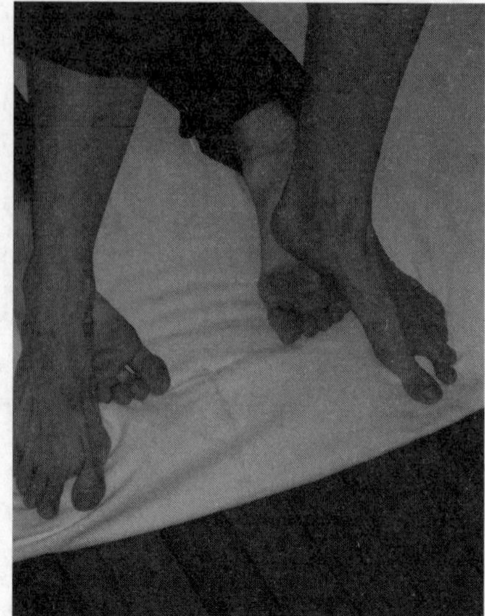

FIGURE 11-67 Foot treading, heel.
The heels provide the strongest pressure. Tread on both soles simultaneously. Do not attempt to mount the heels. If the client's ankles are tight, place a pillow under the ankles.

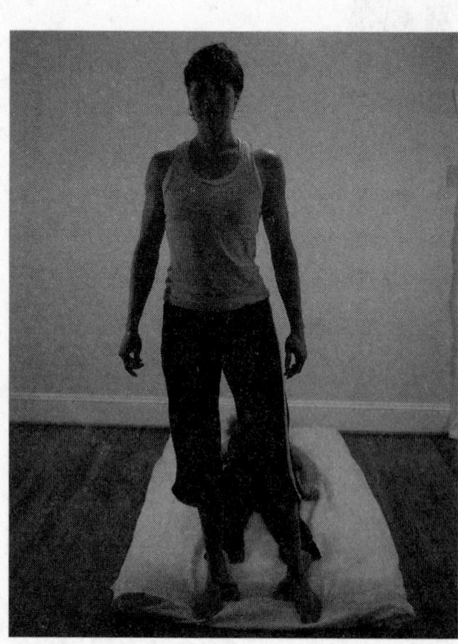

FIGURE 11-68 Foot treading, swaying.
Transfer your weight from side to side for a couple minutes, slightly shifting the location of your heels on the soles of the client's feet.

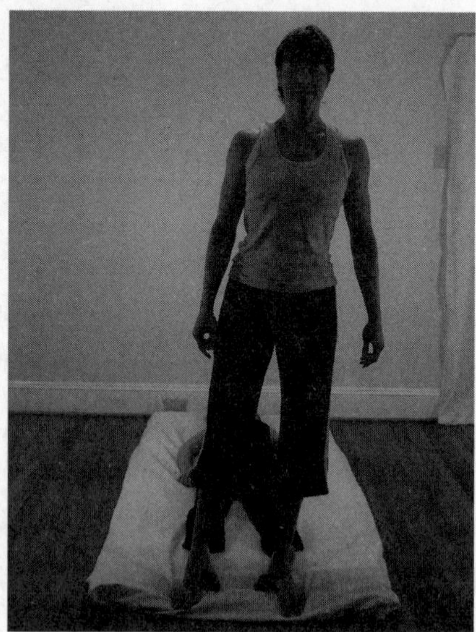

FIGURE 11-69 Foot treading, swaying continued.
If the client's feet are sensitive, omit the heels and use the balls of your feet (gentlest version) or the sides of your feet (moderate version) instead.

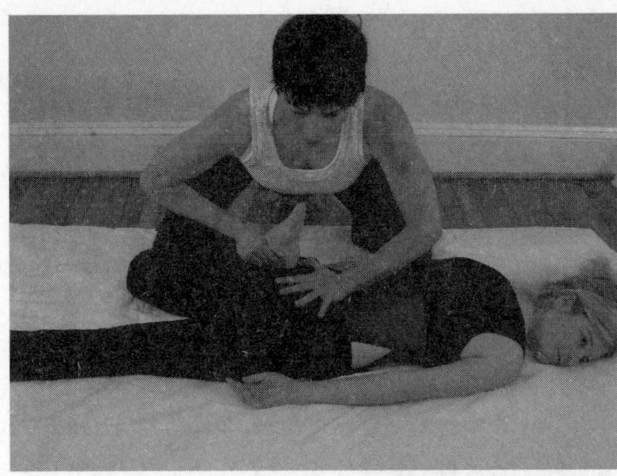

FIGURE 11-70 **Quadriceps/St/Sp stretch.** Grab the client's ankle and bend the knee. Stabilize the client's sacrum and press the heel toward the buttock.

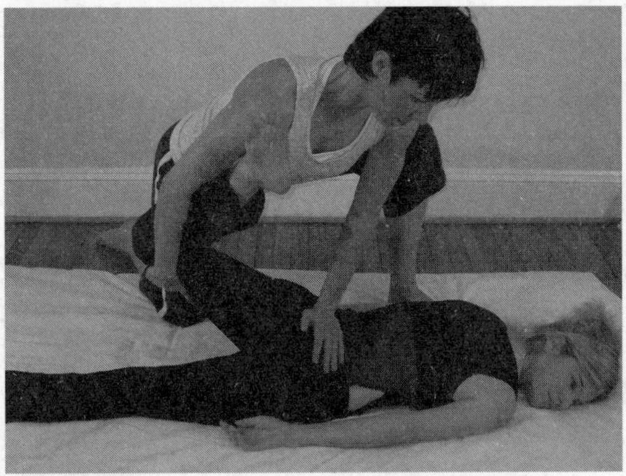

FIGURE 11-71 **Hip flexor/St/Sp stretch.** Scoop one hand under the client's inner thigh just above the knee. Stabilize the client's sacrum. Lift the leg. Switch sides and repeat the quadricep and hip flexor stretches on other leg.

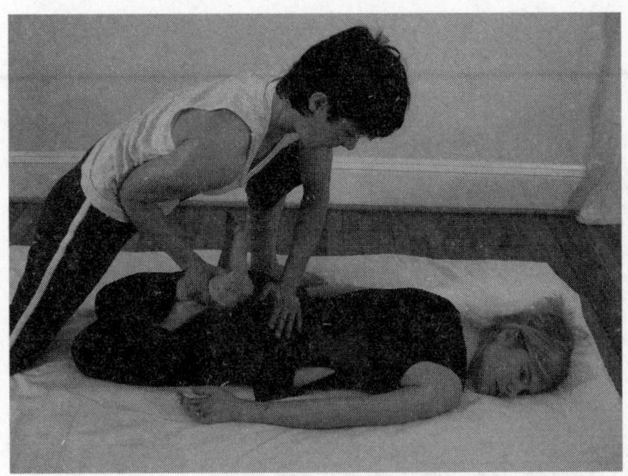

FIGURE 11-72 **Crossed-leg quadriceps stretch.**
Cross one foot over the other and press the heels toward the buttocks while stabilizing the sacrum.

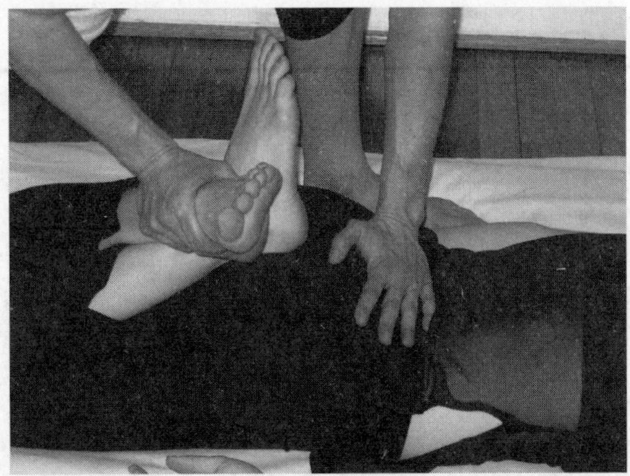

FIGURE 11-73 **Close-up of crossed-leg quadriceps stretch.**
Reverse and repeat.

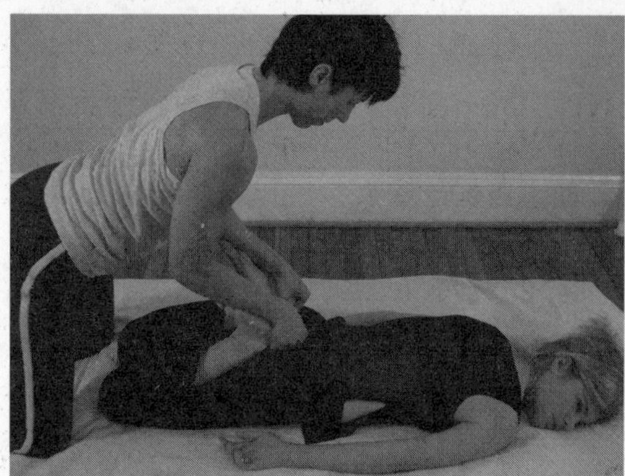

FIGURE 11-74 Double quadriceps and soleus stretch (St/Bl).
Curl your fingers over the client's heels and press your forearms down, flexing the client's feet. Push the heels toward the buttocks.

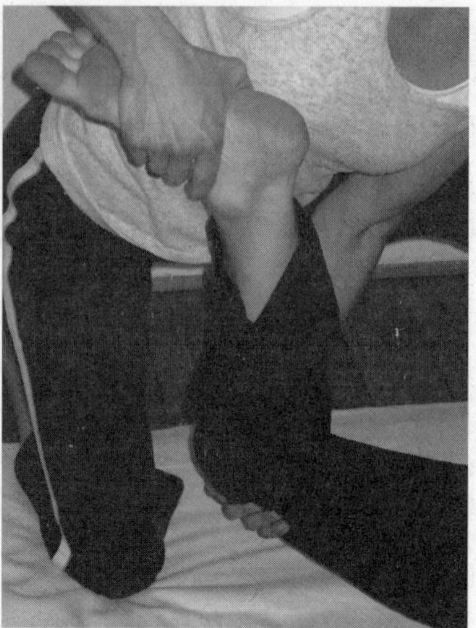

FIGURE 11-75 Adductor/Yin Meridian stretch preparation.
Grab the client's foot with your innermost hand and lift the leg. Place your outer hand above the client's knee and support the thigh.

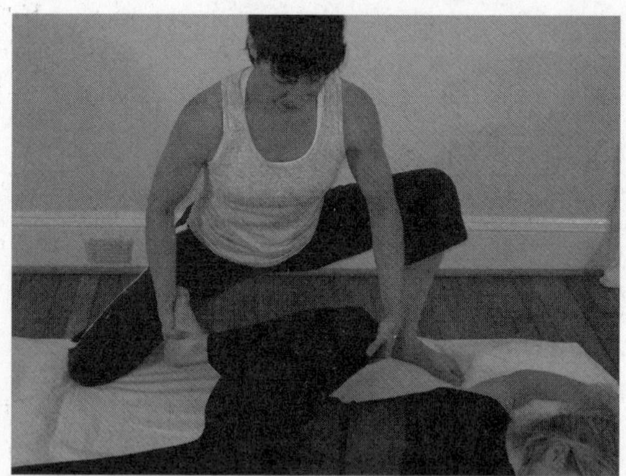

FIGURE 11-76 Adductor/Yin Meridian stretch.
Rotate the client's leg laterally (sideways/outward), and draw the knee to the waist. Retract the leg a little and repeat several times. Switch sides and repeat.

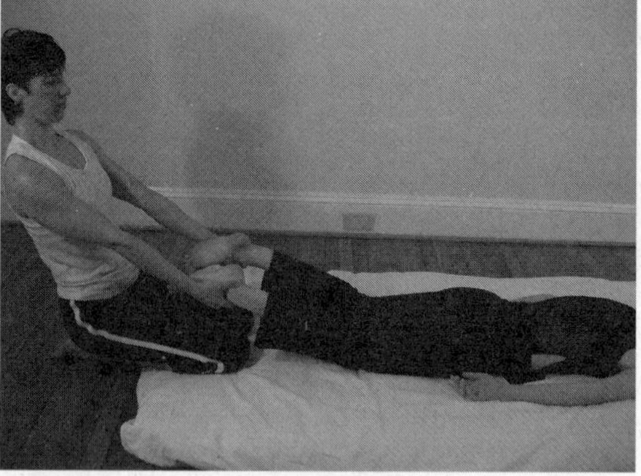

FIGURE 11-77 Final traction.
Cup both hands under the dorsal surface of the client's feet and gently pull. Alternative ending (not shown): Press both thumbs in Ki 1 and hold.

REFERENCE

Gach, M. (1990). *Acupressure' s potent points: A guide to self-care for common ailments.* New York: Bantam.

12

Supine Lower Body Protocol

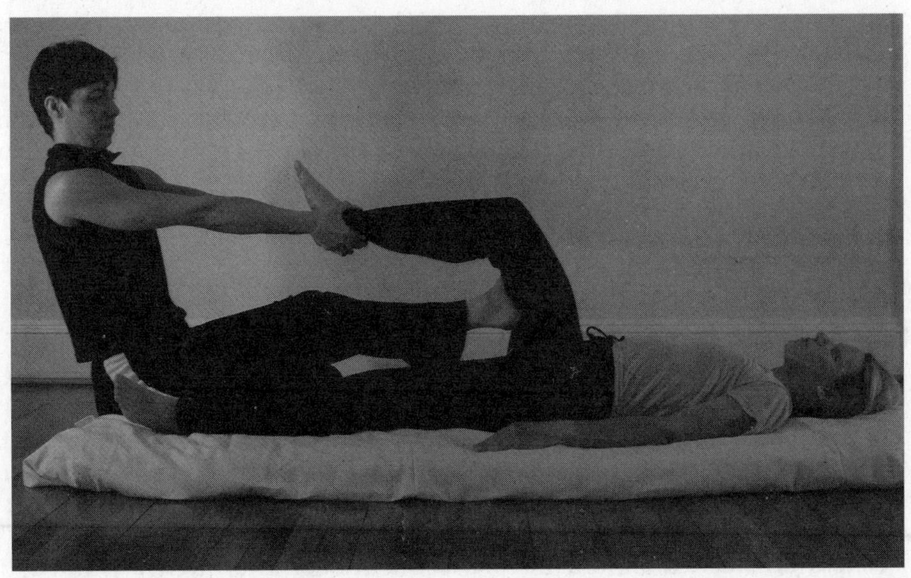

Therapeutic Emphasis

The supine lower body protocol is fairly elaborate and complex, primarily because the supine position allows the practitioner to apply a broad array of stretches and body mobilization techniques (BMTs) to the feet, ankles, legs, and hips that are not possible in other positions. The supine position is also the most comprehensive of positions because every Meridian in the legs, even the Bladder Meridian of the posterior leg, can be accessed to a greater or lesser degree. Becoming proficient at all the techniques shown will enrich and diversify your practice, allowing you to customize and vary your Shiatsu sessions. Nevertheless, some of the stretches and BMTs, especially the more acrobatic ones, may be inappropriate for you or your client, so exercise good judgment and honor your physical boundaries as well as your client's.

The Stomach (St), Spleen (Sp), Liver (Lr), and Kidney (Ki) Meridians of the legs are particularly amenable to treatment in this position. Focused work on these Meridians and key acupressure points can benefit clients who have painful obstruction syndrome—localized muscular soreness and joint aches—in the front and inner thighs, inner and outer lower legs, and tops of the feet; clients whose Meridians assess as Kyo or Jitsu or are otherwise symptomatic; and clients who present physical disorders or psychological disharmonies associated with the corresponding elements.

Causes of Discomfort and Treatment Strategies

Because the muscles of the legs are relatively large and powerful, a client is more likely to develop painful obstruction syndrome in the lower body from vigorous exercise and participation in sports events, performing arts, and outdoor recreational activities than from ordinary manual labor or prolonged or repetitive low-load occupational activities. To disperse blood and fluid stagnation, sore and fatigued muscles should be pressed, squeezed, and rubbed. To clear blockages in energy flow, key acupressure points in the associated muscles should be pressed and held or pressed and subjected to friction. Although the muscles of the front and inner thigh are large—three members of the quadriceps group are named *vastus*, meaning "vast"; one member of the adductors is named *magnus*, meaning "great"; and another is named *longus* meaning "long"—they tend to be sensitive, so use industrial-strength techniques only if appropriate for the client. If soreness extends along the pathway of a Meridian, the entire Meridian should be given Shiatsu. The listed examples target isolated areas of the anterior lower body that can become sore and fatigued from exertion. For photos of point locations on a human model, see Appendix 1. For illustrated charts of acupressure point and Meridian locations, see the Flow of Qi chart in Figure 2–1 and the Anterior Meridians and Associated Musculature Chart on p. 254.

KEY ACUPRESSURE POINTS FOR THE ANTERIOR LOWER BODY

- **Front of Thighs**: The quadriceps (front thigh muscles) can become sore from doing hip flexion and knee extension exercises like squats, lunges, leg presses, and seated knee extensions; from using a stairmaster or elliptical cardio machine or riding a bicycle (especially uphill or out of saddle drills); from climbing and doing step aerobics; from jumping as in basketball, volleyball, and high-impact aerobics; and from leaping and extending the leg to the front or side as in dance, gymnastics, and martial arts. Those clients who complain of knee soreness and aches should have the quadriceps thoroughly worked, with particular attention to the tendinous attachments at and below the knee. Give Shiatsu to the Stomach and Spleen Meridians and acupressure to St 31, St 34, Sp 10, and Sp 11 of the thigh and Sp 9, St 35, St 36, and GB 34 to benefit the knee.
- **Inner Thighs**: The adductors (inner thigh muscles) can become sore from hip adduction exercises that entail drawing or squeezing the inner thighs together or moving one leg across the midline of the body against resistance. Riding a horse requires isometric contraction of the adductors to keep the rider in the saddle. Soccer requires concentric contraction of the adductors to travel kick the ball or pass kick the ball sideways. Give Shiatsu to the Spleen, Liver, and Kidney Meridians.
- **Side of Thighs**: The iliotibial band (band of connective tissue on the side of the thigh) can become sore from leg abduction exercises; lateral traveling movements made in tennis, basketball, and racquetball; and hip stabilization, as when balancing on one leg or breaking the momentum of a swing in golf or baseball. Give Shiatsu to the Gallbladder Meridian and acupressure to GB 31.
- **Back of Thighs**: The hamstrings (posterior thigh muscles) can become sore from doing hip extension and knee flexion exercises like hamstring curls, as well as from running and biking. Give Shiatsu to the Bladder Meridian on the posterior thigh and acupressure to Bl 36, B1 37, and Bl 40.
- **Calves**: The gastrocnemius and soleus (calf muscles) can become sore from doing knee flexion and plantarflexion exercises like heel raises, jumping as in basketball and volleyball, leaping as in dance, and propelling oneself forward as in power walking, walking in sand, hiking uphill, and running. They can also become sore from wearing high heels, which places these muscles in a contracted position for a prolonged period of time. Give Shiatsu to the Bladder Meridian in the calves and acupressure to Bl 40, Bl 56, and Bl 57. Pinch Bl 60 and Ki 3 on either side of the Achilles tendon.
- **Outer Shins**: The anterior tibialis (shin muscle) can become sore from doing ankle flexion exercises like toe taps and toe raises, from hiking uphill in boots,

and from absorbing the shock of running. Those clients with tight ankles or lateral shin splints should have these muscles worked. Similarly, the toe extensors on the dorsal surface (top) of the feet can become sore from dorsiflexion (ankle flexion) and toe extension exercises. Those clients with hammer toes should have these muscles worked. The peroneals (outer shin muscles) can become sore from lateral movements made in skating and from ankle stabilization, as when walking, hiking, or running on uneven surfaces. Give Shiatsu to the Stomach and Gallbladder Meridians in the lower leg and acupressure to St 36, St 41, GB 34, and GB 40.

- **Inner Shins**: The posterior tibialis (inner shin muscle) can become sore from plantarflexion (pointing of the foot) and from the propulsion and impact of running. Those clients who have inner shin splints should have these muscles worked. Give Shiatsu to the Spleen Meridian in the lower leg and acupressure to Sp 6 and Sp 9.
- **Feet**: Giving acupressure to points on the feet is beneficial locally as well as distally. In general, stimulating points on the feet clears obstructions in the associated Meridians and organs and moves energy downward. Press Lr 3 and Ki 1 to reduce excess energy in the upper body contributing to symptoms such as hypertension, headache, migraine, dizziness, vertigo, fatigued inflamed eyes, irritability, mental agitation, and insomnia. Lr 3 also addresses Lower Burner disorders such as irritable bowel syndrome, abdominal bloating and pain, PMS, and dysmenorrhea (painful menstrual cramps), and expedites delayed menses or labor, while Ki 1 also mitigates pain in the lumbar area and sole of the foot. Press Sp 3 to treat Dampness in the Lower Burner contributing to symptoms such as heaviness and edema, abdominal bloating, loose stools, diarrhea, leucorrhea (a white vaginal discharge), and profuse urination. Sp 3 also treats cognitive disturbances associated with the Earth element, especially distractibility, lack of focus, drowsiness, and mental stupor or fogginess. Apply moxa to B1 67 in the 38th week to rotate a breech presentation and during labor to reduce labor pain and facilitate delivery of the child.
- **Here are the key acupressure points in various locations:**
  Anterior thighs: St 31, St 34
  Medial thighs: Sp 10, Sp 11
  Lateral thighs: GB 31
  Knee: St 35, Bl 40
  Outer shin: St 36, GB 34
  Inner shin: Sp 6, Sp 9
  Posterior calves: Bl 56, Bl 57
  Ankles: Bl 60, Ki 3, GB 40, St 41
  Feet: Ki 1, Lr 3, Sp 3, Bl 67

KYO JITSU IMBALANCES

A client with a Meridian that is demonstrably Kyo (empty and deficient) or Jitsu (full and excessive) should be given Shiatsu to the Meridian (see "Meridian Diagnosis" and "Application of Techniques" as well as Table 6-1, in Chapter 6). The Yin Meridians of the leg (the Spleen, Liver, and Kidney Meridians) are placed in the Meridian stretch position by bending the knee, rotating the leg outward, and placing the sole of the client's foot at progressively higher levels next to the client's other leg. The foot is placed at ankle level of the other leg for the Spleen Meridian, at calf level for the Liver Meridian, and at knee level for the Kidney Meridian (see the discussion of

Meridian stretches in Chapter 9). To place the Gallbladder Meridian of the leg in the stretch position, bend the knee and rotate the leg inward across the midline of the body or cross it over the client's other leg. Although a Stomach Meridian stretch position exists, it is not used because Westerners are typically too tight to enter into or rest in the position. The Stomach Meridian stretch position, which entails reclining backward on a folded leg, entails a risk of pulling the quadriceps and straining the lower back and is therefore not recommended. Instead, a facilitated stretch can be applied in the prone position by bending the client's knee and pressing the heel toward the buttock (see Figure 11–70). There is no passive, resting Bladder Meridian stretch position for the leg in the supine position. However, an active, facilitated stretch involving hip flexion and knee extension can be applied instead.

Palpate along the Meridian, feeling the quality of the tissues (see "Qualities of Kyo and Jitsu" and "Meridian Diagnosis" in Chapter 6). Jitsu tissues feel firm and toned, whereas Kyo tissues often feel mushy, flabby, and slack or, alternatively, very hard and tough. A Jitsu Meridian feels resistant but springy, whereas a Kyo Meridian feels bottomless or unyielding and inert. Initially, pressure on a Jitsu Meridian may elicit a lancinating (lightning bolt) sensation that abates with continued therapy, providing pressure remains within the client's pain threshold. The piercing sensation may be accompanied by a groan or exclamation from the client, a startle response like a jerk, or a jump response like a muscle twitch. These reactions are more common on the anterior thighs, especially above the knees, the lateral thighs, and the inner shins, which tend toward hypersensitivity. Pressure on a Kyo Meridian tends to elicit a soothing, dull sensation or no sensation. When the sensation is agreeable, the client may sigh or request the practitioner to remain in the area or repeat the technique.

To sedate a Jitsu Meridian, apply stimulating techniques to disperse stagnation and congestion and to release blocked Qi (see "Application of Techniques" and Table 6-1 in Chapter 6). Two-handed compression can be used to cover more surface area and to intensify the effect. Compression along the Meridian should be moderate to deep, fairly brisk, and rhythmic, following a downward and outward direction or countercurrent to the flow of the Meridian (see "Direction of Movement" in Chapter 6. Additionally, kenbiki (jostling, torsion wringing, and cross-fiber friction) and tapotement (pummeling) can be applied. Specific Jitsu dispersal techniques include dynamic forearm techniques such as "rolling pin" and "sawing" on the quadriceps and leg traction plus foot compression on the hamstrings.

To tonify a Kyo Meridian, apply nurturing techniques to draw and gather Qi to the area of deficiency (see "Application of Techniques" and Table 6-1 in Chapter 6). Specific two-handed Kyo tonification techniques include butterfly hands, double fists, and double forearms, which provide a broad, flat, noninvasive form of compression. The Mother/Son hand technique may be used when the legs present signs of deficiency—lack of tone, emaciation, weakness, coldness, edema (fluid retention), or varicose veins—or are too hyperirritable for Jitsu dispersal techniques. Place the Mother hand like a warm compress on a deficient area like CV 4, the knee, St 36, or Sp 9, or use the Mother hand to hold a key acupressure point like Sp 6 or Lr 3, while the Son hand presses the length of the Meridian (see Practice Exercise 6-1). Pressure should be light to moderate and fairly slow and steady, following an upward and inward direction or concurrent with the flow of the Meridian (see "Direction of Movement" in Chapter 6).

Certain activities, if done to excess, such as standing, sitting, or lying down can stress a Meridian, leading to an energetic disharmony in the Meridian, which should be given Shiatsu. Excessive standing strains the Kidney and Bladder Meridians; excessive physical activity strains the Liver and Gallbladder Meridians, and excessive sitting strains the Stomach and Spleen Meridians (Gach, 1990).

Since sitting is a fact of modern life, it warrants a deeper analysis. The seated position is used when in office and school settings; traveling in a car, train, or airplane;

eating and socializing; and watching television, movies, sports, and entertainment. It is the position used most in the information age and is associated with study and intellectual effort. Aside from the physical position itself, intense and prolonged mental concentration done while sitting can create an energetic imbalance in the Earth element, whose psychological capacity is thinking.

Ideally, those who are earning a living doing desk work or who are studying for a degree should receive acupressure to St 36 and Shiatsu on the Stomach and Spleen Meridians of the legs. The muscles associated with the Stomach and Spleen Meridians should be stretched, particularly the hip flexors (rectus femoris and psoas), which get tight from sitting. Ampuku (abdominal massage) should be given, as well as acupressure to key points on the abdomen (St 25, St 27, and CV 12), since mental preoccupation, worry, and strain are often accompanied by digestive disorders, poor eating habits, or compensatory overindulgence in food (see "The Earth Element: Spleen and Stomach" in Chapter 5 and the abdominal protocol in Chapter 14). Additionally, St 25 and St 27 are good releasing points for the psoas, whose attachments at the lumbar vertebrae can be pressed through the intestines.

In the short term, the push to complete projects by a deadline can often cause the Stomach and Spleen Meridians to assess Jitsu, so dispersal techniques are usually indicated (except on the abdomen), but the client may be sensitive, at least initially. On the other hand, long-term strain may cause these Meridians to assess Kyo from depletion, in which case tonifying techniques are in order. Finally, because excess thinking draws excess energy up toward the head, contributing to headaches, giving Shiatsu and acupressure to the feet, especially Lr 3 and Ki 1, is helpful to draw energy back down (see "Principle 2" on distal points on the feet and "Superior/Inferior Point Combination" in Chapter 7).

ELEMENT TYPE IMBALANCES

Clients who present a constellation of physical disorders or psychological disharmonies associated with a particular element should be given Shiatsu to the Yang and Yin Meridians of that element. The Spleen and Stomach Meridians are associated with the Earth element type and the Spleen and Stomach organ functions. The Kidney and Bladder Meridians are associated with the Water element type and the Kidney and Bladder organ functions. The Liver and Gallbladder Meridians are associated with the Wood element type and the Liver and Gallbladder organ functions. When a client, especially a Yang element type (Wood, Fire, and driven Water), manifests symptoms of stress disorders in the head, neck, and shoulders, acupressure to the lower body, especially the feet, is helpful to draw energy downward. Lr 3 and Ki 1 lower Qi that flares upward toward the head.

For a profile on the element types, see Chapter 4, and for a description of element imbalances, see Chapter 5. Additionally, Table 4-1 summarizes correspondences for each of the Five Elements; Table 7-4 summarizes physical disorders associated with each element's organ pair, and Table 7-5 summarizes psychological disharmonies associated with each element.

CLIENT COMFORT

Be sure the futon or other surface is well padded to cushion the client's sacrum (triangular-shaped bone at the base of the spine) and spinous processes of the vertebrae while lying down and while receiving BMTs. If the client has lower back issues or a history of sciatica, place a bolster under the knees to increase client comfort during compression techniques. Remove the bolster to do stretches and BMTs so it does not obstruct your work.

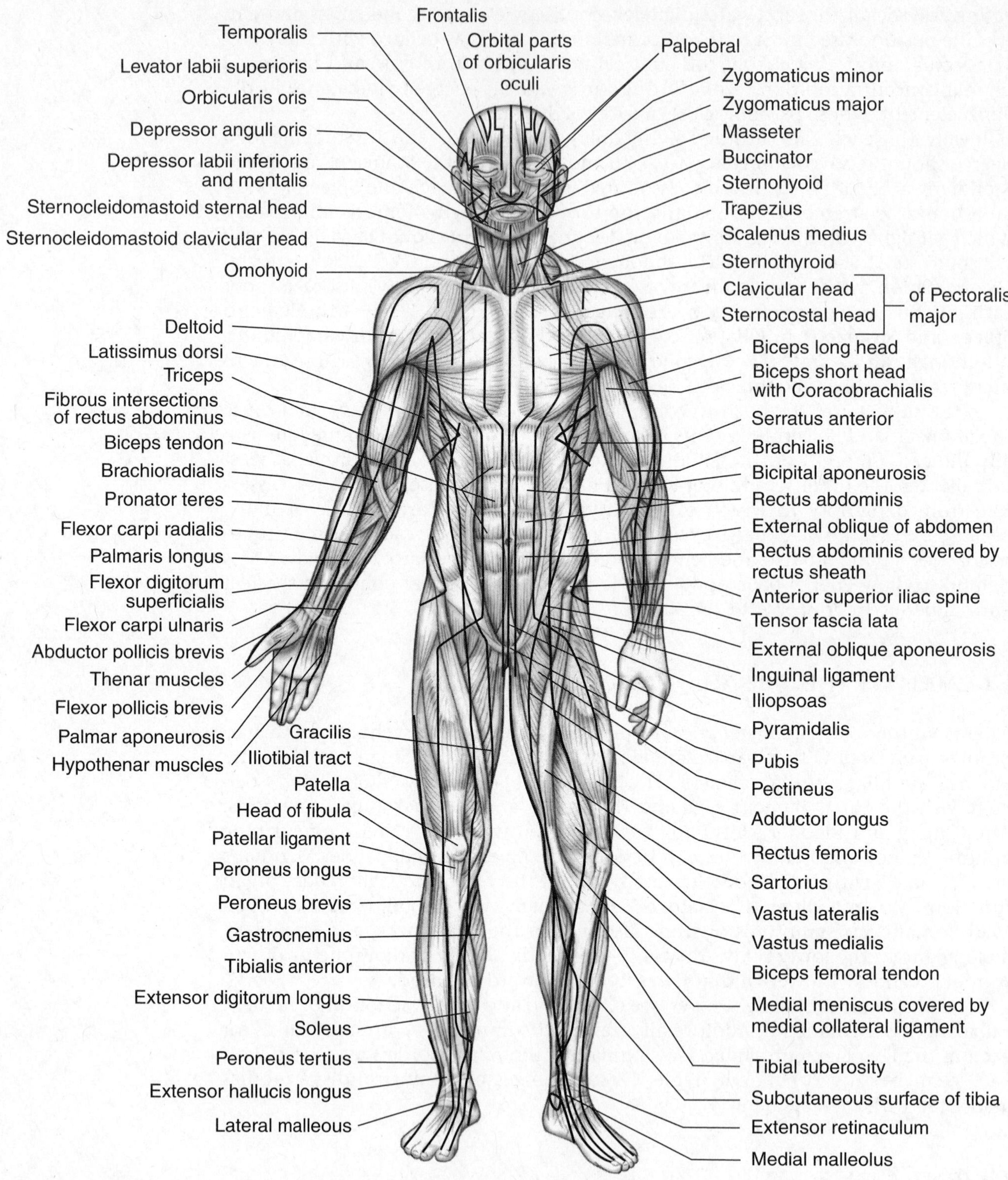

Anterior Meridian and Associated Musculature. (See Color Plate 6.)

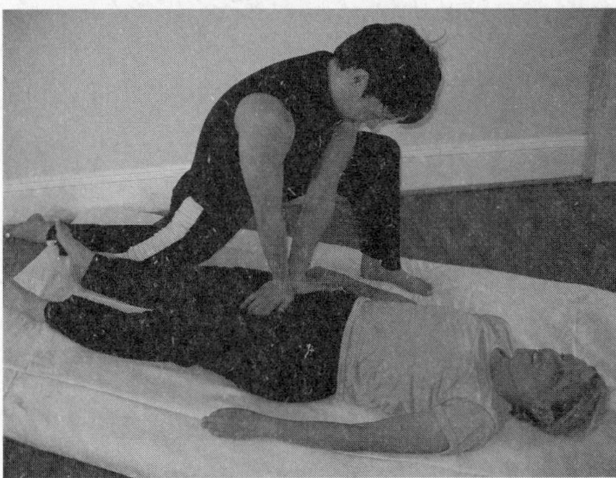

FIGURE 12-1 Butterfly down the Stomach and Spleen Meridian.
Move from hip to knee.

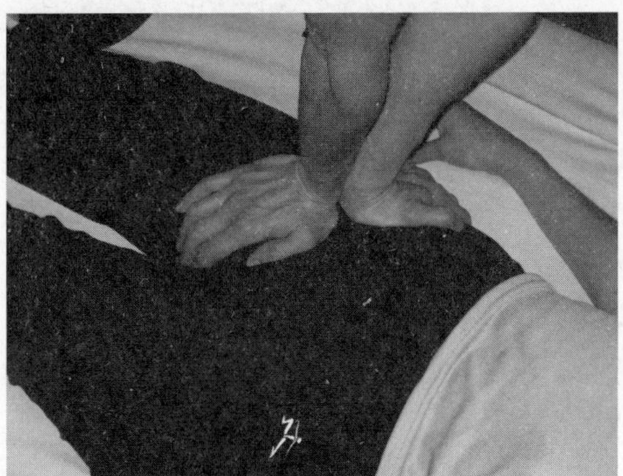

FIGURE 12-2 Close-up of butterfly.

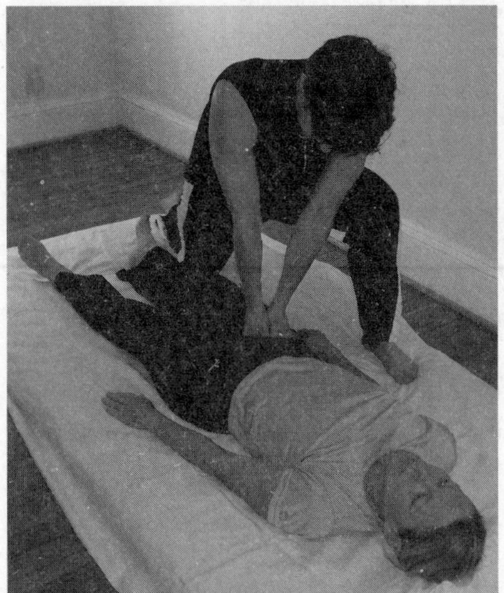

FIGURE 12-3 Double fists down the Stomach and Spleen Meridian.
Move from hip to knee.

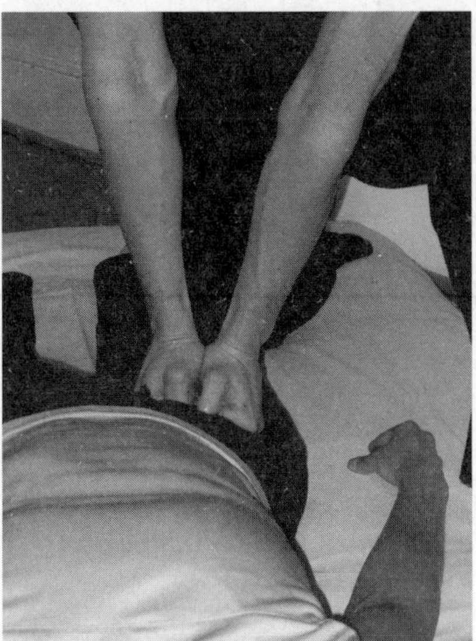

FIGURE 12-4 Close-up of double fists.
Palms face one another. This technique may be oriented sideways, if preferred.

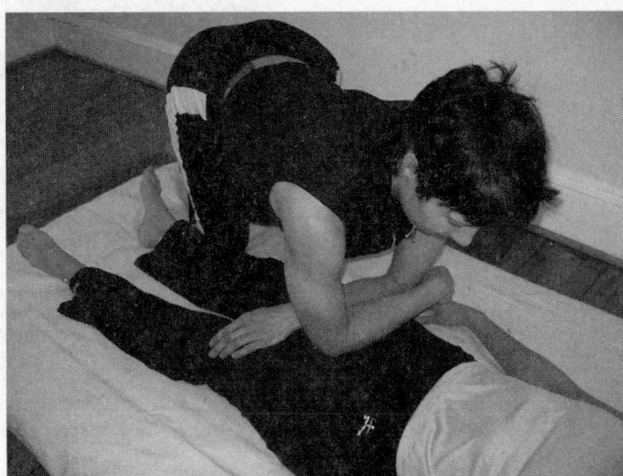

FIGURE 12-5 Double forearms down the Stomach and Spleen Meridians.
Move from hip to knee.

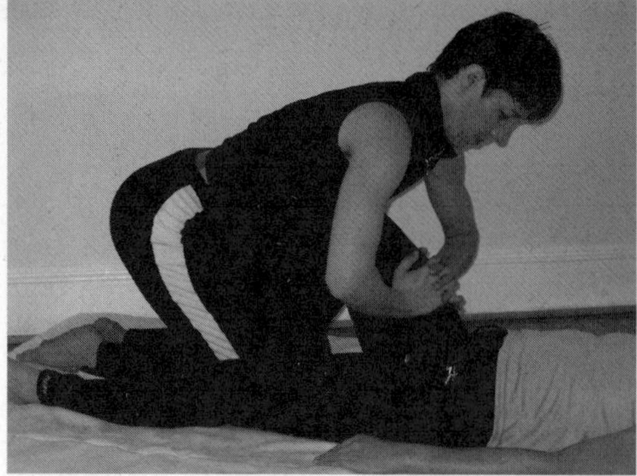

FIGURE 12-6 **Double hand clasp down the Stomach and Spleen Meridians.**
Sandwich the client's foot between your knees.

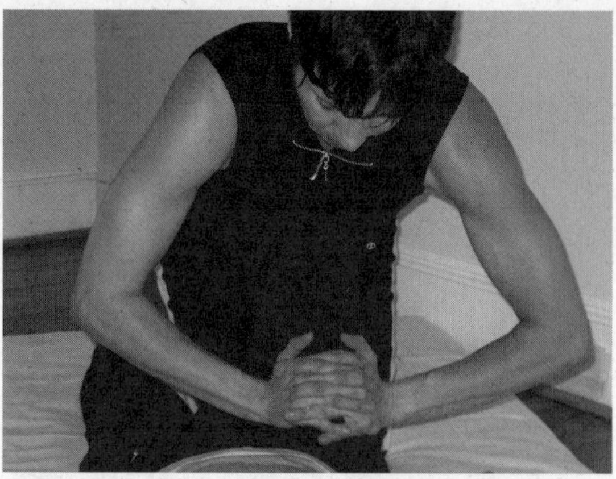

FIGURE 12-7 **Close-up of double hand clasp.**
Squeeze inward. Move from hip to knee.

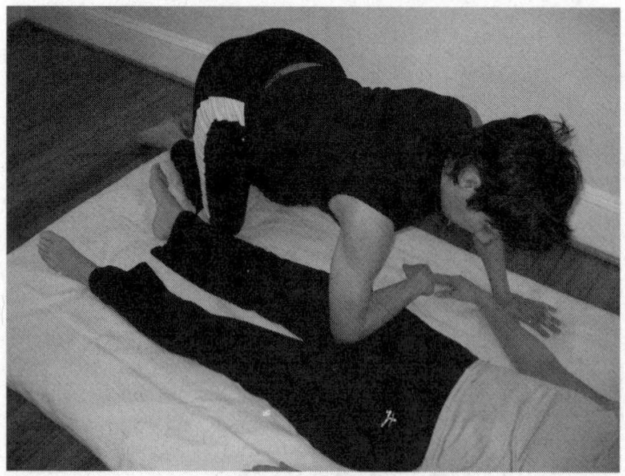

FIGURE 12-8 **Rolling pin forearm, palm down.**
Compress the muscles against the bone.

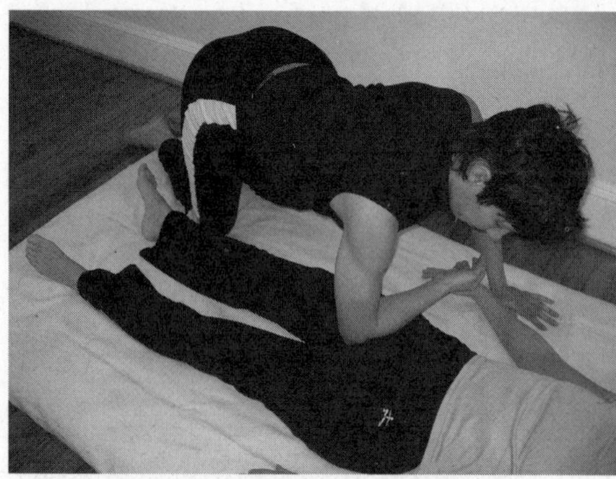

FIGURE 12-9 **Rolling pin forearm, palm up.**
Roll and flatten the muscles.

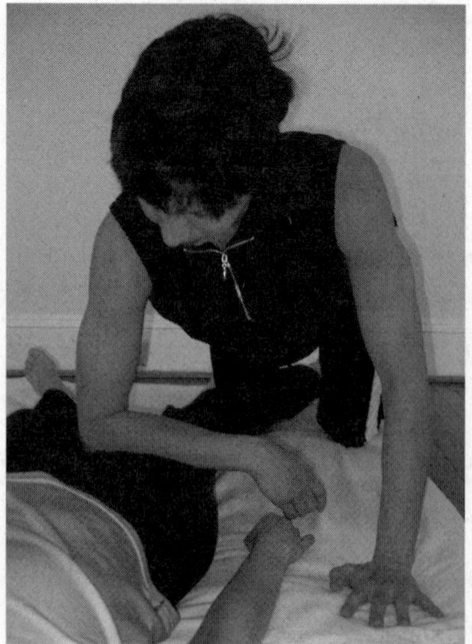

FIGURE 12-10 **Close-up of rolling pin, palm down.**
Alternate forearm pronation and supination, rolling in place.

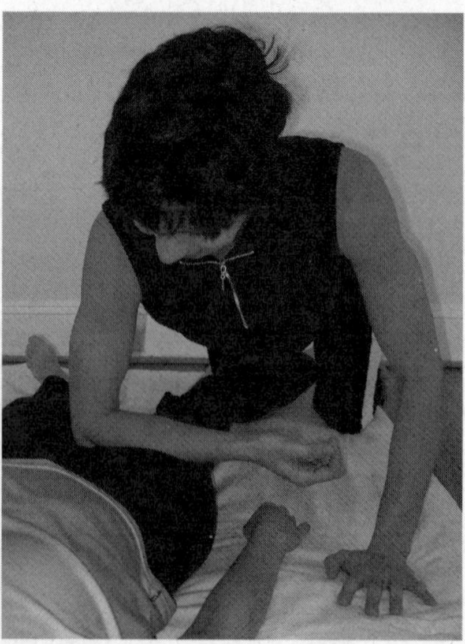

FIGURE 12-11 **Close-up of rolling pin, palm up.**
Relocate the forearm, moving down the Stomach and Spleen Meridians to the knee.

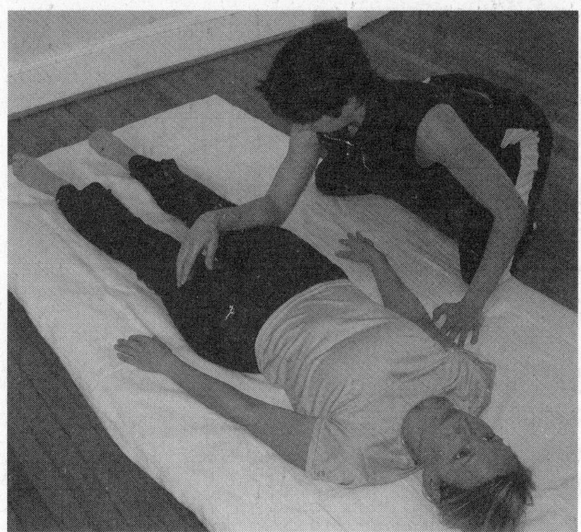

FIGURE 12-12 Sawing forearm, medial push.

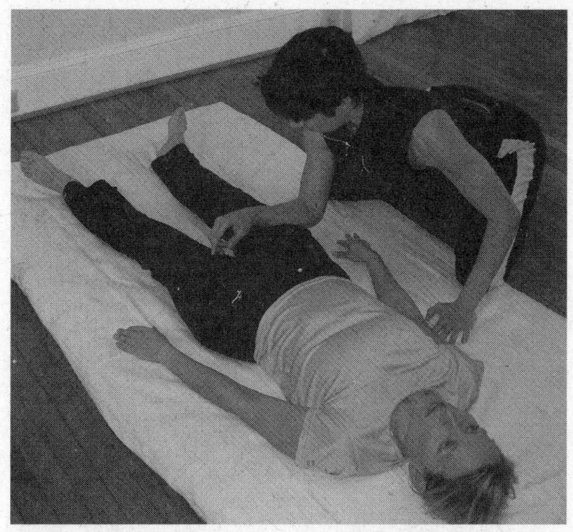

FIGURE 12-13 Sawing forearm, lateral pull.

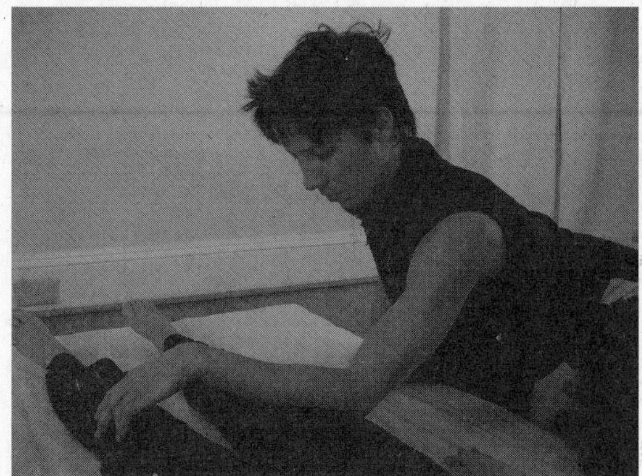

FIGURE 12-14 Close-up of sawing forearm, medial push.
Compress the muscles against the bone and push. The client's leg should rotate inward.

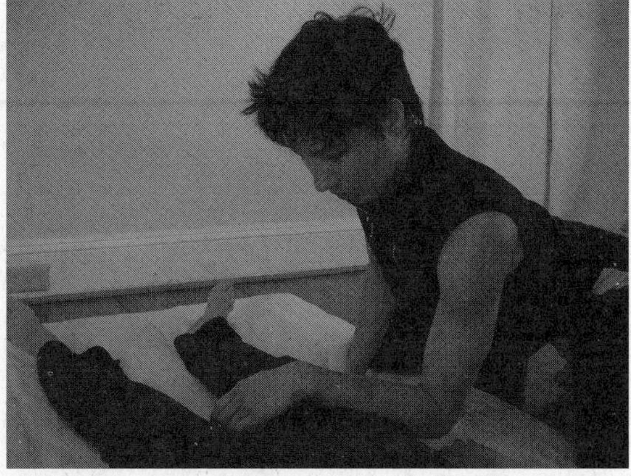

FIGURE 12-15 Close-up of sawing forearm, lateral pull.
Compress the muscles against the bone and pull. The client's leg should rotate outward. Saw down the Stomach and Spleen Meridians from hip to knee.

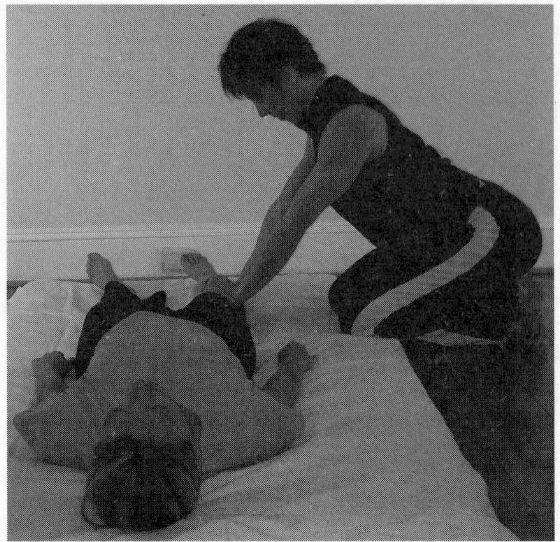

FIGURE 12-16 Heels of the hands press the Stomach Meridian.
Move from knee to foot.

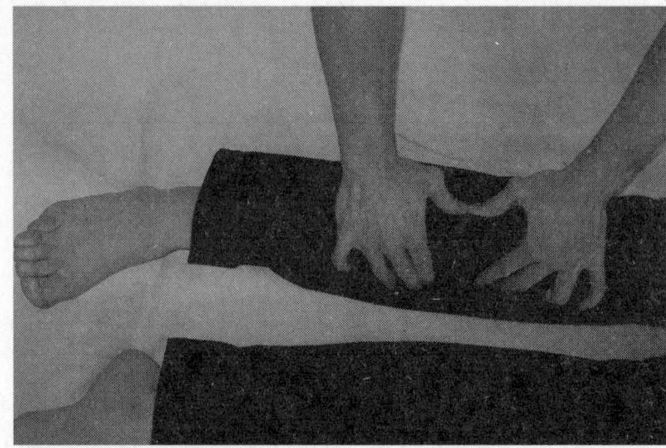

FIGURE 12-17 Double thumbs press the Stomach Meridian.
Move from knee to foot.

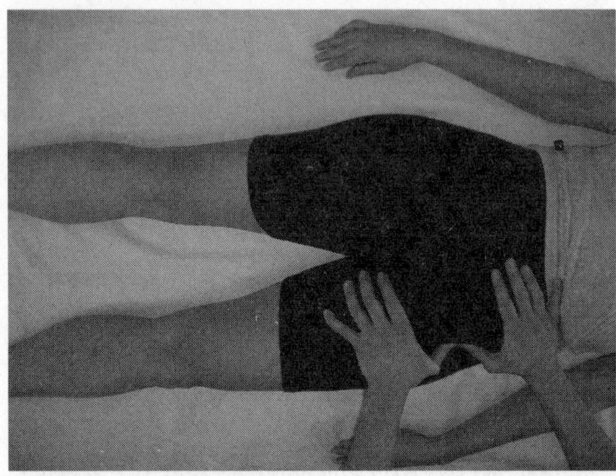

FIGURE 12-18 St 31.
Below the ASIS (pelvic bone), between the sartorious and tensor fascia latae tendons.

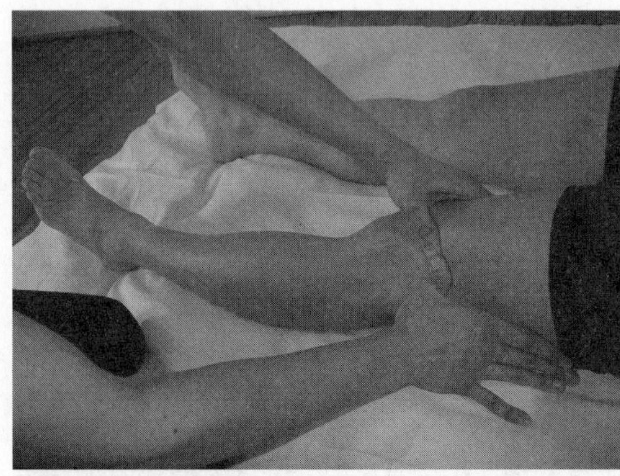

FIGURE 12-19 St 34.
Between the rectus femoris and vastus lateralis (middle and outer quadriceps).

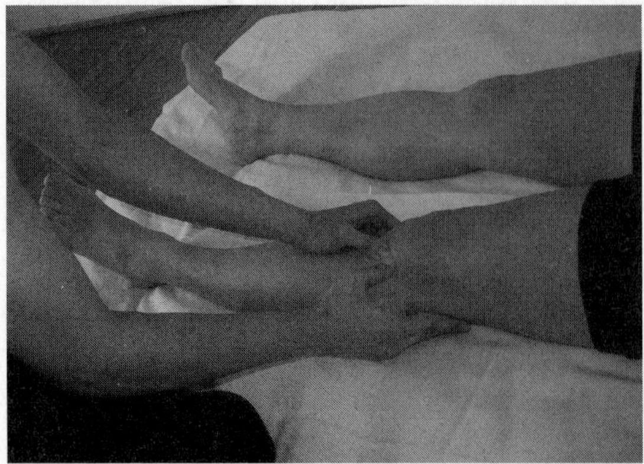

FIGURE 12-20 St 35.
On the outer, lower border of the patella (kneecap).

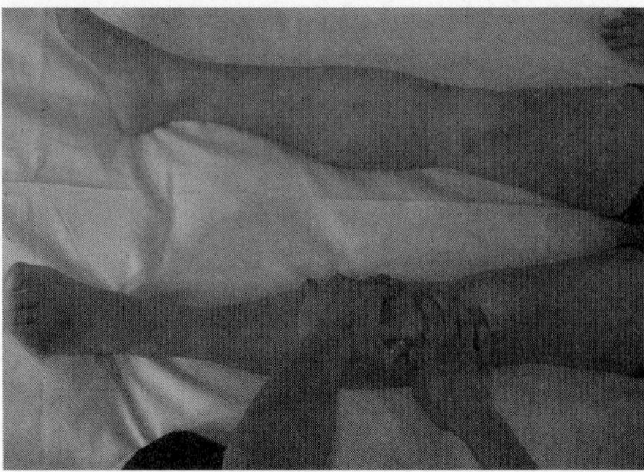

FIGURE 12-21 St 36.
Three cun (4 fingers widths) below the patella (kneecap) against the tibia (shinbone).

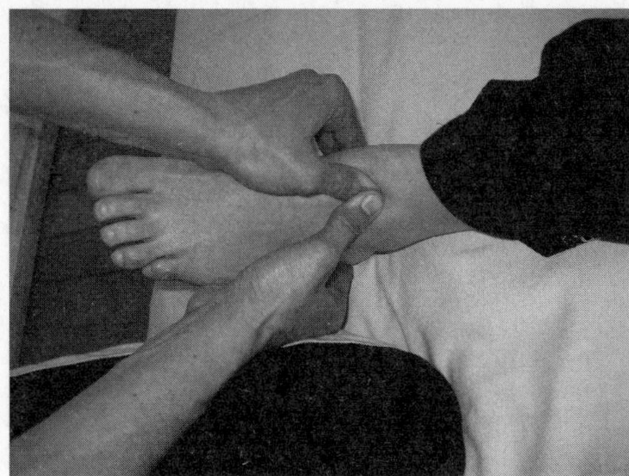

FIGURE 12-22 **St 41.**
At ankle level between the extensor hallucis longus (big toe tendon) and extensor digitorum longus (tendon of the other toes). To define these tendons, ask client to flex the foot.

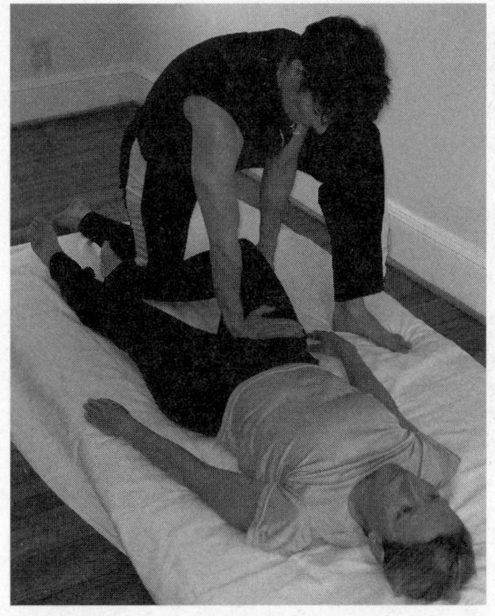

FIGURE 12-23 **Palm press down the Spleen Meridian to the knee.**
Bend the client's knee; rotate the leg laterally (outward) and set the foot above ankle level to access the Spleen Meridian. Support the knee or prop the leg with a pillow. Palm press down the Spleen Meridian to the knee.

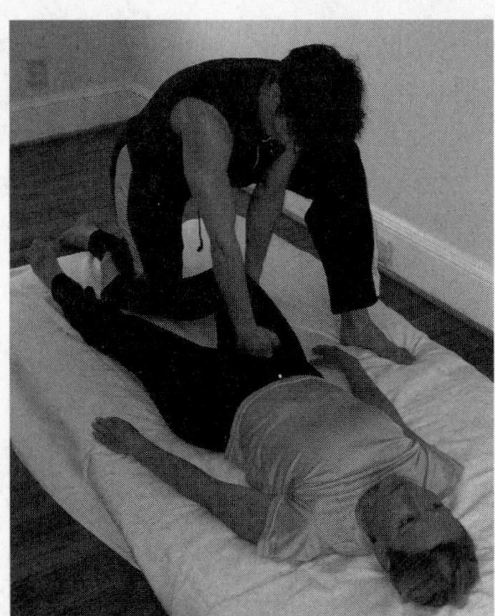

FIGURE 12-24 **Fist press down the Spleen Meridian to the knee.**

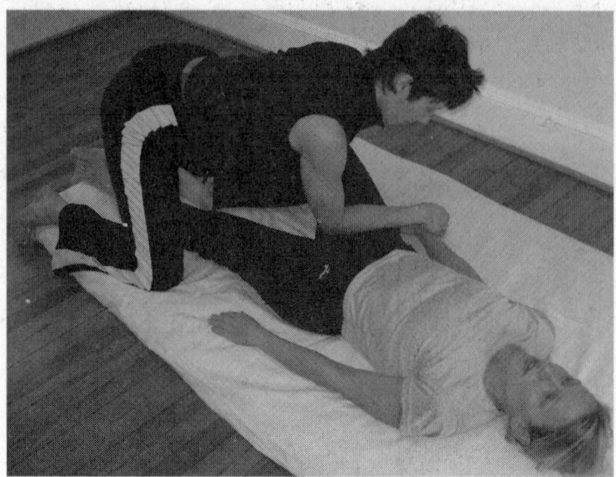

FIGURE 12-25 Forearm press down the Spleen Meridian to the knee.

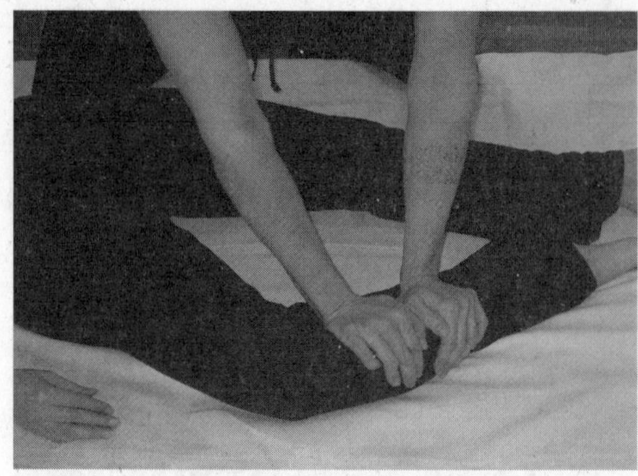

FIGURE 12-26 Heels of the hand press the inner shin.
Press the Yin Meridians from knee to ankle.

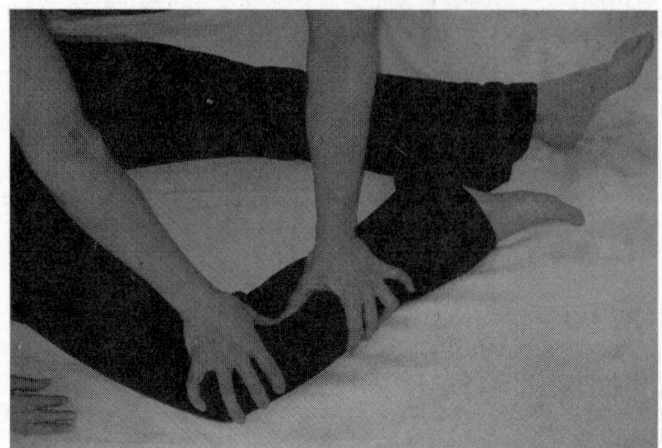

FIGURE 12-27 Double thumbs press the Spleen Meridian from knee to ankle.

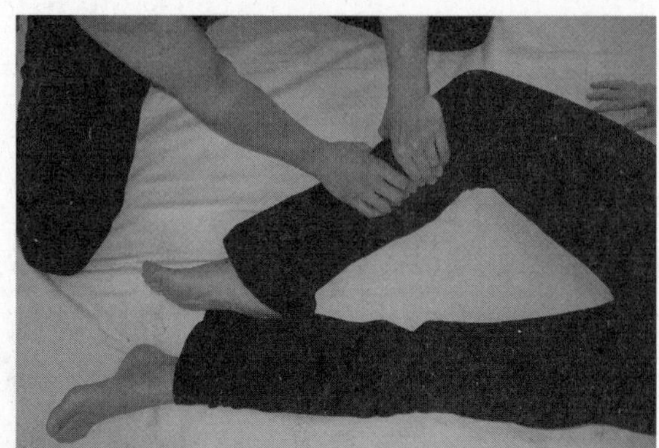

FIGURE 12-28 Fingertips squeeze.
Alternative position: The Spleen Meridian can also be treated from a different orientation, as shown.

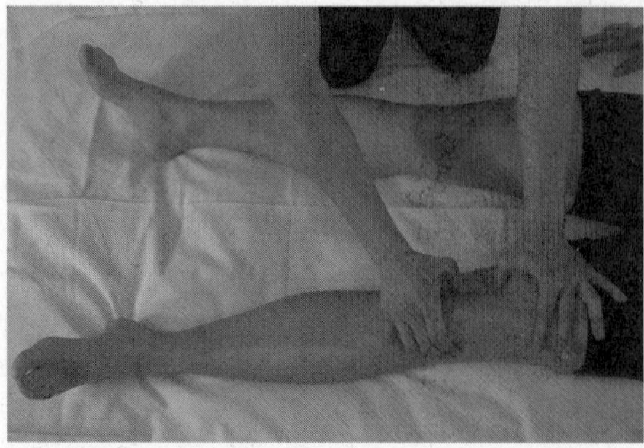

FIGURE 12-29 Sp 10.
Above the patella (kneecap) on the vastus medialis (inner quadriceps).

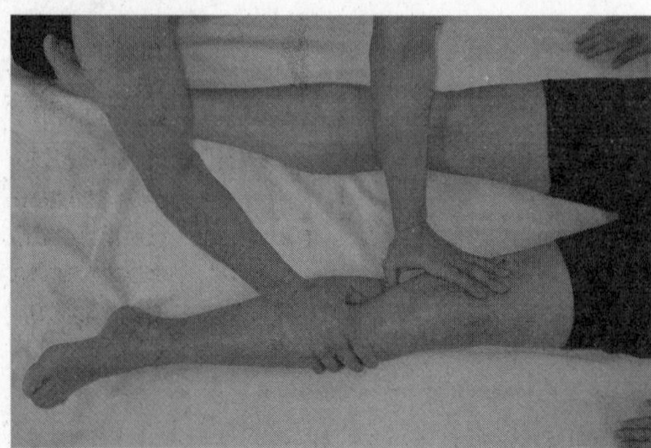

FIGURE 12-30 Sp 9.
Below the patella (kneecap) in the bony hollow against the tibia (shinbone).

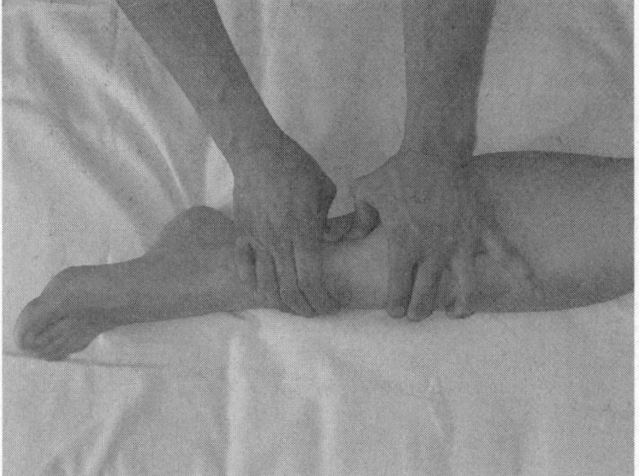

FIGURE 12-31 **Sp 6.**
Three cun above the medial malleolus (inner anklebone) against the tibia (shinbone).

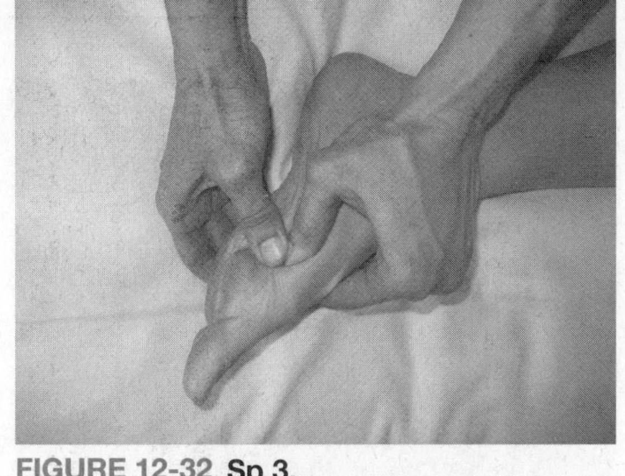

FIGURE 12-32 **Sp 3.**
On the medial arch, at the juncture of the first metatarsal and big toe, which forms a bunion on some clients.

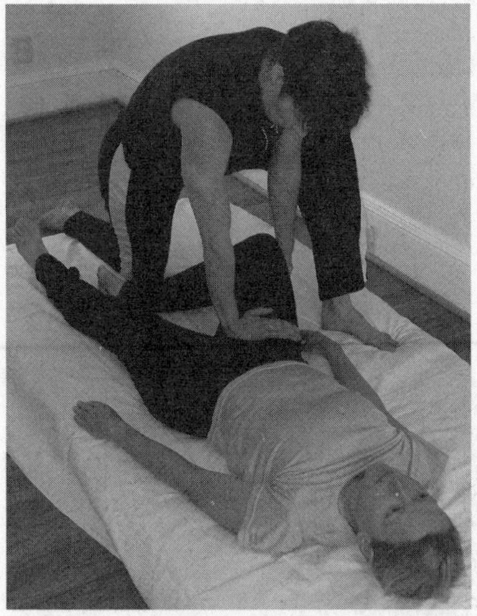

FIGURE 12-33 **Palm press down the Liver Meridian.**
Set the client's foot at calf level to access the Liver Meridian. Palm press down the Liver Meridian to the knee.

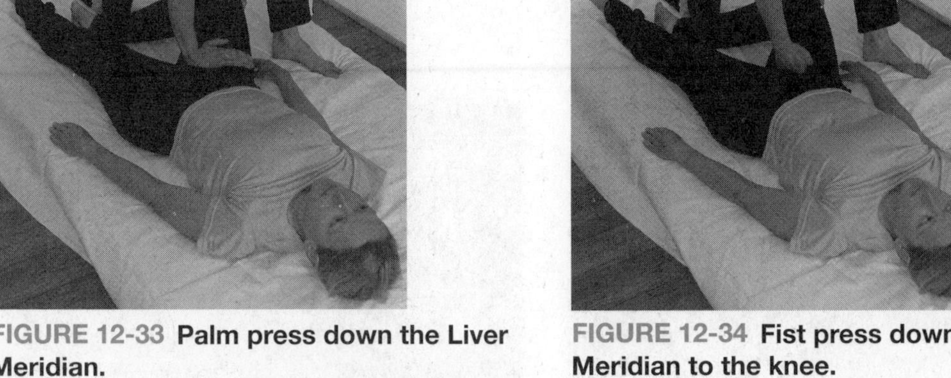

FIGURE 12-34 **Fist press down the Liver Meridian to the knee.**

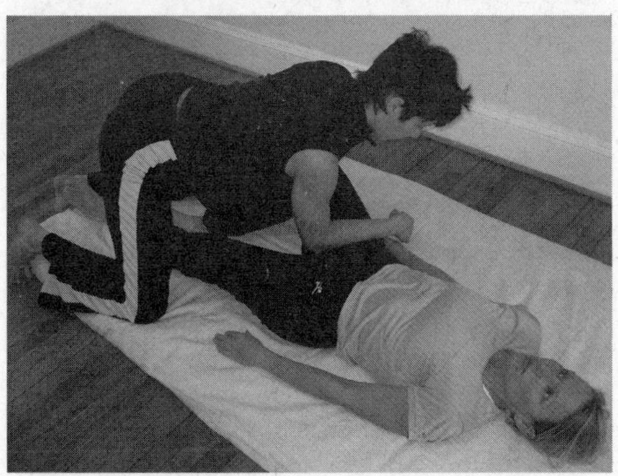

FIGURE 12-35 **Forearm press down the Liver Meridian to the knee.**

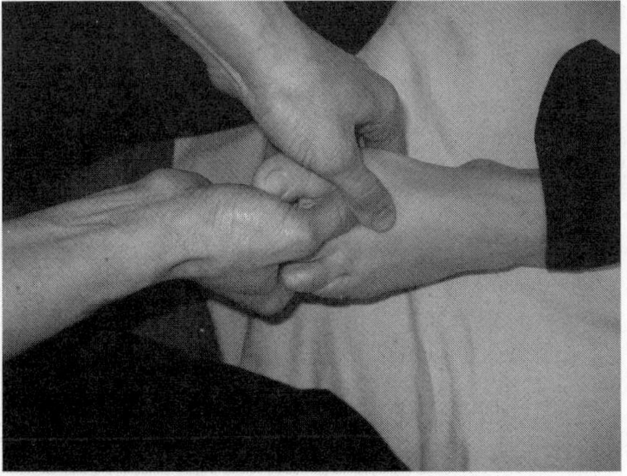

FIGURE 12-36 **Lr 3.**
On the web of flesh in the bony hollow between the first and second metatarsals (bones aligned with the big and second toes).

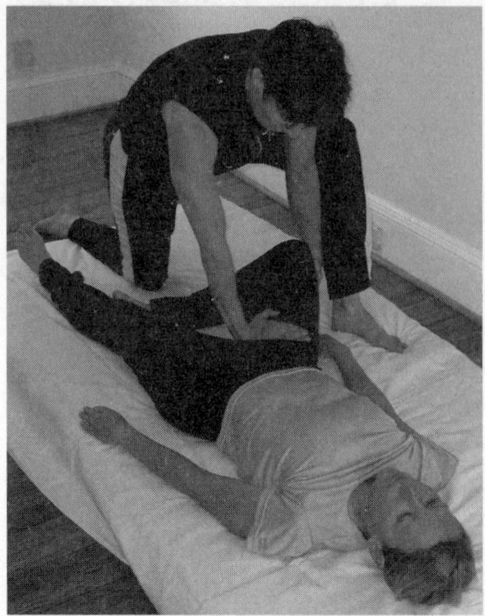

FIGURE 12-37 **Palm press down the Kidney Meridian to the knee.**
Set the client's foot at knee level to access the Kidney Meridian. Palm press down the Kidney Meridian to the knee.

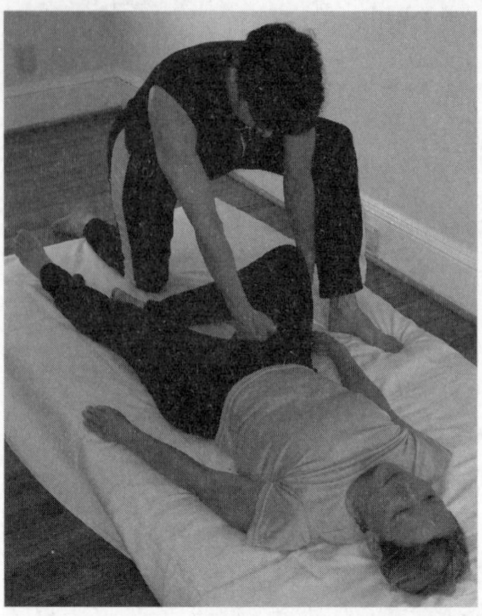

FIGURE 12-38 **Fist press down the Kidney Meridian to the knee.**

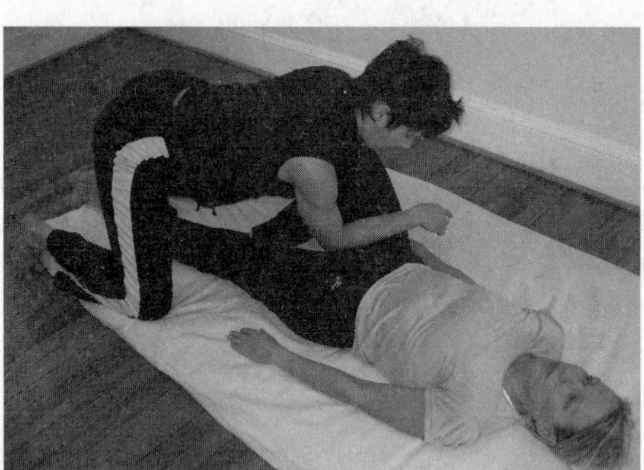

FIGURE 12-39 **Forearm press down the Kidney Meridian to the knee.**

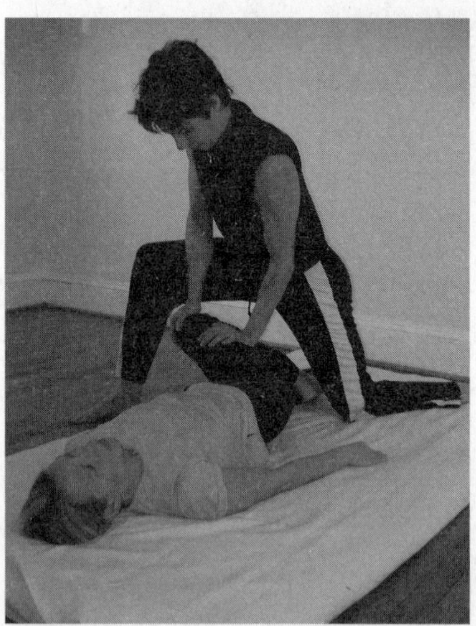

FIGURE 12-40 **Heel of the hand press down the Gallbladder Meridian to the knee.**
Rotate the client's leg medially (inward). Hook the heel of your hand under the iliotibial band. Stabilize the client's knee with counterresistance, if necessary.

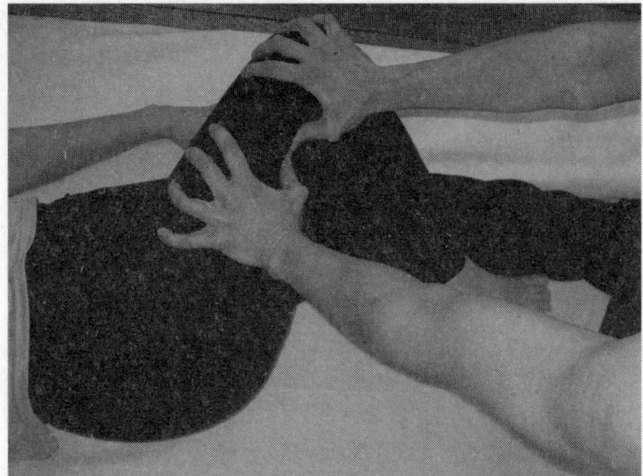

FIGURE 12-41 Double thumbs press down the Gallbladder Meridian to the knee. Hook your thumbs under the iliotibial band.

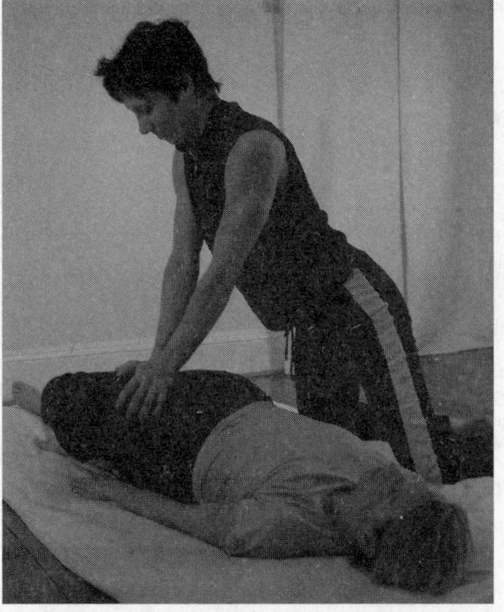

FIGURE 12-42 Butterfly down the Gallbladder Meridian to the knee. Compress the muscles against the bone.

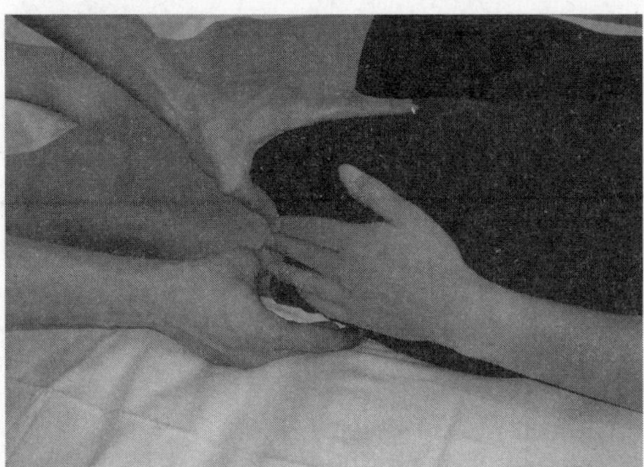

FIGURE 12-43 GB 31. Half way down the outer thigh, where the tip of the client's middle finger touches.

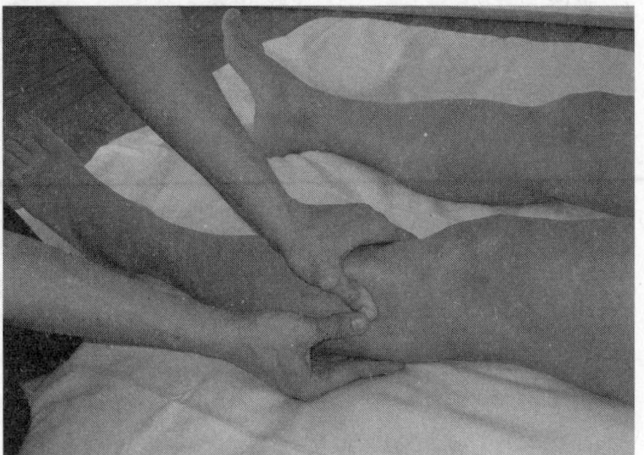

FIGURE 12-44 GB 34. Just in front of and below the head of the fibula (feel for the bony knob at the side of the lower leg).

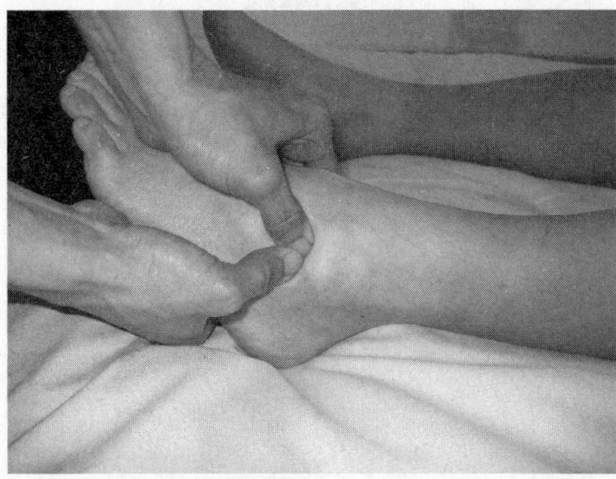

FIGURE 12-45 GB 40. In the bony hollow in front of and below the lateral malleolus (outer anklebone).

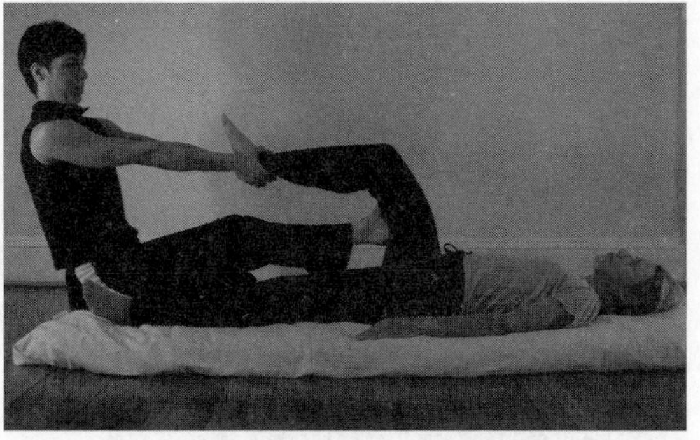

FIGURE 12-46 Foot press down the Bladder Meridian from hip to knee. For stability and effectiveness, flex the client's hip at a 90-degree angle so that the thigh is perpendicular to the floor.

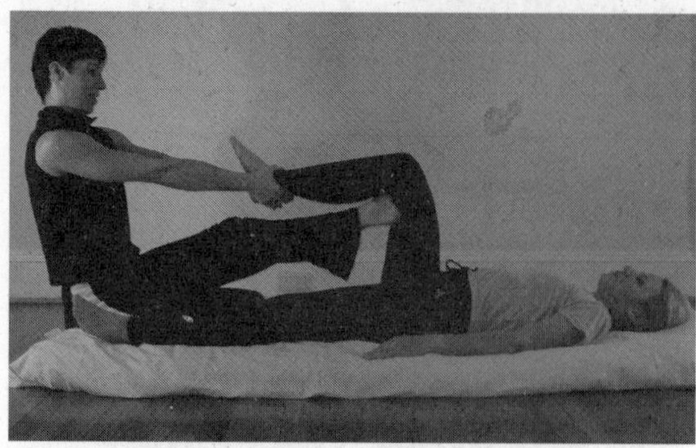

FIGURE 12-47 Foot press continued.
Simultaneously pull the client's ankle and push with your foot.

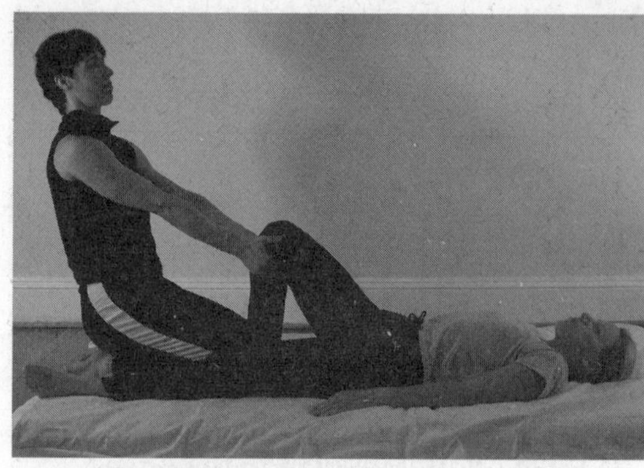

FIGURE 12-48 Finger pads press down the Bladder Meridian from knee to ankle.

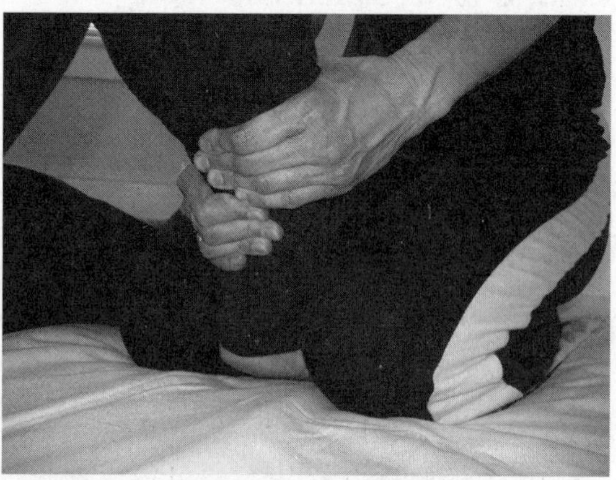

FIGURE 12-49 Close-up of finger pad press.
Sandwich the client's foot between your knees; press your finger pads into the calf and lean backward.

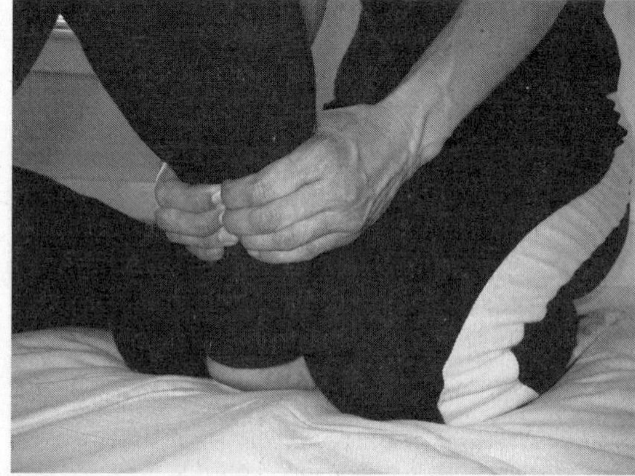

FIGURE 12-50 Fingertip press.
The fingertips provide a sharper, more intense sensation than the finger pads.

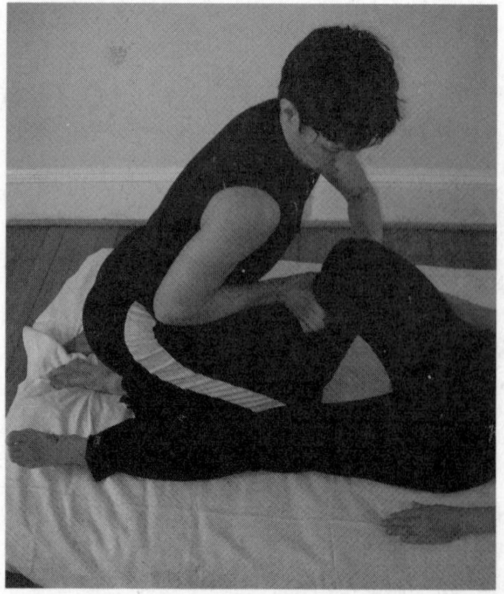

FIGURE 12-51 Kenbiki torsion wring of the calf, medial (inward) rotation.

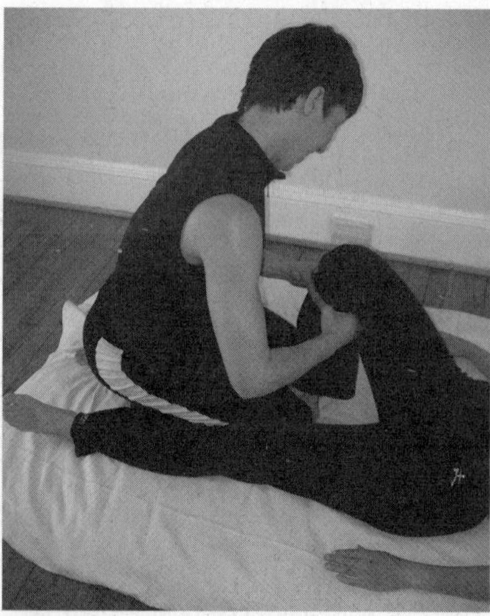

FIGURE 12-52 Kenbiki torsion wring of the calf; lateral (outward) rotation.

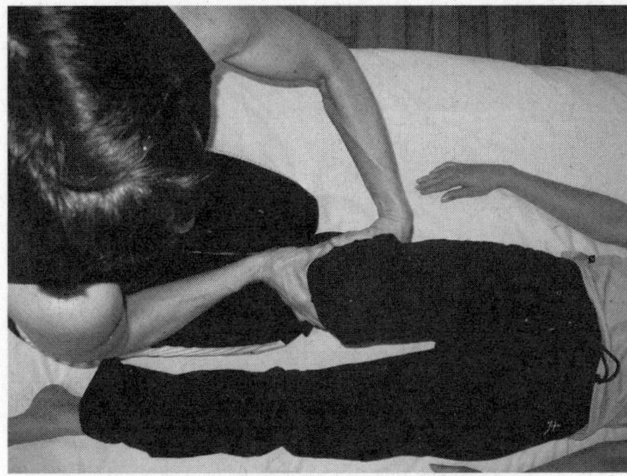

FIGURE 12-53 **Kenbiki, aerial view.** Sandwich the client's foot between your knees; compress the muscle against the bone and twist inward.

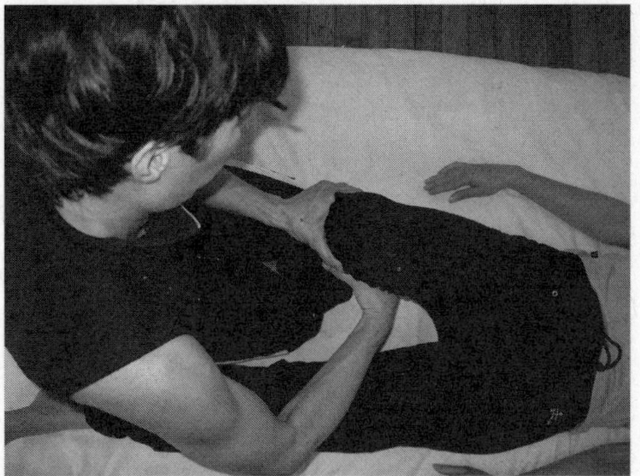

FIGURE 12-54 **Kenbiki, aerial view.** Compress and twist outward. Work down the Bladder Meridian, wringing the calf. Repeat Figures 12–1 through 12–54 on the other leg.

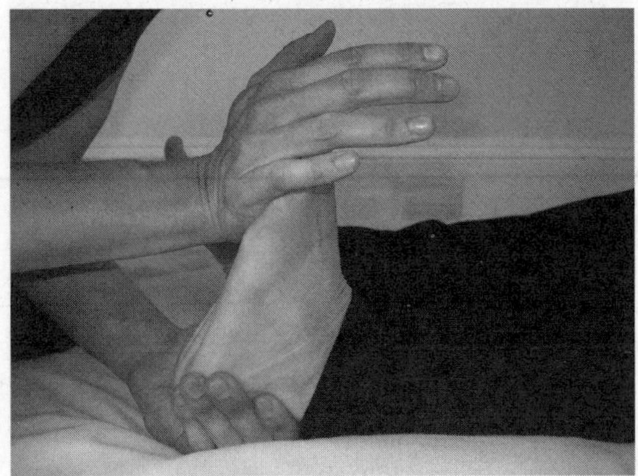

FIGURE 12-55 **Dorsiflexion.** Stabilize the heel and push the ball of the foot upward.

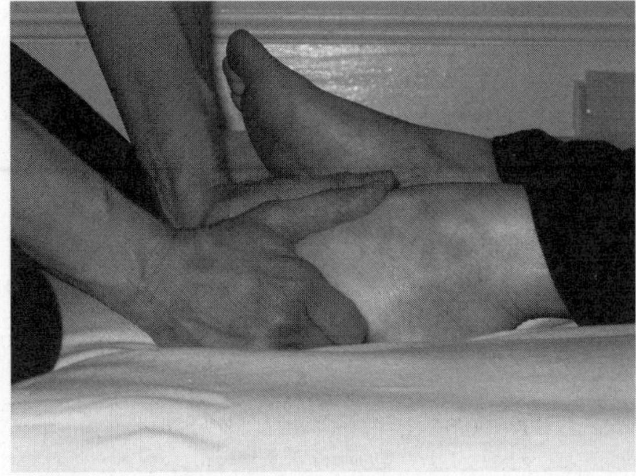

FIGURE 12-56 **Plantarflexion.** Place the heels of your hands on the dorsal surface of the foot and press downward.

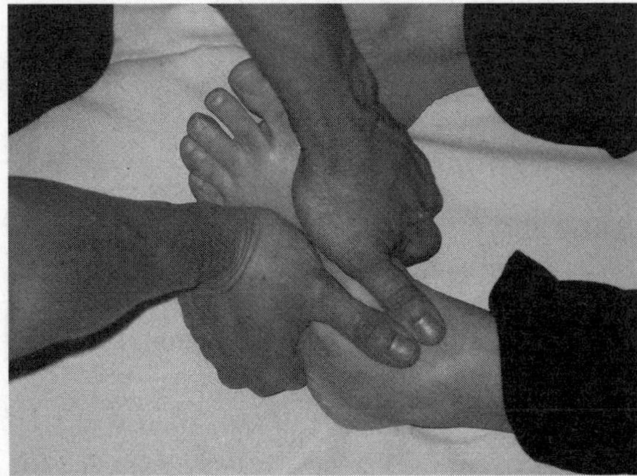

FIGURE 12-57 **Inversion, aerial view.** Wrap your hands around the foot and twist inward.

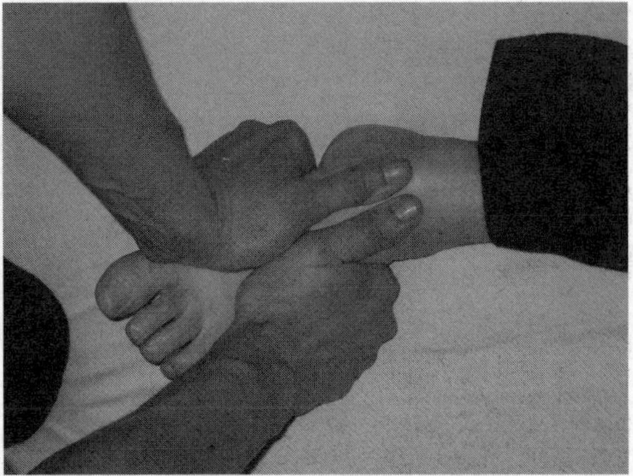

FIGURE 12-58 **Eversion, aerial view.** Twist the foot outward. Alternate several times.

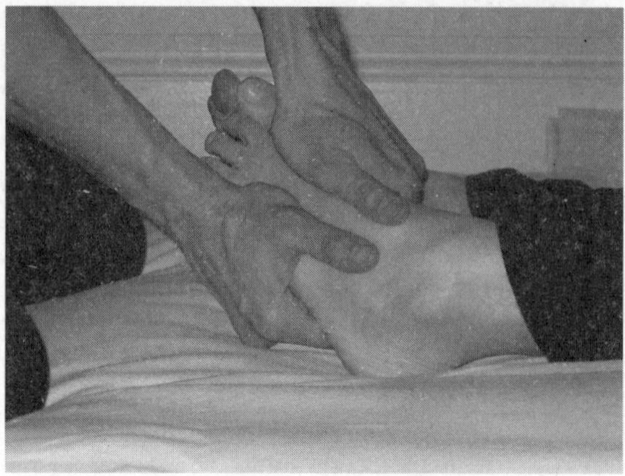

FIGURE 12-59 Inversion, side view.

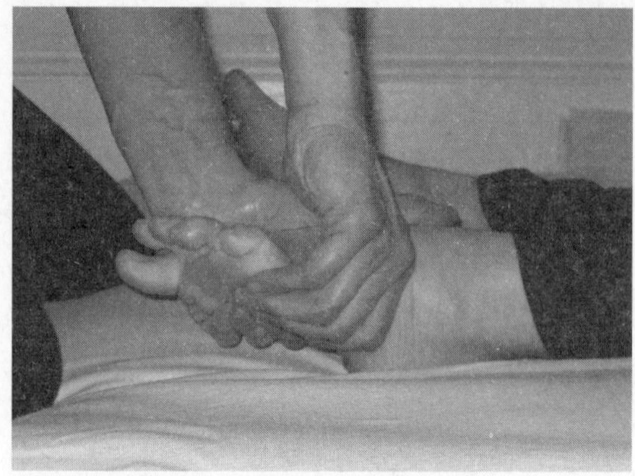

FIGURE 12-60 Eversion, side view.

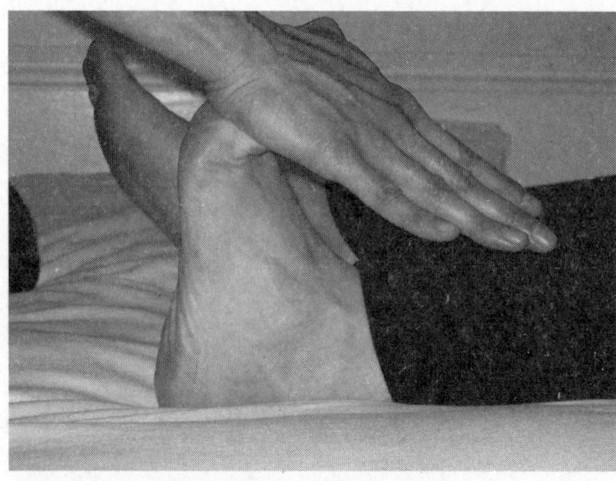

FIGURE 12-61 Toes, extension.
Press the toes backward.

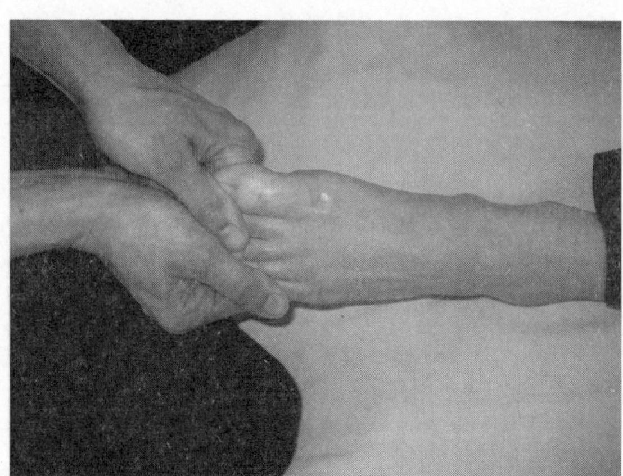

FIGURE 12-62 Toes, traction.
Pull the toes.

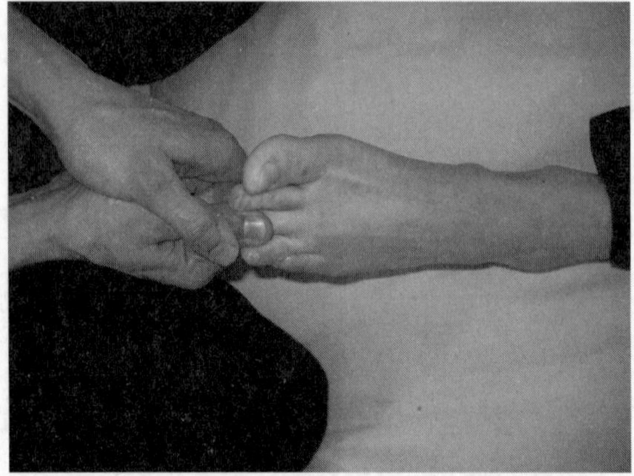

FIGURE 12-63 Individual toe traction.
(Toes may crack.)

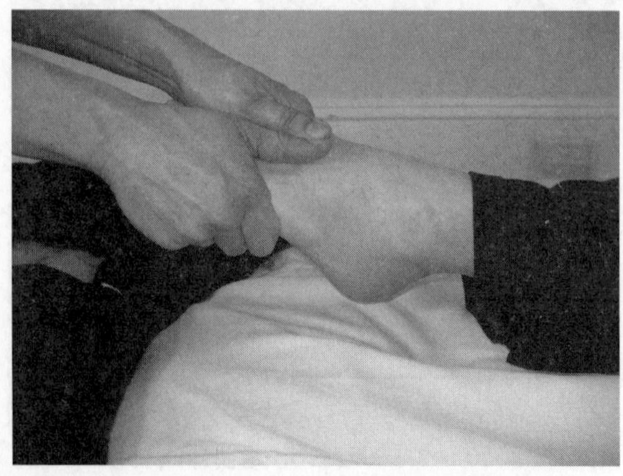

FIGURE 12-64 Foot and leg traction.
Pull slowly and firmly to release the hip.

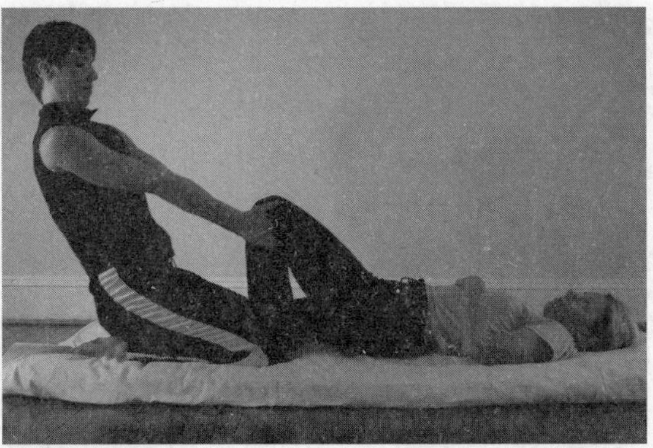

FIGURE 12-65 Lumbar traction.
Sandwich the client's foot between your knees; lean back so that the client's hip lifts off the ground. Release and repeat several times.

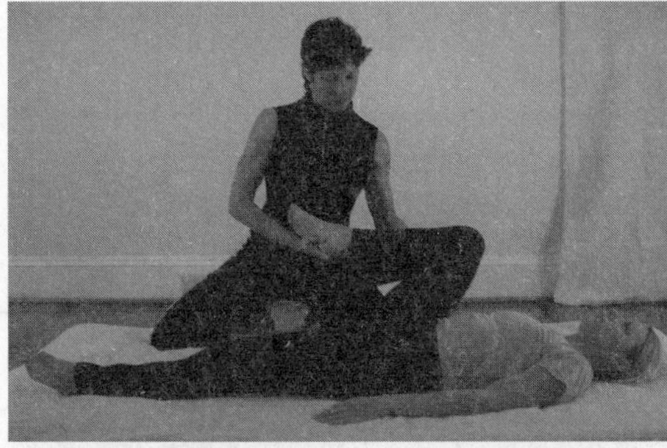

FIGURE 12-66 Cradle swing, up phase.
Support the client's leg under the knee and heel. Flex the client's knee and hip.

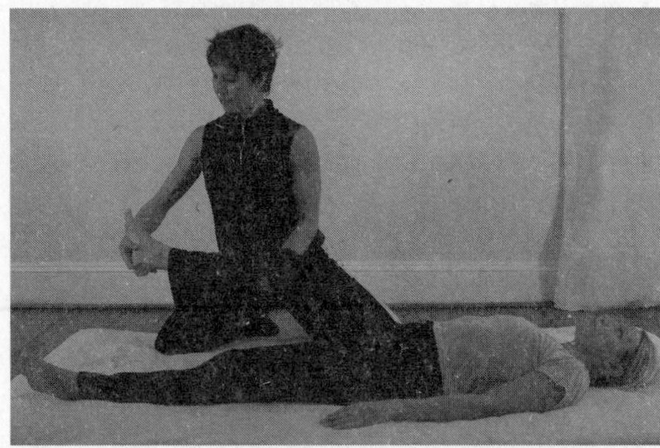

FIGURE 12-67 Cradle swing, down phase.
Extend the client's knee. Gently swing the leg up and down several times.

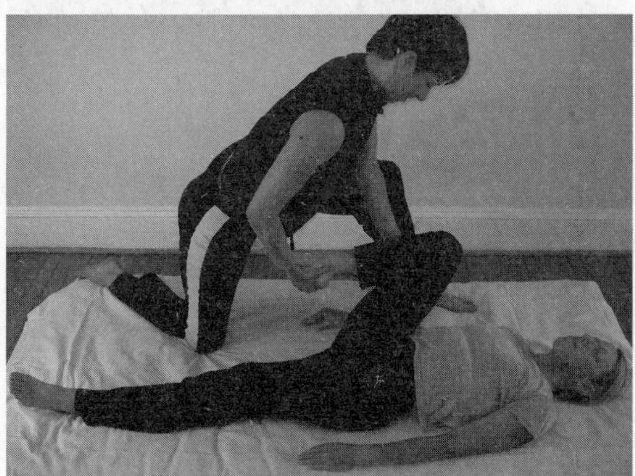

FIGURE 12-68 Hip rotation, preparation.
Support the client's leg under the heel and at the side of the knee.

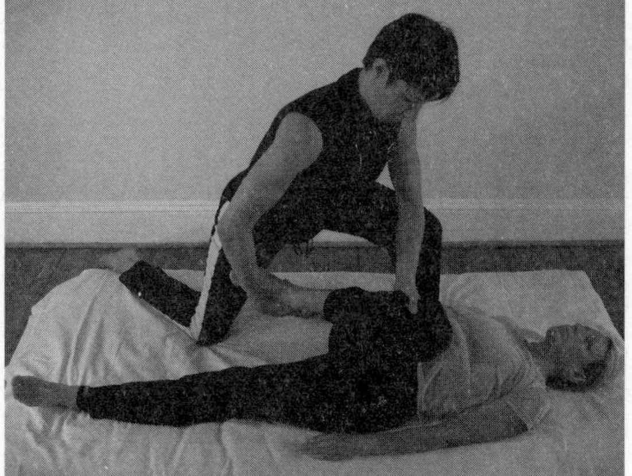

FIGURE 12-69 Hip rotation.
Rotate the leg medially (inward) and laterally (outward) several times.

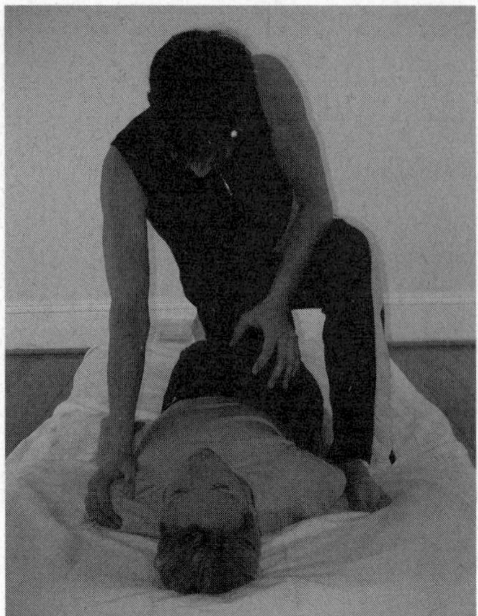

FIGURE 12-70 **Knee to chest press.**
In a kneeling lunge, place the client's foot in the crease of your thigh (groin); hold the client's knee and stabilize the opposite shoulder; lean in.

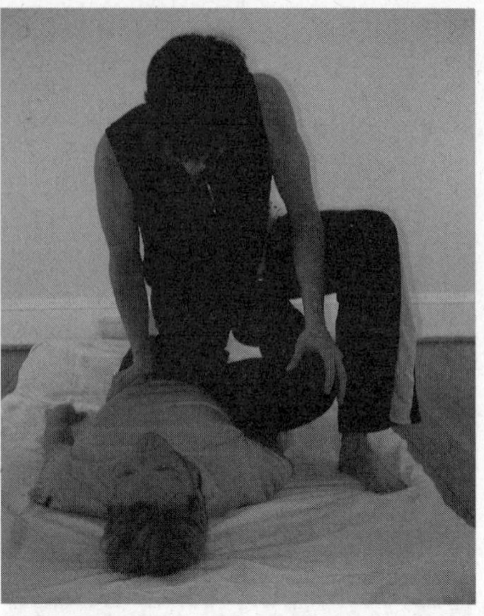

FIGURE 12-71 **Knee to side press, 45 degrees.**
Rotate the client's leg outward and repeat.

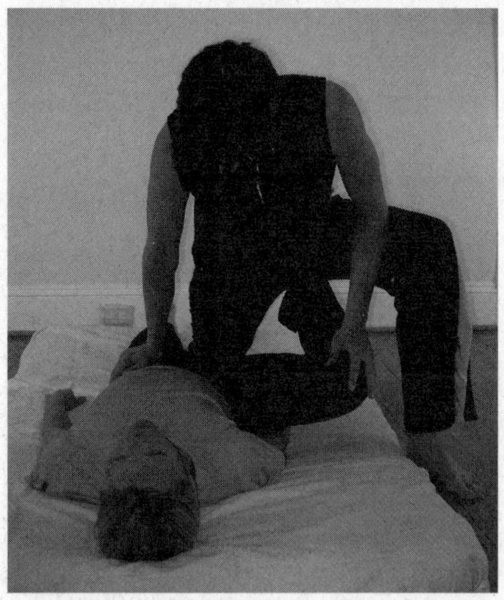

FIGURE 12-72 **Knee to floor press, 90 degrees.**
Rotate the client's leg further and repeat.

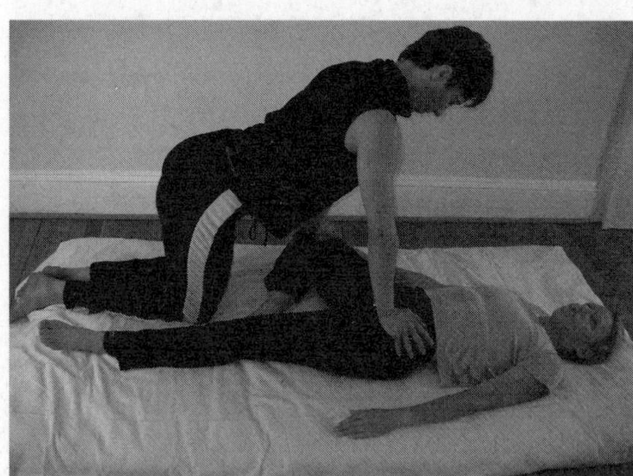

FIGURE 12-73 **Bent leg Yin Meridian/adductor stretch.**
Press the client's knee down and stabilize the opposite hip.

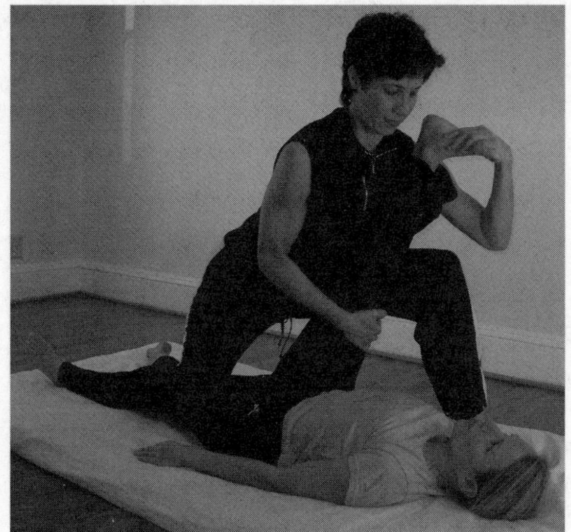

FIGURE 12-74 **Bl/Hamstring stretch.** In a kneeling lunge, prop the client's heel between your neck and shoulder; clasp your hands above the client's knee to straighten the leg and lean forward. If the client is limber, dorsiflex the foot with one hand while the other braces the thigh, as shown.

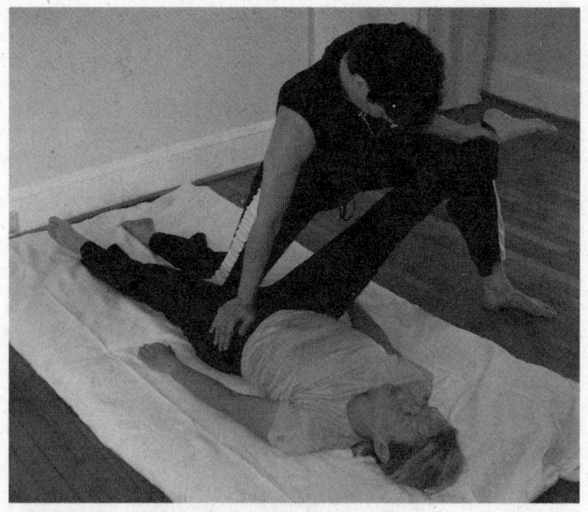

FIGURE 12-75 **Straight leg Yin Meridian/adductor stretch.** Prop the client's leg on your thigh. Stabilize the opposite hip.

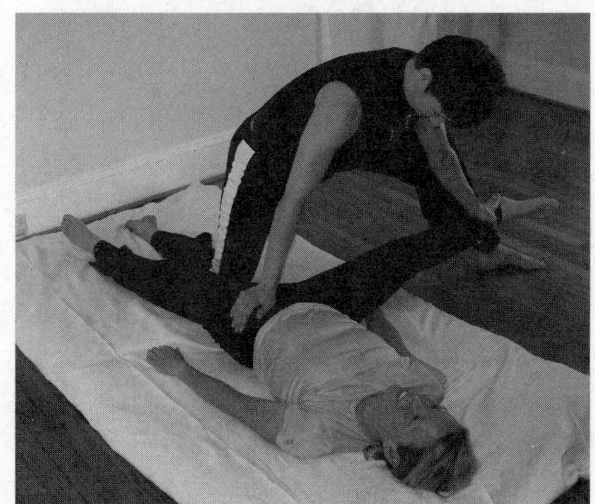

FIGURE 12-76 **Straight leg Yin Meridian/adductor stretch continued.** If the client is limber, slide the client's leg down to your ankle.

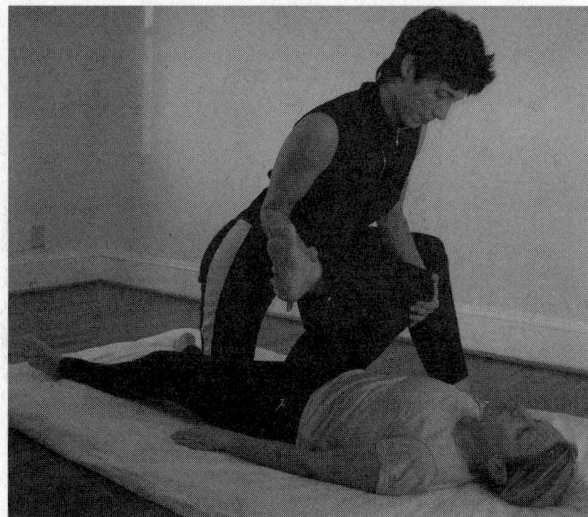

FIGURE 12-77 **GB/gluteal stretch 1.** Hold the client's ankle and knee. Rotate the client's leg laterally (outward). Press the client's shin toward the chest.

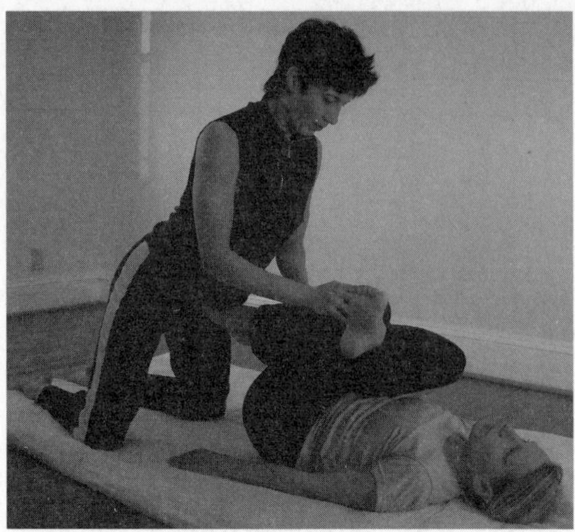

FIGURE 12-78 **GB/gluteal stretch 2.** Cross and hook the client's laterally rotated leg over the client's bent leg; press the shin toward the chest.

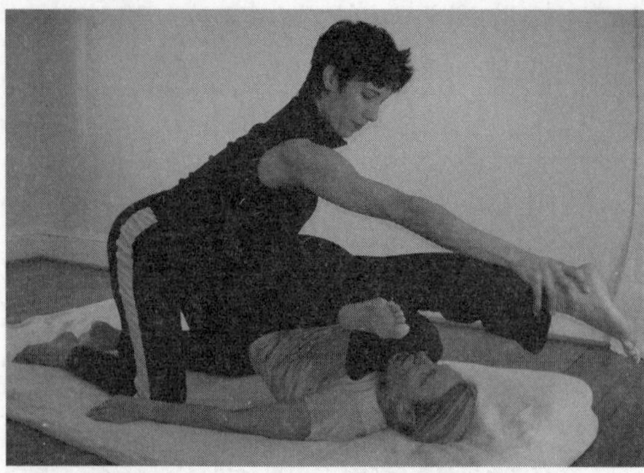

FIGURE 12-79 **Overhead leg extension.** Hold the client's ankle and extend the bent leg overhead; your other hand supports the sacrum (triangular-shaped bone at the base of the spine).

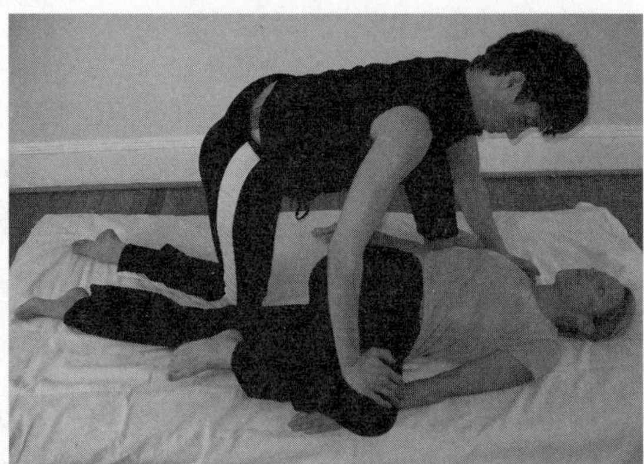

FIGURE 12-80 **Crossed bent-leg twist.** Press down on the side of the knee and stabilize the opposite shoulder.

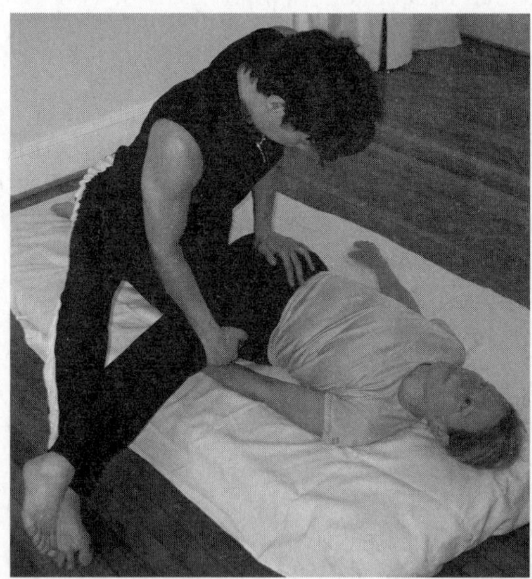

FIGURE 12-81 **Crossed straight-leg twist.** In a kneeling lunge between the client's legs, extend the client's leg and hook the client's ankle above your ankle. Stabilize the opposite hip and press down on the client's thigh to straighten the leg.

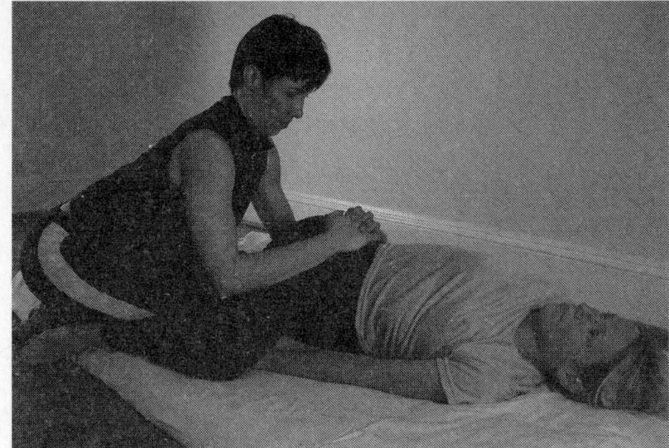

FIGURE 12-82 **Crossed bent-leg hip traction.**
Kneeling between the client's legs, clasp your hands above the client's pelvic crest; pull toward you and release several times.

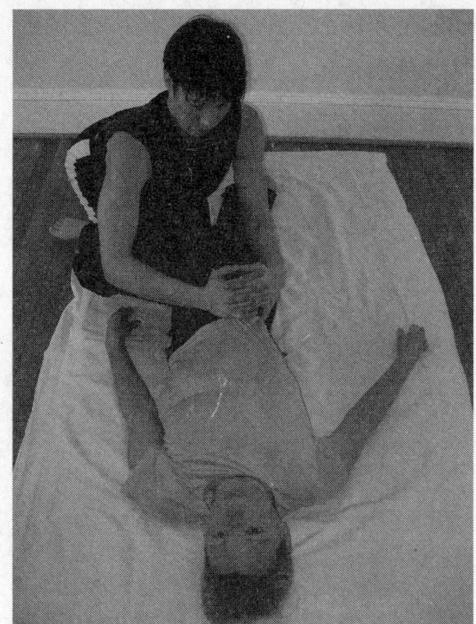

FIGURE 12-83 **Crossed bent-leg hip traction, front view.**

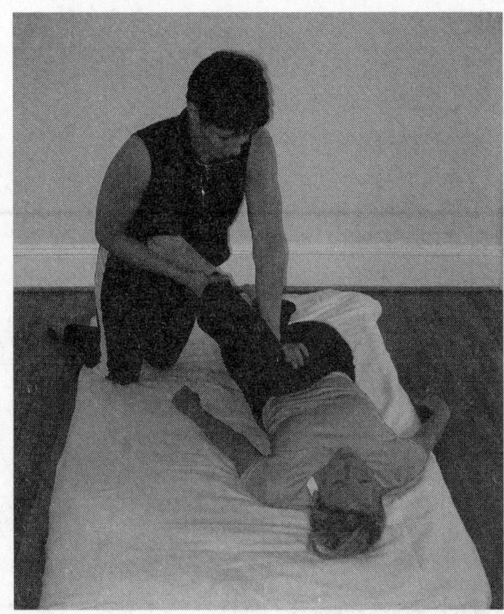

FIGURE 12-84 **Hip traction: flexion phase, front view.**
Hold the client's ankle and press down on the back of the client's thigh.

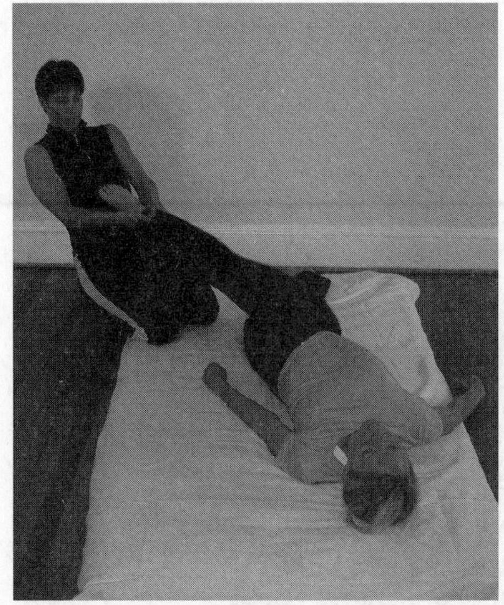

FIGURE 12-85 **Hip traction, extension phase, front view.**
Grab the client's ankle with both hands and lean back. Repeat several times.

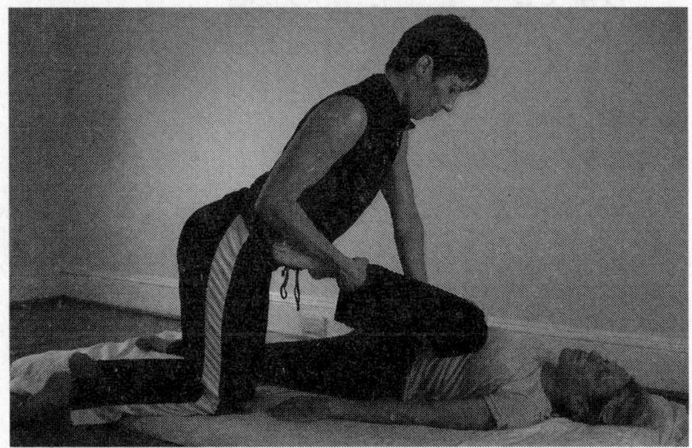

FIGURE 12-86 **Hip traction, flexion phase, side view.**

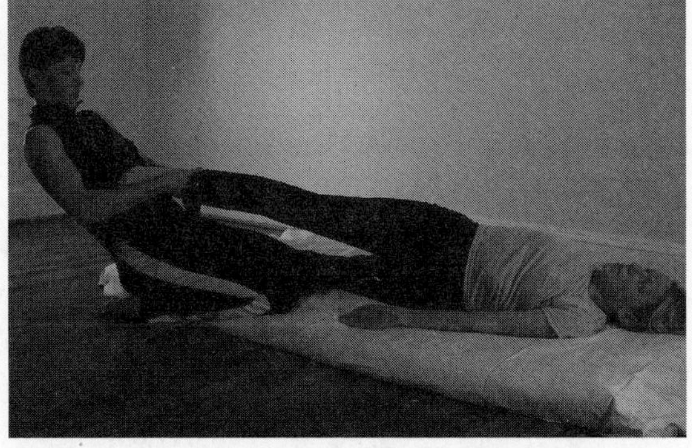

FIGURE 12-87 **Hip traction, extension phase, side view.**

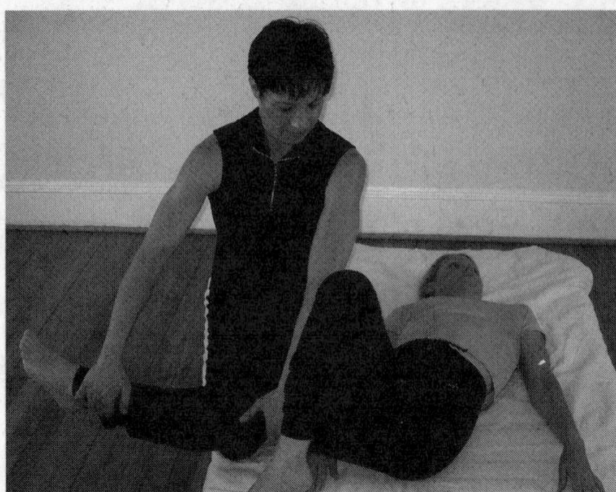

FIGURE 12-88 **Crossed bent-leg GB/abductor stretch.**
Kneel beside the client's straight leg. Hold the client's leg at the knee and ankle; gradually scoot backward. Repeat Figures 12–55 through 12–88 on the other leg.

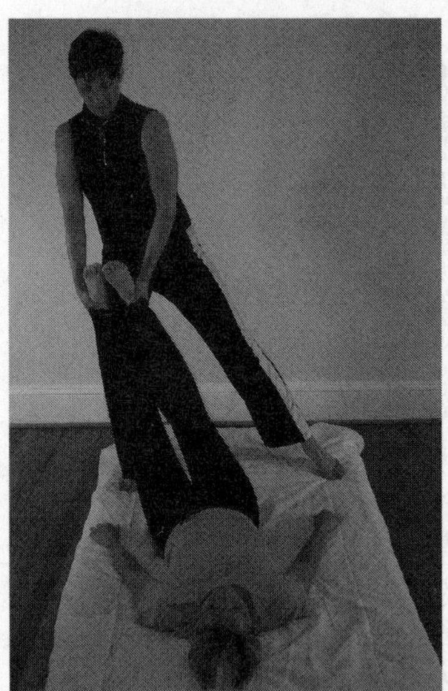

FIGURE 12-89 **Double leg pendulum swing, left.**
Hold the client's ankles; lunge and sway from side to side, swinging the client's legs.

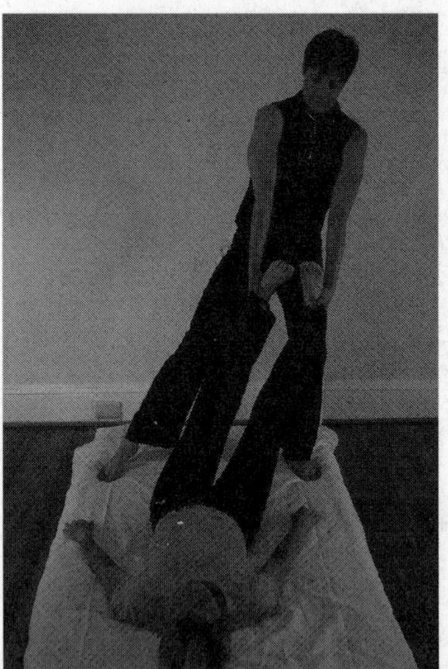

FIGURE 12-90 **Double leg pendulum swing, right.**
Alternate three or four times.

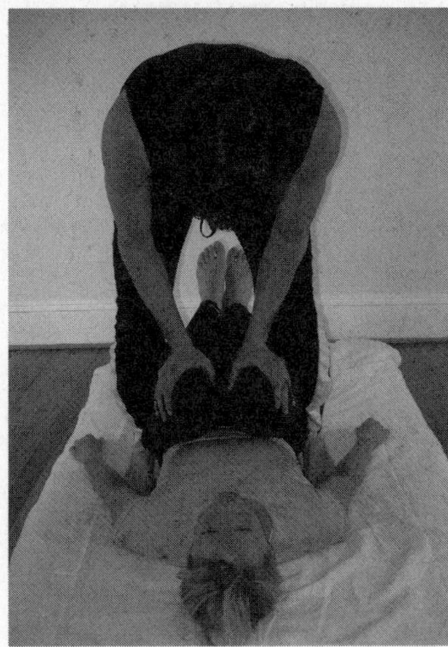

FIGURE 12-91 **Double bent-knee chest press.**
Bend the client's knees; straddle the client and press both knees into the chest.

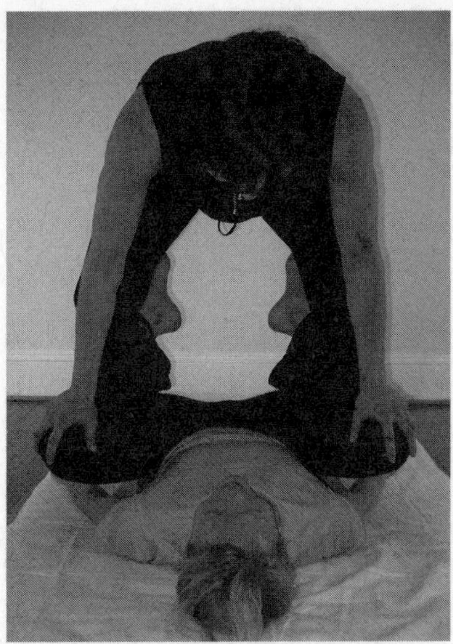

FIGURE 12-92 **Double bent-knee side press/frog pose.**
Splay the client's legs outward and press both knees toward the floor.

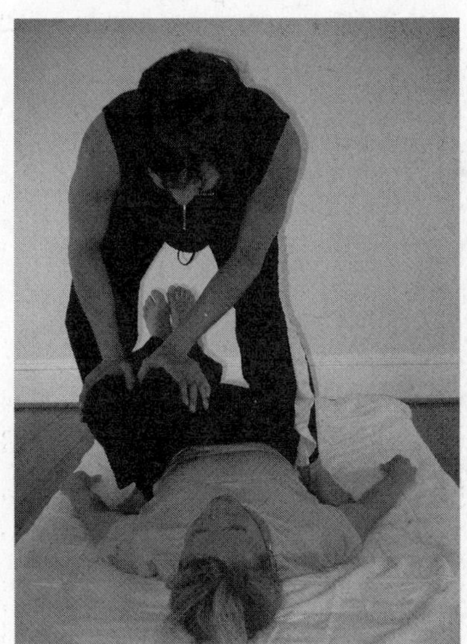

FIGURE 12-93 **Double bent-knee circumduction to the left.**
Rotate the legs in small circles several times.

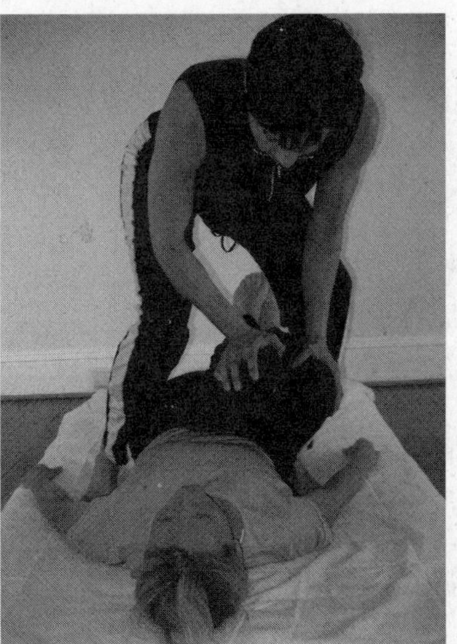

FIGURE 12-94 **Double bent-knee circumduction to the right.**
Reverse the direction of the rotation.

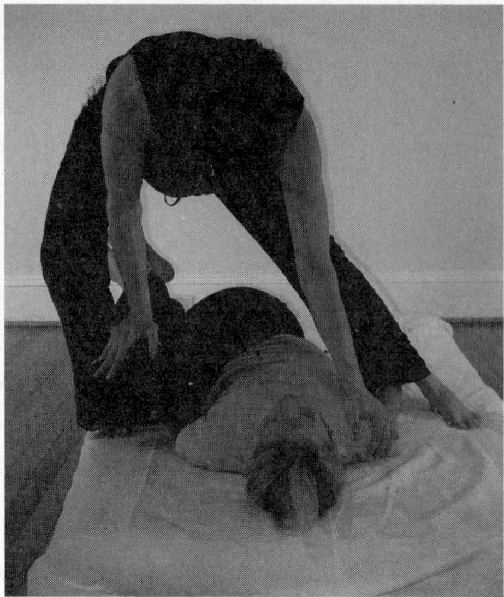

FIGURE 12-95 **Double bent-knee spinal twist, left.**
Slide the client's shins down your leg to the floor; stabilize the knee and opposite shoulder.

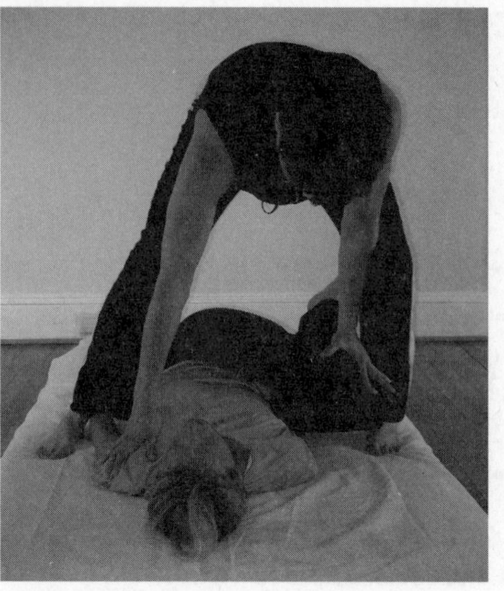

FIGURE 12-96 **Double bent-knee spinal twist, right.**
Reverse sides.

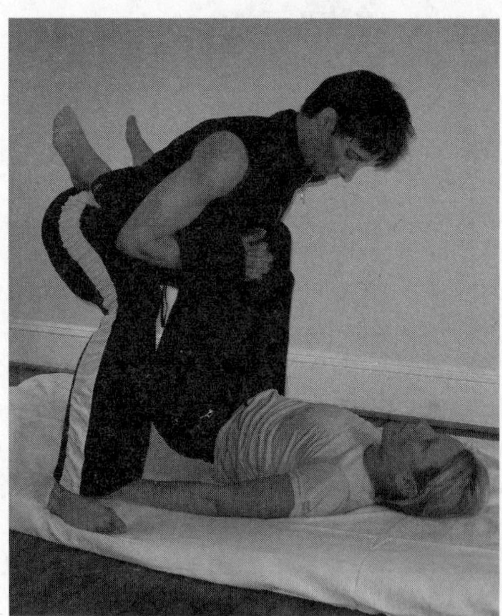

FIGURE 12-97 **Wheelbarrow lift, side view.**
Squat; drape the client's legs over yours; tuck your arms under the client's legs and clasp your hands; prop your elbows on your thighs; squat deeper to lift the client's hips.

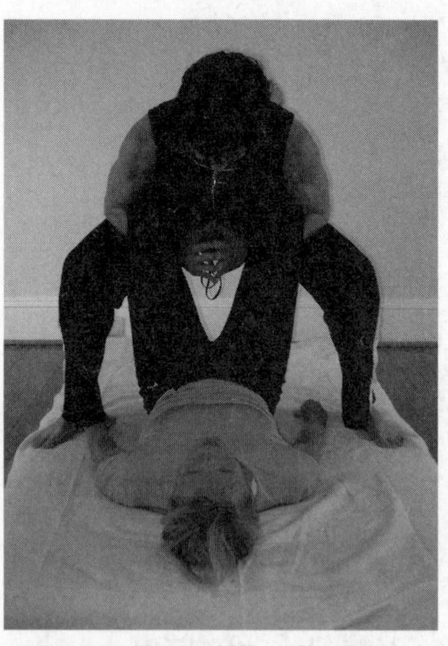

FIGURE 12-98 **Wheelbarrow lift, front view.**
Omit this technique if the client is larger and heavier than you.

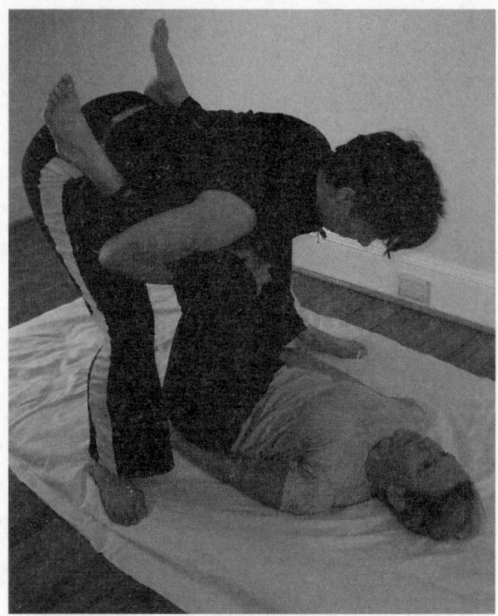

FIGURE 12-99 **Wheelbarrow pelvic rock to the left.**
Jiggle the client's hips side to side.

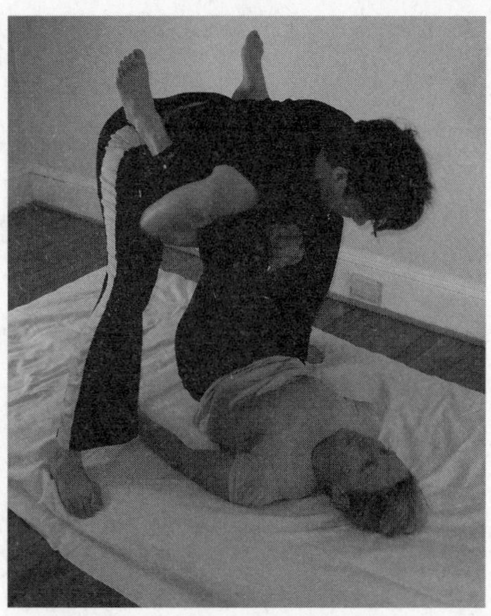

FIGURE 12-100 **Wheelbarrow pelvic rock to the right.**
Repeat several times.

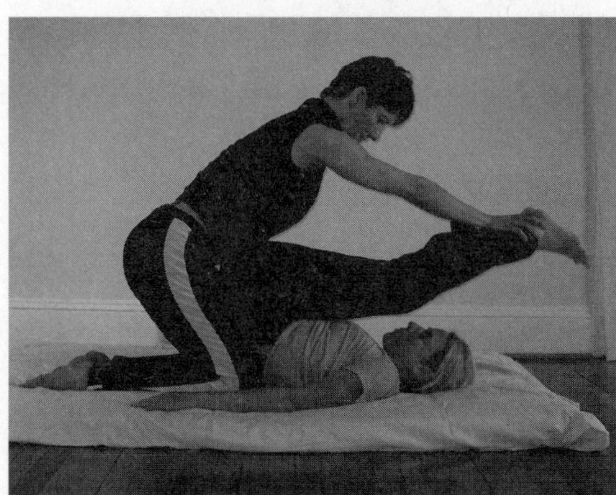

FIGURE 12-101 **Kneeling lumbar-sacral rock, preparation 1.**
Grab the client's ankles and push them overhead while supporting the client's sacrum with your other hand; scoot your knees under the client's hips.

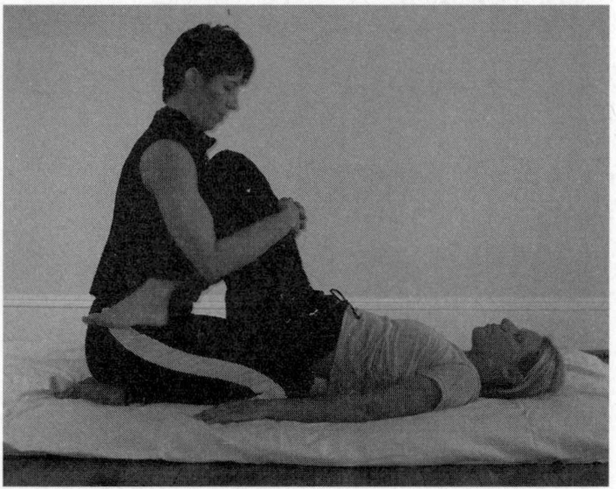

FIGURE 12-102 **Kneeling lumbar-sacral rock, preparation 2.**
Lower the client's legs and set the client's feet beside your hips; wrap your arms around the client's legs and clasp your hands.

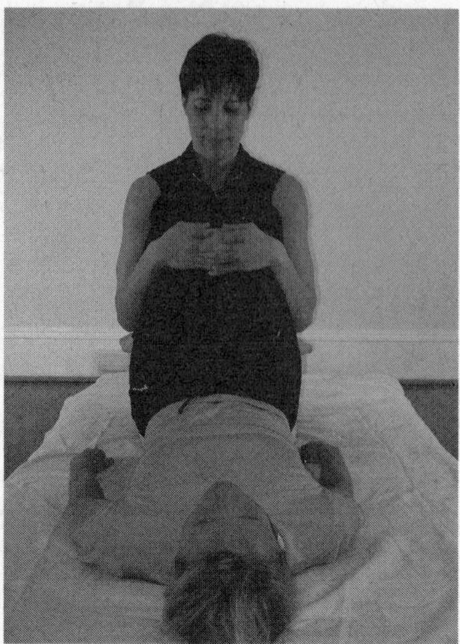

FIGURE 12-103 **Kneeling lumbar-sacral rock, preparation 2, front view.**

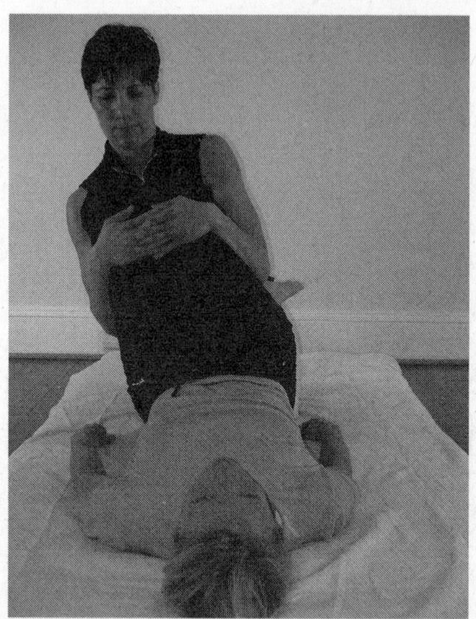

FIGURE 12-104 **Kneeling lumbar-sacral rock to the left.**
Rock side to side several times.

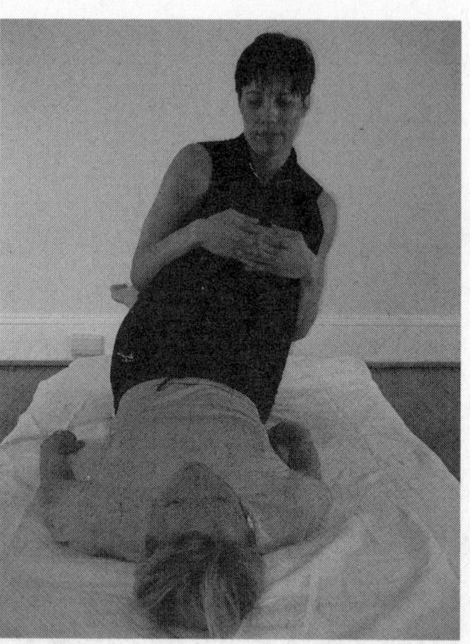

FIGURE 12-105 **Kneeling lumbar-sacral rock to the right.**
To exit, gradually scoot backward while rocking.

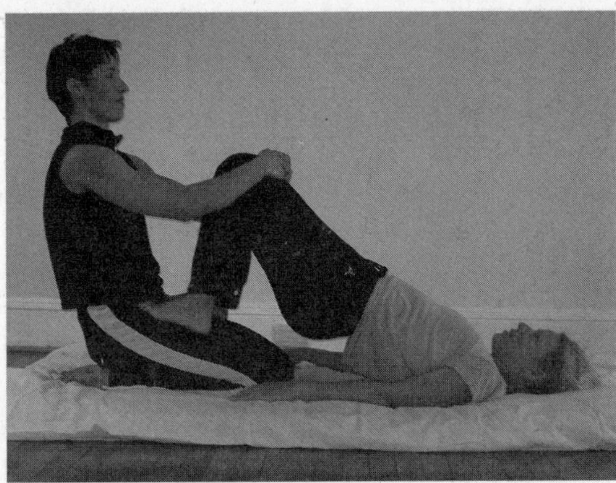

FIGURE 12-106 Bridge pose.
Set the client's feet on your thighs. Clasp your hands above the client's knees. Lean back to lift the client's hips off the floor.

REFERENCES

Alicia, M. (Director and Producer). (1997). *The stretching process* [video cassette].

Jarmey, C. & Mojay, G. (1991/1999). *Shiatsu: The complete guide,* Great Britain: Thorsons.

Gach, M. (1990). *Acupressure's potent points: A guide to self-care for common ailments.* New York: Bantam.

13

SUPINE UPPER BODY PROTOCOL

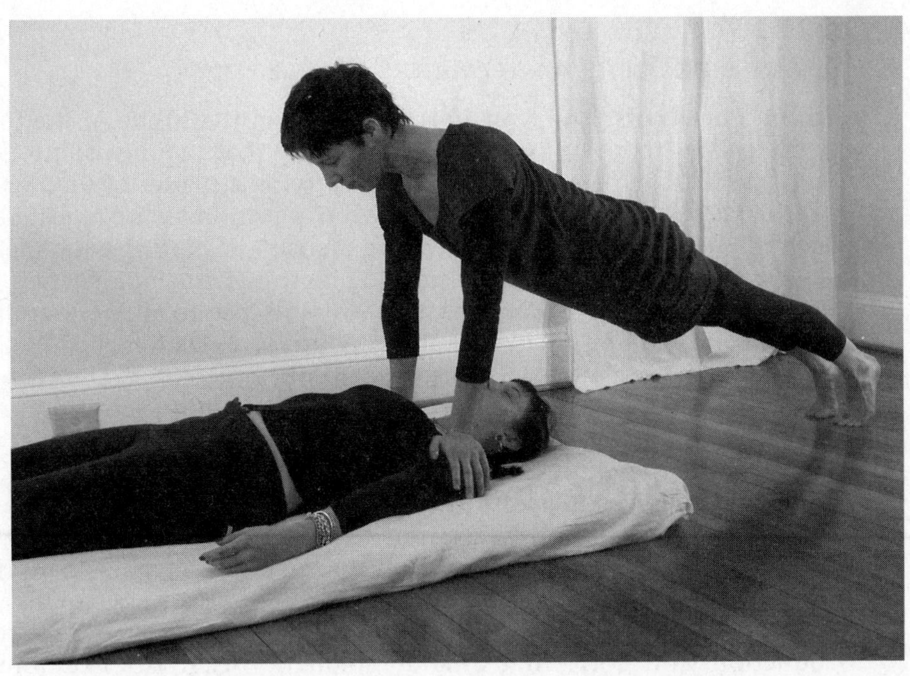

THERAPEUTIC EMPHASIS

The supine upper body protocol is fairly extensive because the supine position is ideal for tractioning, stretching, and mobilizing the wrist, arm, shoulder, and neck. Additionally, a great number of acupressure points can be accessed, especially on the face, neck, chest, and inner arms. The Yin Meridians of the arm—the Lung (Lu), Pericardium (PC), and Heart (Ht) Meridians—are especially amenable to treatment in this position, though the Yang Meridians of the arm can also be worked. Focused work on these Meridians and key acupressure points can benefit clients who have painful obstruction syndrome—localized muscular soreness and joint aches—in the arms and chest; clients whose Meridians assess as Kyo or Jitsu or are otherwise symptomatic; and clients who present physical disorders or psychological disharmonies associated with the corresponding elements.

CAUSES OF DISCOMFORT AND TREATMENT STRATEGIES

A client can develop painful obstruction syndrome from hard manual labor, vigorous exercise, participation in sports events or performing arts, or any unaccustomed activity that subjects the body to a stress load to which it has not adapted. Even customary but prolonged low-load activities or repetitive low-load activities such as those required by most occupations can cause painful obstruction syndrome. To disperse blood and fluid stagnation, sore and fatigued muscles should be pressed, squeezed, and rubbed. To clear blockages in energy flow, key acupressure points in the associated muscles should be pressed and held or pressed and subjected to friction. If soreness extends along the pathway of a Meridian, the entire Meridian should be given Shiatsu. The listed examples target isolated areas of the anterior upper body that can become sore and fatigued from exertion. For photos of point locations on a human model, see Appendix 1. For illustrated charts of acupressure points and Meridian locations, see the Flow of Qi chart in Figure 2-1 and the Anterior Meridians and Associated Musculature chart on p. 280.

KEY ACUPRESSURE POINTS FOR THE ANTERIOR UPPER BODY

- **Inner Forearms**: The wrist flexor muscles on the inside of the forearm can become sore from wrist curls, or any activity that requires controlling a load with the wrist hyperextended, such as carrying a platter of food or balancing on the hands, or any activity that requires prolonged or repeated grasping, such as holding a power tool, cleaning utensil, or sporting equipment; pulling weeds; kneading dough; hand washing clothing; stocking shelves; and scanning and bagging consumer products. Give Shiatsu to all Yin Meridians of the forearm and acupressure to wrist flexor points Lu 5, Lu 7, Lu 9, PC 6, PC 7, Ht 3, Ht 5, and Ht 7 (treating SI 8 is also beneficial).
- **Inner Upper Arms**: The biceps (inner upper arm muscle) and brachioradialis (forearm muscle) can become sore from doing elbow flexion exercises like dumbbell, barbell, and cable curls; shoveling dirt; and lifting and carrying heavy boxes. Give Shiatsu to the Lung, Pericardium, and Heart Meridians in the arm and forearm and acupressure to Lu 3, Lu 4, Lu 5, Lu 6, PC 2, and PC 3.
- **Front of Shoulders and Chest**: The biceps and coracobrachialis (upper arm muscles), anterior deltoid (front shoulder muscle), and pectoralis major and minor (chest muscles) can become sore from doing shoulder flexion, shoulder adduction, and horizontal shoulder adduction exercises like dumbbell and barbell bench presses, flies, and push-ups; from arm wrestling; and from participating in sports like tennis, racquetball, and squash, which involve swinging the arm across the chest to strike a ball with force, and sports like boxing and martial arts, which use hook and upper-cut punches. Even everyday activities like picking up and carrying a baby or a 5-gallon jug of water can fatigue these muscles. Give Shiatsu to the chest, upper shoulders, and arms, and acupressure to Kidney Meridian points along the sternum, especially Ki 27, as well as St 13, St 14, St 15, Lu 1, Lu 2, and Lu 3.
- **Postpartum Chest Points**: Stimulate GB 21, Lu 1, St 13, St 16, and CV 17 to encourage lactation or milk letdown in nursing mothers (see "Pregnant Women" in Chapter 9).
- **Head points**: In general, stimulating head points draws energy upward and clears Qi blockages that cause local disorders, and especially of the sense organs. B1 1, 2, and 10 alleviate inflamed, fatigued eyes. B1 1 and 2 ease frontal headaches, while B1 10 eases occipital headaches and relaxes neck tension. GB 1 sharpens vision. LI 20 and St 3 open the nasal passages, clear obstruction, dispel congestion, and improve nostril breathing and the sense of smell. TH 17, GB 2, and SI 19 mitigate various ear disorders, including earache, ear infection, and tinnitus (a shrill, droning noise in the ears), and improve the sense of hearing. Additionally, TH 17 reduces the loss of balance and equilibrium associated with Meniere's disease, eases facial pain and paralysis, relaxes jaw tension, and facilitates swallowing and speaking in cases of difficulty. St 6 and 7 relax jaw and neck tension, mitigate toothache, facial pain, and paralysis, and reduce symptoms associated with temporomandibular joint syndrome (TMJ) or jaw dysfunction (pain and difficulty opening and/or closing the jaw) and bruxism (clenching and/or grinding of the teeth). St 8 and Tai

Yang alleviate temporal headaches or unilateral migraines, dispel mental fogginess and improve clarity and focus, ease dizziness, and clear blurred vision. GV 20 relieves headaches and raises sinking Qi, and especially in cases of chronic loose stools or diarrhea, hemorrhoids, organ prolapse, or mental exhaustion.

- **Here are the key acupressure points in various locations:**

  Hand: PC 8, Ht 9
  Wrist: Lu 9, PC 7, Ht 7
  Forearm: Lu 5, Ht 3
  Upper arm: PC 3
  Front shoulder: Lu 2
  Chest: Lu 1, St 13, St 14, St 15, Ki 27, PC 17
  Neck: GV 16, Bl 10, GB 20
  Eyes: Bl 1, Bl 2, GB 1
  Nose: LI 20, St 3
  Ears: TH 17, GB 2, SI 19
  Jaws: St 6, St 7
  Temples: St 8, Tai Yang
  Crown of head: GV 20

KYO JITSU IMBALANCES

A client with a Meridian that is demonstrably Kyo (empty and deficient) or Jitsu (full and excessive) should be given Shiatsu to the Meridian. The Yin Meridians of the arm (the Lung, Pericardium, and Heart Meridians) are placed in the Meridian stretch position by turning the palm up and positioning the arm at a 45 degree angle away from the body for the Lung Meridian, at a 90 degree angle for the Pericardium Meridian, and at a 120 degree angle for the Heart Meridian (see the discussion of Meridian stretches in Chapter 9). The Yang Meridians of the arm (the Large Intestine, Triple Heater, and Small Intestine Meridians) can also be worked in the supine position, though not as easily as in the prone position. To place the Yang Meridians of the arm in the Meridian stretch position, turn the palm down and position the arm at a 45 degree angle away from the body for the Large Intestine Meridian. Cross the forearm over the belly for the Triple Heater Meridian, and cross the forearm over the chest for the Small Intestine Meridian. Usually, less pressure is applied when working the Triple Heater and Small Intestine Meridians in the supine position, since compressions on the arm will also depress the belly or the breasts, unless the practitioner wraps his hands around the arm and squeezes from both sides.

Palpate along the Meridian, feeling the quality of the tissues (see "Qualities of Kyo and Jitsu" and "Meridian Diagnosis" in Chapter 6). Jitsu tissues feel firm and toned or even hypertonic (tense), whereas Kyo tissues often feel mushy, flabby, limp, and slack or, alternatively, very hard and tough. Additionally, Jitsu tissues may feel warm or hot to the touch and may look red, in contrast with Kyo tissues, which may feel cool or cold and may look pale. A Jitsu Meridian rebuffs pressure in a bouncy way, whereas a Kyo Meridian feels bottomless, engulfing, and void or, conversely, unyielding, inert, and shut.

Initially, pressure on Jitsu may elicit a sharp or painful sensation that mellows and dissipates with continued therapy. The sensation may be noted by the client's groan or exclamation, a startle response like a jerk, or a jump response like a muscle twitch. These reactions are more common on the chest at the sternal and clavicular attachments, on the front of the shoulder at the coracoid process, and on the bicep at the elbow attachment. Delayed onset muscle soreness can render the tissues squeamish to touch. In spite of this skittishness, Jitsu tension tends to relax quickly if therapy is given within the pain threshold. By contrast, Kyo is relatively impassive (nonresponsive). Unlike Jitsu, pressure on Kyo does not initiate immediate change. Kyo tissues need prolonged holding, like a block of ice that needs to thaw. Pressure on a Kyo Meridian tends to elicit a soothing, dull sensation or no sensation. When the sensation is agreeable, the client may sigh or request the practitioner to remain in the area or repeat the technique.

To sedate a Jitsu Meridian, apply stimulating techniques to disperse stagnation and congestion and to release blocked Qi (see "Application of Techniques" and Table 6-1 in Chapter 6). Two-handed compression can be used to cover more surface area and to intensify the effect. Compression along the Meridian should be moderate to deep, fairly brisk, and rhythmic, following a downward and outward direction or countercurrent to the flow of the Meridian (see "Direction of Movement" in Chapter 6). Additionally, kenbiki (jostling, torsion wringing, and cross-fiber friction) and tapotement (pummeling) can be applied. Specific Jitsu dispersal techniques include treading on the pectorals and anterior deltoids with the heels and sides of the hands, treading on the upper shoulders with the feet, and scrubbing CV 17 to stimulate Qi flow in the chest.

To tonify a Kyo Meridian, apply nurturing techniques to draw and gather Qi to the area of deficiency (see "Application of Techniques" and Table 6-1 in Chapter 6). A specific Kyo tonification technique is palmar compression, which offers a broad, flat, noninvasive surface. The Mother/Son hand technique may be used when the arms present signs of deficiency—lack of tone, emaciation, weakness, coldness, or edema (fluid retention)—or are too hyperirritable for Jitsu dispersal techniques. Place the Mother hand like a warm compress on a deficient area like CV 17, Ki 27, or Lu 1, or use the Mother hand to hold a key acupressure point like Ht 7, PC 6, or Lu 9, while the Son hand presses the length of the Meridian (see Practice Exercise 6-1). Pressure should be light to moderate and fairly slow and steady, following an upward and inward direction or concurrent with the flow of the Meridian (see "Direction of Movement" in Chapter 6).

Certain activities, if done to excess, such as standing, sitting, or lying down, can tax a Meridian, leading to an energetic imbalance in the Meridian (Gach, 1990). Prolonged lying down, as when convalescing from an injury or illness, strains the Large Intestine and Lung Meridians, adversely affecting breathing and bowel movements. Give Shiatsu to these Meridians.

ELEMENT TYPE IMBALANCES

Clients who present a constellation of physical disorders or psychological disharmonies associated with a particular element should be given Shiatsu to the Yang and Yin Meridians of that element. The Lung Meridian is associated with the Metal element and the Lung and Large Intestine organ functions. The Pericardium and Heart Meridians are associated with the Fire element and the Pericardium, Heart, Triple Heater, and Small Intestine organ functions. When a client, especially a Yin element type such as Earth, manifests symptoms of deficiency disorders in the lower body, acupressure to the upper body, especially the chest, shoulders, and head, is helpful to draw energy upward. GV 20 raises sinking Qi.

For a profile on the element types, see Chapter 4, and for a description of element imbalances, see Chapter 5. Additionally, Table 4-1 summarizes correspondences for each of the Five Elements, Table 7-4 summarizes physical disorders associated with each element's organ pair, and Table 7-5 summarizes psychological disharmonies associated with each element.

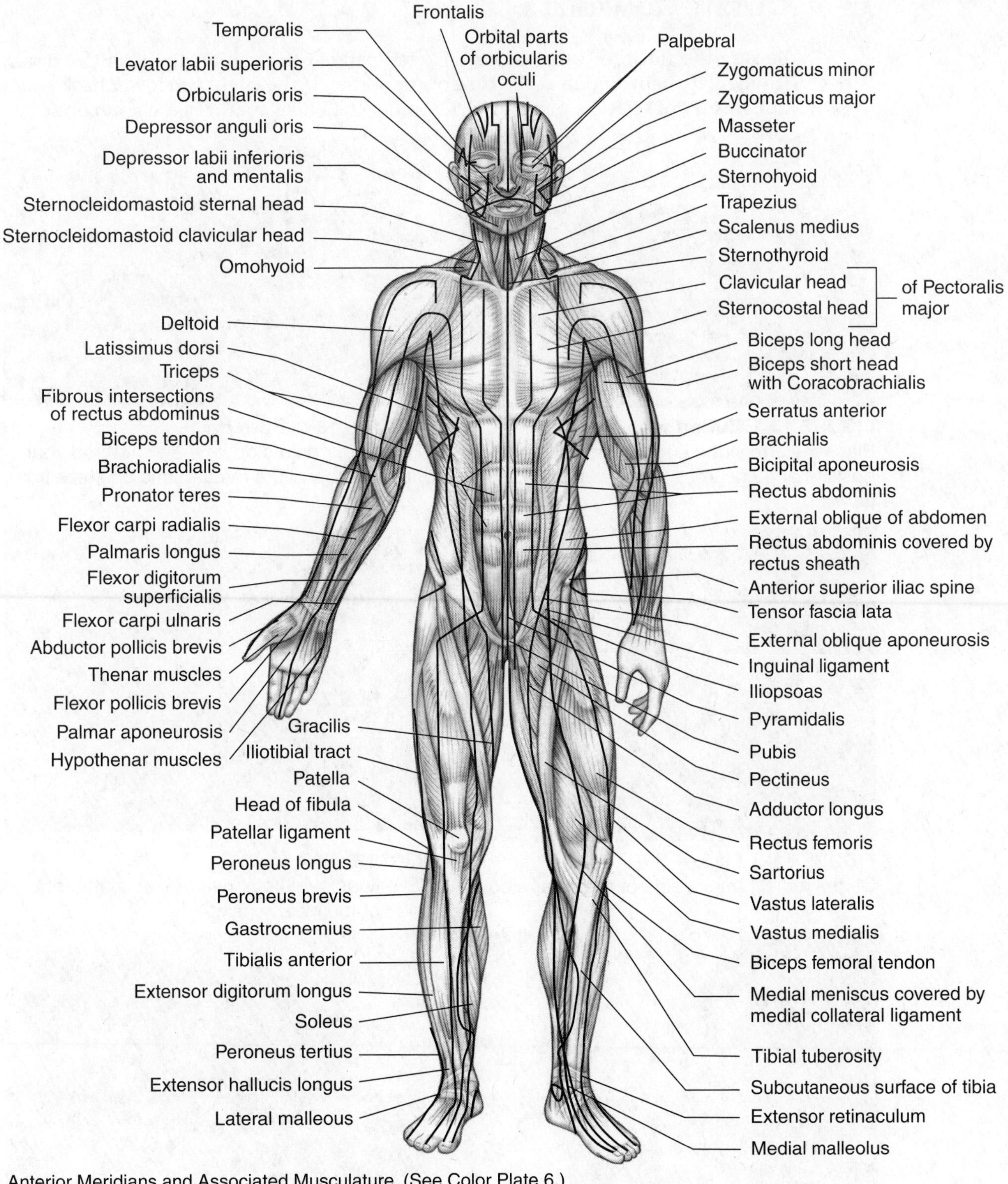

Anterior Meridians and Associated Musculature. (See Color Plate 6.)

CLIENT COMFORT

Be sure the futon or other surface is well padded to cushion the client's sacrum (triangular-shaped bone at the base of the spine). If the client has lower back issues or a history of sciatica, place a bolster under the knees to increase client comfort.

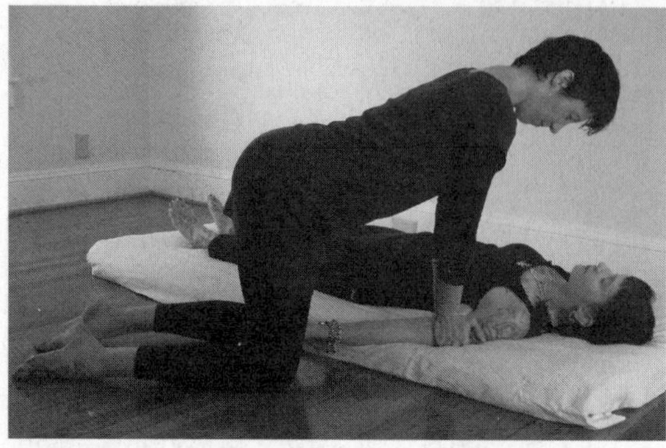

FIGURE 13-1 **Butterfly.**
Place the arm in the Lung Meridian stretch position at 45 degrees away from body, palm up.

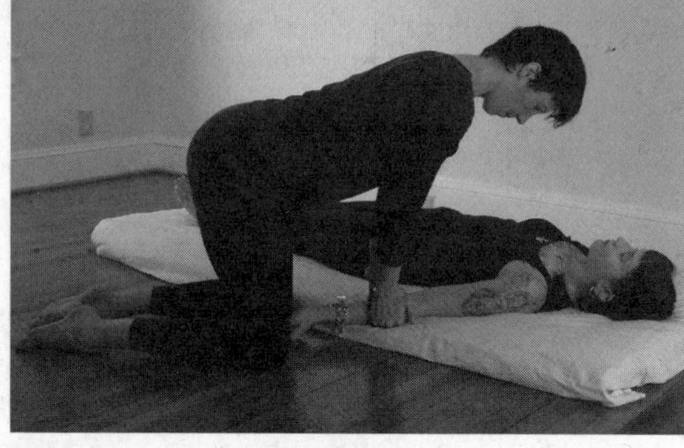

FIGURE 13-2 **Butterfly.**
Press your palms down the arm. Wrap your fingers around the forearm and squeeze from both sides.

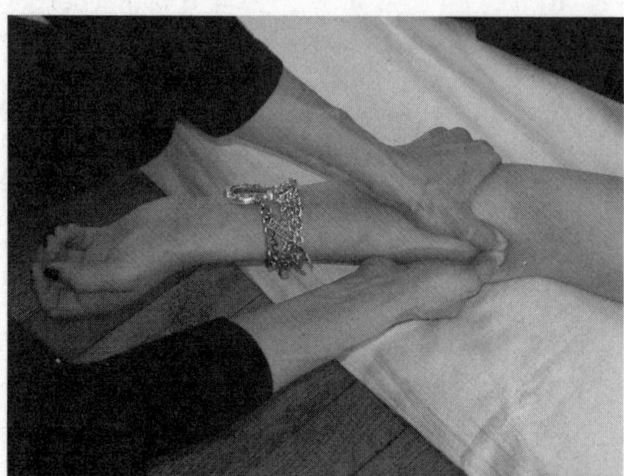

FIGURE 13-3 **Lu 5.**
On the radial (thumb) side of the inner elbow.

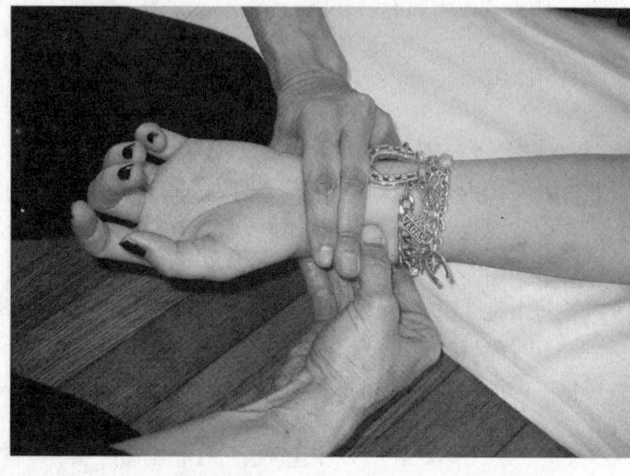

FIGURE 13-4 **Lu 7.**
Two finger widths above the radial (thumb) side of the inner wrist.

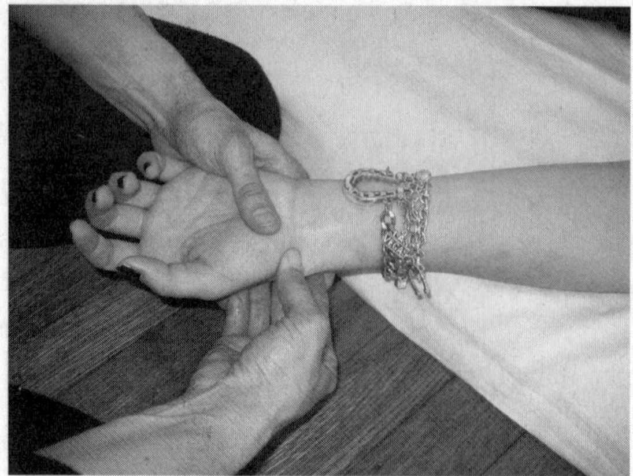

FIGURE 13-5 **Lu 9.**
On the radial (thumb) side of the inner wrist.

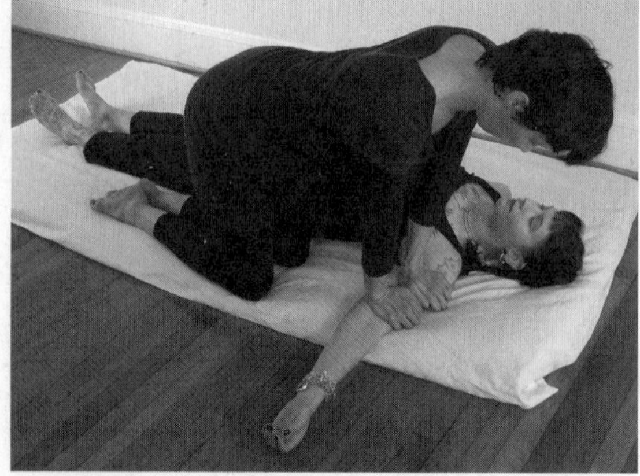

FIGURE 13-6 **Heel of the hand compression.**
Place the arm in the Pericardium Meridian stretch position at 90 degrees away from body, palm up.

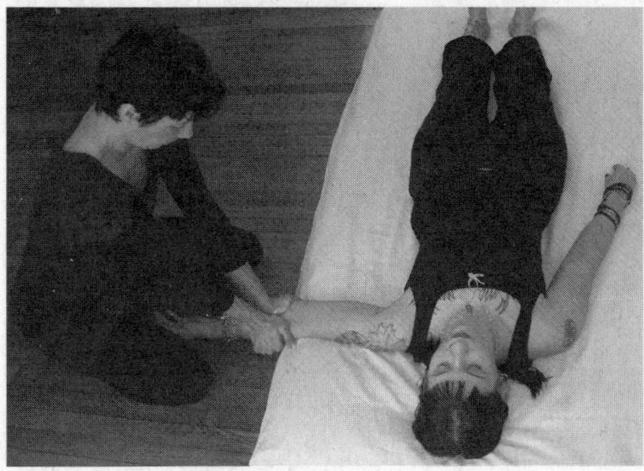

FIGURE 13-7 **Butterfly.**
Wrap your fingers around the forearm and squeeze from both sides.

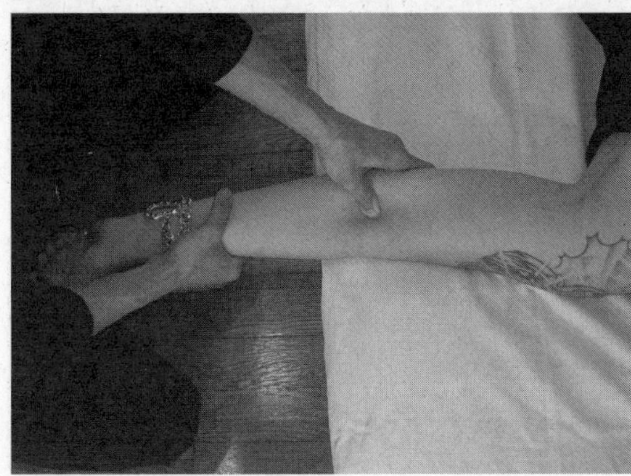

FIGURE 13-8 **PC 3.**
On the bicep tendon, above the inner elbow.

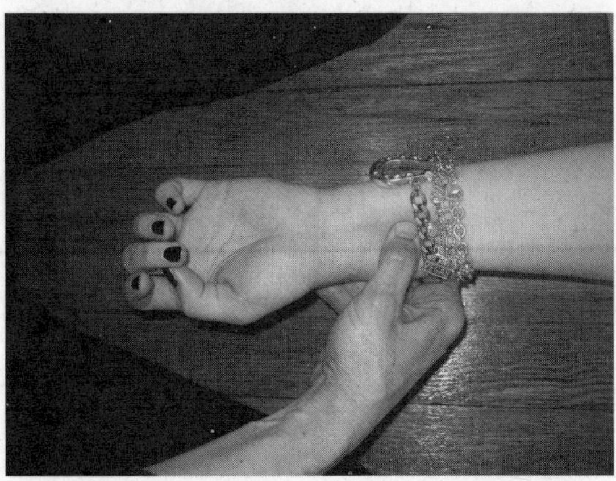

FIGURE 13-9 **PC 6.**
Two and a half finger widths above the inner wrist between the two wrist flexor tendons.

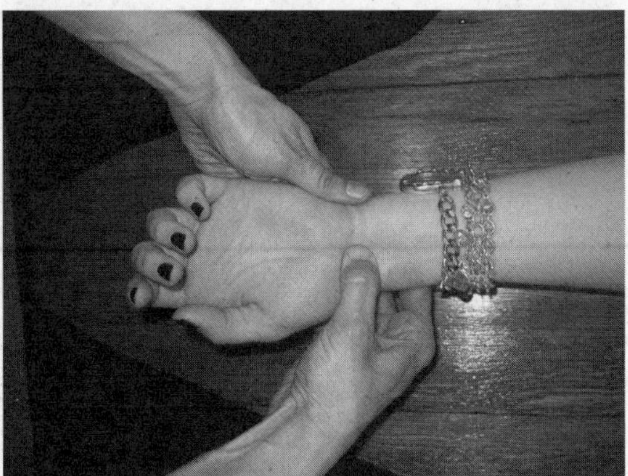

FIGURE 13-10 **PC 7.**
At the inner wrist between the two wrist flexor tendons.

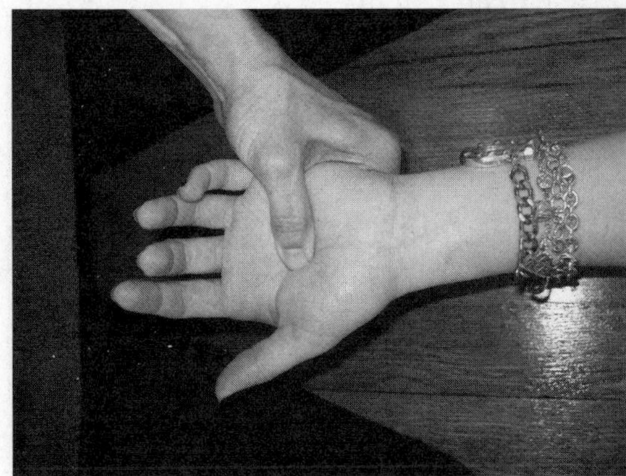

FIGURE 13-11 **PC 8.**
Near the center of the palm.

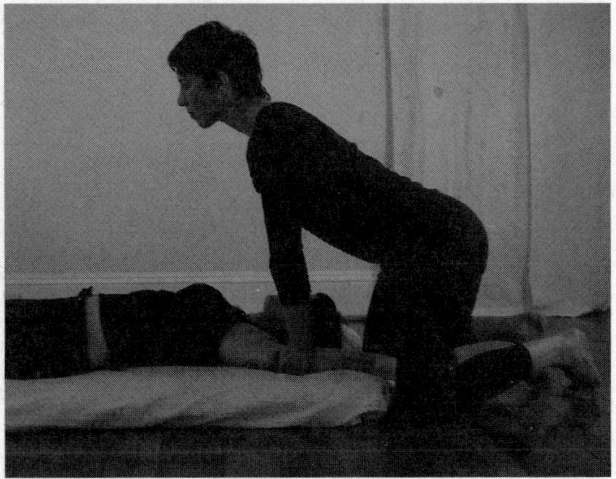

FIGURE 13-12 **Butterfly.**
Place the arm in the Heart Meridian stretch position at 120 degrees away from body, palm up.

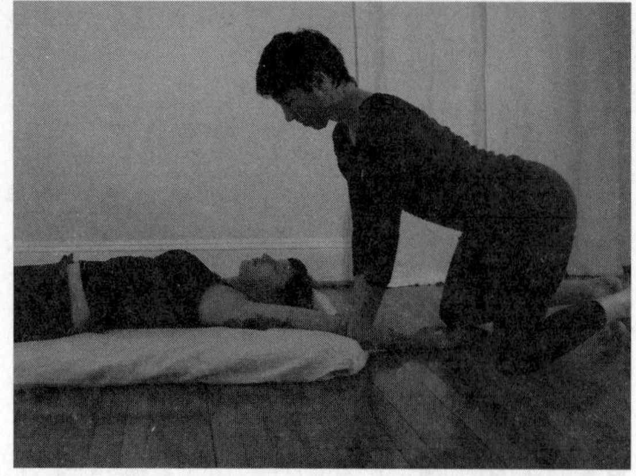

FIGURE 13-13 Butterfly.

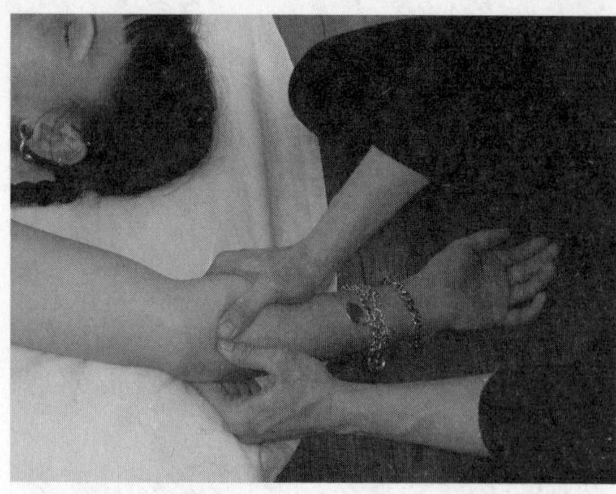

FIGURE 13-14 Ht 3.
On the ulnar (little finger) side of the inner elbow.

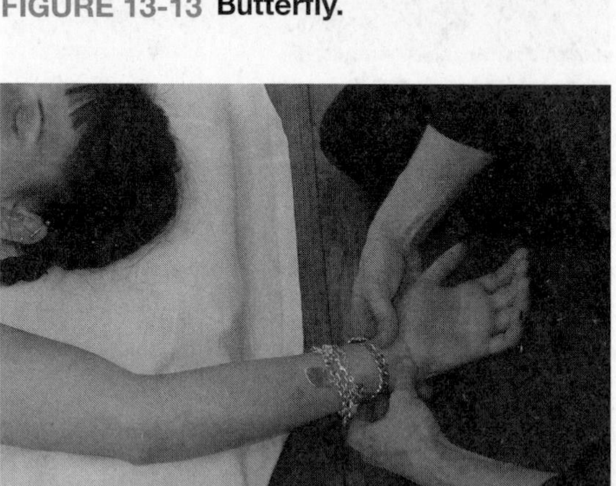

FIGURE 13-15 Ht 7.
On the ulnar (little finger) side of the inner wrist.

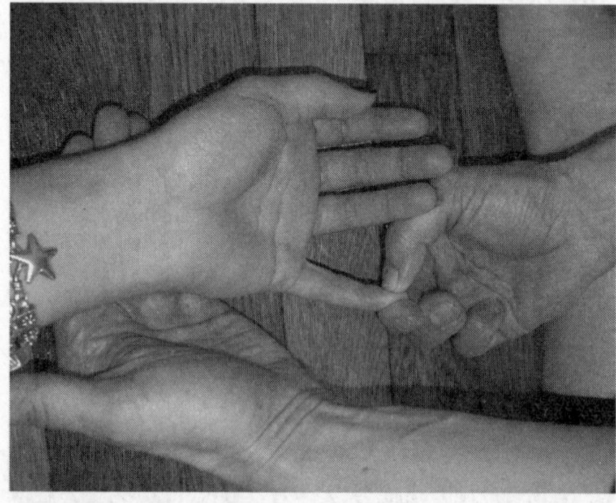

FIGURE 13-16 Ht 9.
At the corner of the inner nailbed of the little finger. Repeat Figures 13–1 through 13–16 on the other side.

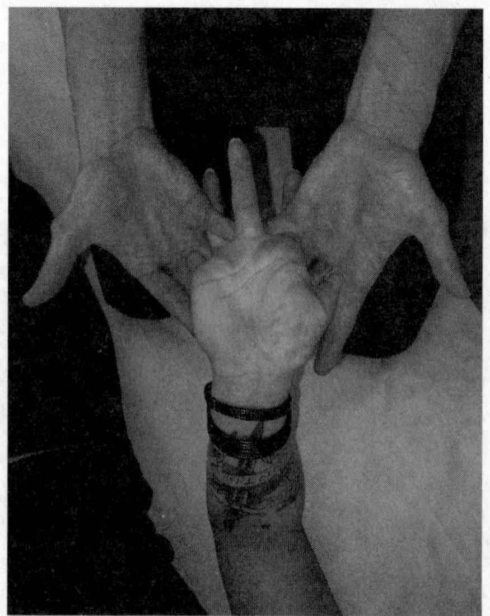

FIGURE 13-17 Interlacing fingers.
Insert the middle and ring fingers of one hand between the client's thumb and pointer finger; insert the little and ring fingers of your other hand between the client's middle and ring fingers; rest your thumbs on the client's palm.

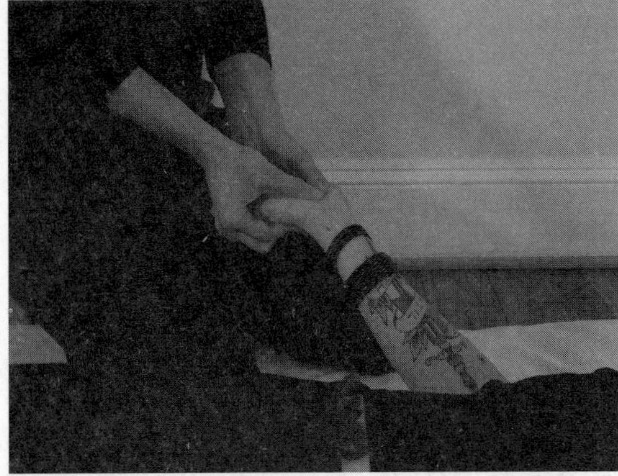

FIGURE 13-18 **Wrist flexor rotation, lax phase.**
Rotate the client's wrist, palm up, by moving the client's forearm in wide circles several times.

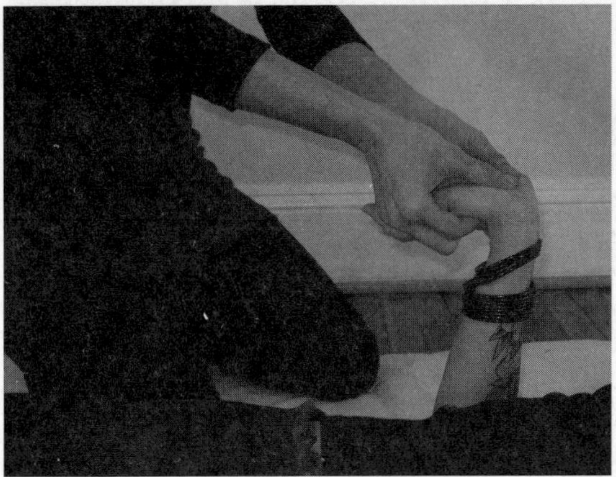

FIGURE 13-19 **Wrist flexor rotation, stretch phase.**
Reverse directions.

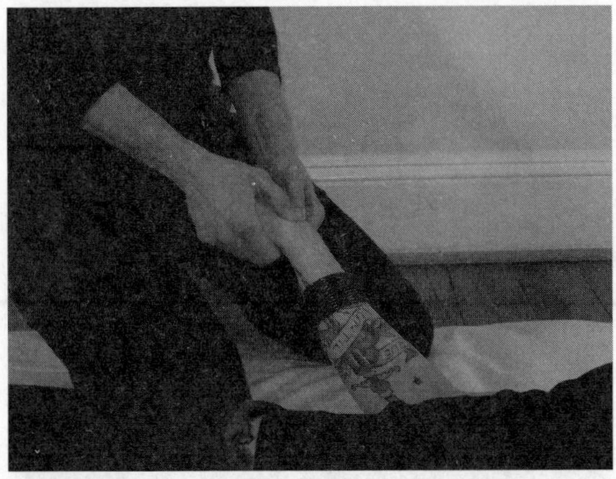

FIGURE 13-20 **Wrist extensor rotation, lax phase.**
Release your interlaced hands; turn the client's hand over and hold the wrist at TH 4. Rotate the client's wrist, palm down, by moving the client's forearm in wide circles several times.

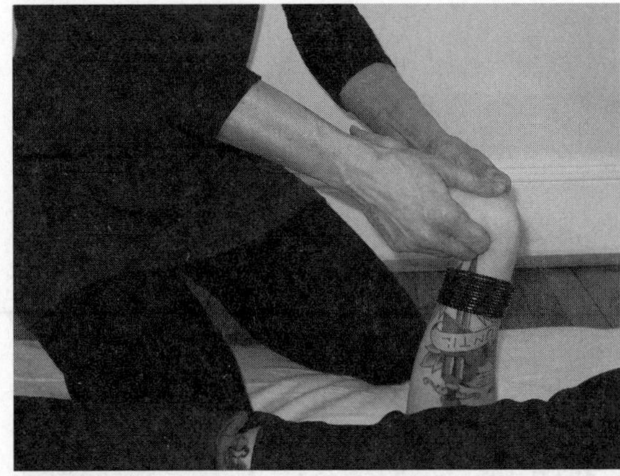

FIGURE 13-21 **Wrist extensor rotation, stretch phase.**
Reverse directions.

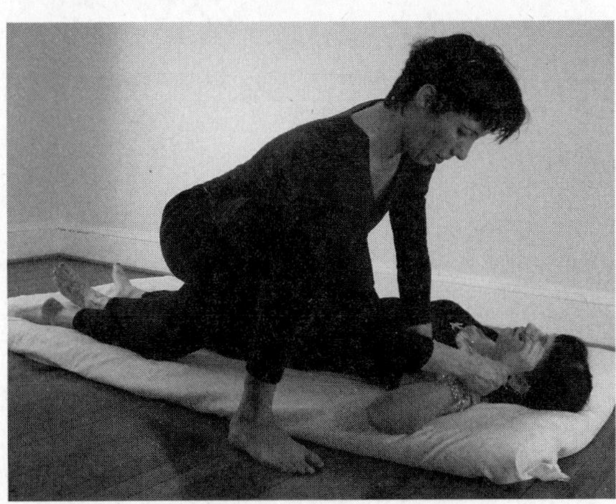

FIGURE 13-22 **Forearm rotation, flexion phase.**
Stabilize the shoulder by pressing the heel of your hand at Lu 1. Hold the wrist and rotate the forearm outward.

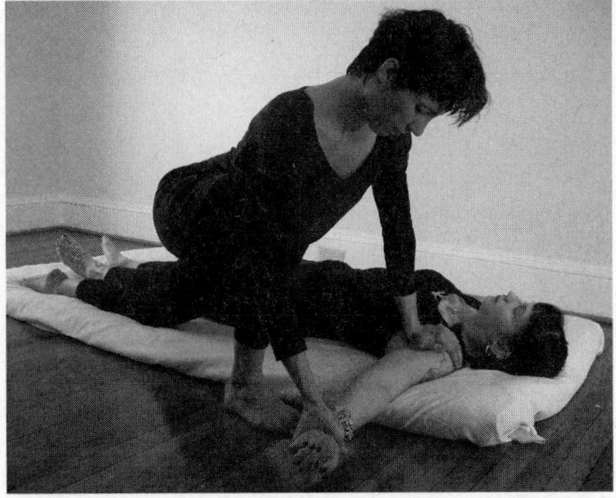

FIGURE 13-23 **Forearm rotation, extension phase.**
Repeat several times; on the final rotation, traction the arm by pressing Lu 1 inward and pulling the arm outward.

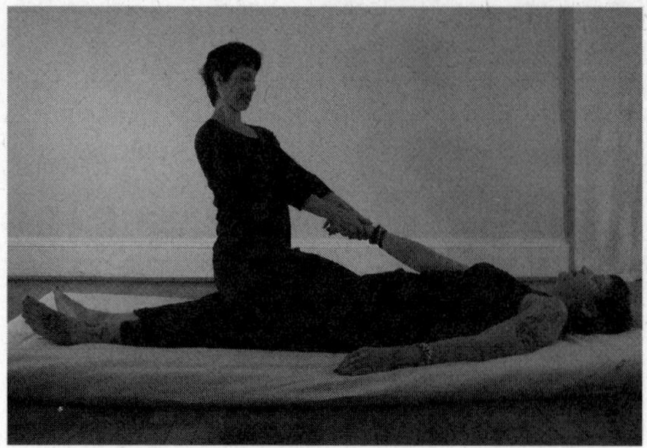

FIGURE 13-24 **Kneeling arm traction, 45 degree abduction.**
Hold the client's wrist and lean back.

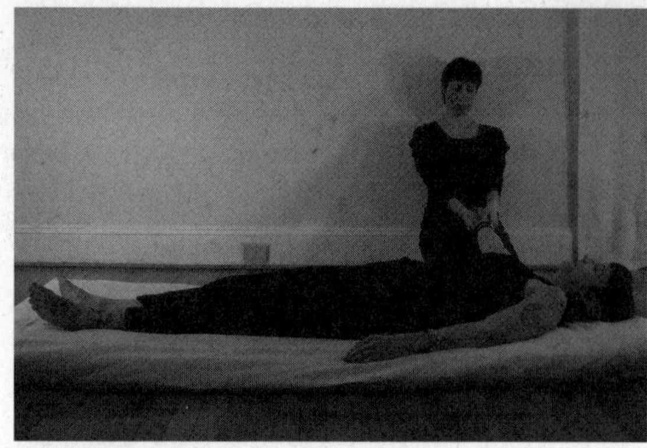

FIGURE 13-25 **Kneeling arm traction, 90 degree abduction.**
Hold the client's wrist and lean back.

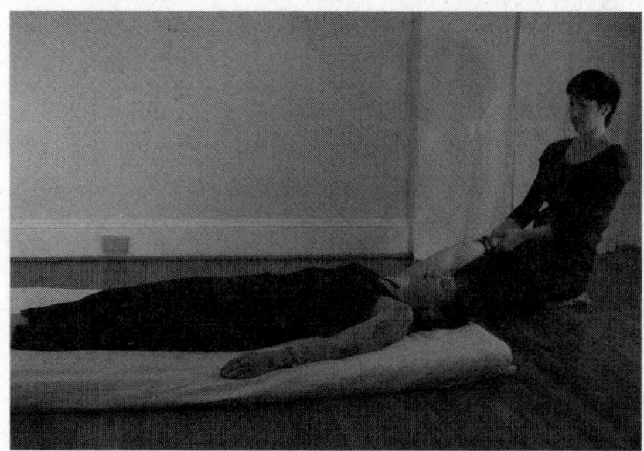

FIGURE 13-26 **Kneeling arm traction, 180 degree abduction.**
If the client experiences discomfort at 180 degrees due to shoulder restrictions, reduce the range of motion within the client's comfort zone.

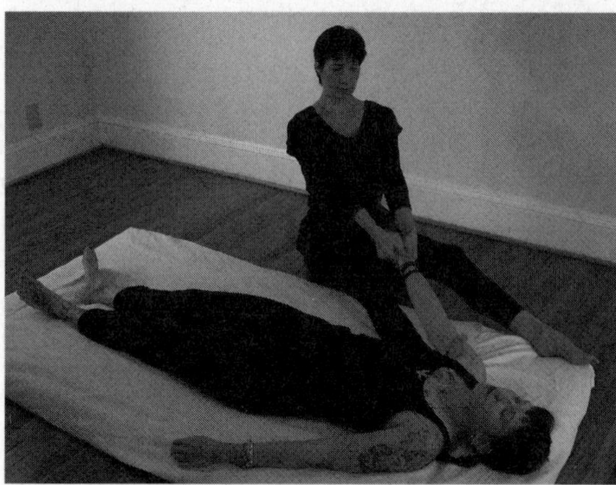

FIGURE 13-27 **Foot in axilla arm traction, 45 degree abduction.**
Gingerly place your foot in the client's armpit, carefully avoiding breast tissue.

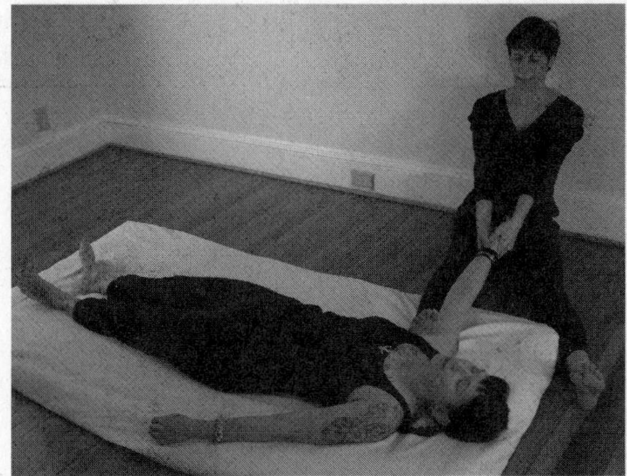

FIGURE 13-28 **Foot in axilla arm traction, 90 degree abduction.**
Do not actively push with your foot; only provide passive resistance for arm traction.

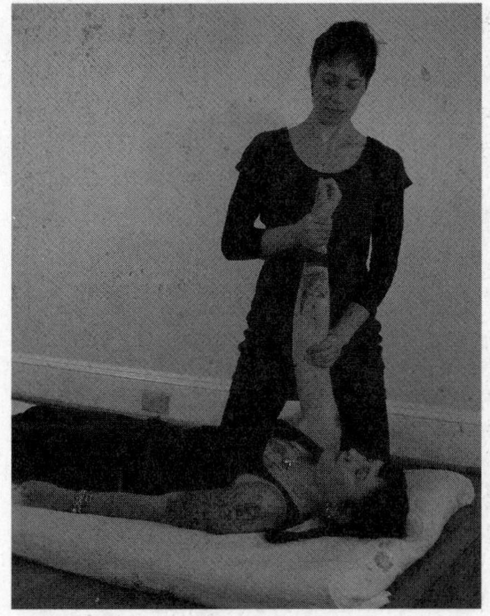

FIGURE 13-29 **Arm traction, 90 degree flexion.**
In an upright kneeling position, brace the client's arm above the wrist and elbow and pull straight up. Release and repeat several times.

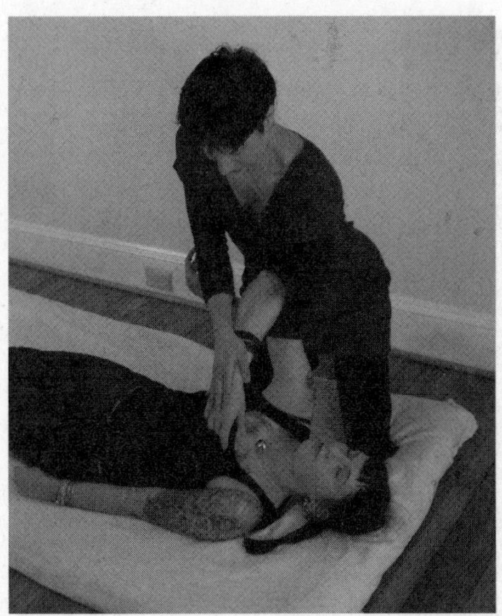

FIGURE 13-30 **Hooked forearm lateral traction, phase 1.**
Face the client at a right angle. Hook your forearm under the client's; stabilize by pressing down on the client's wrist with your other hand. Rise into an upright kneeling position.

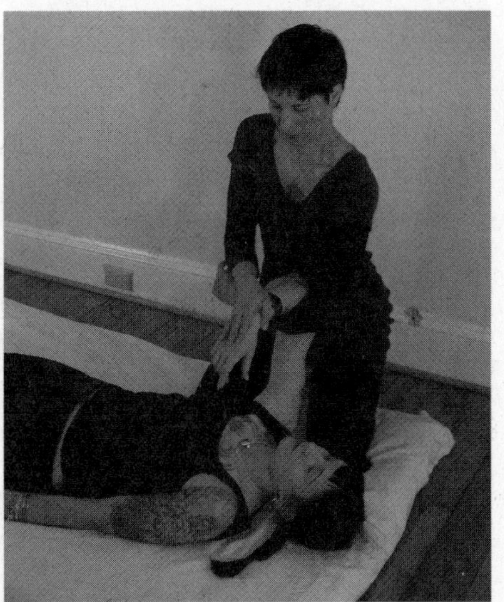

FIGURE 13-31 **Hooked forearm lateral traction, phase 2.**
Pull outward and sit back. Repeat several times consecutively: lifting up, pulling out, and sitting back.

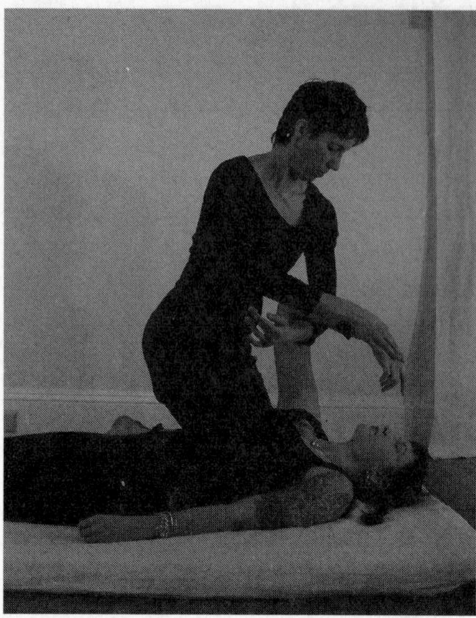

FIGURE 13-32 **Hooked forearm inferior traction, phase 1.**
Reposition yourself at a 45 degree angle. Lift up.

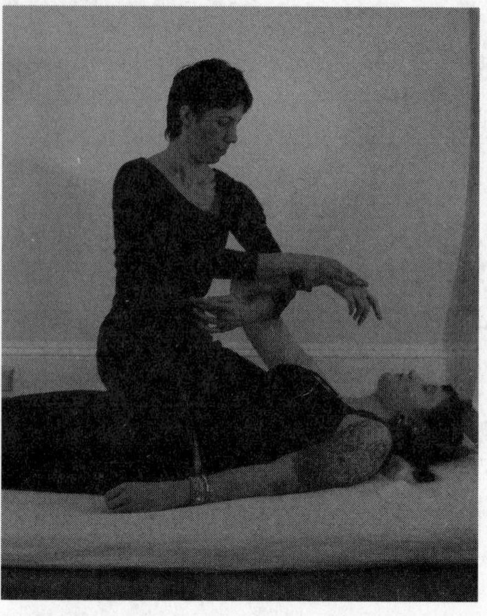

FIGURE 13-33 **Hooked forearm inferior traction, phase 2.**
Pull downward and sit back. Repeat several times consecutively: lifting up, pulling down, and sitting back.

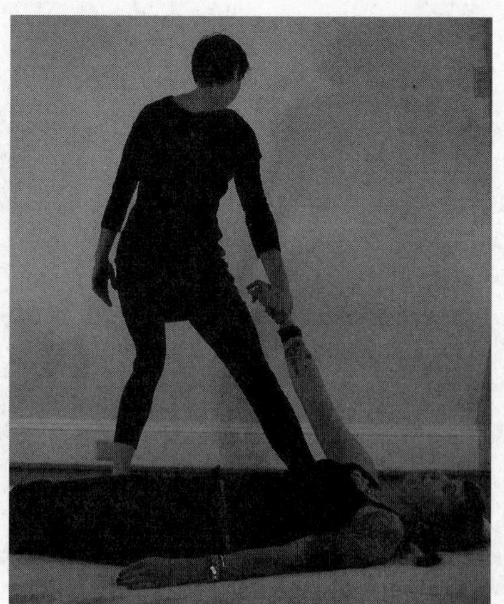

FIGURE 13-34 **Standing arm traction, 45 degrees.**
Hold the client's wrist; rise to a standing lunge and pull down toward the feet.

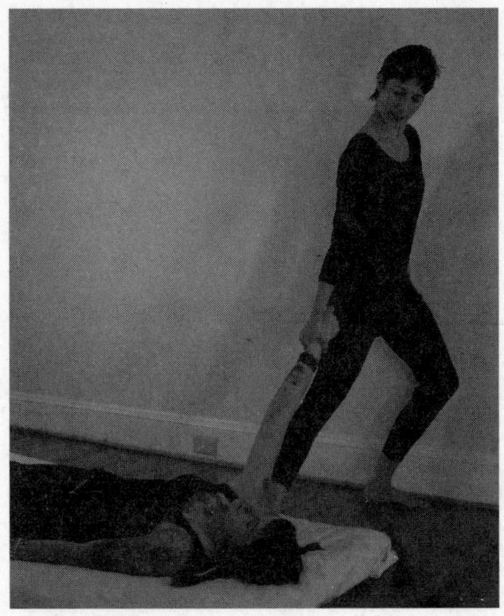

FIGURE 13-35 **Standing arm traction, 90 degrees.**
Walk to the client's side and pull outward.

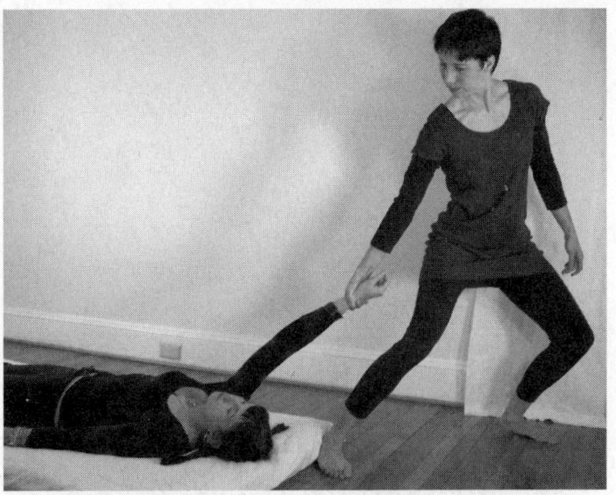

FIGURE 13-36 **Standing arm traction, 180 degrees.**
Walk to the client's head and pull upward.

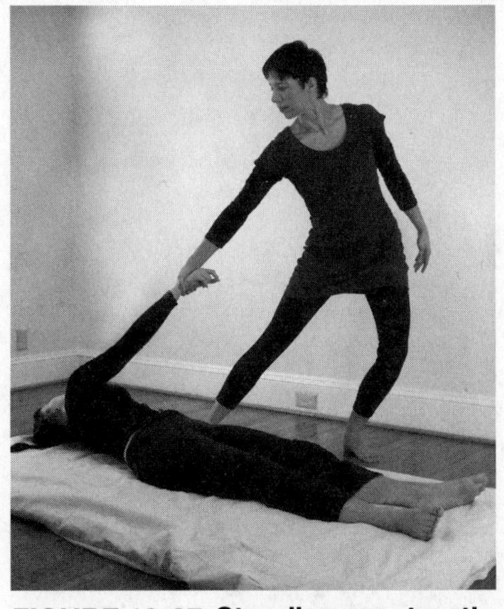

FIGURE 13-37 **Standing arm traction, crossover.**
Walk to the client's opposite side and pull across.

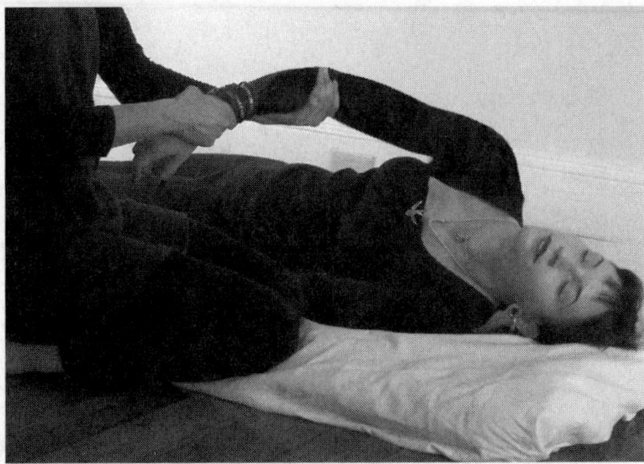

FIGURE 13-38 **Crossover arm traction.**
Descend to a kneeling position and brace the client's arm above the wrist and elbow. Pull toward you and release several times.

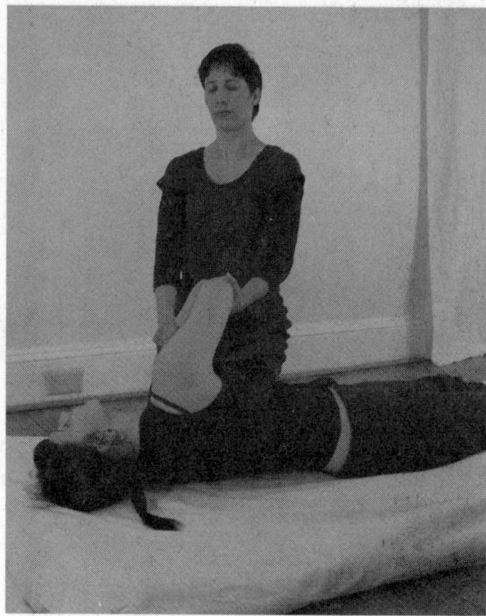

FIGURE 13-39 Crossover arm traction.
The client's shoulder and upper back should lift off the ground.

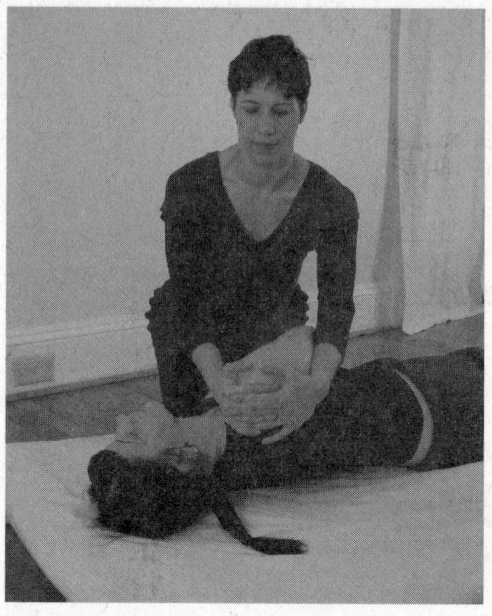

FIGURE 13-40 Clasped-hand shoulder traction.
Clasp your hands around the client's shoulder; pull toward you and release several times.

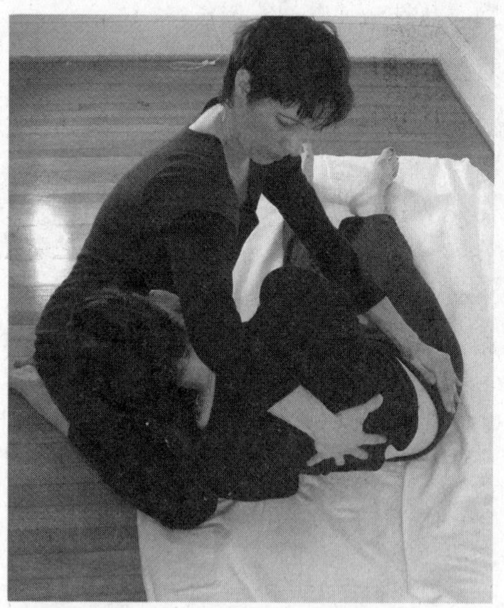

FIGURE 13-41 Torso torque.
Scoop your uppermost forearm under the client's shoulder and back. Plant your lowermost hand on the client's ASIS (front hipbone). Shift your weight back and pull client with you. The Client's torso should lift off the ground in a twist. Repeat Figures 13–17 through 13–41 on the other side.

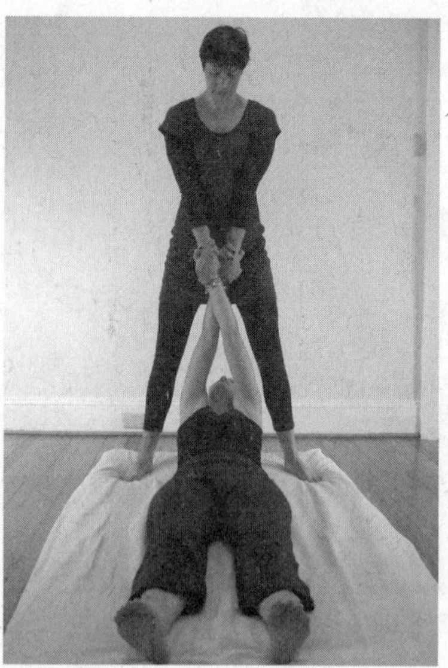

FIGURE 13-42 Crossed-arm traction, center.
Straddle the client and direct her to cross her arms and actively grasp your wrists. Lift straight up.

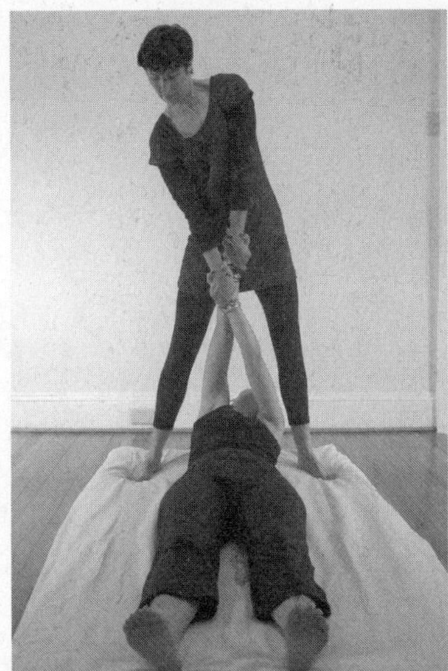

FIGURE 13-43 **Crossed-arm shoulder traction, right.**
Lean to one side to pull one arm higher.

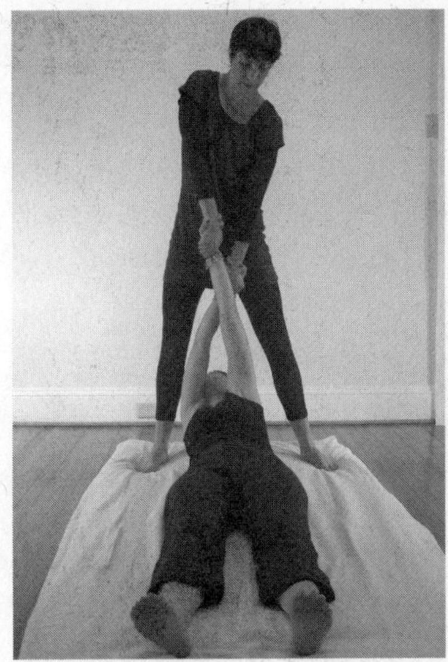

FIGURE 13-44 **Crossed-arm shoulder traction, left.**
Lean to the other side to pull the other arm higher. Repeat several times.

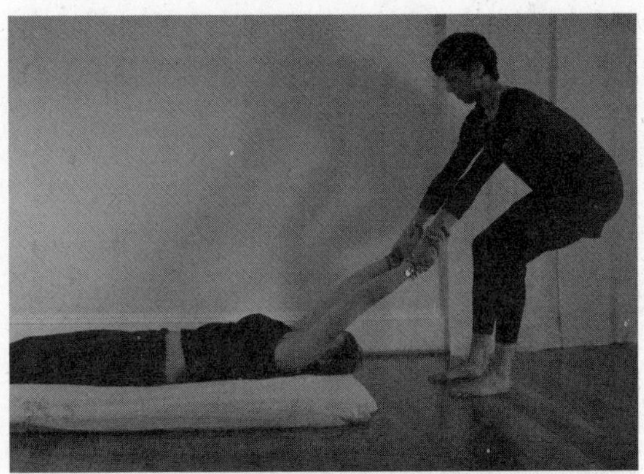

FIGURE 13-45 **Double arm traction, phase 1.**
Hold the client's wrists, walk backward as far as you can, and begin to squat.

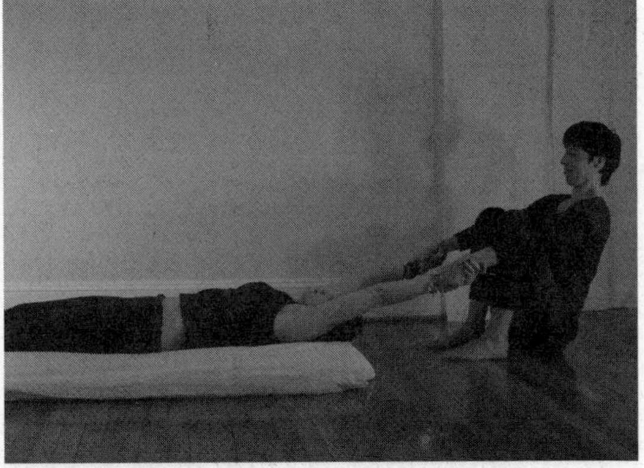

FIGURE 13-46 **Double arm traction, phase 2.**
Slowly lower into a seated squat, pulling the arms overhead.

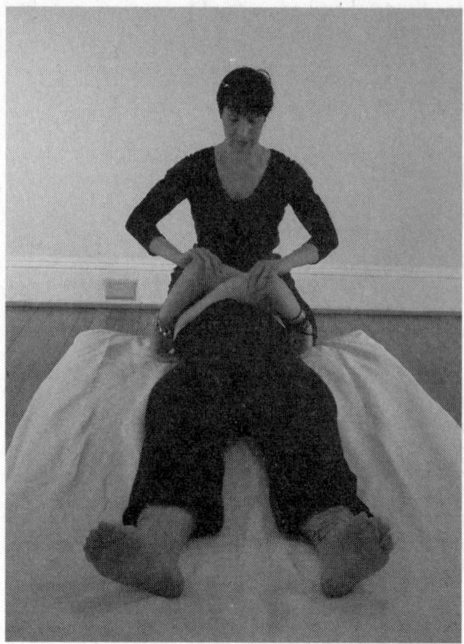

FIGURE 13-47 **Crossed-arm shoulder stretch, left.**
Cross one arm over the other and press the elbows down toward the floor.

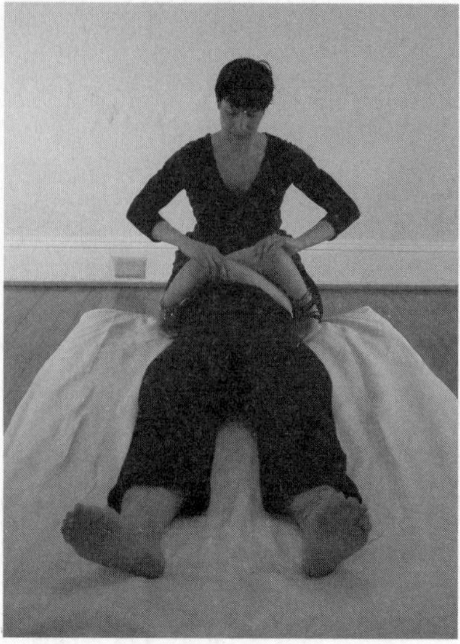

FIGURE 13-48 **Crossed-arm shoulder stretch, right.**
Reverse and repeat.

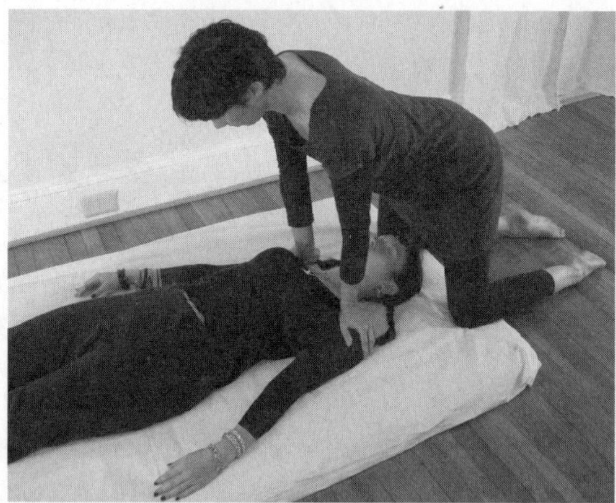

FIGURE 13-49 **Heel of the hand compression.**
Press the heels of your hands down on the pectorals (chest) and anterior deltoids (front of the shoulders). Press both hands simultaneously or alternately, padding around the upper chest like a cat.

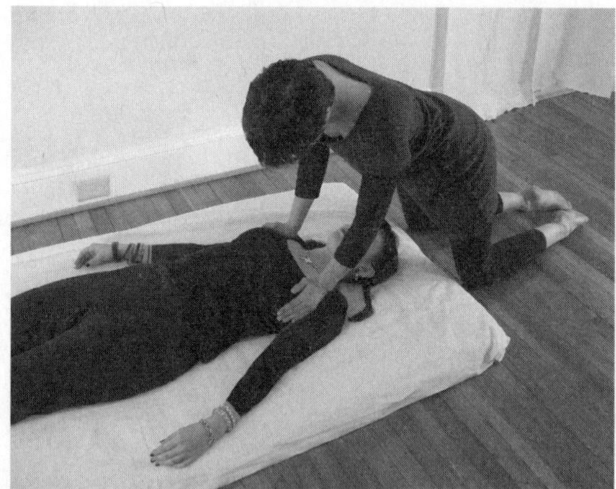

FIGURE 13-50 **Side of the hand compression.**
Repeat with the side of your hand in the groove between the chest and shoulders

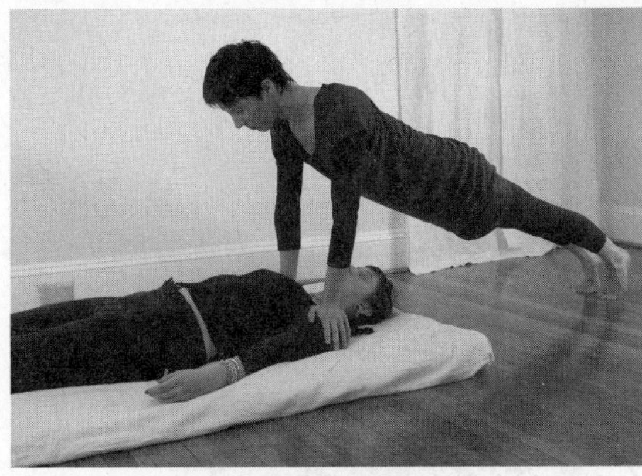

FIGURE 13-51 **Heel of the hand compression, intensified.**
For those clients who like deeper pressure, lean more of your body weight into the client by rising into a push-up or plank position and holding.

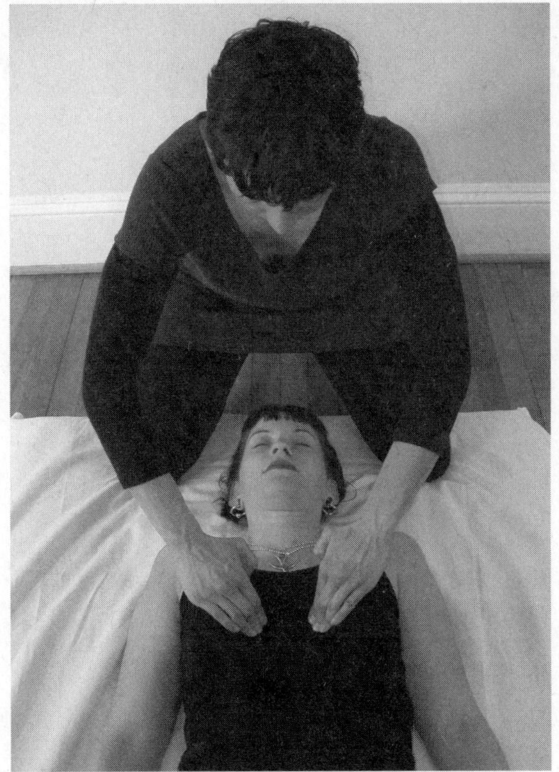

FIGURE 13-52 **Fingertip friction along the sternum.**
Apply circular or cross-fiber friction to the pectoral attachments on either side of the breastbone.

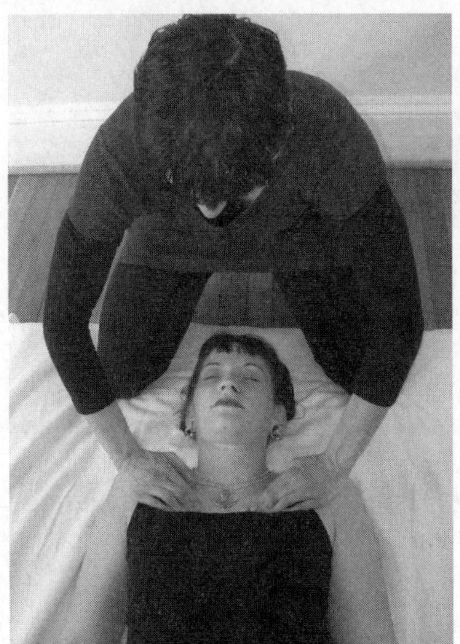

FIGURE 13-53 **Fingertip friction at Ki 27.**
Apply friction to the pectorals at the juncture of the sternum (breastbone) and clavicle (collarbone).

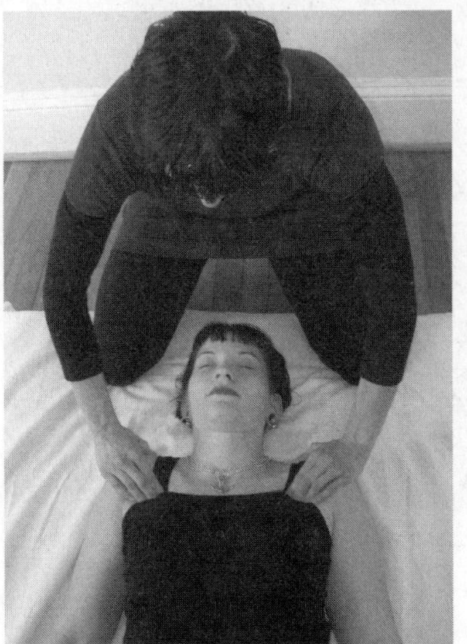

FIGURE 13-54 **Fingertip friction at Lu 1.**
Apply friction to the pectorals at about 2 cun below the outer end of the clavicle (collarbone).

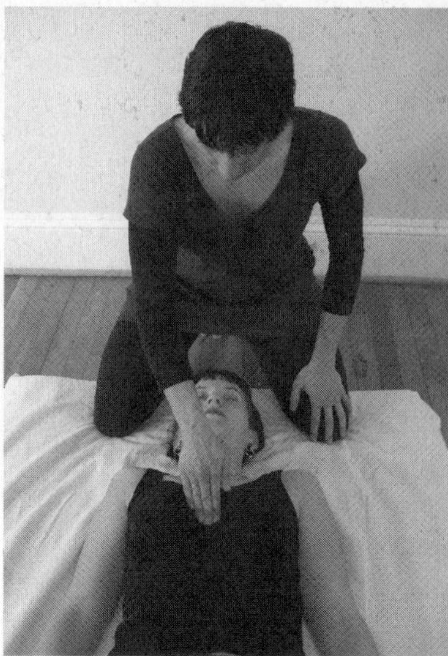

FIGURE 13-55 Fingertip friction at CV 17 and on sternum.
Apply friction in the center of the breastbone as the nipple line.

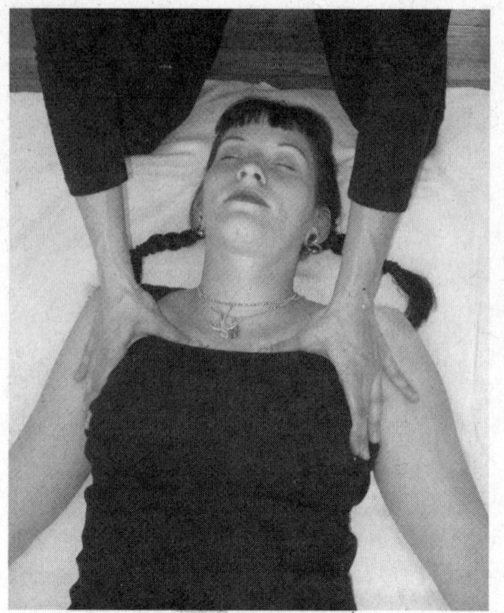

FIGURE 13-56 Thumb press at Ki 27.

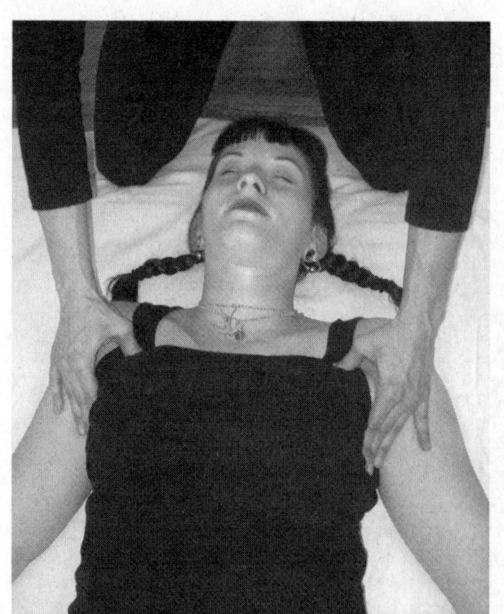

FIGURE 13-57 Thumb press at Lu 1.

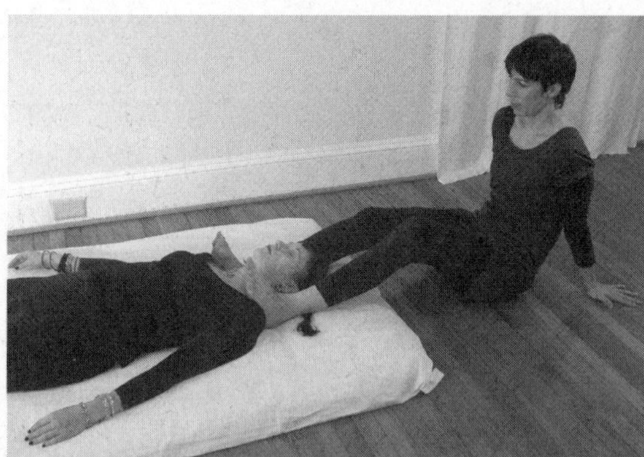

FIGURE 13-58 Bicycling the shoulders.
Sit back and plant your feet on the client's upper trapezius (shoulders). Alternately press each foot downward. If the client's shoulders are broad, walk your feet in and out, covering the entire surface.

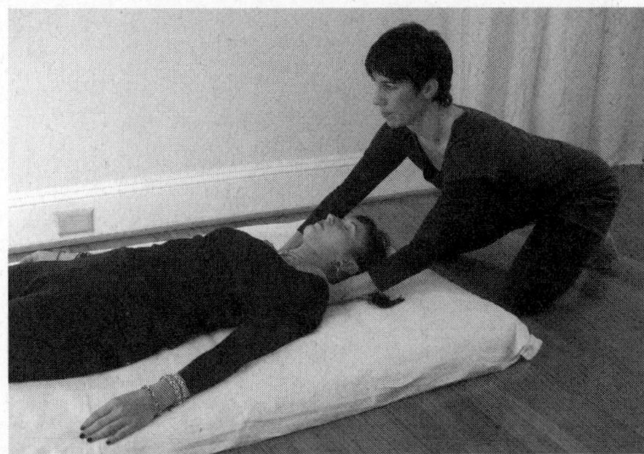

FIGURE 13-59 **Palm press the upper trapezius.**
Return to an open kneeling position and press your palms on the client's upper shoulders. Press both hands simultaneously or alternately.

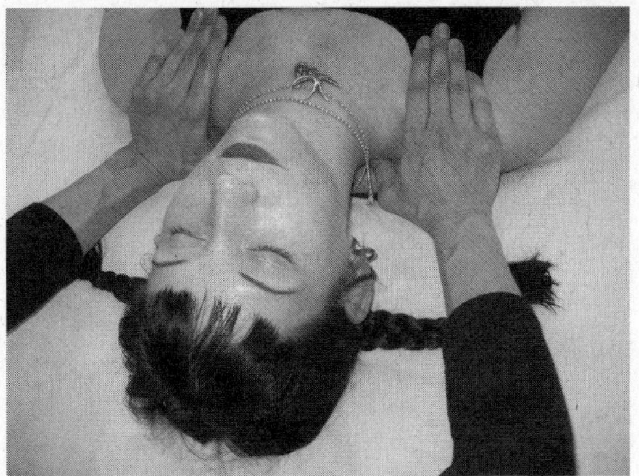

FIGURE 13-60 **Thumb press the upper trapezius.**
Work from the midline outward and pause at GB 21, on the belly of the upper trapezius.

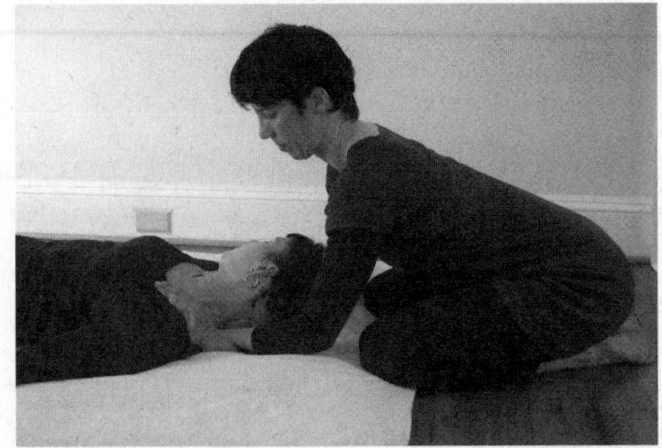

FIGURE 13-61 **Neck rotation plus palm press.**
Scoop your right hand under the nape of the neck to support the occiput (bony ridge at the base of the skull). Rotate the client's head right and palm press the upper trapezius, mildly stretching the neck.

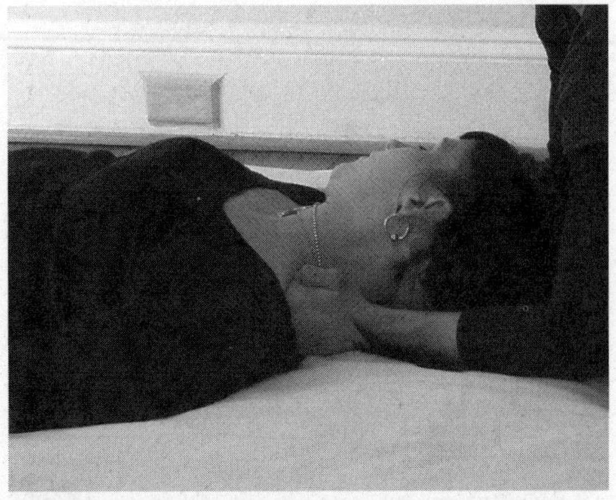

FIGURE 13-62 **Neck rotation plus fist press.**
Repeat with fist press or twist.

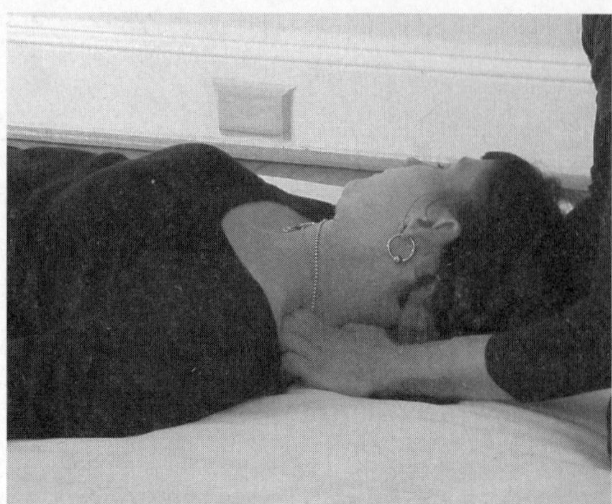

FIGURE 13-63 Neck rotation plus knuckle press.
Repeat with knuckle press or friction.

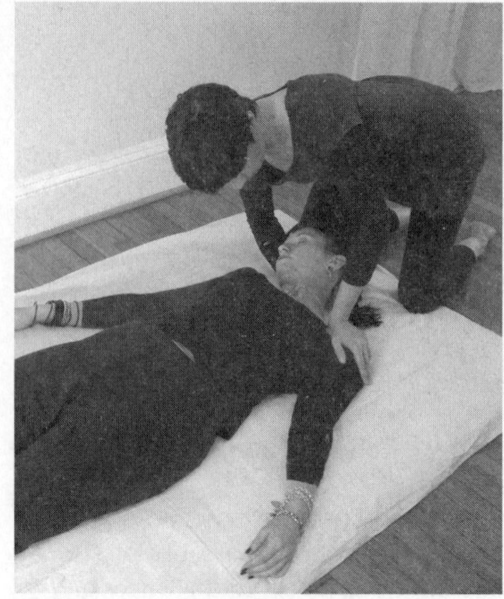

FIGURE 13-64 Neck stretch.
With the neck still rotated, plant your left hand on Lu 1 and rise up to press down on the shoulder while pulling the neck. Repeat Figures 13–61 through 13–64 on the other side.

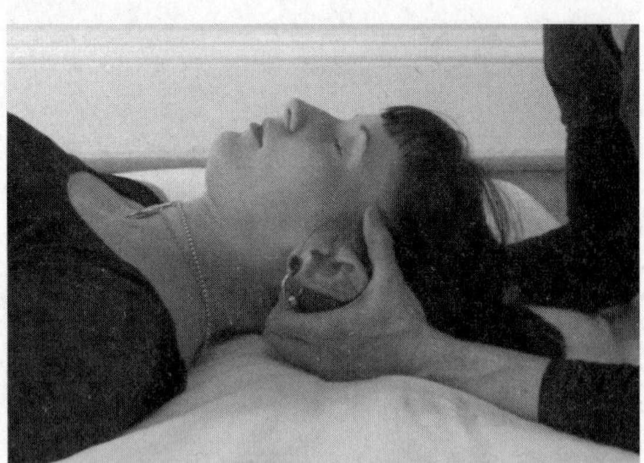

FIGURE 13-65 Fingertip neck traction.
Hook your fingers under the client's occiput and pull upward.

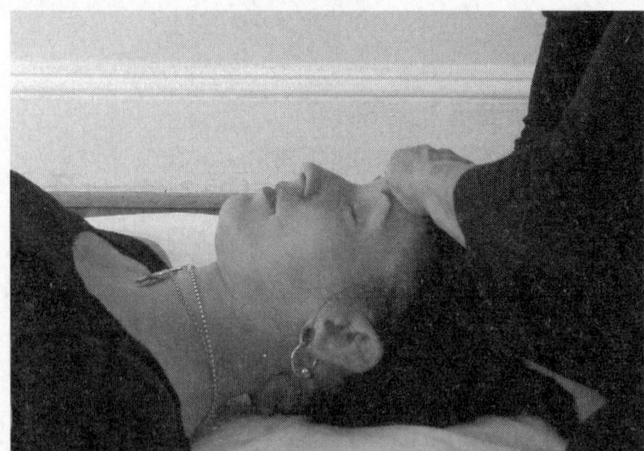

FIGURE 13-66 Palm neck traction.
Scoop one hand under the occiput, plant the other on the forehead, and pull upward.

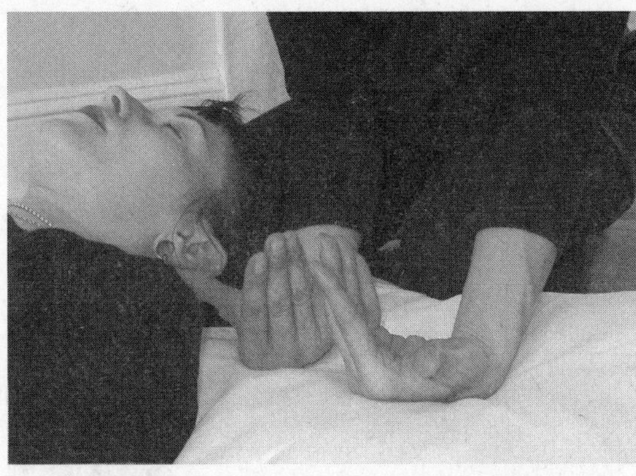

FIGURE 13-67 Fingertip press beside the cervicals.
Place your fingers as shown here, pads or tips pointing upward, on either side of the cervicals (neck bones) at the nape of the neck.

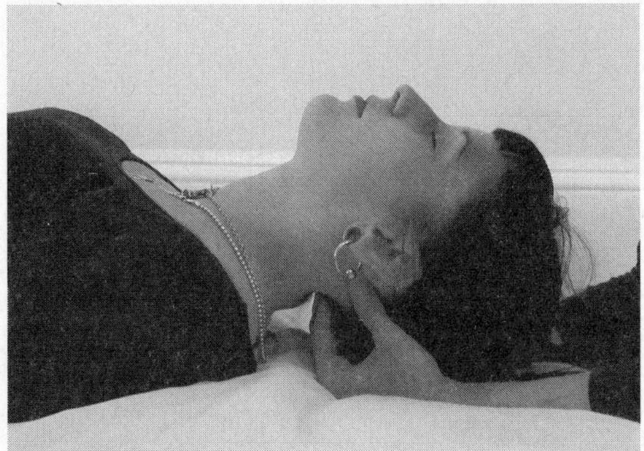

FIGURE 13-68 Fingertip press under the occiput.
Press upward, hold, and release. Inch down and repeat, moving from C-1 to C-7. Each time, the client's head should tilt backward slightly and the chin should lift.

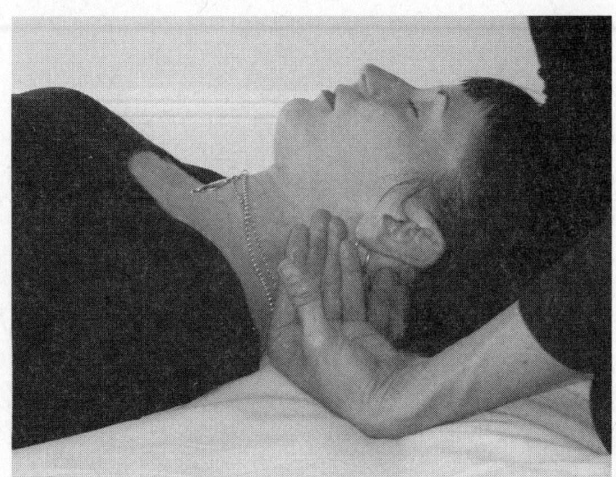

FIGURE 13-69 Thumb and fingertips straddling the cervicals.
Scoop one hand under the nape of the neck to support the occiput. Place your fingers on one side of the cervicals and your thumb on the other side, as shown here, pads or tips pointing upward.

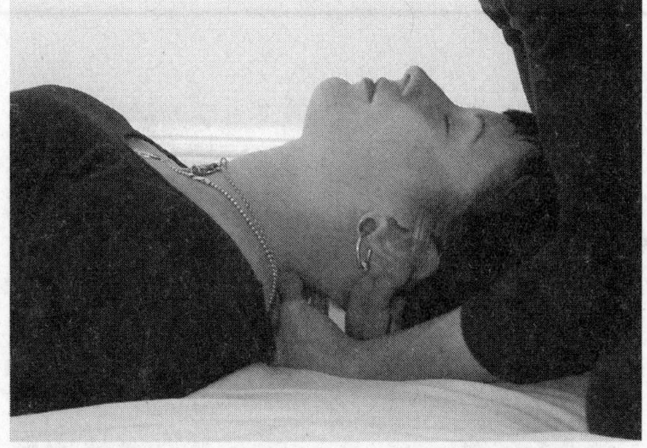

FIGURE 13-70 Thumb and fingertips straddling cervicals.
With your fingers and thumb, press upward and hold while your supporting hand gently tilts the client's head backward, arching the neck in extension. Inch down and repeat, moving from C-1 to C-7. Switch hands and repeat (the thumb is the stronger instrument).

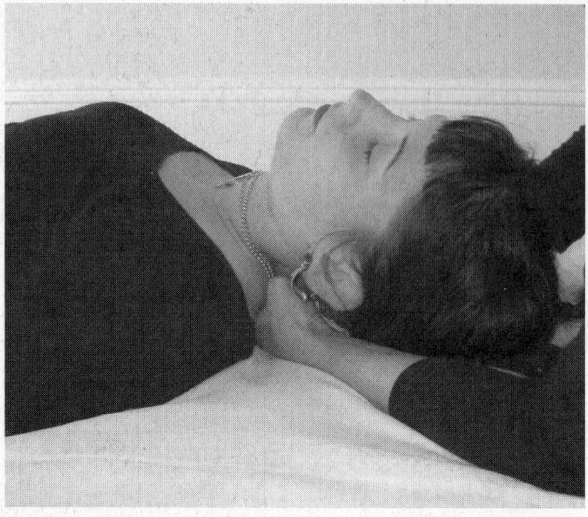

FIGURE 13-71 **Thumb press and rotation, phase 1.**
Support the client's occiput with your right hand. Plant your left thumb on the scalenes (muscles at the front/side of neck).

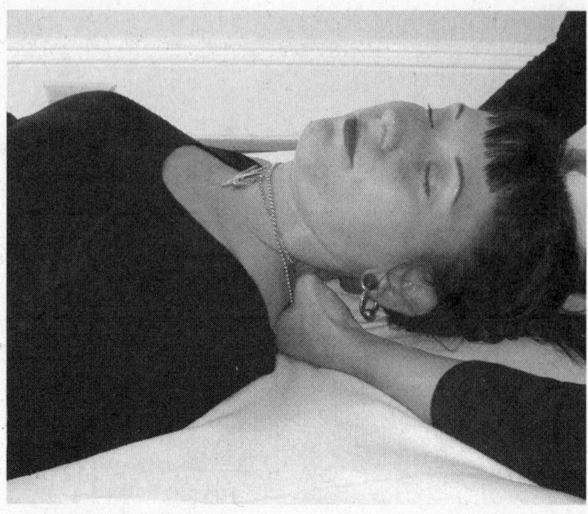

FIGURE 13-72 **Thumb press and rotation, phase 2.**
While applying thumb pressure, rotate the client's head to the left, swiveling the chin toward the shoulder. Relocate your thumb and repeat, covering the muscles on the side of neck, including the levator scapula and rectus capitus.

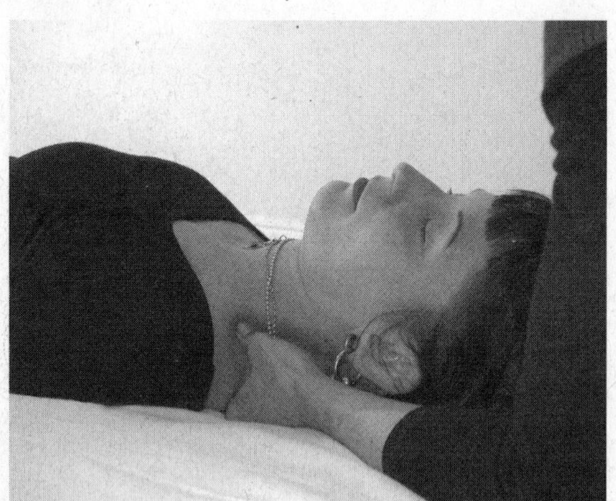

FIGURE 13-73 **Thumb press and lateral flexion, phase 1.**
Support the client's occiput with your right hand. Plant your left thumb on the scalenes (muscles at the front/side of neck).

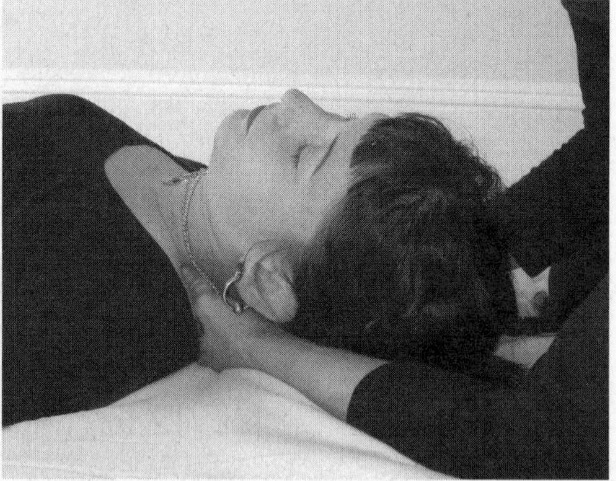

FIGURE 13-74 **Thumb press and lateral flexion, phase 2.**
While applying thumb pressure, bend the client's neck to the left side, drawing the ear toward the shoulder. Relocate your thumb and repeat, covering the muscles on the side of the neck, including levator scapula and rectus capitus.

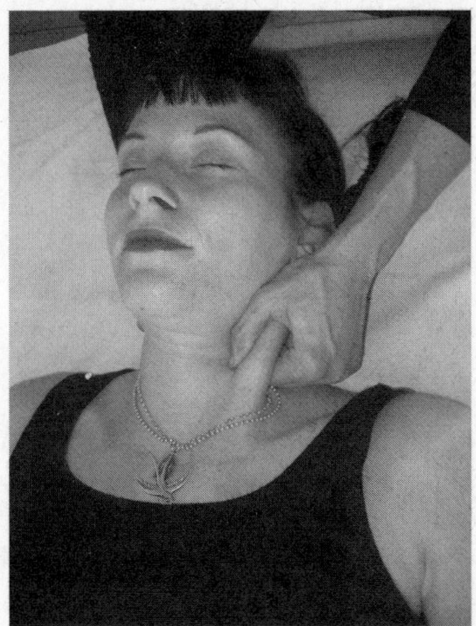

FIGURE 13-75 **Sternocleidomastoid (SCM) squeeze.**
Grab and pinch the length of the SCM, the prominent neck muscle that runs from the mastoid process (the corner of the skull just behind the jawbone) to the sternum (breastbone) and clavicle (collarbone). Repeat with friction, rolling the muscle in between your thumb and fingers. Repeat Figures 13–71 through 13–75 on the other side.

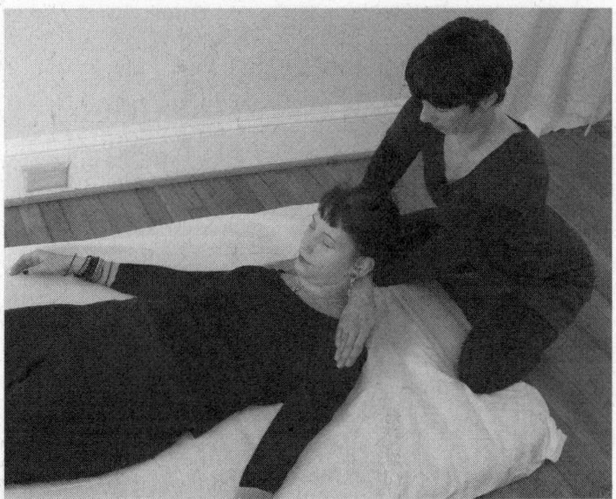

FIGURE 13-76 **Crossed-arm neck flexion.**
Slide your right forearm under the client's occiput; cross and plant your right hand on the client's left shoulder. Slide your left forearm under your right forearm; cross and plant your left hand on the client's right shoulder. Slowly lift the client's head into forward flexion, pressing the chin toward the chest.

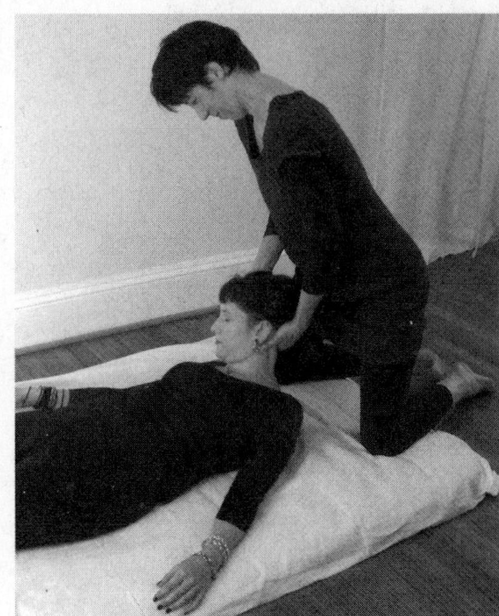

FIGURE 13-77 **Neck rotation, right.**
Place your hands under the client's occiput; in an upright kneeling position, slowly rotate the client's head.

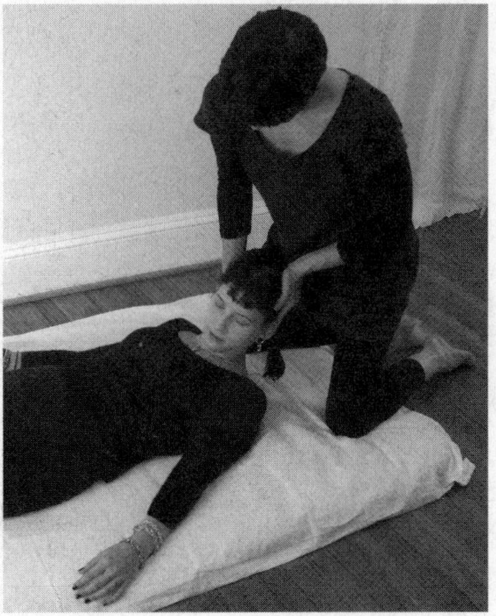

FIGURE 13-78 **Neck rotation, left.**
Reverse directions and repeat.

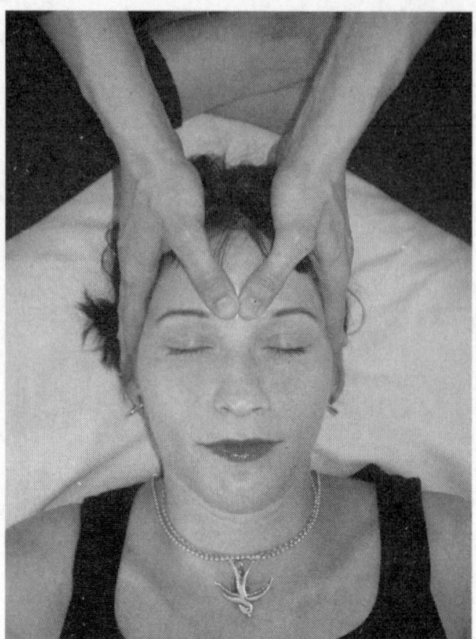

FIGURE 13-79 **Horizontal forehead sweep, phase 1.**
Thumb press GV 24.5 at the third eye.

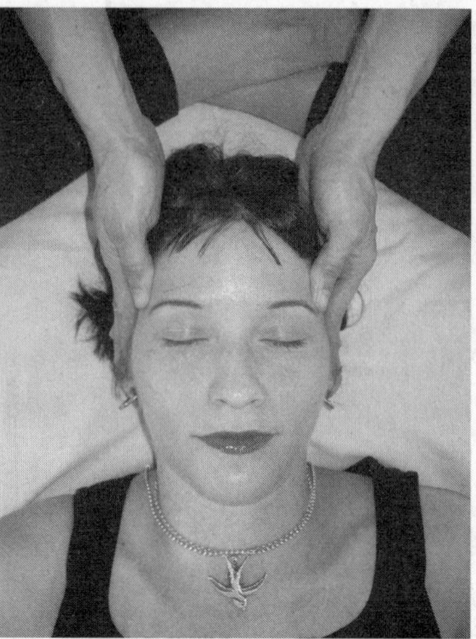

FIGURE 13-80 **Horizontal forehead sweep, phase 2.**
Glide outward toward the temples. Repeat, covering the forehead.

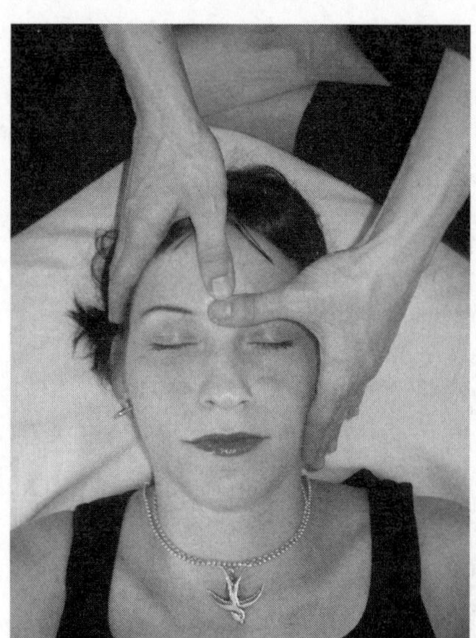

FIGURE 13-81 **Vertical forehead sweep, phase 1.**
Thumb press GV 24.5 at the third eye.

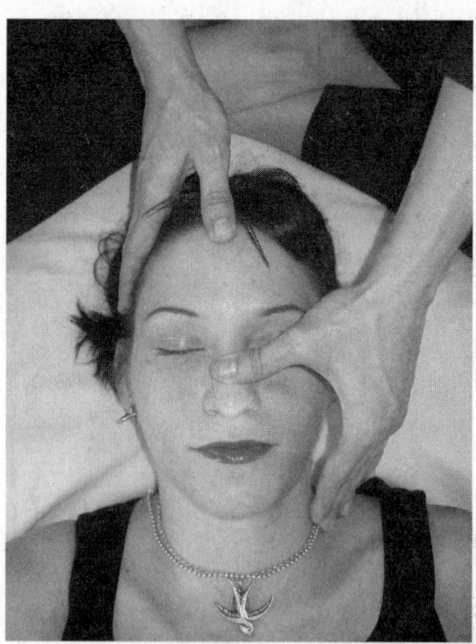

FIGURE 13-82 **Vertical forehead sweep, phase 2.**
Glide up over the forehead and down on the bridge of the nose. Repeat several times.

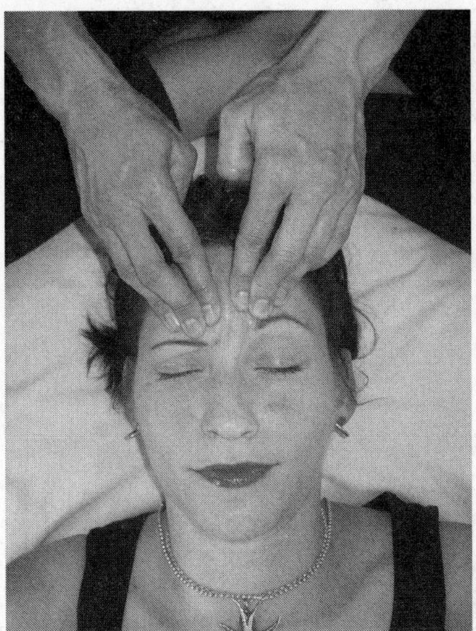

FIGURE 13-83 **Forehead scrunch, phase 1.** Bunch and wriggle the skin of the forehead, scooting the fingers of each hand in opposite directions.

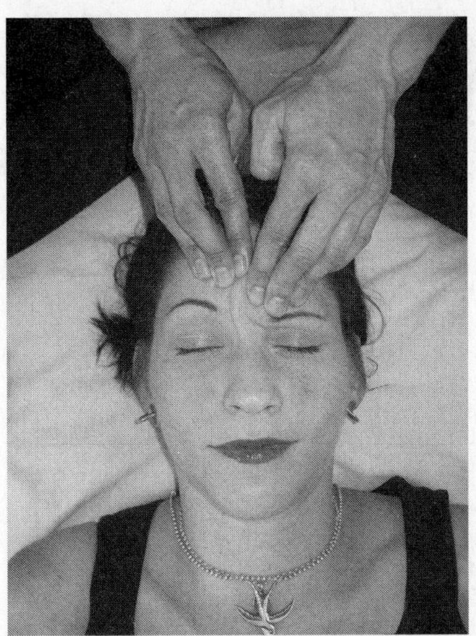

FIGURE 13-84 **Forehead scrunch, phase 2.** Relocate and repeat, covering the entire forehead.

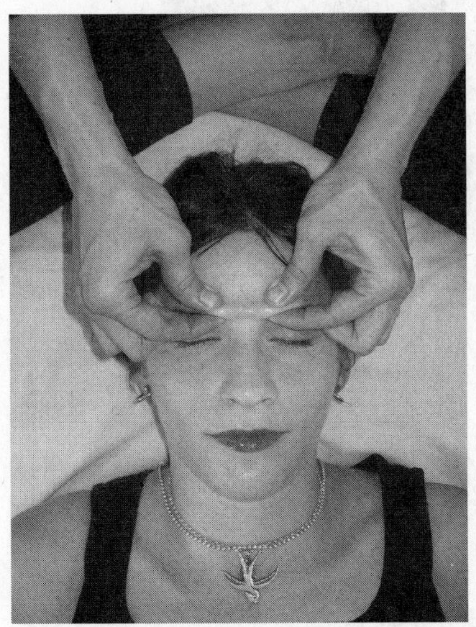

FIGURE 13-85 **Eyebrow squeeze.** Pinch along the entire length of the eyebrows.

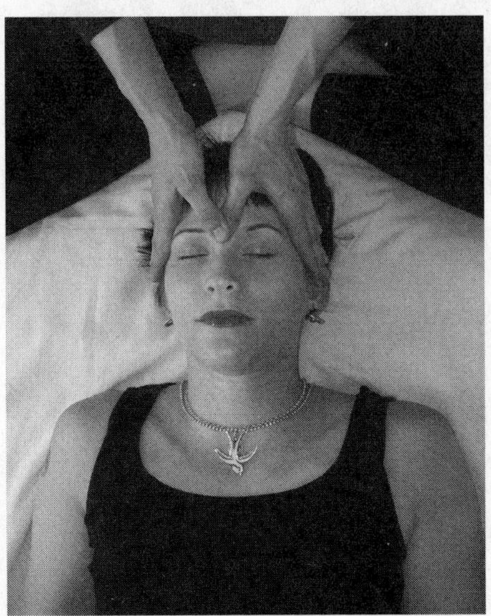

FIGURE 13-86 **Pause at GV 24.5.**

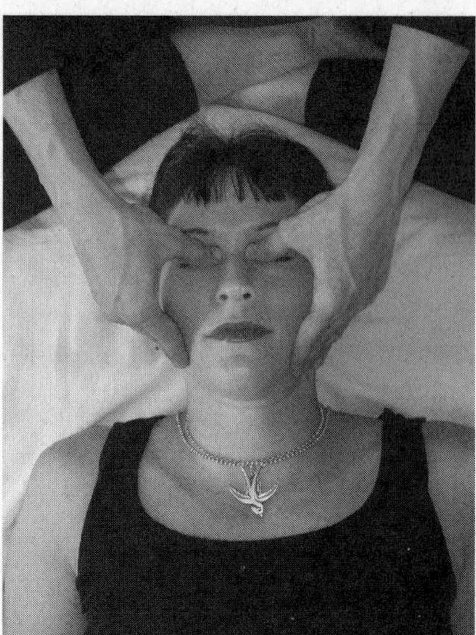

FIGURE 13-87 **Bl 1.**
At the inner corners of the eyes.

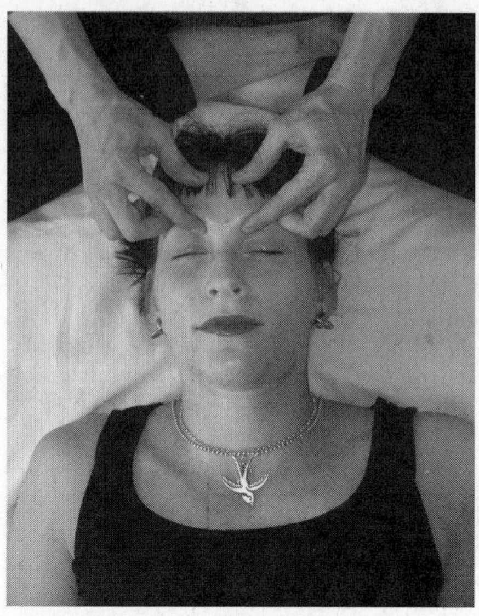

FIGURE 13-88 **Bl 2.**
At the inner corners of the eyebrows, pressing up against the frontal bone of the forehead.

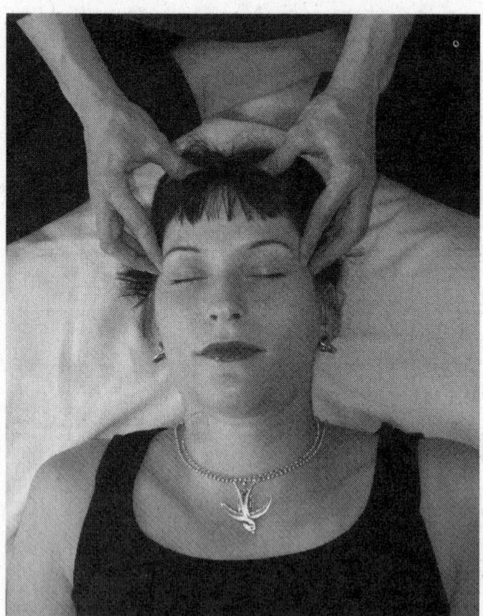

FIGURE 13-89 **GB 1 and Tai Yang.**
At the outer corners of the eyes and temples.

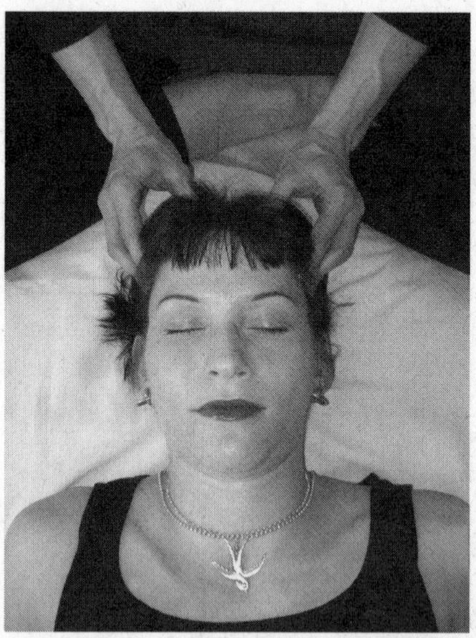

FIGURE 13-90 **St 8.**
On the temporalis just inside the hairline (to locate, ask the client to clench the jaws; this chewing muscle will bulge).

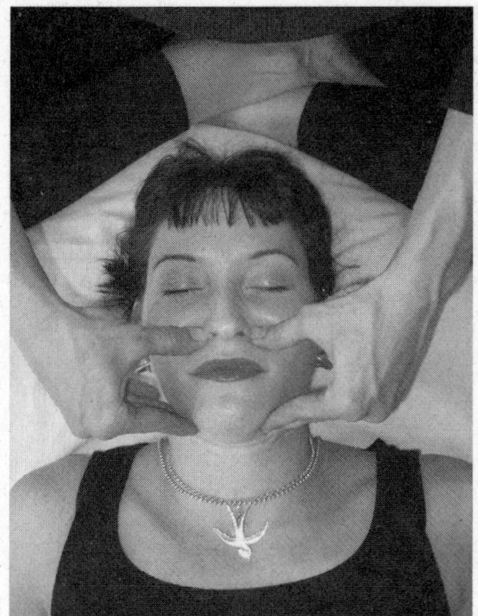

FIGURE 13-91 **LI 20.**
Beside the nostrils.

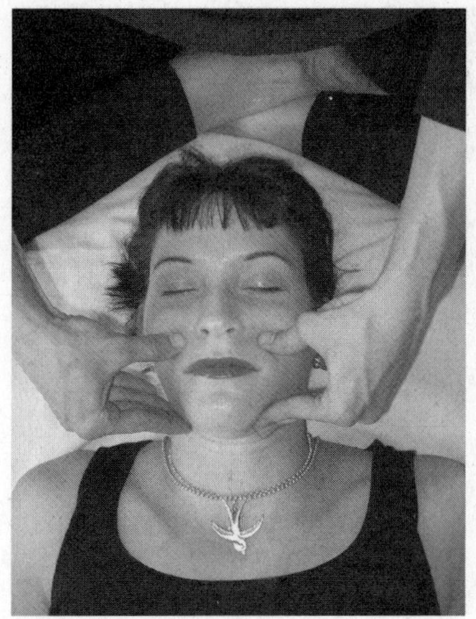

FIGURE 13-92 **St 3.**
On the zygomatic arches (cheekbones) in line with the pupils of the eyes.

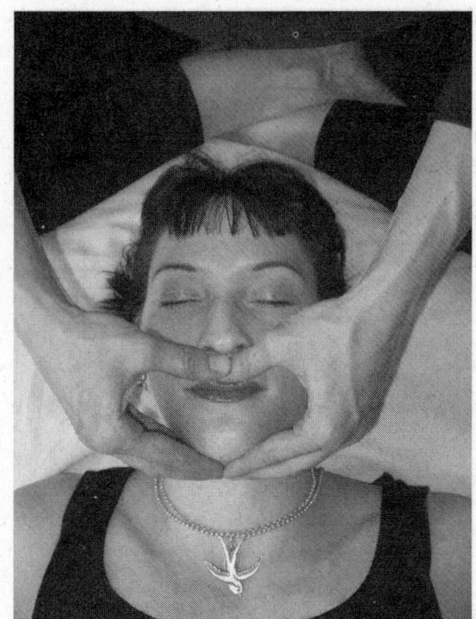

FIGURE 13-93 **GV 26.**
On the maxilla between the nose and upper lips.

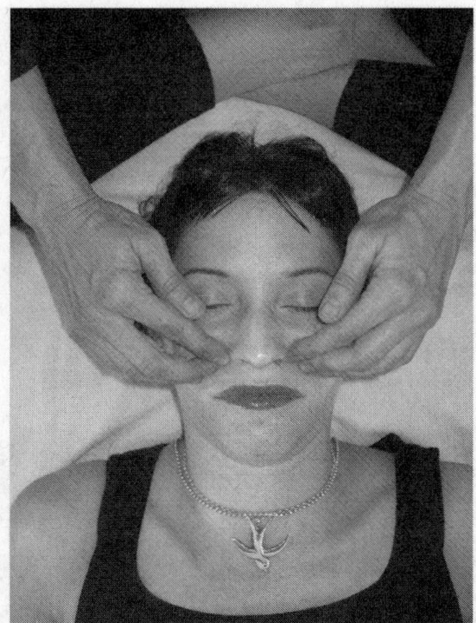

FIGURE 13-94 **Zygomatic arch sweep, phase 1.**
Hook your fingers under the cheekbones.

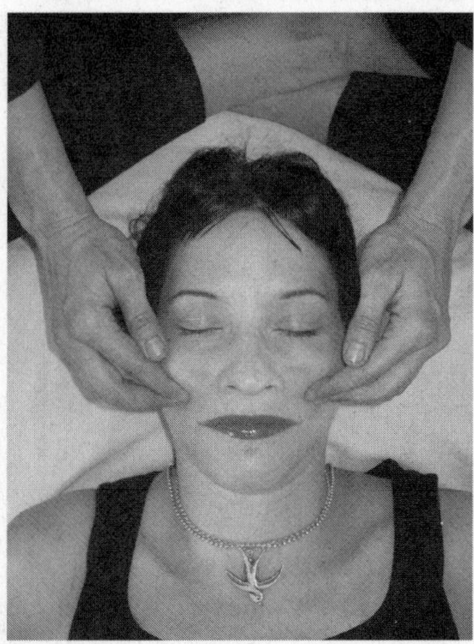

FIGURE 13-95 **Zygomatic arch sweep, phase 2.**
Glide outward. Repeat several times.

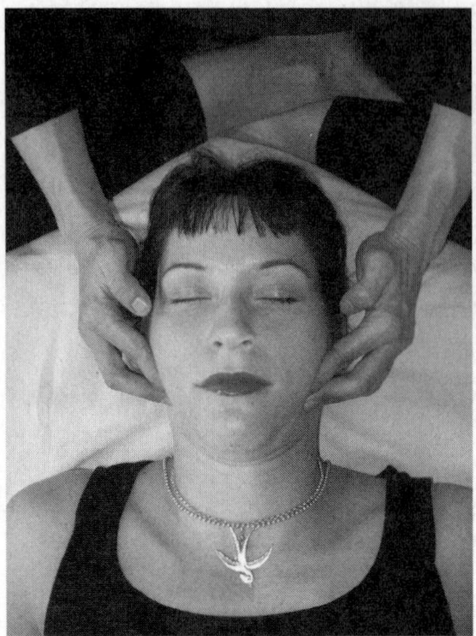

FIGURE 13-96 **St 6.**
On the lower aspect of the masseter (jawbone muscle).

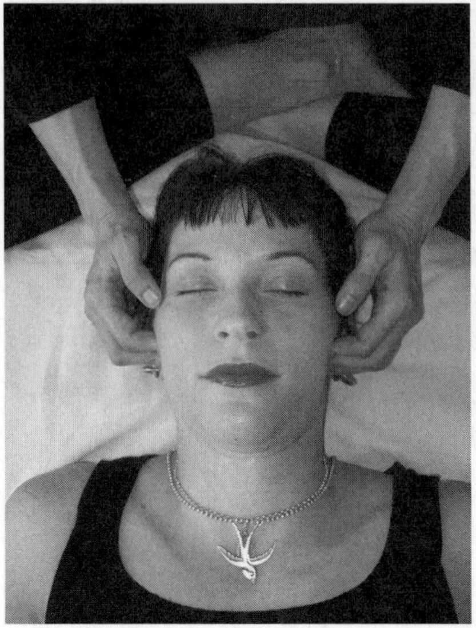

FIGURE 13-97 **St 7.**
On the upper aspect of the masseter (jawbone muscle), where the mandible (jawbone) attaches to the cranium.

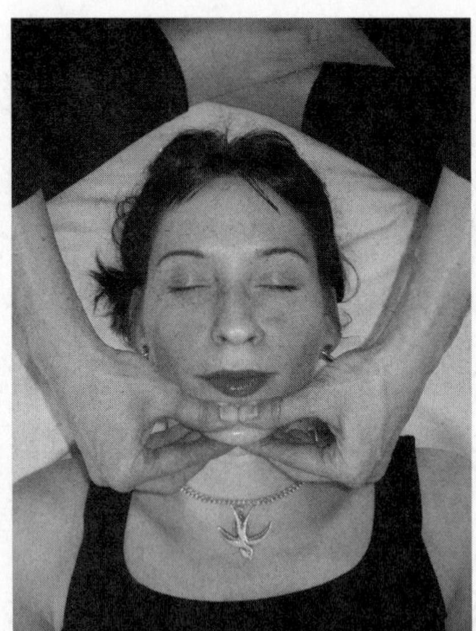

FIGURE 13-98 **Mandible sweep, phase 1.**
Pinch the chin.

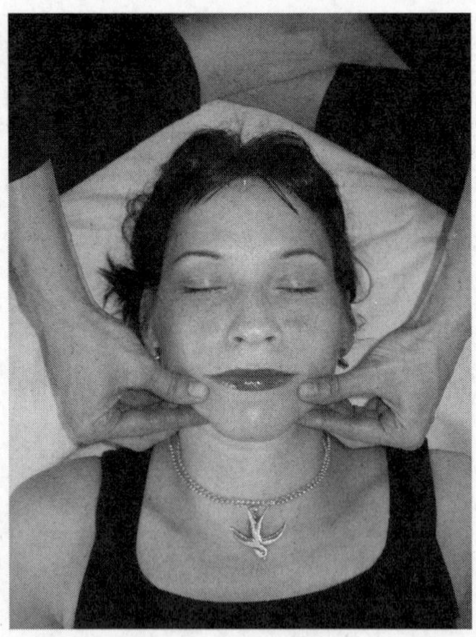

FIGURE 13-99 **Mandible sweep, phase 2.**
Glide outward. Repeat several times.

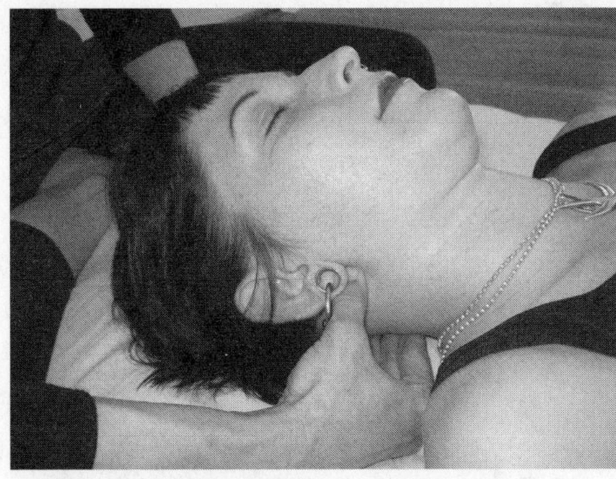

FIGURE 13-100 **TH 17.**
In the bony hollow just behind the mandible and below the earlobe.

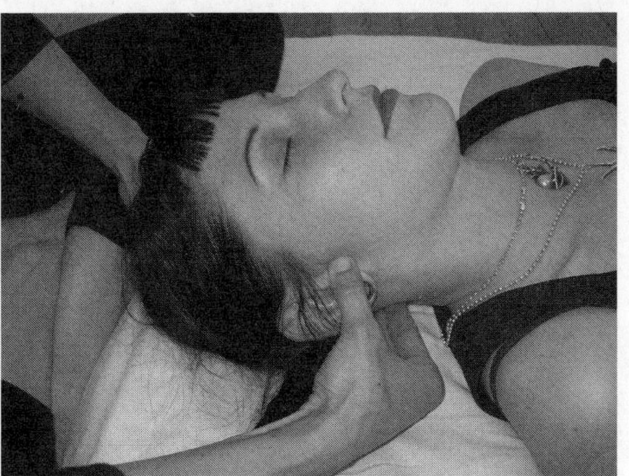

FIGURE 13-101 **GB 2.**
In front of the earlobe.

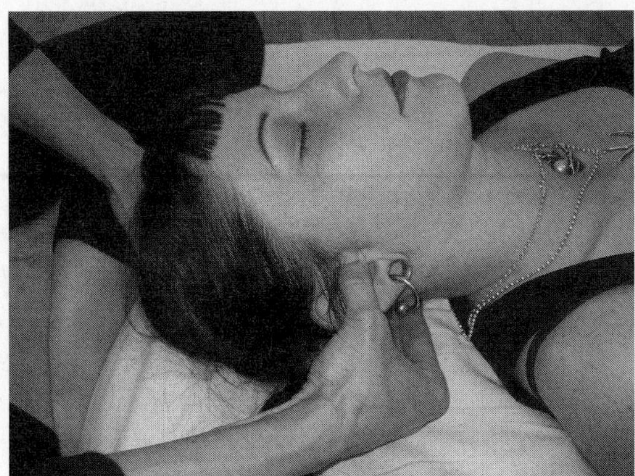

FIGURE 13-102 **SI 19.**
In the notch between the tragus and earlobe (to locate, ask the client to open the jaw slightly, which enlarges the bony hollow where the point is located). Repeat Figures 13–100 through 13–102 on the other side.

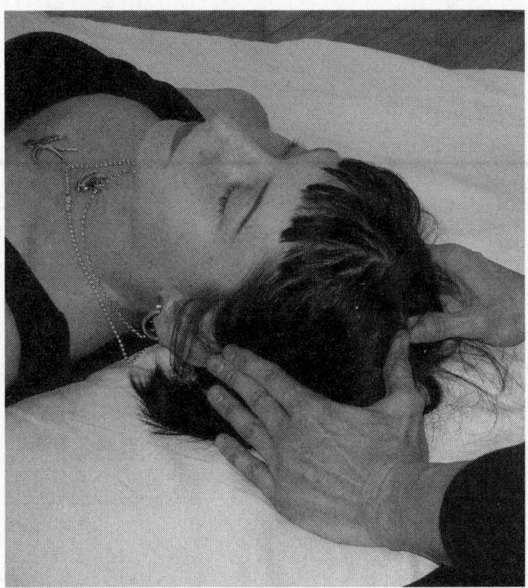

FIGURE 13-103 **GV 20.**
On the crown of the head in line with the tops of the ears.

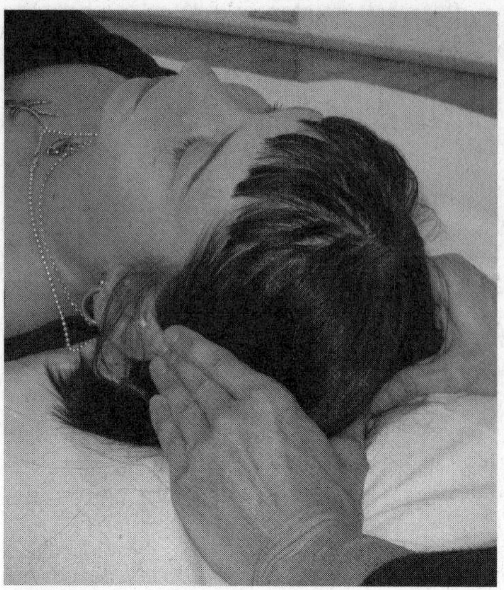

FIGURE 13-104 GV 19.
Just behind the crown of the head. On some clients, the skull forms a trough-like gully at this point.

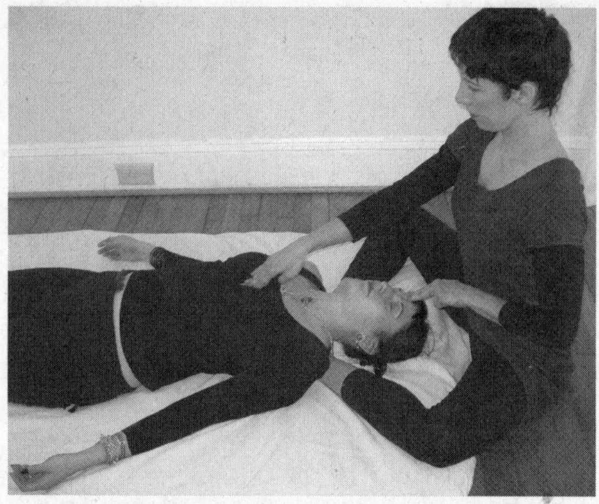

FIGURE 13-105 Relaxation hold.
Scoot the dorsal surface of your feet under the client's upper back on either side of the spine. Rotate your legs outward so that the soles of your feet are pressed together in prayer position and the arches of your feet lift the client's chest upward. Place the fingers of one hand on CV 17 and those of the other on GV 24.5. Hold for a few minutes.

REFERENCES

Alicia, M. (Director & Producer). (1997). The Stretching Process [video cassette].

Esher, B. (2001). Asian healing arts: Transformation. *Massage Today, 1* (11), 21.

Gach, M. (1990). *Acupressure's potent points: A guide to self-care for common ailments*. New York: Bantam.

Garmey, C. & Mojay, G. (1991/1999). *Shiatsu: The complete guide*. Great Britain: Thorson's.

14

Ampuku

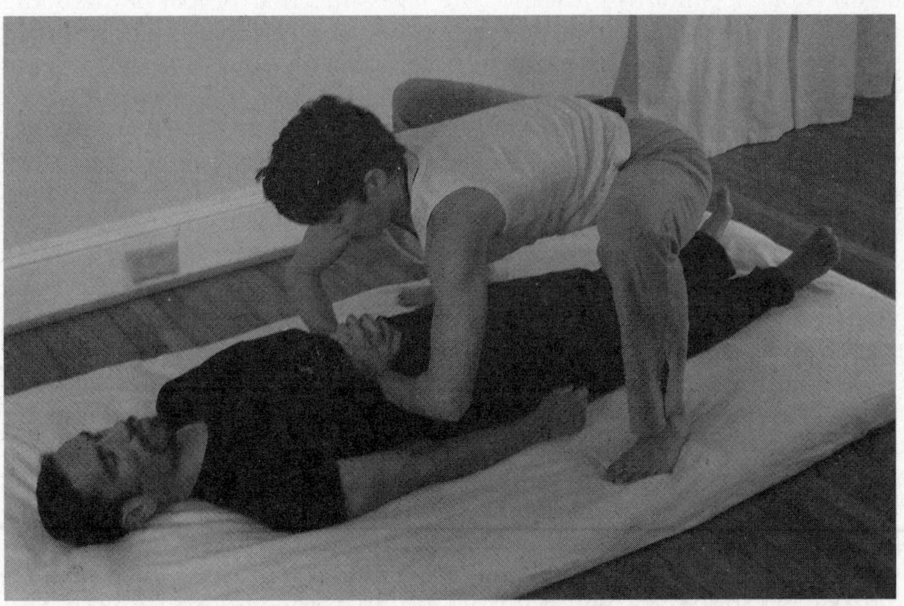

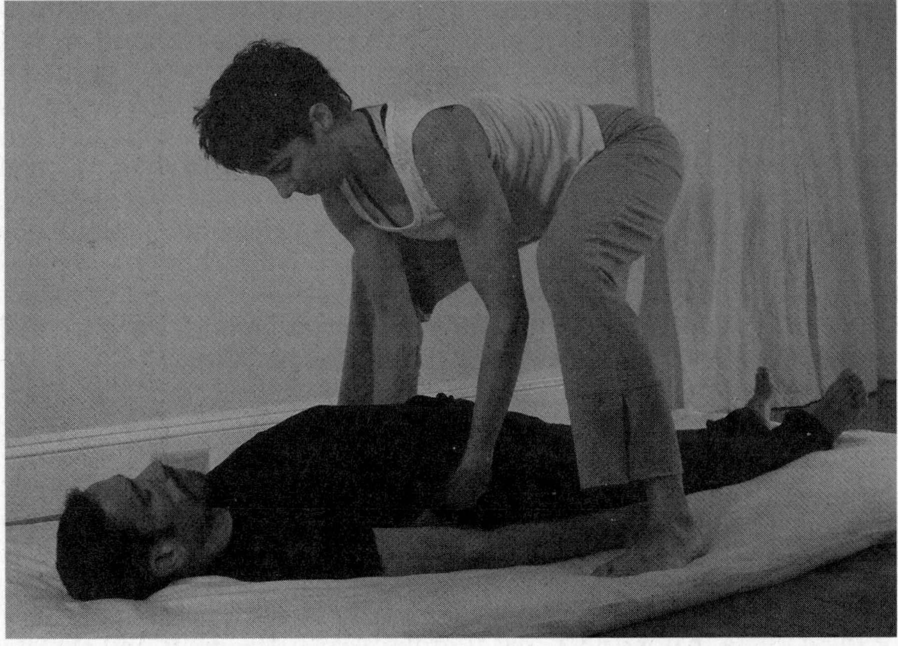

Therapeutic Emphasis

This protocol introduces abdominal massage, called Ampuku in Japanese and Chi Nei Tsang in Chinese. In Japan and China, abdominal massage is a medical specialty that involves the diagnosis and treatment of organ maladies and gynecological and obstetric conditions, but these medical applications require a level of expertise beyond the scope of the conventional Shiatsu practice. Nevertheless, even a basic form of abdominal massage enhances organ functioning and promotes good health by stimulating the flow of blood and lymph and the movement of the smooth muscle of the viscera, facilitating the passage of solids, liquids, and gases through the alimentary tract.

Abdominal massage manually stimulates intestinal peristalsis, the undulating contractions of the smooth muscle of the intestines that propel partially digested food and waste through the alimentary tube. This facilitates the resorption of nutrients and water and the expulsion of wastes through bowel movements. Abdominal massage manually clears obstructions and blockages at junctions prone to congestion, stagnation, and backup, especially the ileocecal valve—the juncture of the Small and Large Intestines in the lower right quadrant of the abdomen—and the sigmoid colon—the last segment of the Large Intestine and the fecal repository in the lower left quadrant of the abdomen. Abdominal massage can alleviate constipation by activating a sluggish bowel, and it can remedy diarrhea by relaxing a tense bowel. It can also relieve or mitigate menstrual cramps.

Abdominal massage increases circulation of blood in the abdomen. This, in turn, dissipates heat in conditions of Excess and generates warmth in conditions of Deficiency. Abdominal massage also releases accumulated gas, which, if chronic, can deform the ribs and twist the vertebrae. While it may seem odd or improbable that something as insubstantial and intangible as air could deform bony structures of the body, air under pressure does indeed have the power to distort solid structures. Consider the analogy of filling a bicycle tire with too much air by using an air pump designed for a car tire, not a bicycle tire. Within seconds, the extreme air pressure will blast a hole in the tire and warp the bicycle frame. Although chronic retention of abdominal gas will not blast a hole in the gut, over time it can bend and torque bones.

Abdominal massage has a pacifying effect on negative emotions. Negative emotions, whether caused by chemical imbalances, hormonal fluctuations, or stress can impair the function of the bowel, especially the Small Intestine. Impaired bowel function often manifests as disturbed digestion, spastic contortions and defensive hardening of the abdomen, and irregular stool patterns, though it can also generate headaches. In Chinese medicine, the Small Intestine is referred to as the "abdominal brain" because it processes emotions (for further explanation, see the discussion of the Small Intestine in Chapter 5). When the abdominal brain is upset, abdominal massage can soothe it, disentangling knots of nerves, lymph nodes, and blood vessels that aggregate and impair healthy exchange. Abdominal massage can, for example, alleviate or reduce the severity of premenstrual symptoms such as irritability and weepiness, abdominal bloating, and constipation or diarrhea.

Cautions and Contraindications

Certain cautions and contraindications apply to abdominal massage. Abdominal massage is contraindicated in the case of a hernia, a bulge in the intestinal wall. It is also contraindicated in the case of a thrombus, a blood clot attached to a blood vessel wall, and in the case of an aortic aneurysm, a blood-filled bulge in the weakened wall of the aorta, a major artery (see "Cardiovascular Disorders and Diseases" in Chapter 9). Abdominal massage, especially on the midline of the body, where the aorta runs and where a pulse can be felt, could dislodge a blood clot or rupture an aneurysm. Overweight or obese clients have an increased risk of thrombosis or aortic aneurysm, so avoid abdominal massage when their medical history is unknown.

Deep abdominal massage is contraindicated during pregnancy; however, it can be applied postpartum to induce uterine involution—the shrinking of the uterus to its former size and the return of the uterus to its subumbilical location (for more information on postpartum Shiatsu, see "Pregnant Women" in Chapter 9). Deep work on the iliopsoas (a hip flexor muscle) of a client who has an artificial hip is also contraindicated. Avoid deep, probing acupressure or friction to the psoas lumbar attachments, beside and beneath the rectus abdominus (the six-pack muscle on bodybuilders), the psoas femur attachment on the thigh near the groin, and the iliacus attachment, inside the bony prominence of the pelvis. For those clients who have had only one hip replacement, work on the iliopsoas of the opposite hip to generate a sympathetic healing response on the side with the artificial hip (for an explanation, see "Right/Left Point Combination" in Chapter 7).

Exercise caution or abstain from abdominal massage when the client has an implanted intrauterine device (IUD); pressure could puncture the uterus (at the time of this writing, this type of IUD is outdated in the United States). Exercise caution or observe a local contraindication on extremely tender surgical scars and extremely painful, inflamed or impacted areas due to severe constipation or someother disorder such as diverticulitis. If possible, work around the area or on opposite the area to create a sympathetic healing response.

KEY THERAPEUTIC AREAS AND ACUPRESSURE POINTS

Some clients may have very strong, hypertoned abdominal muscles from working out, especially from doing torso flexion exercises like curls, reverse curls, twisting curls, pelvic thrusts, and leg lowers or raises. Bodybuilders, dancers, gymnasts, Yoga and Pilates practitioners, martial artists, and boxers are examples of clients who could benefit from having their hypertonic abdominal muscles massaged. Give Shiatsu to the Kidney and Stomach Meridians to relax the rectus abdominus, the main torso flexor, which runs from the sternum to the pubic bone. General abdominal massage to the rest of the abdomen will relax the obliques, which are engaged in torso rotation (twisting) and lateral flexion (side-bending) movements, and the transverse abdominus, which supports the spine and abdominal contents and which is engaged by sucking in the gut or drawing the navel toward the spine.

For clients who complain of lower back discomfort or pain, especially those who have exaggerated lumbar lordosis (swayback), supplement Shiatsu to the Bladder Meridian in the lower back with Shiatsu to the Stomach Meridian in the abdomen. Give deep, probing acupressure to St 25, St 26, and St 27 to release tension in the psoas muscle. A hypertonic (tense) psoas can cause the pelvis to tilt forward in a swayback posture, increasing the compressive load and strain on the soft tissues and intervertebral disks in the lumbar area.

Various acupressure points on the abdomen and rib cage, called Bo in Japanese and Mu in Chinese, correspond to the condition of internal organs. These points have both assessment and therapeutic value. Tenderness, hypersensitivity, sharp pain, or any other abnormal sensation elicited by palpation of a Mu/Bo point may indicate an acute condition in the associated organ that can be positively influenced by acupressure (see Figure 7-7 for the location of Mu/Bo points and Table 7-4 for organ correspondences of Mu/Bo points; figures at the end of this protocol show locations on a live model). A few disorders and associated points are listed below for easy reference:

Stomach disorders: CV 12
Large Intestine disorders: St 25
Small Intestine disorders: CV 4
Bladder disorders: CV 3

KYO JITSU IMBALANCES

The Ampuku protocol offers a good opportunity to practice hara diagnosis if desired (see the Hara reflex zones illustration below). Before doing the protocol, take time to lightly palpate the various reflex zones of the abdomen to identify the most deadened Kyo and the most lively Jitsu zones. Make note of your findings and palpate the corresponding Meridians in the body to verify the accuracy of your assessment. For example, suppose you find that the Gallbladder reflex zone, under the client's right rib cage, ejects your touch and the U-shaped Kidney reflex zone, under and around the navel, feels vapid or vacuous. Compare these results with those on the Meridians of the leg. If you discover that the Gallbladder Meridian is Jitsu and the Kidney Meridian Kyo, you have confirmed your findings. During a regular full-body Shiatsu session, you would want to emphasize sedating the Gallbladder Meridian and tonifying the Kidney Meridian.

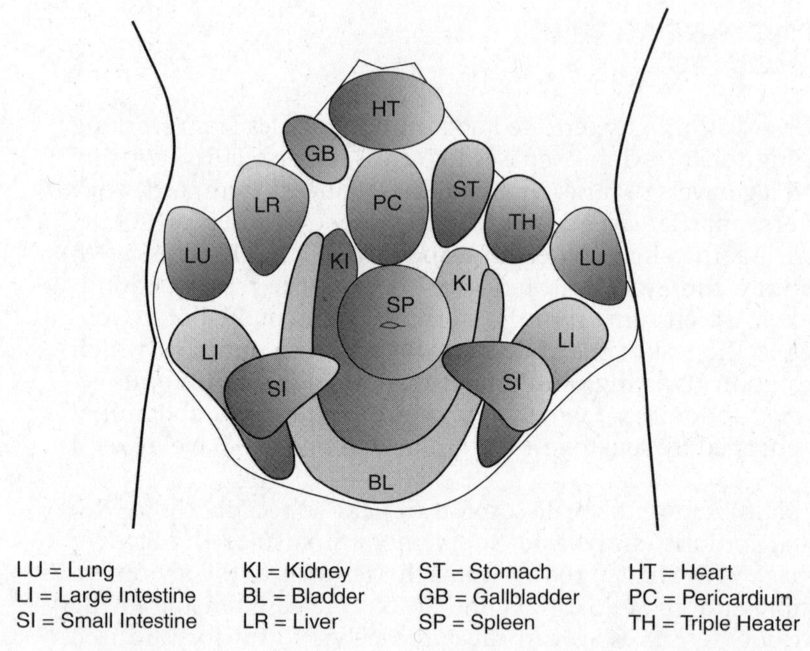

Hara Reflex Zones

CLIENT AND PRACTITIONER COMFORT

Be sure the futon or other surface is well padded to cushion the client's sacrum (triangular-shaped bone at the base of the spine). A bolster can be placed under the client's knees to relax the abdomen and to increase the comfort of a client who has lower back issues or a history of sciatica.

This protocol shows the practitioner straddling the client in a squatting position so that the practitioner's hara is directly over the client's hara. The advantages of this position are that it does not entail torquing of the practitioner's torso, which reduces the risk of strain for the practitioner, and that pressure can be applied at a perpendicular rather than oblique angle, which is more effective for contacting and influencing Qi flow. Also, the lower back mobilizations can be administered only from a straddling position. Nevertheless, some practitioners may prefer kneeling beside the client if the straddling squat is uncomfortable or impracticable due to weakness in the hip flexors or back extensors, tightness in the adductors, hamstrings, or back extensors, injury, or some other reason. However, the side kneeling position entails twisting the torso and delivering pressure at an oblique angle, and the lower back mobilizations must be omitted.

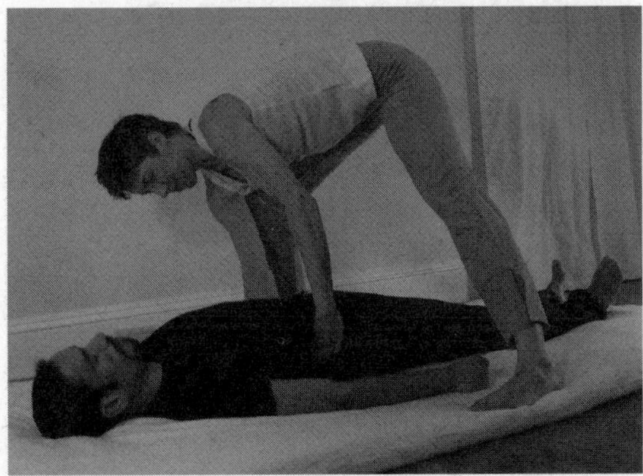

FIGURE 14-1 **Lumbar release, pulling left.** Straddle the client and slide your hands under the client's lower back. Lean and pull from side to side.

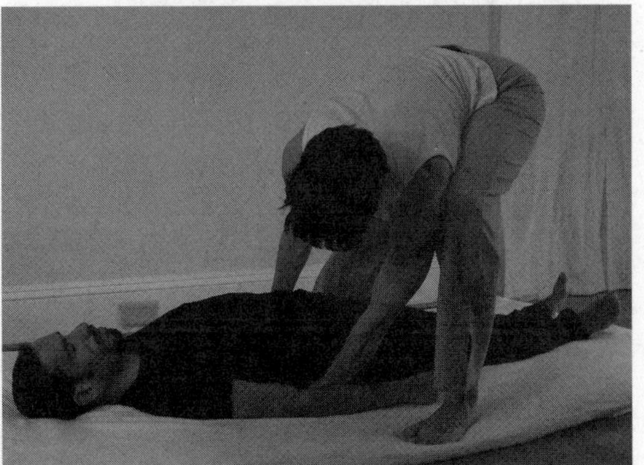

FIGURE 14-2 **Lumbar release, pulling right.** Repeat several times, alternately lifting the client's hips.

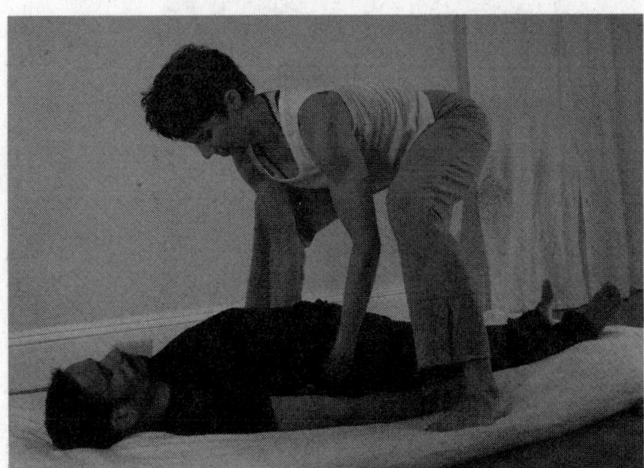

FIGURE 14-3 **Lumbar release, pulling up.** Squat down and lift the client's waist several times. Omit if you have lower back problems or if the client is substantially heavier than you.

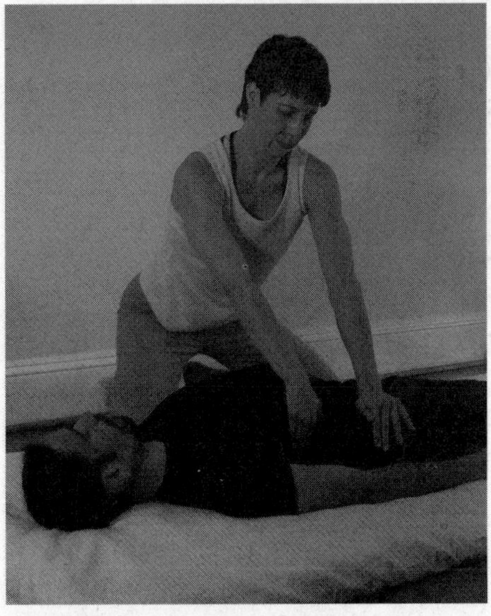

FIGURE 14-4 **Waist twist.** Kneel beside the client. Pull up on the client's rib cage with one hand and push down on the client's hip with the other.

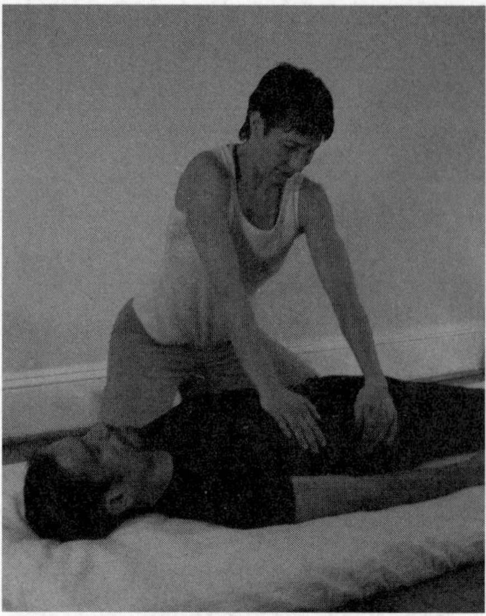

FIGURE 14-5 **Waist twist reversal.** Push down on the client's rib cage with one hand and pull up on the client's hip with the other. Repeat several times and then switch sides.

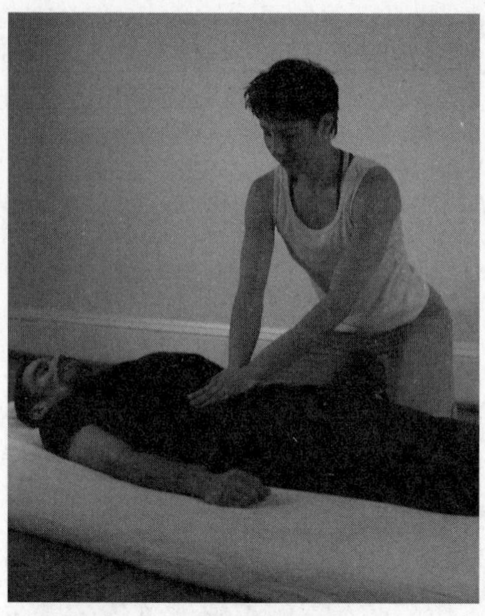

FIGURE 14-6 **Hara rock.** Place your hands on the client's abdomen and rock back and forth.

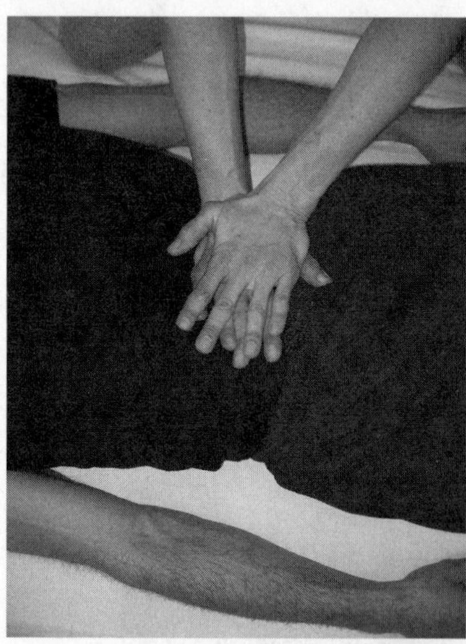

FIGURE 14-7 **Hara push/pull, phase 1.** Beginning at the side of the abdomen closest to you, push the client's abdomen away toward the other side.

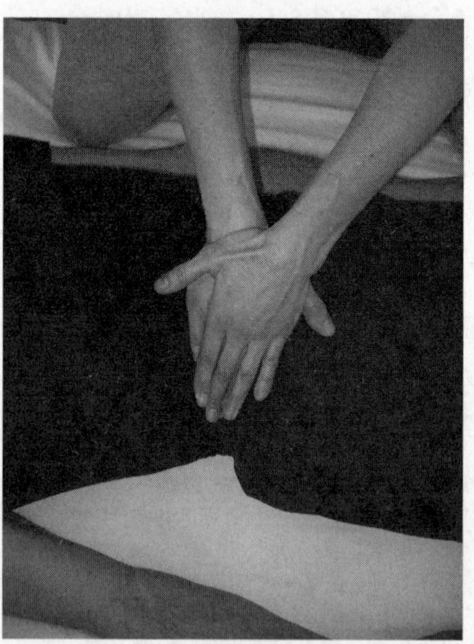

FIGURE 14-8 **Hara push/pull, phase 2.** Scoop and pull the client's abdomen toward you. Repeat several times.

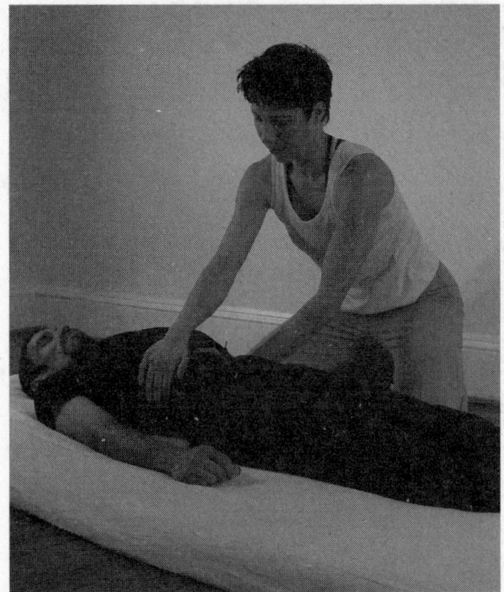

FIGURE 14-9 **Hara wringing, phase 1.** Reach over to the opposite side and pull one hand toward you while the other pushes away from you.

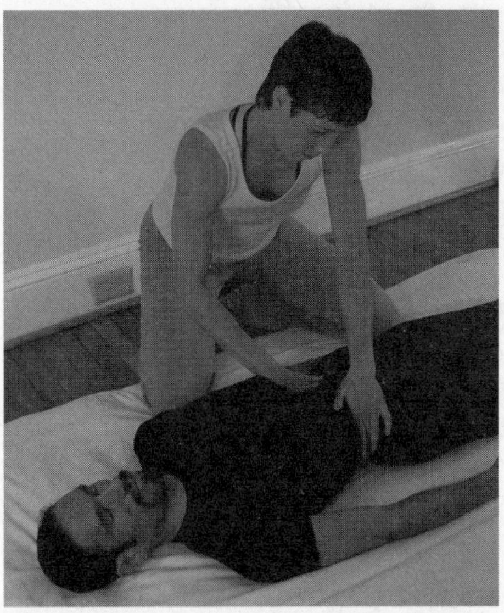

FIGURE 14-10 **Hara wringing, phase 2.** Repeat several times, switching hands.

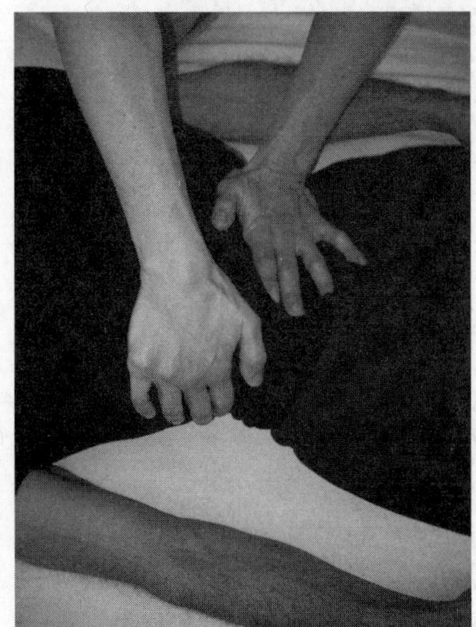

FIGURE 14-11 **Close-up of hara wringing.**

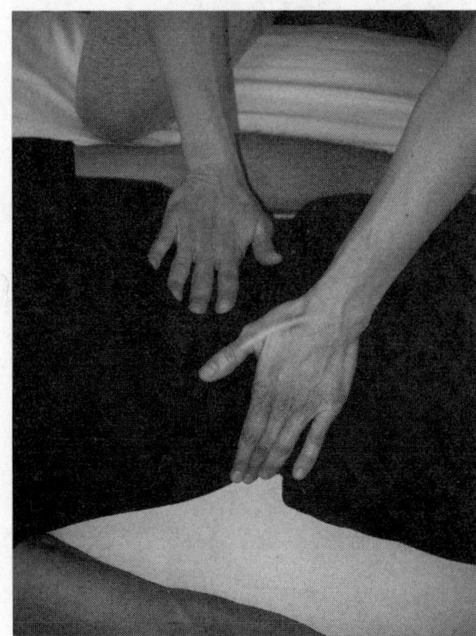

FIGURE 14-12 **Close-up of hara wringing.**

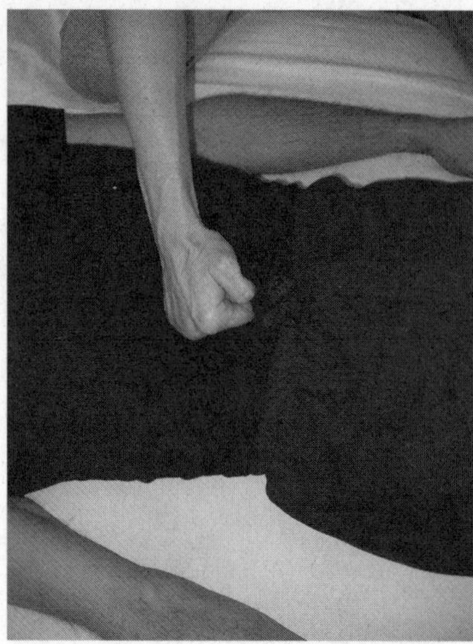

FIGURE 14-13 Fist roll, phase 1. Plant your fist on the client's navel. Rotate sideways toward your fifth metacarpal.

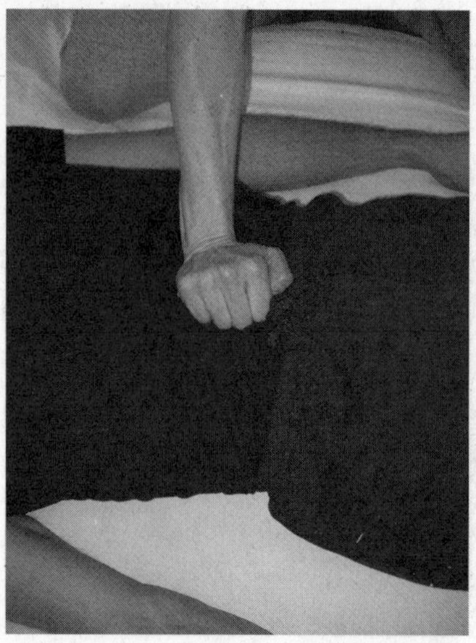

FIGURE 14-14 Fist roll, phase 2. Rotate backward, extending your wrist.

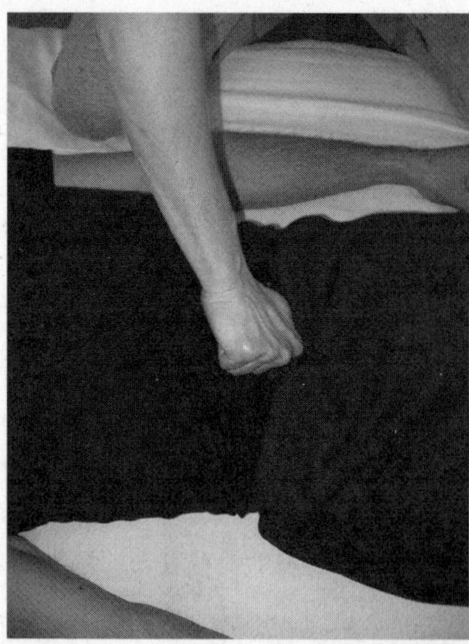

FIGURE 14-15 Fist roll, phase 3. Rotate sideways toward your first metacarpal.

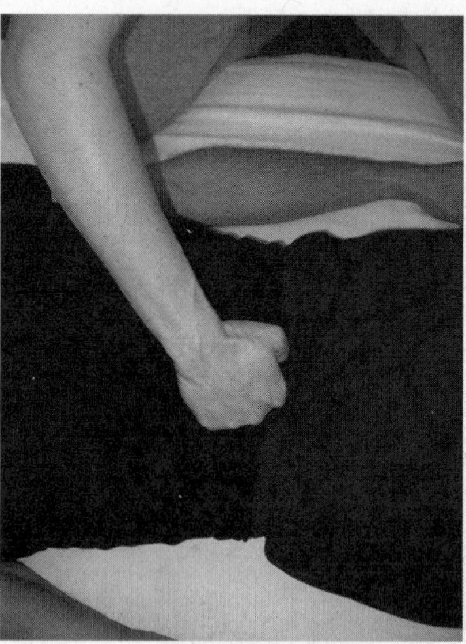

FIGURE 14-16 Fist roll, phase 4. Rotate forward, flexing your wrist. Repeat several times.

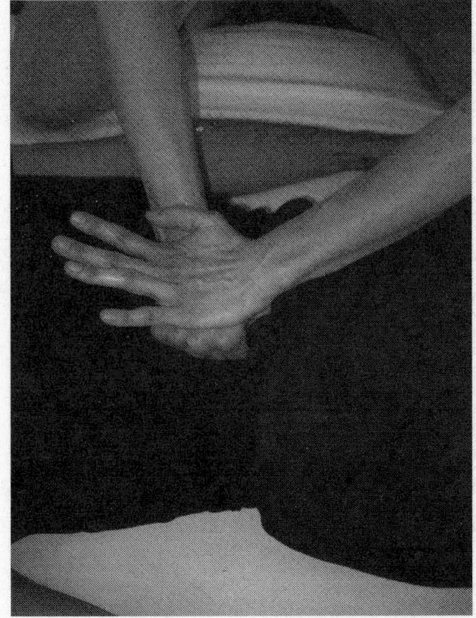

FIGURE 14-17 **Fist roll reinforced.**
For deeper work, place your free hand over your rotating fist and push down a little farther. Cover the entire abdomen with fist rolls.

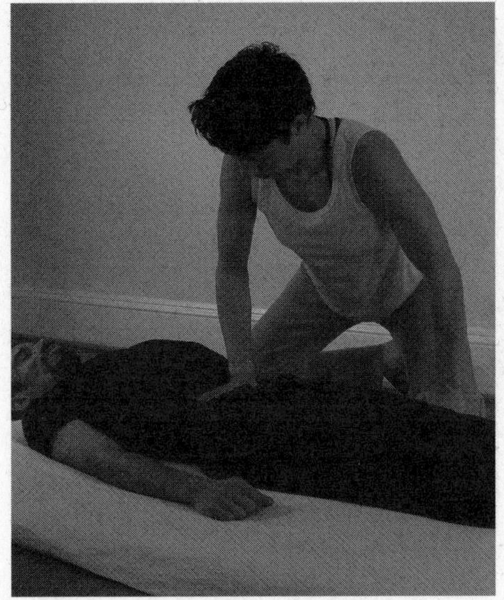

FIGURE 14-18 **Spiraling down.**
Using a rotary motion, gradually press the client's navel toward floor.

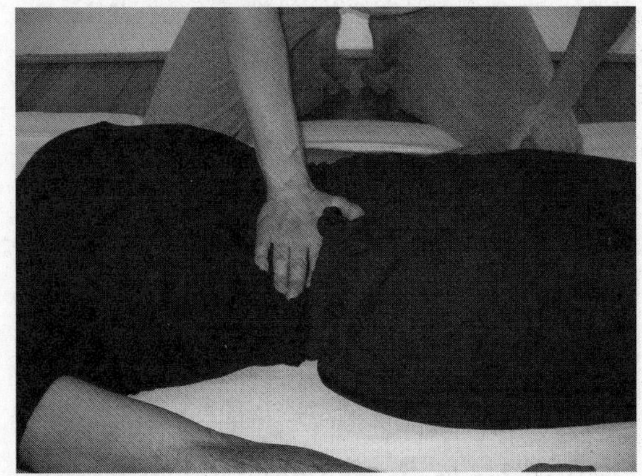

FIGURE 14-19 **Vibrating.**
Release the pressure slightly, and rapidly jiggle the client's navel side to side or up and down.

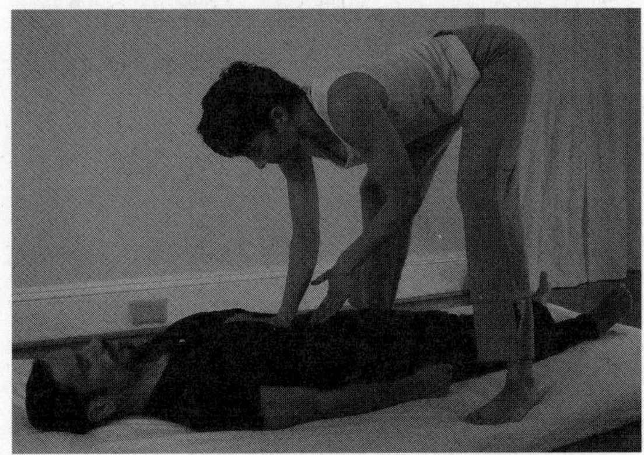

FIGURE 14-20 **Palm stroke, phase 1.**
Palm stroke down the midline and stop above the pubic bone.

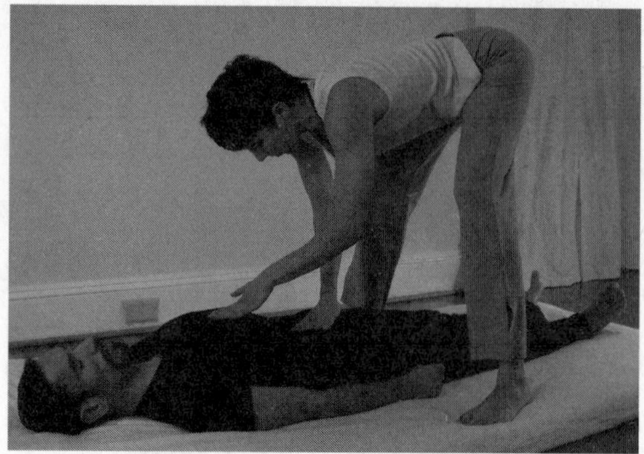

FIGURE 14-21 **Palm stroke, phase 2.** Repeat several times, alternating hands.

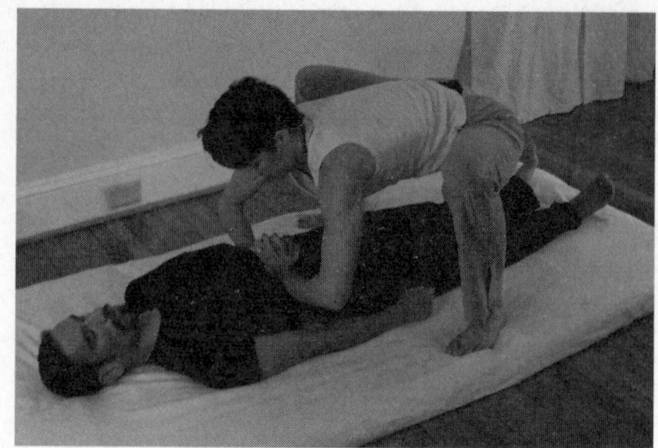

FIGURE 14-22 **Hand clasp.** Straddle the client; squat down; clasp your hands and squeeze the heels of your hands toward the midline. Work down the rectus abdominus.

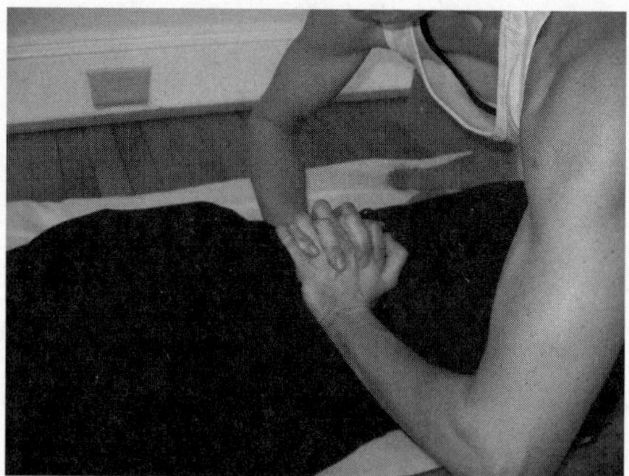

FIGURE 14-23 **Close-up of hand clasp.**

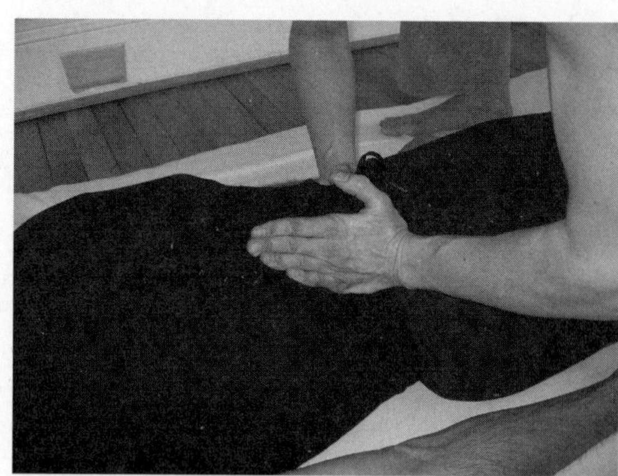

FIGURE 14-24 **Side of the hand squeeze.** Repeat, using the sides of your hands.

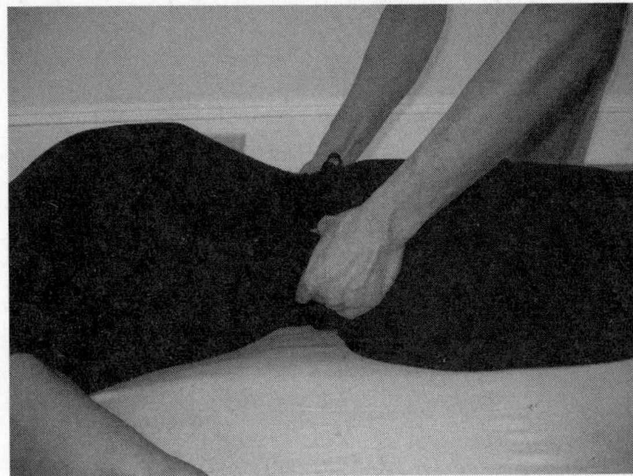

FIGURE 14-25 Pinching the waist from overhead.
Wrap your fingers around the sides of the waist and clamp down. Relocate your hands and repeat, covering the area between the rib cage and pelvis.

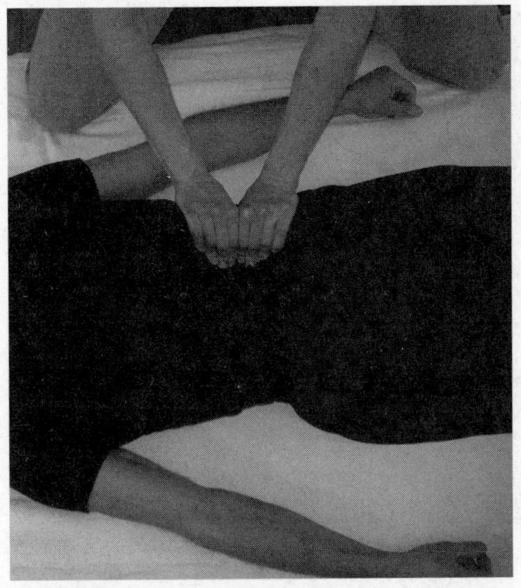

FIGURE 14-26 Pinching the waist from the side, left.
Wrap your hands around one side of the waist and clamp down.

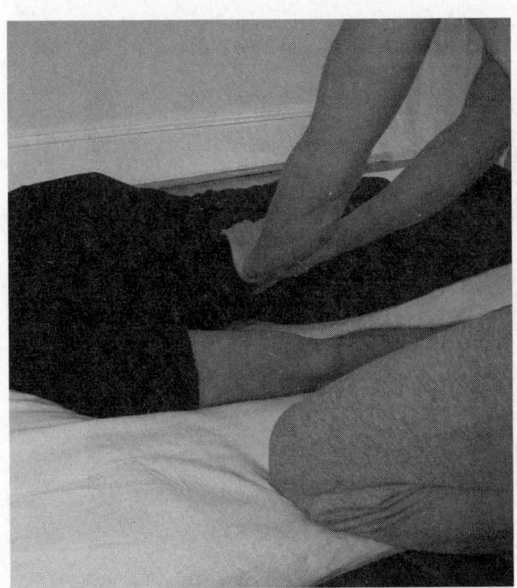

FIGURE 14-27 Pinching the waist from the side, right.
Repeat on the other side.

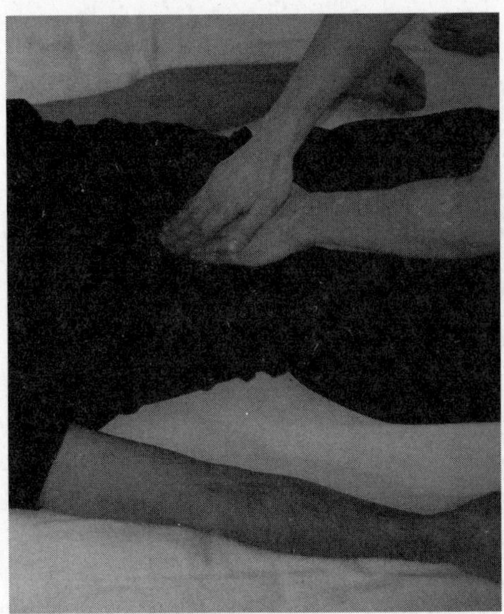

FIGURE 14-28 Fingertip press down the Conception Vessel.
Follow the path of the Conception Vessel along the midline from the xiphoid process (below the breastbone) to the pubic bone.

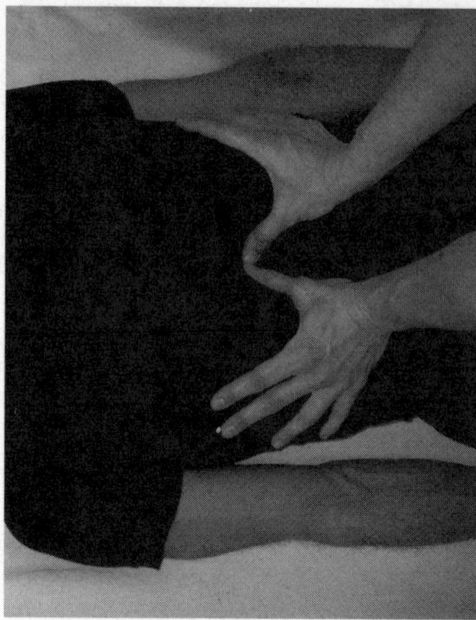

FIGURE 14-29 **Thumbs press down the Conception Vessel.**
Repeat, covering the Ht, PC, Sp, Ki, and Bl reflex zones.

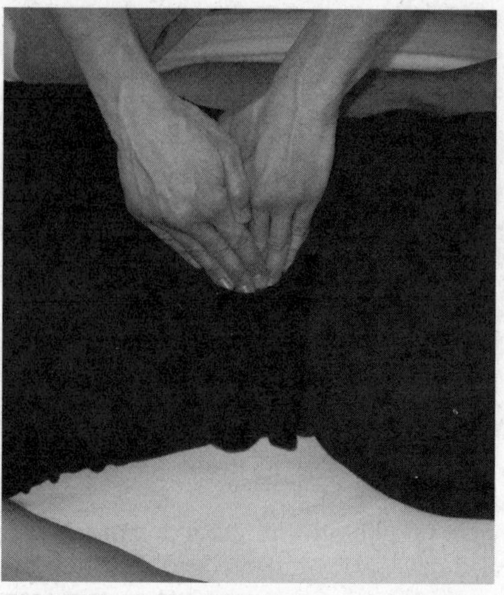

FIGURE 14-30 **Fingertip press down the Stomach Meridian.**
Follow the path of the Stomach Meridian alongside the rectus abdominus. This Meridian can be worked unilaterally (one side at a time), as shown.

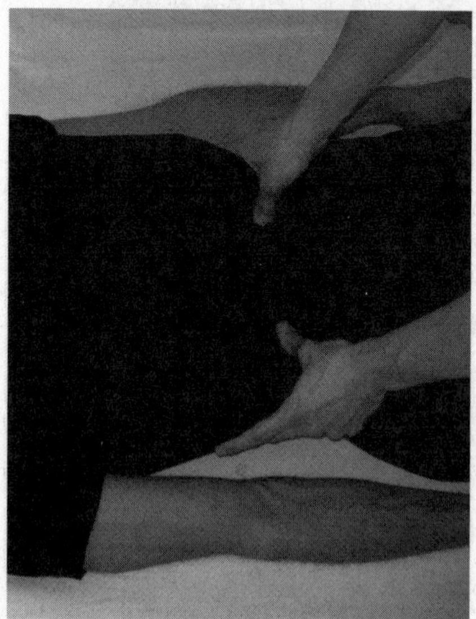

FIGURE 14-31 **Thumb press down the Stomach Meridian.**
Alternatively, the Stomach Meridian can be worked bilaterally (simultaneously on both sides), as shown.

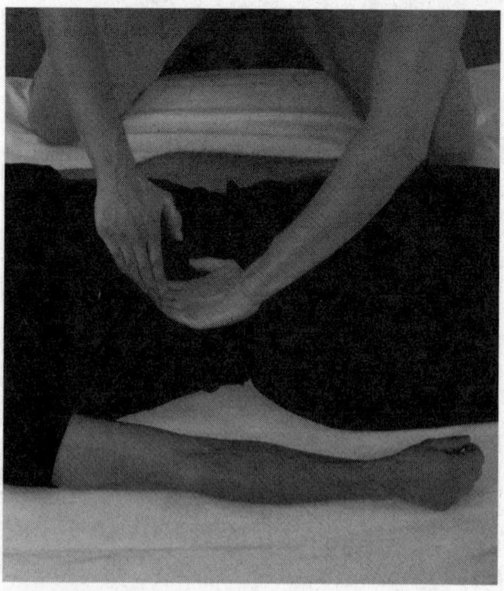

FIGURE 14-32 **Side of the hands under the rib cage.**
Press the side of your fingers under the right rib cage.

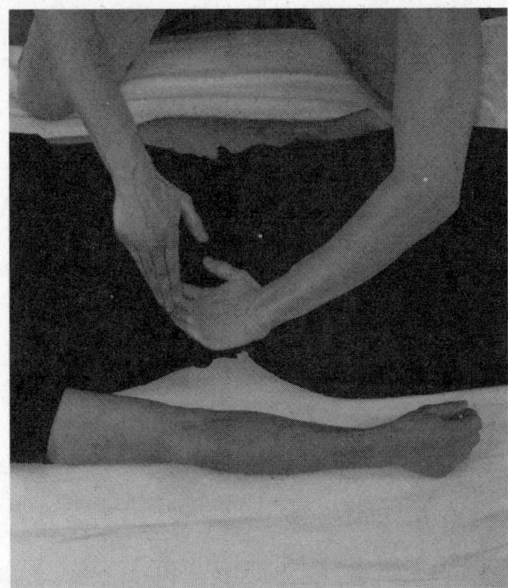

FIGURE 14-33 Side of the hands under the rib cage.
Move laterally and repeat.

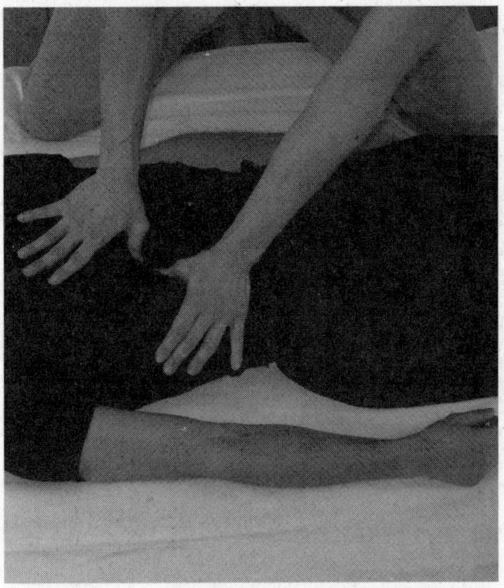

FIGURE 14-34 Thumbs, Ht reflex zone.
Apply static pressure or transverse friction under the xiphoid process.

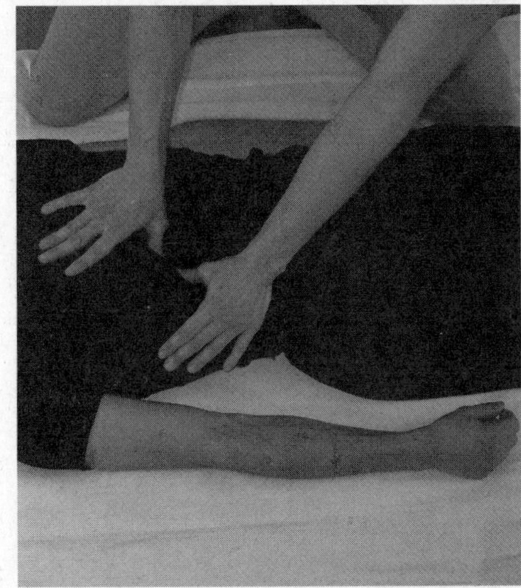

FIGURE 14-35 Thumbs, GB reflex zone.
Move laterally. Apply static pressure or transverse friction under the rib.

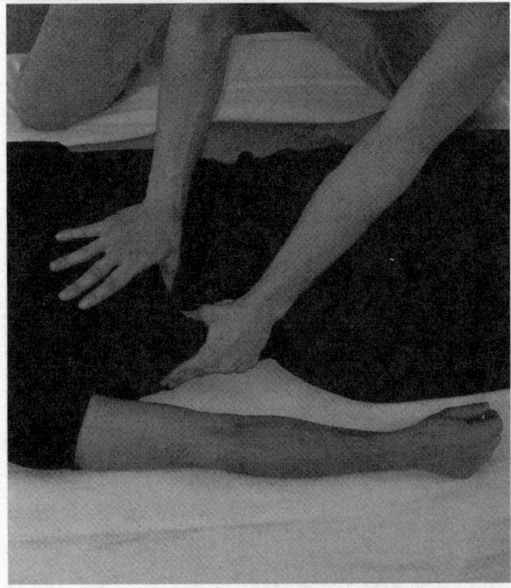

FIGURE 14-36 Thumbs, Lr reflex zone.
Move laterally. Apply static pressure or transverse friction under the rib.

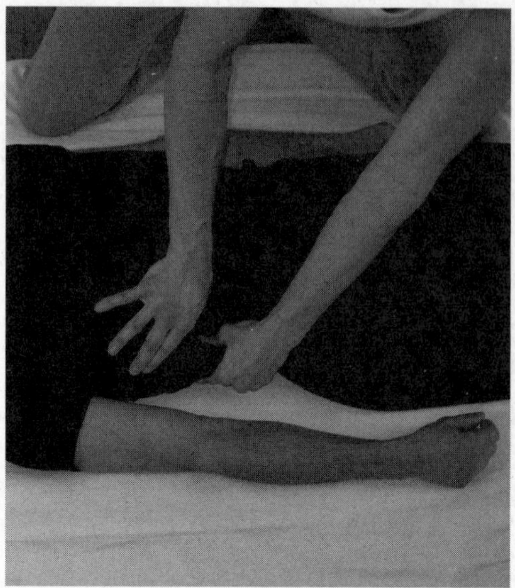

FIGURE 14-37 **Thumbs, Lu reflex zone.** Move laterally. Apply static pressure or transverse friction under the rib.

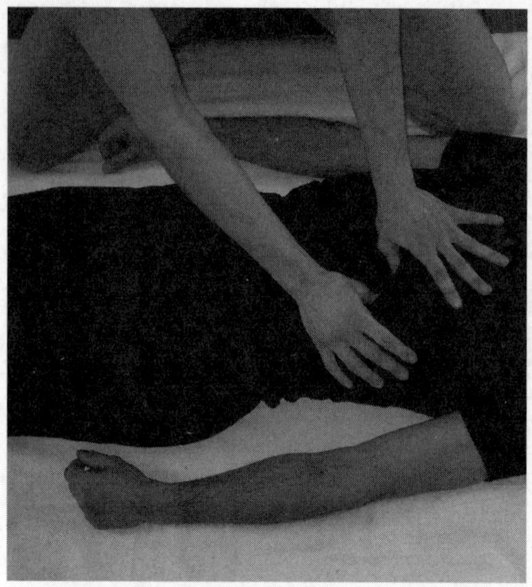

FIGURE 14-38 **Thumbs, Ht reflex zone.** Switch sides to work the left side of the rib cage. Warm up by pressing the side of the hands under the ribcage, as in Figures 14-32 and 14-33; then add thumbs.

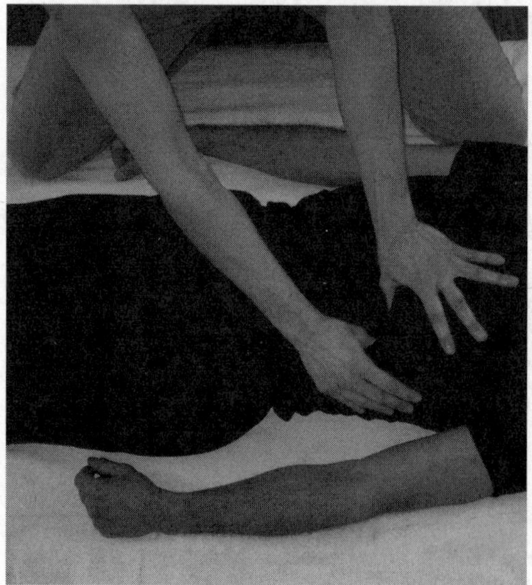

FIGURE 14-39 **Thumbs, St reflex zone.**

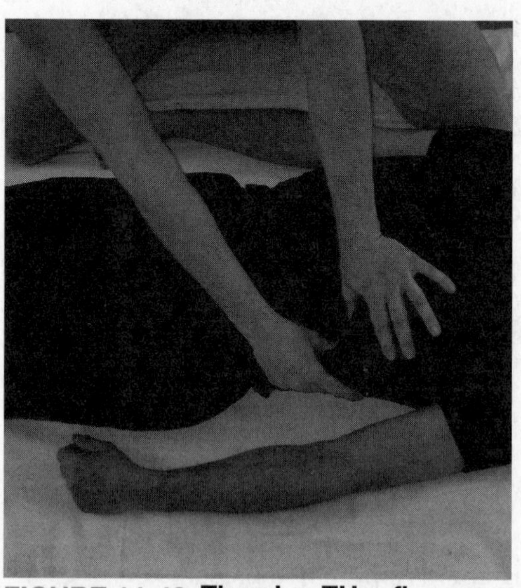

FIGURE 14-40 **Thumbs, TH reflex zone.**

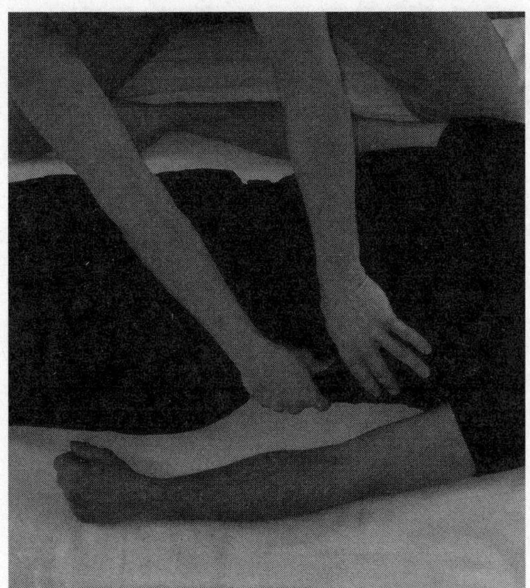

FIGURE 14-41 **Thumbs, Lu reflex zone.**

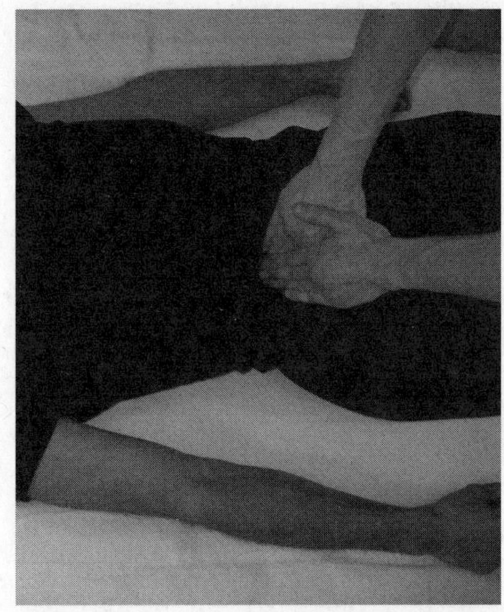

FIGURE 14-42 **Friction, Sp reflex zone.**
Apply circular pressure with your fingertips around the Sp reflex zone, encircling the navel.

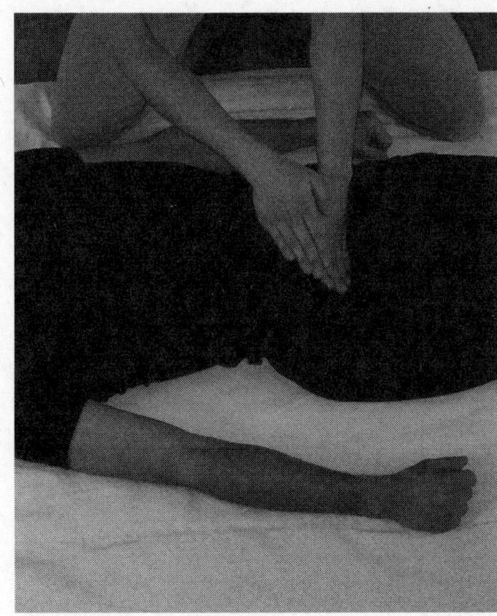

FIGURE 14-43 **Friction, Ki and Bl reflex zones.**
Apply circular friction with your fingertips on the horseshoe-shaped Ki and Bl reflex zones.

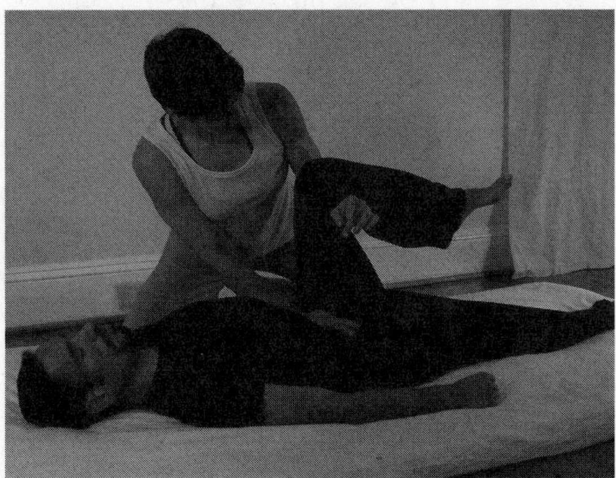

FIGURE 14-44 **Hara press plus leg lift.**
Hook your forearm under the client's knee. Simultaneously press down on the abdomen and pull up on the leg. Relocate your hand and repeat, palpating the entire abdomen.

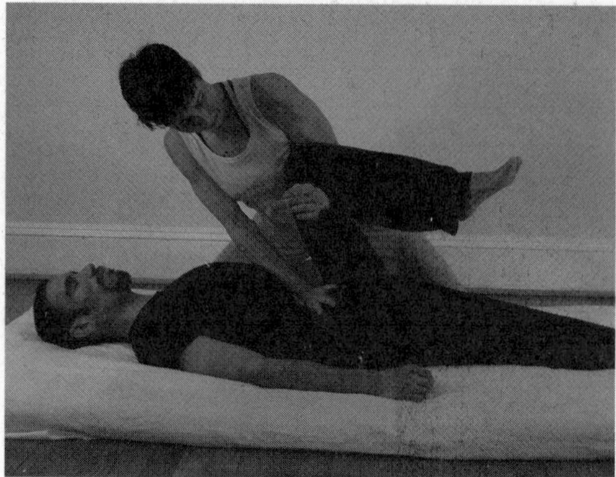

FIGURE 14-45 Hara press plus leg lift.
This technique can be used to finish Ampuku or in lieu of Ampuku when doing a full-body session. Alternative positioning (not shown): In a kneeling lunge, face the client's head; use your inner hand to press the shin toward the chest and your outer hand to press down on the abdomen.

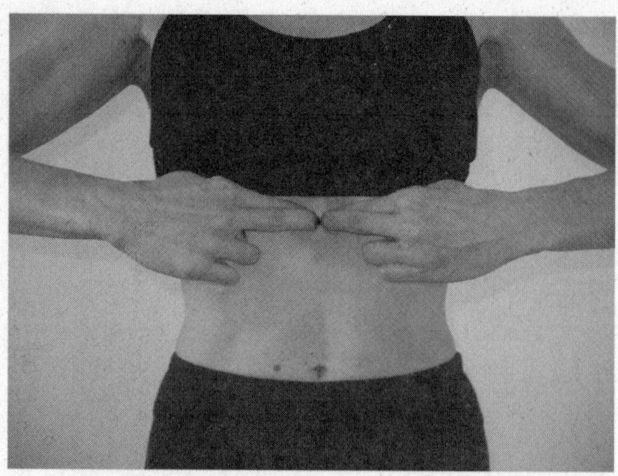

FIGURE 14-46 CV 14.
On the upper abdomen, 6 cun above the navel; Mu/Bo point for the Heart.

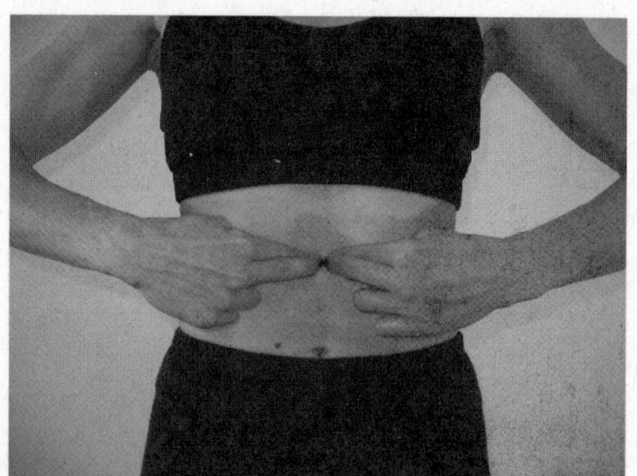

FIGURE 14-47 CV 12.
On the upper abdomen, halfway between the navel and xiphoid process of the sternum (notch of the breastbone) or 4 cun above the navel; Bo/Mu point for the Stomach.

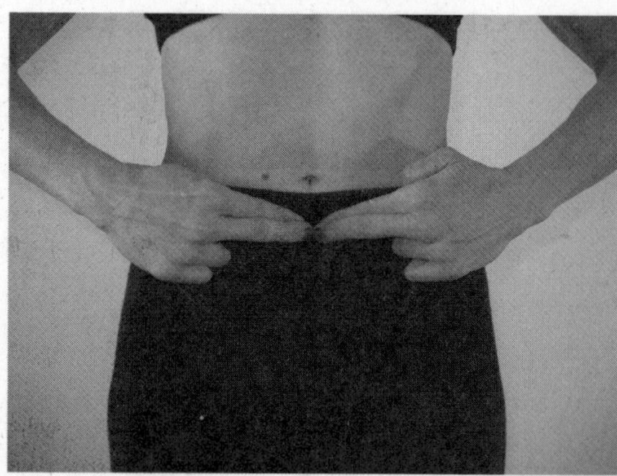

FIGURE 14-48 CV 6.
On the lower abdomen, 1.5 cun below the navel.

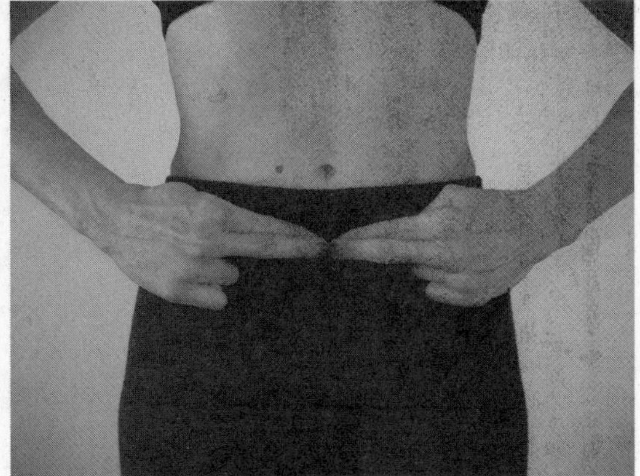

FIGURE 14-49 **CV 5.**
On the lower abdomen, 2 cun below the navel; Mu/Bo point for the Triple Heater.

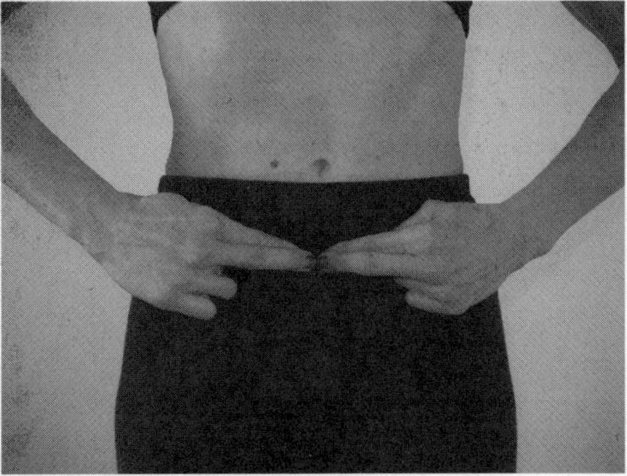

FIGURE 14-50 **CV 4.**
On the lower abdomen, 3 cun below the navel; Mu/Bo point for the Small Intestine.

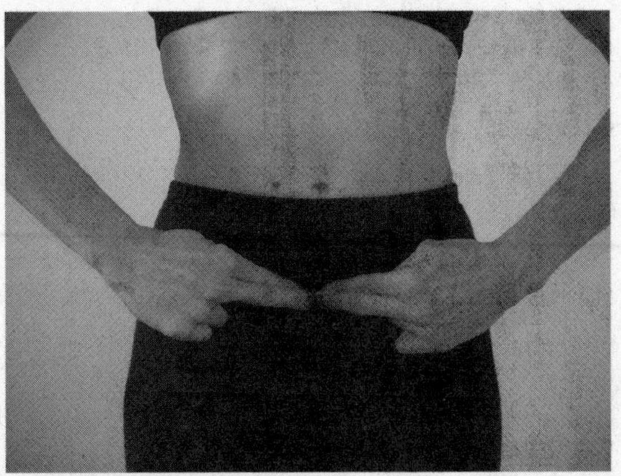

FIGURE 14-51 **CV 3.**
On the lower abdomen, 4 cun below the navel; Mu/Bo point for the Bladder.

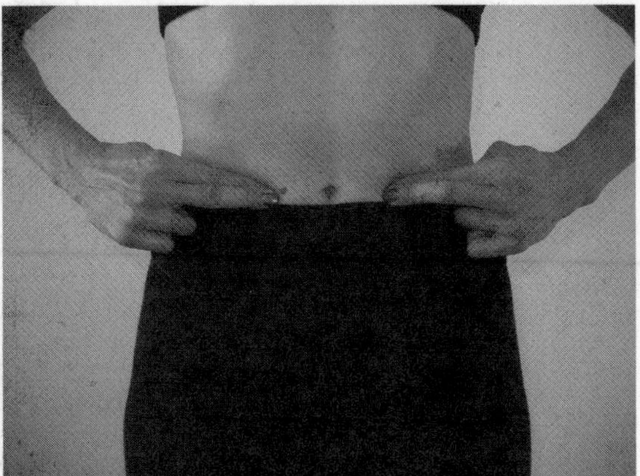

FIGURE 14-52 **St 25.**
On the abdomen, 2 cun lateral to the navel; Mu/Bo point for the Large Intestine.

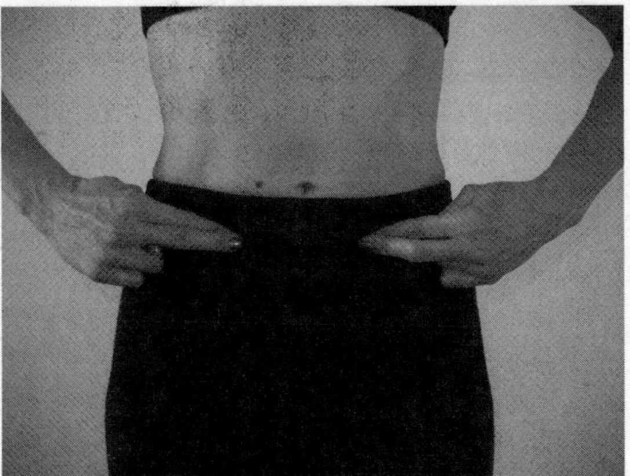

FIGURE 14-53 **St 27.**
On the abdomen, 2 cun lateral and 2 cun inferior to the navel.

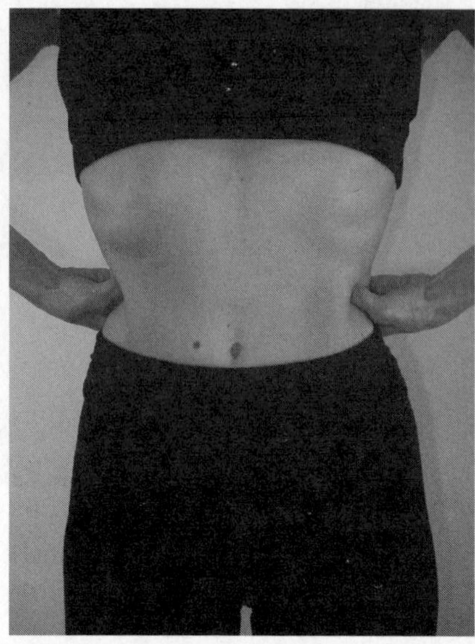

FIGURE 14-54 **Lr 13.**
On the lateral waist, inferior to the end of the eleventh floating rib; Mu/Bo point for the Spleen.

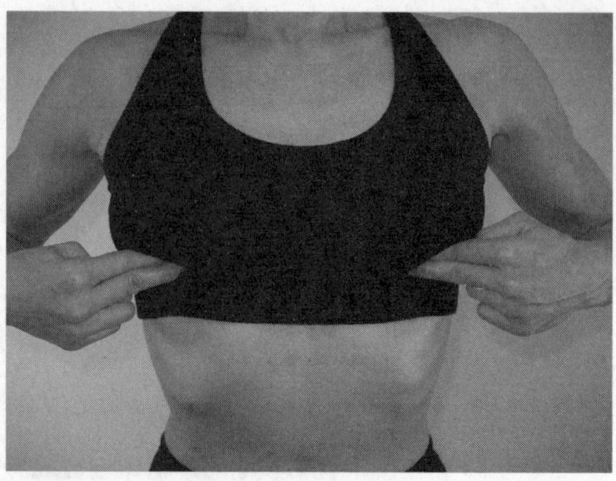

FIGURE 14-55 **Lr 14.**
On the rib cage, in the sixth intercostal space (between the sixth and seventh ribs) in vertical alignment with the nipple; Mu/Bo point for the Liver.

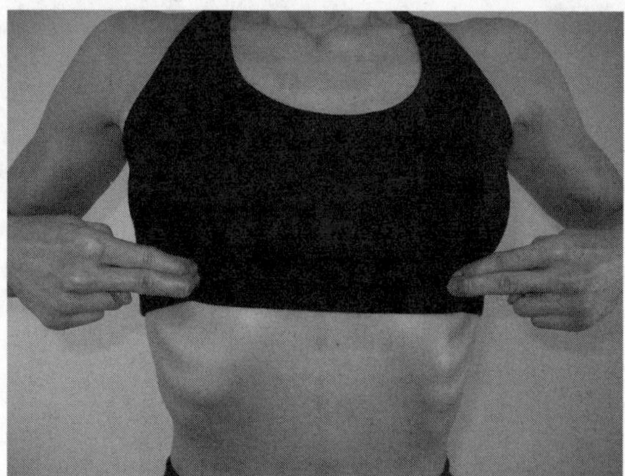

FIGURE 14-56 **GB 24.**
On the rib cage, in the seventh intercostal space (between the seventh and eighth ribs) in vertical alignment with the nipple; Mu/Bo point for the Gallbladder.

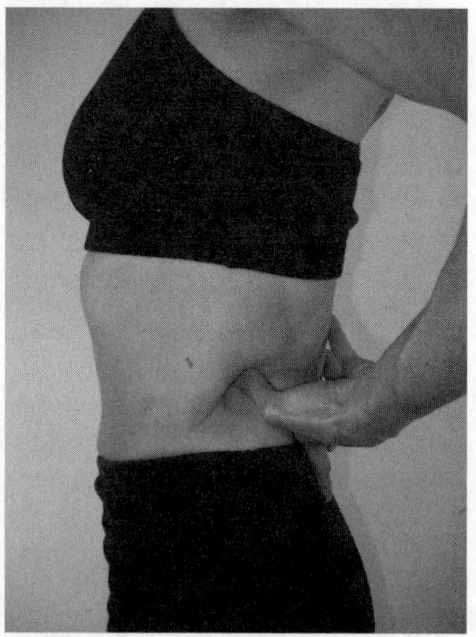

FIGURE 14-57 **GB 25.**
On the lateral waist, inferior to the end of the twelfth floating rib; Mu/Bo point for the Kidneys.

15

SIDELYING PROTOCOL

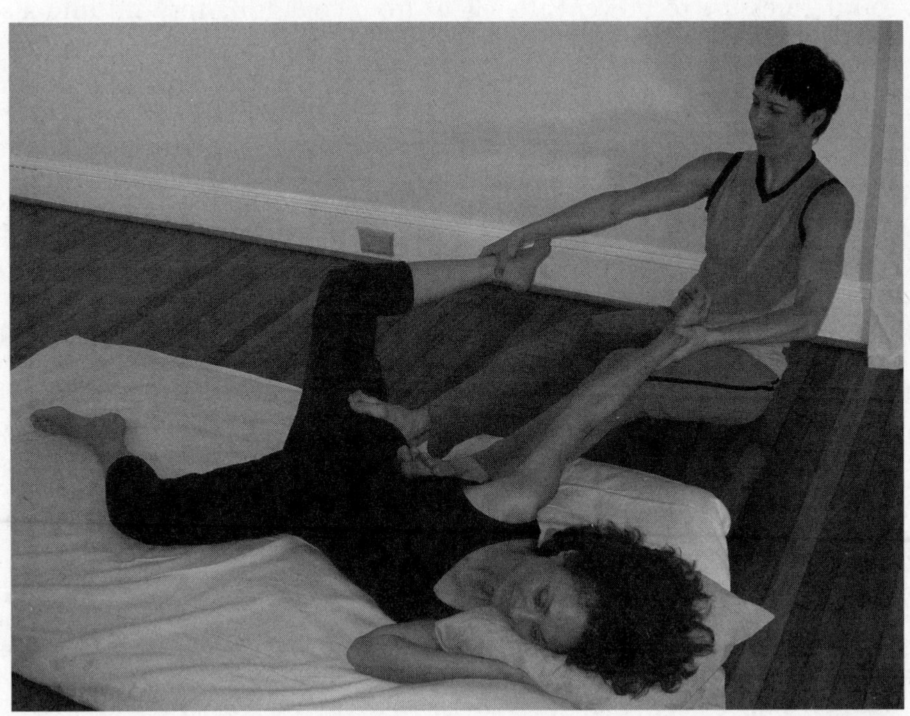

THERAPEUTIC EMPHASIS

The sidelying position has many uses. It is a practical alternative to the prone and supine positions when those positions are uncomfortable or contraindicated for the client, as, for example, when neck rotation is limited or painful in the prone position, when the lower back feels unsupported or strained and the lumbar curve is accentuated in the prone position, when resting on a distended abdomen or sore breasts feels awkward and unpleasant in the prone position, or when lying supine would aggravate sciatica or obstruct the venous return during the second and third trimester of pregnancy (see "Pregnant Women" in Chapter 9). For clients who have no problems with the prone and supine positions, sidelying adds another dimension to the Shiatsu experience.

Since most Meridians are accessible in the sidelying position, it can be used exclusively to give full-body Shiatsu. Some Meridians, however, are easier to access and treat than others. The Gallbladder Meridian on the outside of the torso and legs and the Yin Meridians—the Spleen, Liver, and Kidney Meridians—on the inside of the legs are easy to treat in the sidelying position. Consequently, sidelying is a good choice for addressing certain Wood element imbalances with compression techniques, though the supine position is preferable for facilitated stretching of the Gallbladder and Liver Meridians.

By contrast, the Bladder Meridian of the back is relatively difficult to treat due to the spatial orientation of the client and the practitioner. The practitioner must deliver pressure sideways into the client's back rather than straight down. This constitutes a logistical disadvantage for the practitioner, who has no natural leverage and cannot harness the power of gravity to sink the body weight into the client. Instead, the practitioner must create leverage, for example, by bracing the working arm against his or her body to provide firm resistance against which to push. Obviously, pushing requires more effort than leaning. Moreover, because the client's hips and shoulders are stacked on top of each other, the practitioner must brace and stabilize the client with counterpressure to prevent the client from collapsing forward into a semi-prone position. While working the upper back, the client's shoulder is braced; while working the lower back and hip, the hip is braced. Clearly, stabilizing the client adds to the practitioner's workload. Because of this, sidelying is not the best choice when the client needs Jitsu dispersal techniques on the back.

For simiar reasons, sidelying is not preferred for applying Jitsu dispersal techniques on the petoralis (chest) muscles, deltoids (outer shoulder muscles), rotator cuff (posterior shoulder muscles), and arms, particularly if the client has dense muscle mass, requires deep pressure, or experiences numbness while lying on (and thereby compressing) the shoulder and chest. The practitioner must expend more energy to deliver pressure at an oblique rather than perpendicular angle, and to stabilize the client's shoulder in order to work the chest, or to stabilize the client's chest in order to work the shoulder. Additionally, the positioning of the client's arm—draped alongside the torso, or draped overhead, or propped on the practitioner's thigh—prevents the practitioner from delivering maximum pressure, either because another part of the client's body could get squashed or because the client's arm is suspended in midair. Clearly, if the client requires sedation in these target areas, the prone and supine positions are better.

Although the sidelying protocol introduces a few new stretches, it reviews many compression techniques and acupressure points. It also challenges the practitioner to become more adept at transitioning, since the practitioner must frequently change work positions or angles.

CLIENT COMFORT

Place a pillow under the client's head to align the cervical vertebrae, another under the uppermost leg to stack the hips, and another under the uppermost arm for additional comfort and support, if desired.

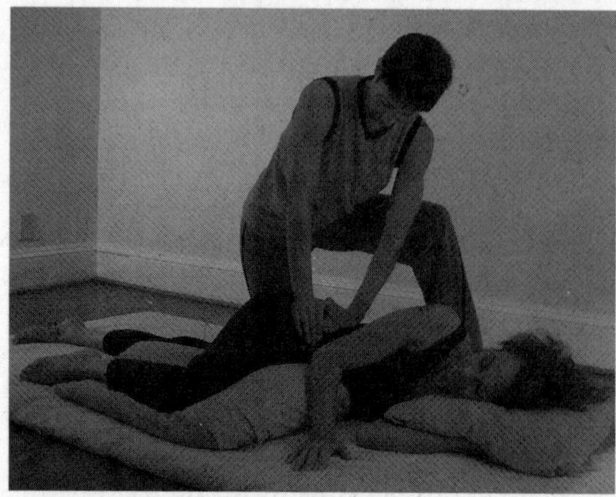

FIGURE 15-1 Palm press. This general technique prepares the tissues for deeper work.

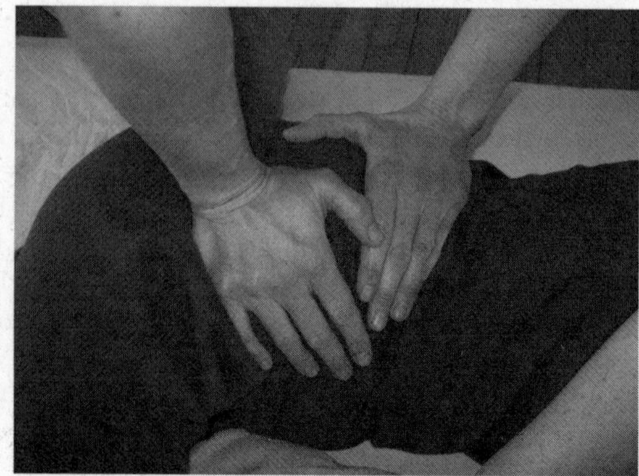

FIGURE 15-2 Close-up of palm press.

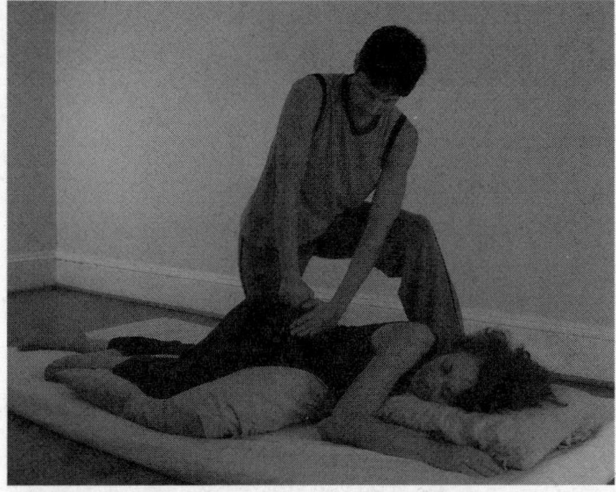

FIGURE 15-3 Fist press or twist.
Stabilize the client's hip by bracing the ASIS (front pelvic bone) or ilium (pelvic crest). Sink into the deeper layers of muscle.

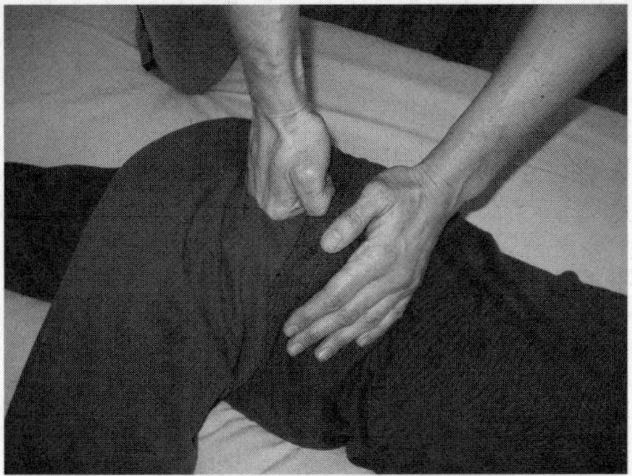

FIGURE 15-4 Close-up of fist twist.
Do not merely slip over clothing or slide over surface tissues; engage the deeper layers of muscle by wringing them.

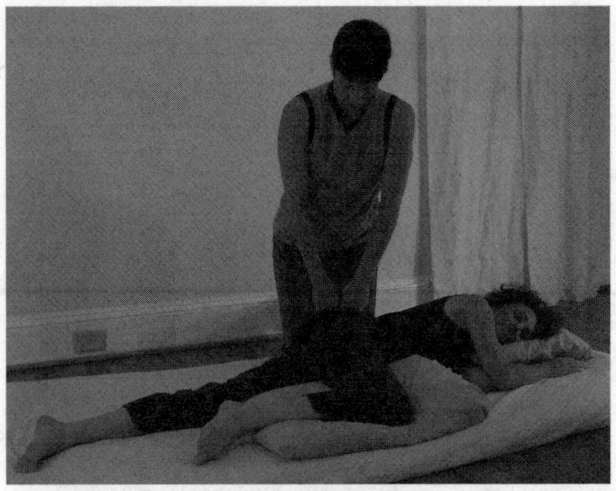

FIGURE 15-5 Knuckle press.
Press or apply friction to the muscle attachments around the greater trochanter of the femur (hipbone), along the ilium (pelvic crest), and along the sacrum (triangular bone at the base of the spine).

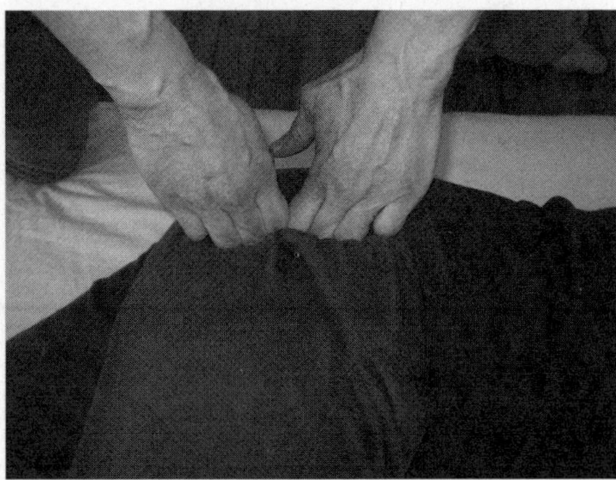

FIGURE 15-6 Close-up of knuckles.
To create friction, combine circular rotations or side-to-side movements with knuckle compression.

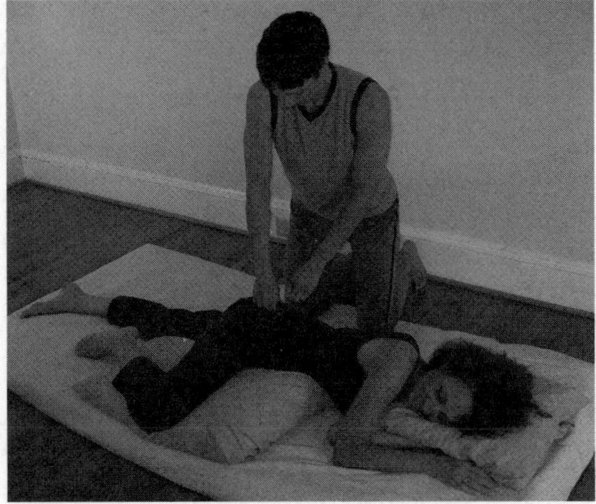

FIGURE 15-7 Alternating knuckles: "cat paws."
Rhythmically press the knuckles of one hand and then the other, repeatedly.

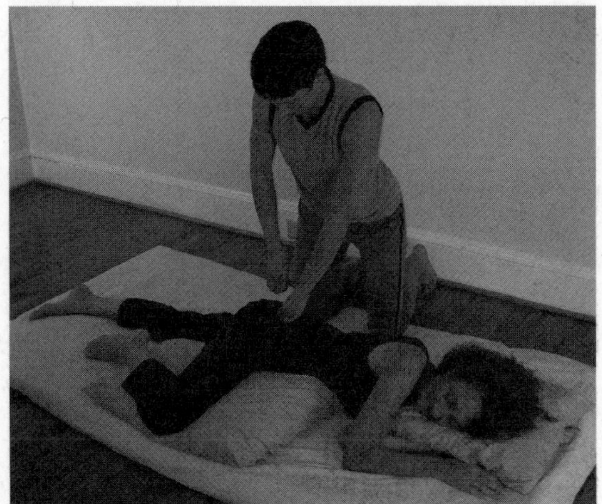

FIGURE 15-8 Alternating knuckles: "cat paws."
The client's hips will jostle slightly.

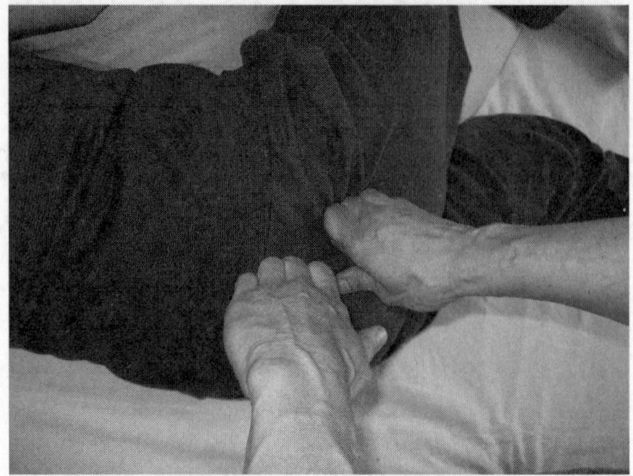

FIGURE 15-9 **Close-up of alternating "cat paw" knuckles.**

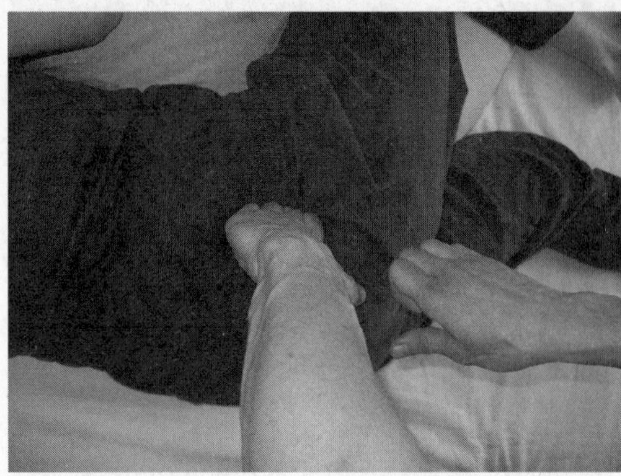

FIGURE 15-10 **Close-up of alternating "cat paw" knuckles.**

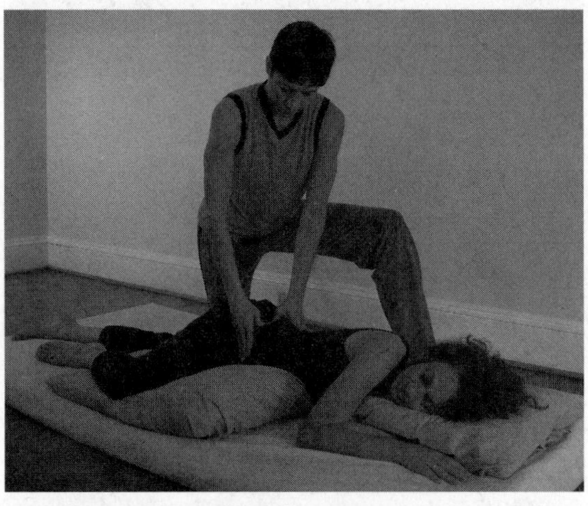

FIGURE 15-11 **Thumb press.**
Press or apply friction to the muscle attachments along the ilium and sacrum.

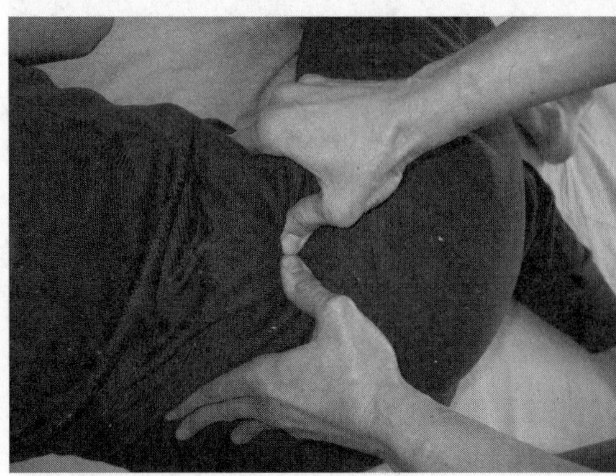

FIGURE 15-12 **Close-up of thumb press.**

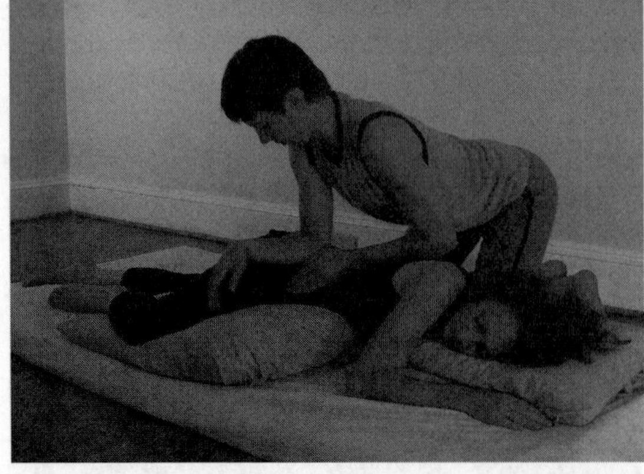

FIGURE 15-13 **Elbow press.**
Work the entire gluteal surface (buttock) but hold pressure at GB 30, Bl 53, and Bl 54.

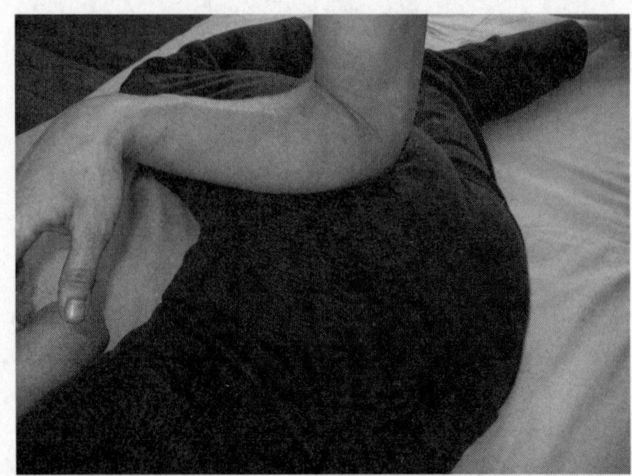

FIGURE 15-14 **GB 30.**
On the gluteal surface (buttock), two-thirds of the distance between the sacrum and greater trochanter of the femur (hipbone).

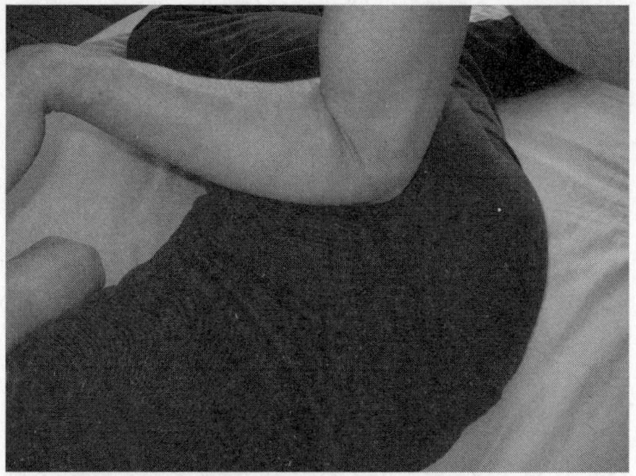

FIGURE 15-15 **Bl 53.**
On the gluteal surface (buttock) at the level of the second sacral foramen (notch).

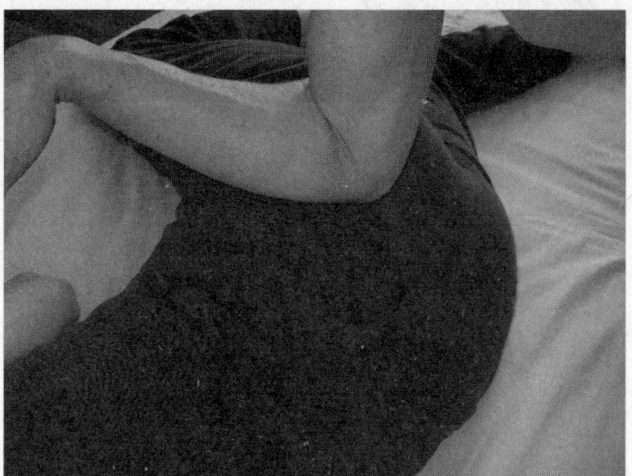

FIGURE 15-16 **Bl 54.**
On the gluteal surface (buttock) at the level of the fourth sacral foramen (notch).

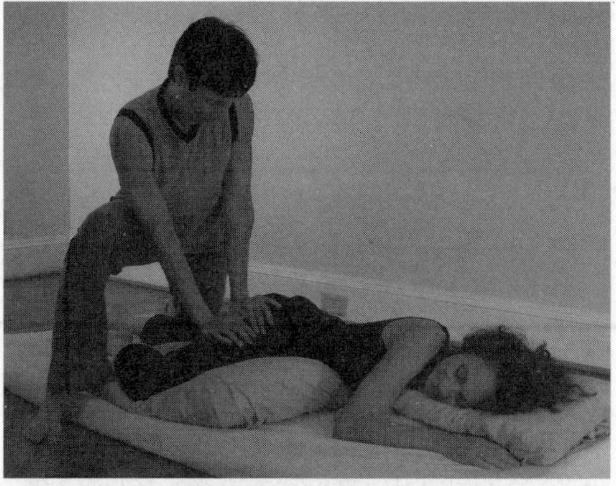

FIGURE 15-17 **Heels of the hands press the Gallbladder Meridian.**
Hook the heels of your hands under the iliotibial (IT) band.

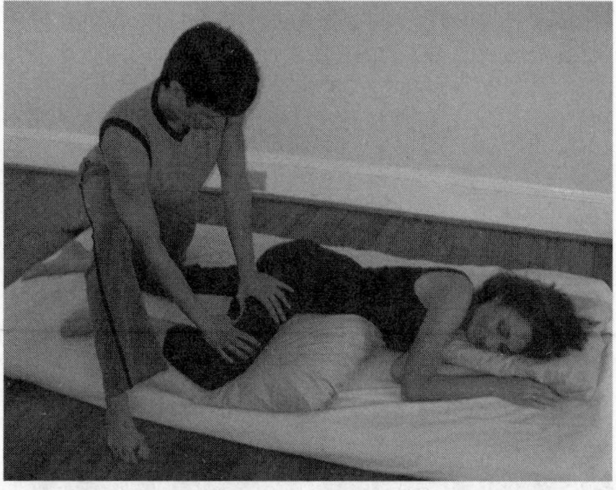

FIGURE 15-18 **Thumbs press the Gallbladder Meridian.**
Hook your thumbs under the IT band.

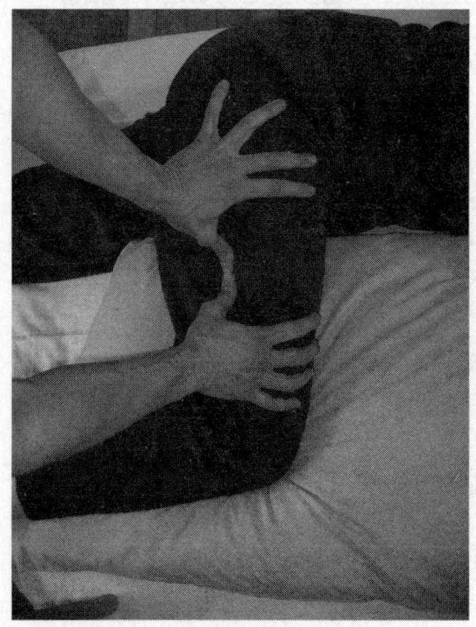

FIGURE 15-19 **GB 31.**
About half way down the lateral (outer) aspect of the leg.

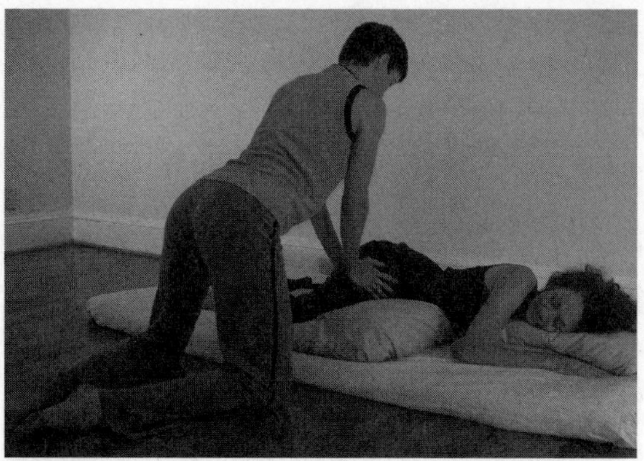

FIGURE 15-20 **Butterfly on the Gallbladder Meridian.**
Compress the IT band and vastus lateralis (outer quadriceps) against the femur (thighbone).

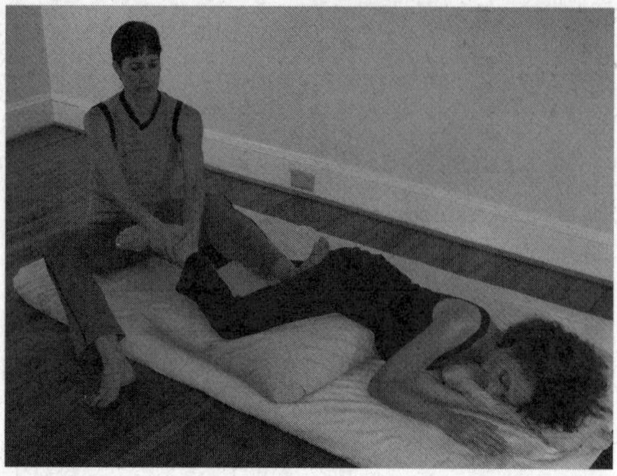

FIGURE 15-21 **Foot press on the Bladder Meridian.**
Hold the client's ankle and press the sole of your foot on the hamstrings, starting at Bl 36.

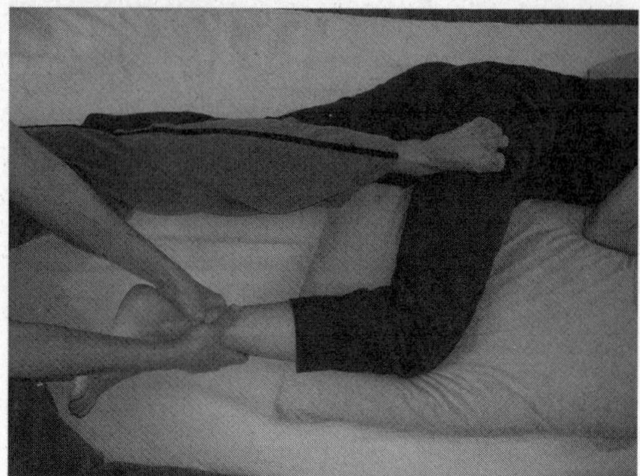

FIGURE 15-22 **Close-up of Bl 36.**
On the hamstring (back of the thigh) attachment at the ischial tuberosity (sit bone).

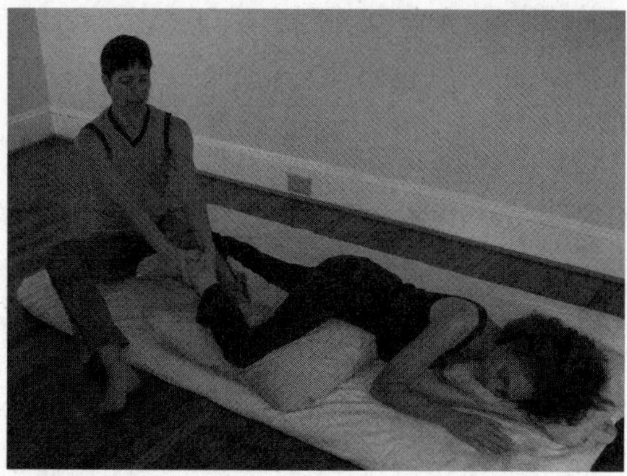

FIGURE 15-23 **Foot press on the Bladder Meridian.**
The client's leg should be bent at a 90 degree angle to maximize pressure and stability.

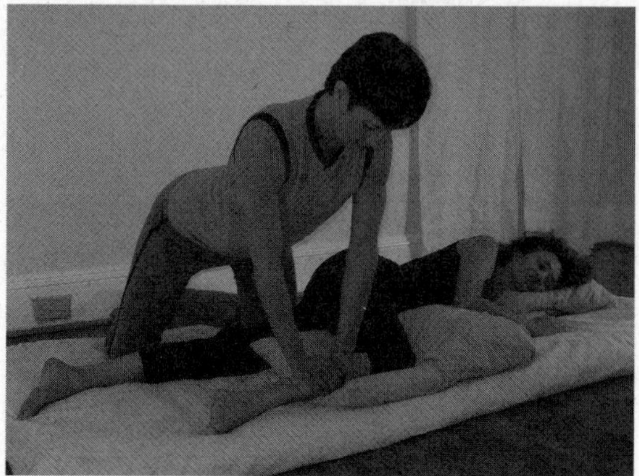

FIGURE 15-24 **Heels of the hands press on the Stomach and Gallbladder Meridians.**
You can also orient yourself on the opposite side, if preferred.

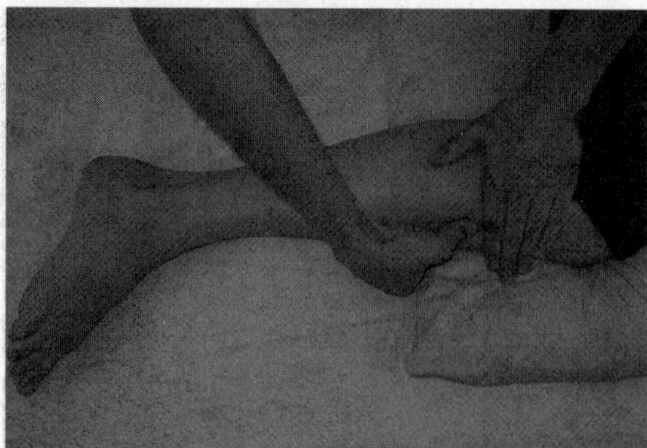

FIGURE 15-25 **St 36.**
Three cun (or four finger widths) below the patella (kneecap) against the tibia (shin).

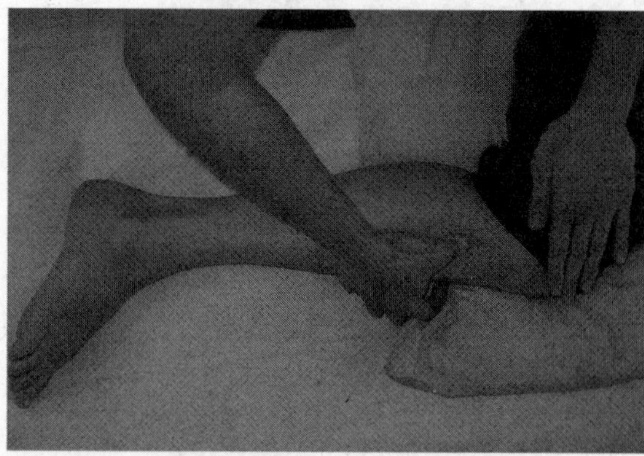

FIGURE 15-26 **GB 34.**
In front of and below the head of the fibula. To locate, feel for the bony knob beside the tibia (shinbone).

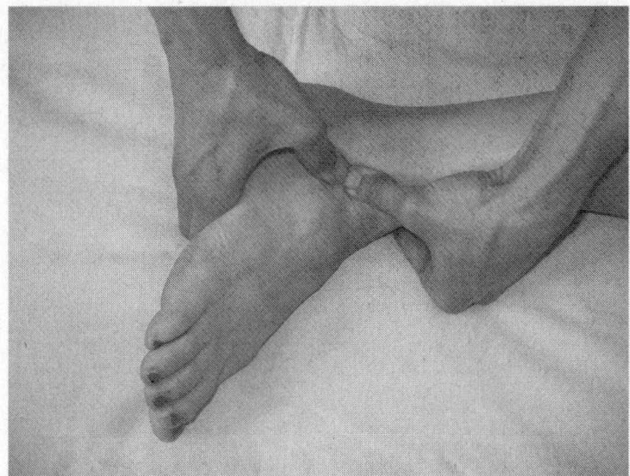

FIGURE 15-27 **GB 40.**
In the bony hollow in front of the lateral malleolus (outer anklebone).

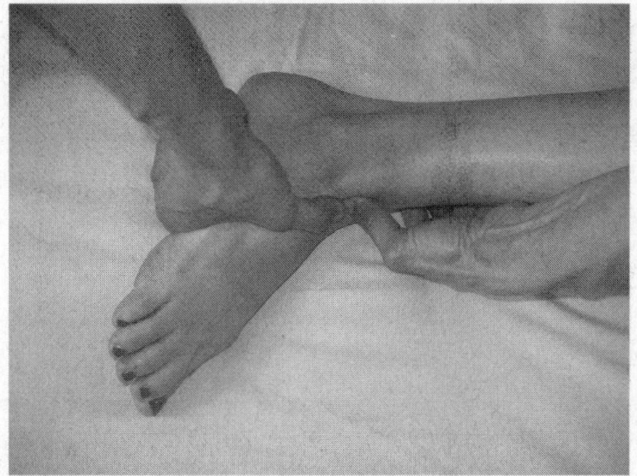

FIGURE 15-28 **St 41.**
Between the extensor hallicus longus (big toe tendon) and extensor digitorum longus (tendon of other toes) on the dorsal surface of the foot.

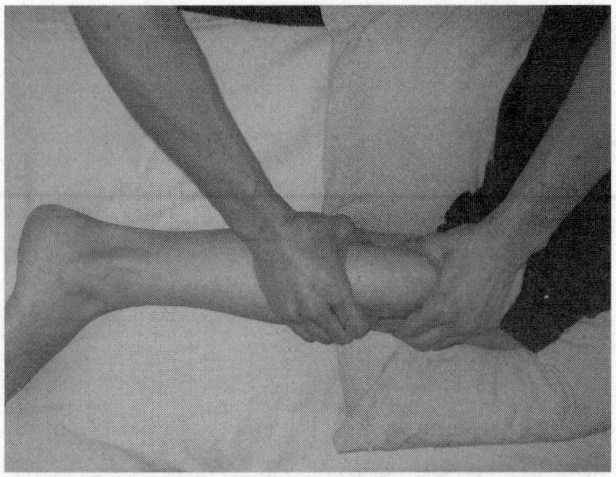

FIGURE 15-29 **Fingertip and thumb squeeze.**
Compress the anterior tibialis (shin muscle) and triceps surae (calf) simultaneously.

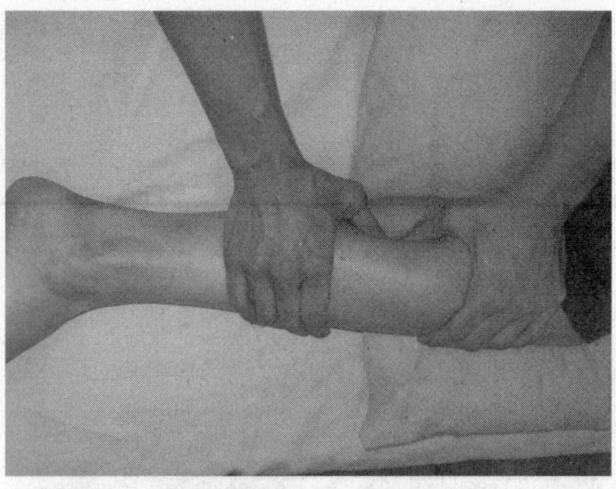

FIGURE 15-30 **Bl 56.**
On the belly of the calf, where the muscle is plumpest.

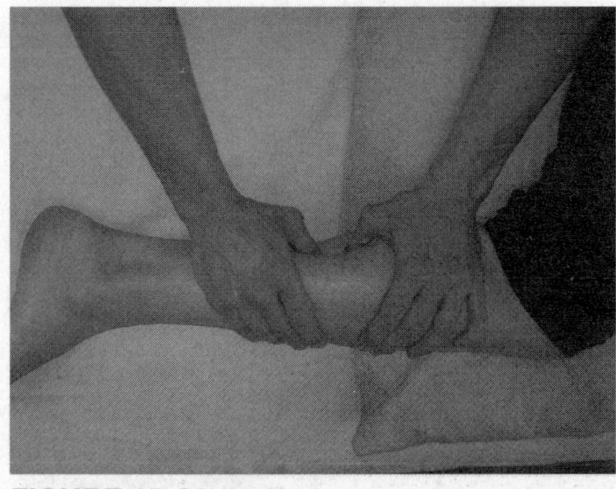

FIGURE 15-31 **Bl 57.**
Below the belly of the calf, where the muscle tapers.

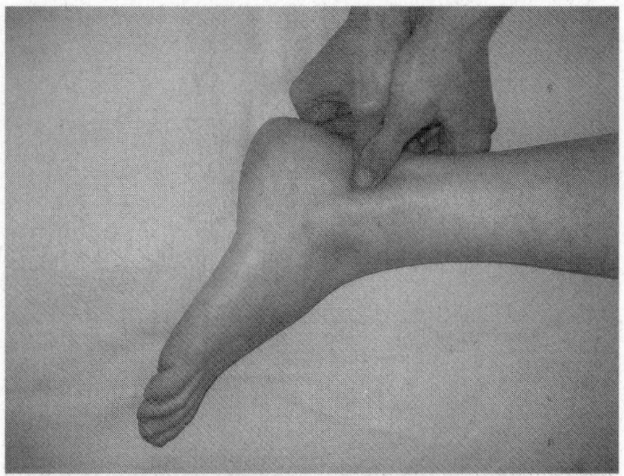

FIGURE 15-32 **Bl 60 (and Ki 3 on the opposite side).**
Bl 60: between the Achilles tendon and lateral malleolus (outer anklebone). Pinch and apply friction (wriggle).

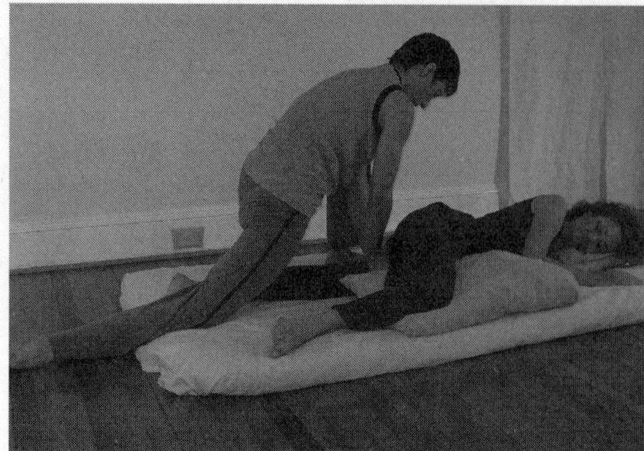

FIGURE 15-33 **Butterfly on the Yin Meridians.**
Straddle the client's leg in a kneeling lunge.

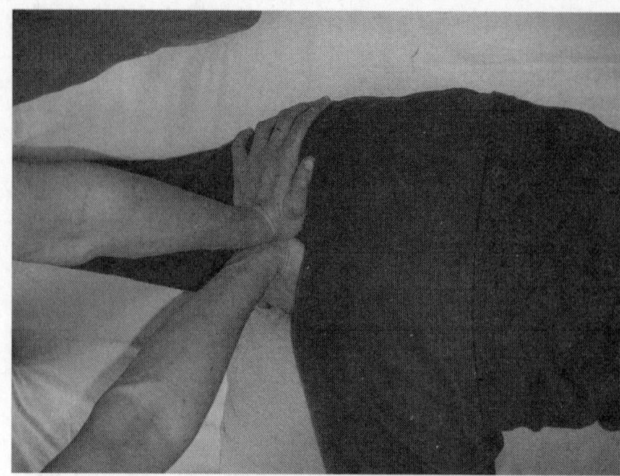

FIGURE 15-34 **Close-up of butterfly.**
Start as high as possible on the thigh while avoiding the client's genitals.

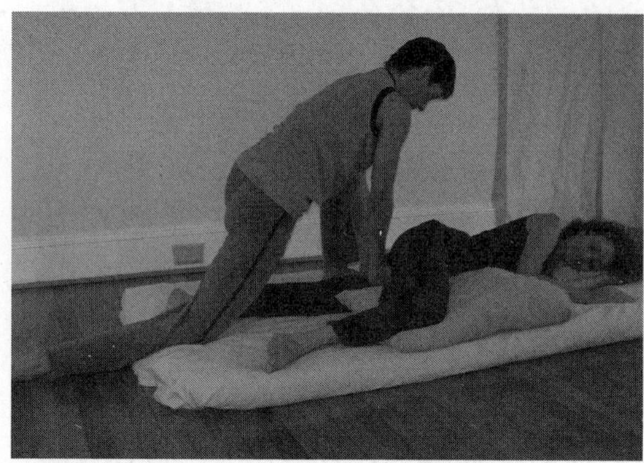

FIGURE 15-35 **Double fists on the Yin Meridians.**

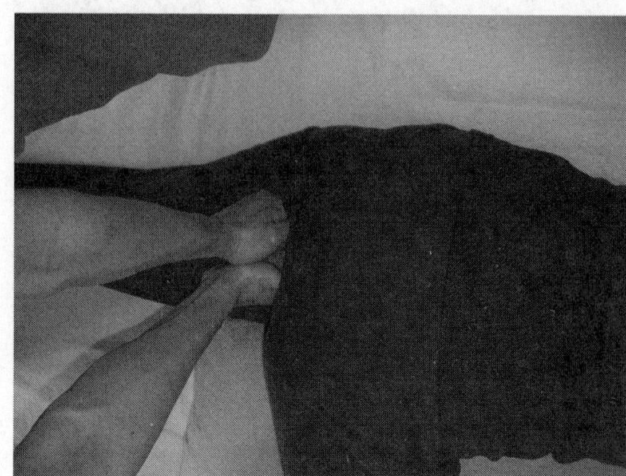

FIGURE 15-36 **Close-up of double fists.**

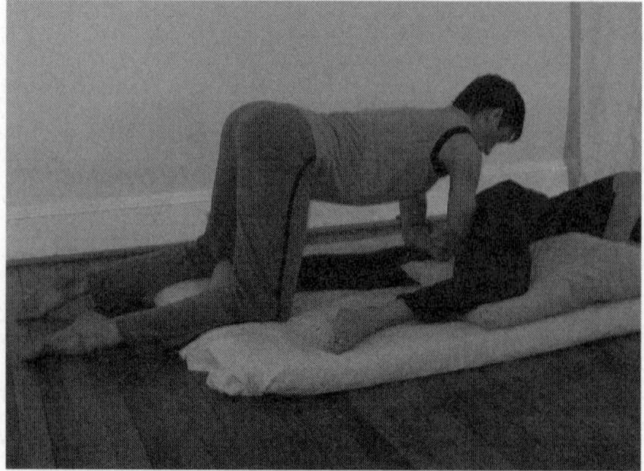

FIGURE 15-37 **Double forearms on the Yin Meridians.**
Straddle the client's leg in the crawl position.

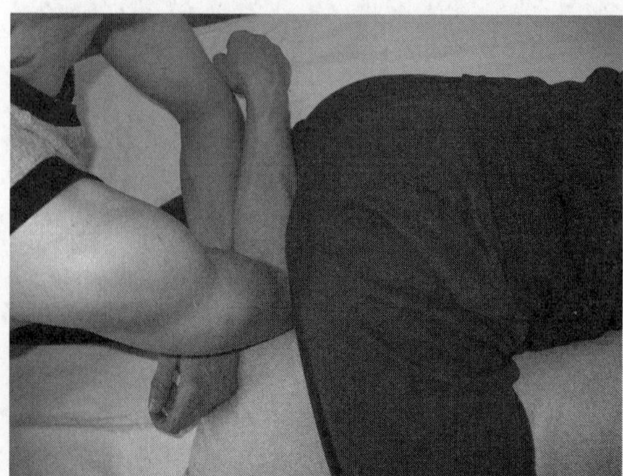

FIGURE 15-38 **Close-up of double forearms.**

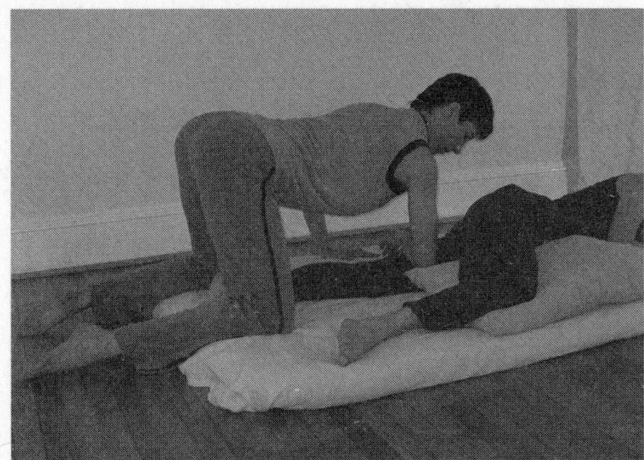

FIGURE 15-39 **Rolling pin, palm down.** Sink your forearm, palm down, into the adductors (inner thigh).

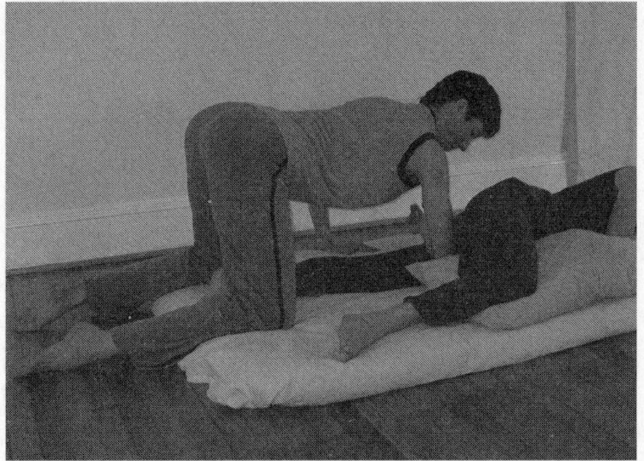

FIGURE 15-40 **Rolling pin, palm up.** Maintaining pressure, rotate your forearm, palm up. Alternate forearm pronation (palm down), and supination (palm up), rolling in place several times.

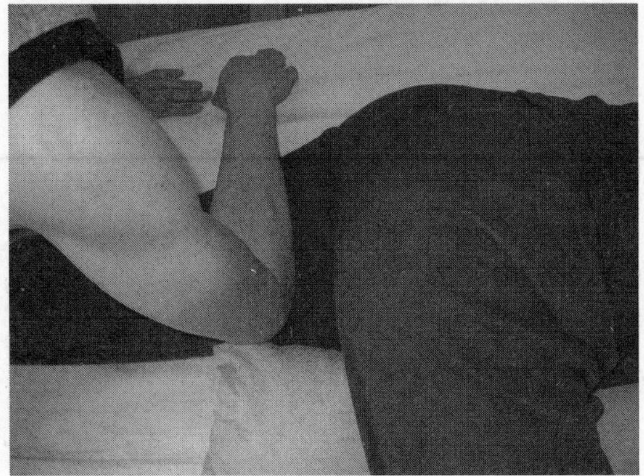

FIGURE 15-41 **Close-up of rolling pin, palm down.** Relocate your forearm and repeat, traversing the length of the adductors.

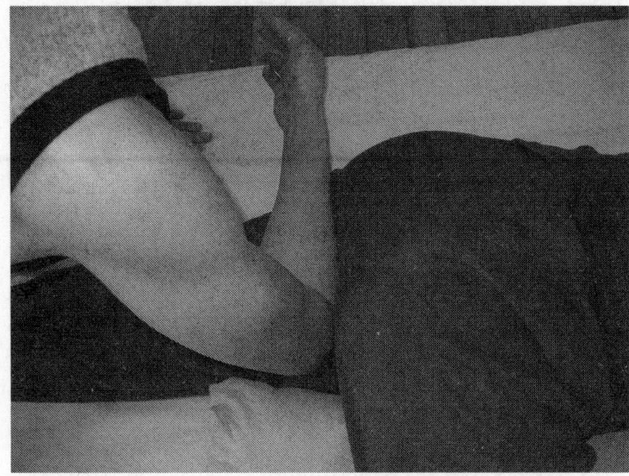

FIGURE 15-42 **Close-up of rolling pin, palm up.**

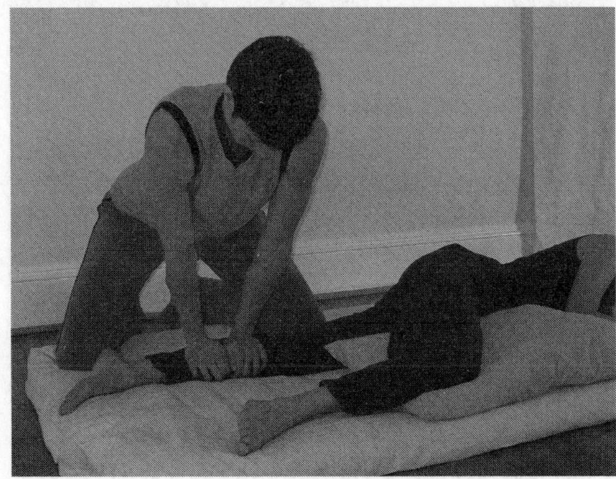

FIGURE 15-43 **Heels of the hands press on the Spleen and Liver Meridians.**

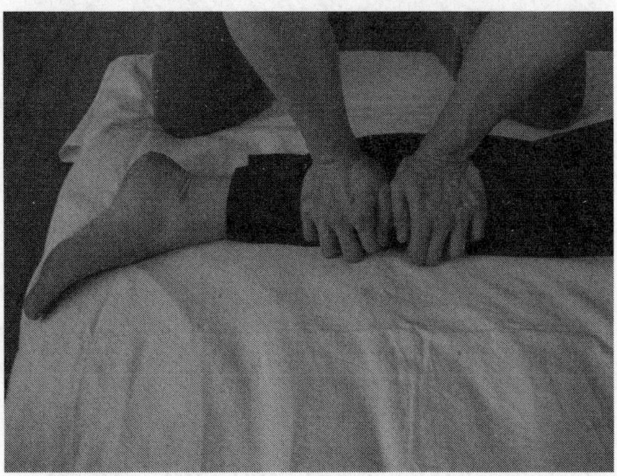

FIGURE 15-44 **Close-up of heel of the hand press.**

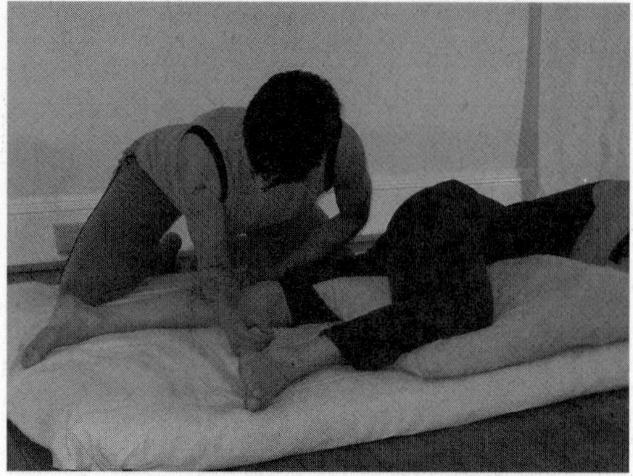

FIGURE 15-45 **Forearm press on the Yin Meridians.**
Use the fleshy part of your forearm and avoid pressing on the shinbone.

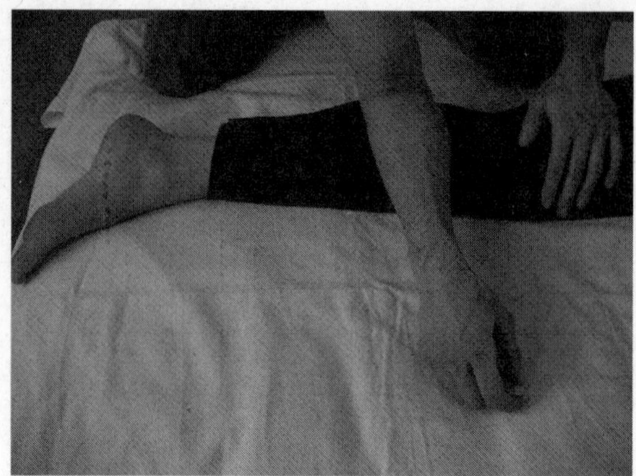

FIGURE 15-46 **Close-up of forearm press.**

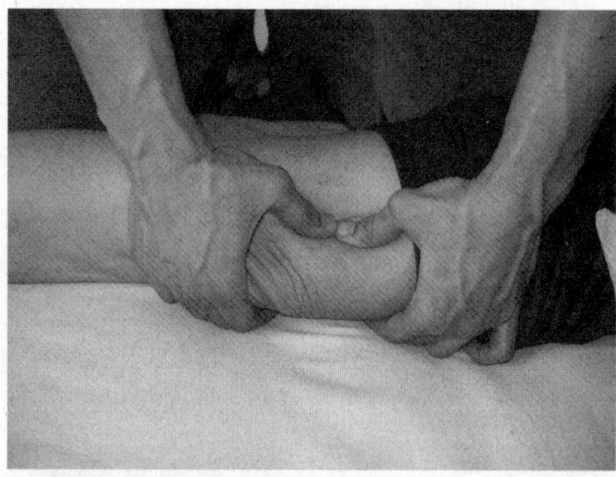

FIGURE 15-47 **Sp 10.**
On the vastus medialis (inner quadriceps) above the patella (kneecap).

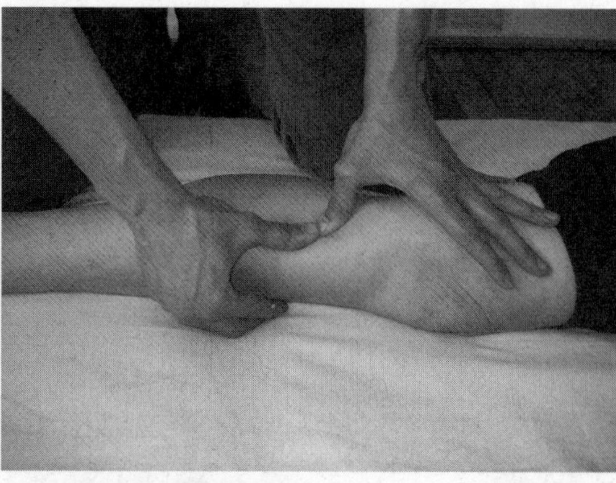

FIGURE 15-48 **Sp 9.**
In the bony hollow of the tibia (shin) below the patella (kneecap).

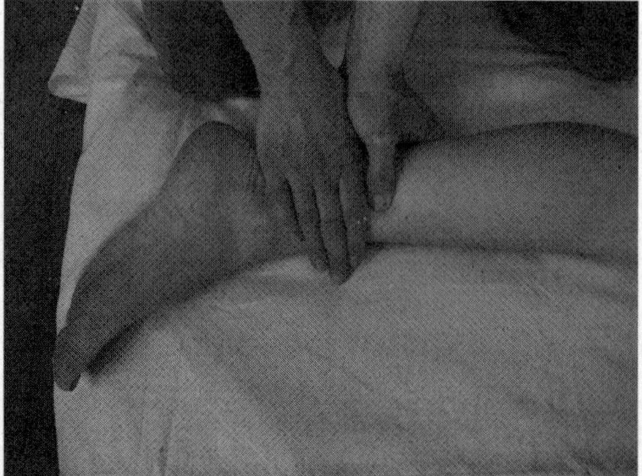

FIGURE 15-49 **Sp 6.**
Three cun (or four finger widths) above the medial malleolus (inner anklebone) against the tibia (shinbone).

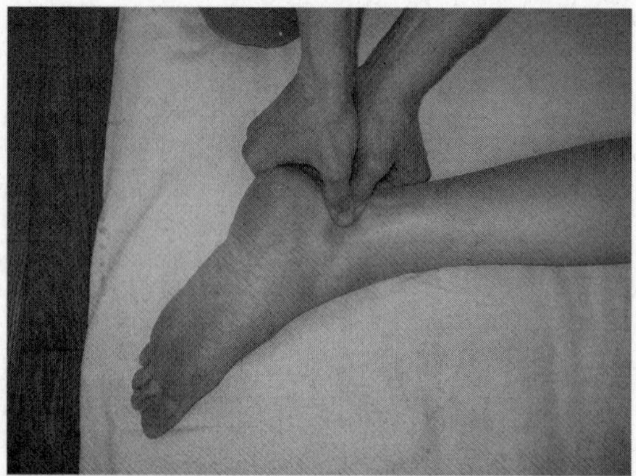

FIGURE 15-50
Ki 3 (and Bl 60 on the opposite side).
Ki 3: between the Achilles tendon and medial malleolus (inner anklebone).
Pinch and apply friction (wriggle).

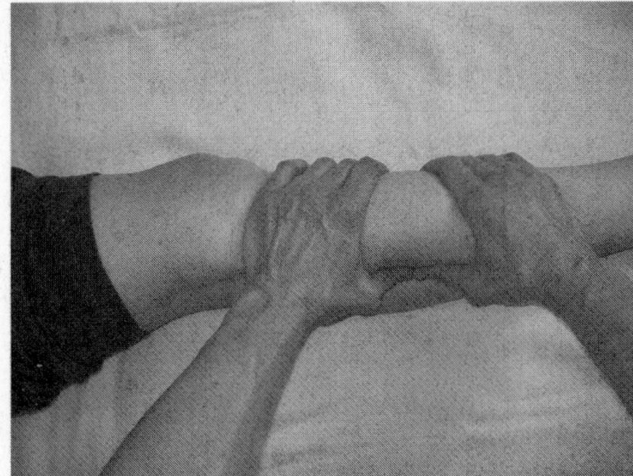

FIGURE 15-51 **Bl 56.**
On the belly of the calf, where the muscle is plumpest.

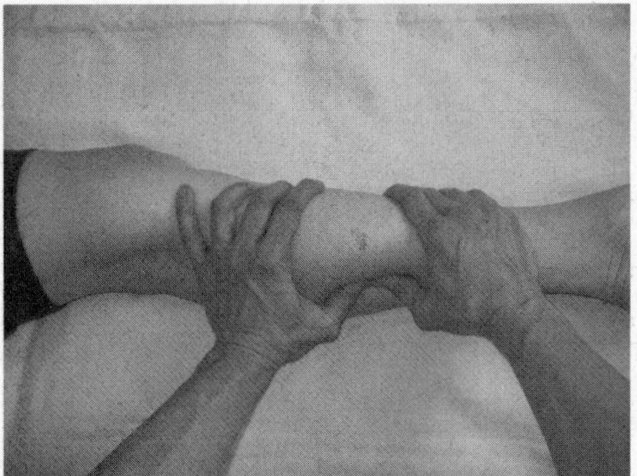

FIGURE 15-52 **Bl 57.**
Below the belly of the calf, where the muscle tapers.

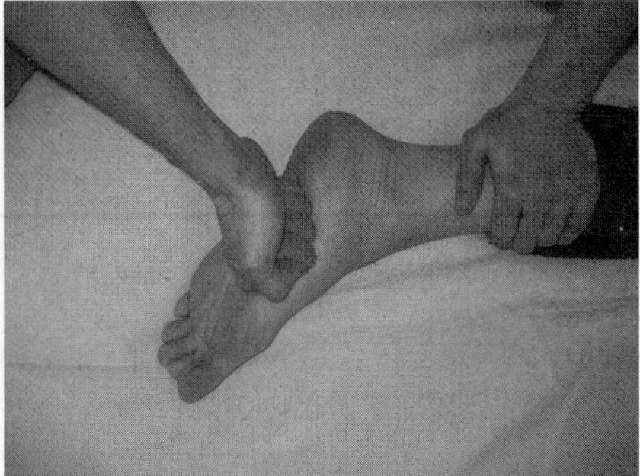

FIGURE 15-53 **Fist twist.**
Work the entire sole of the foot.

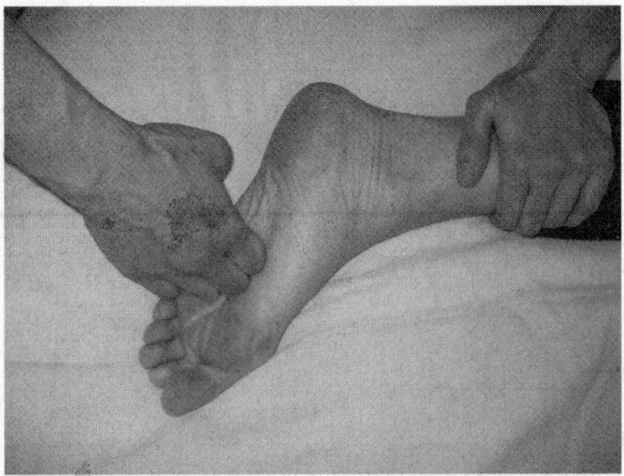

FIGURE 15-54 **Knuckle press or apply friction.**
Work the entire sole of the foot.

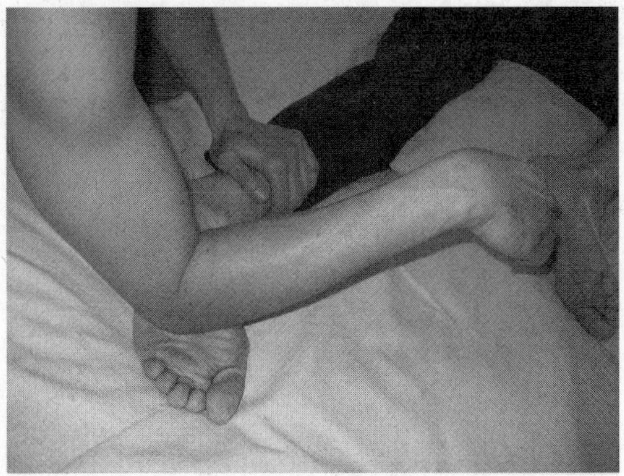

FIGURE 15-55 **Elbow press.**

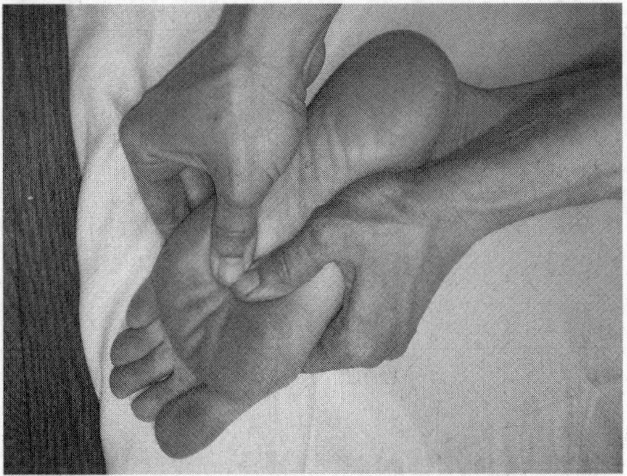

FIGURE 15-56 **Ki 1.**
Above the calloused ball of the foot between the second and third metatarsals. Use knuckles instead of thumbs to press or apply friction, if preferred.

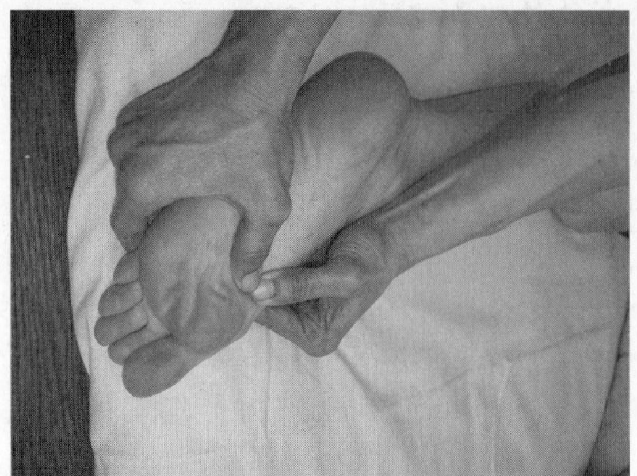

FIGURE 15-57 **Sp 3.**
On the inner arch under the first metatarsal.

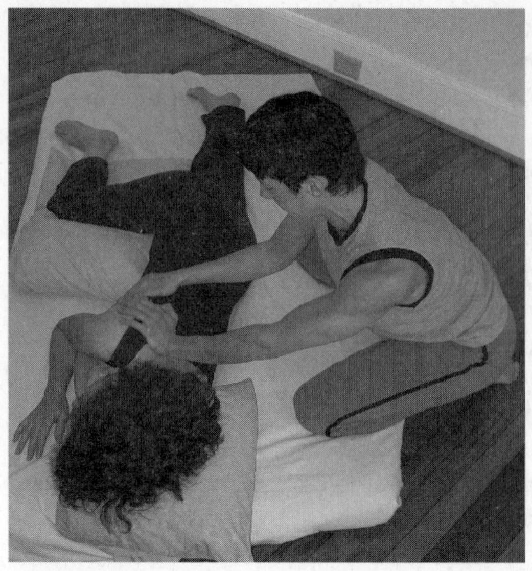

FIGURE 15-58 **Palm press on the Bladder Meridian, side view.**
When compressing the client's back, stabilize by counter-pulling on the client's ribcage or hip to prevent the client from collapsing forward into a semi-prone position.

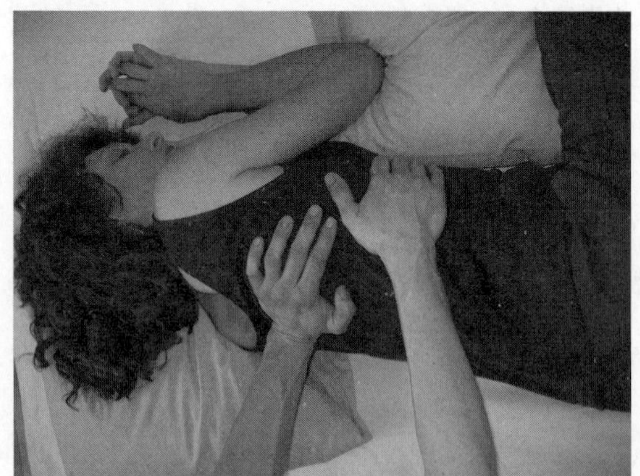

FIGURE 15-59 **Palm press, middle back.**

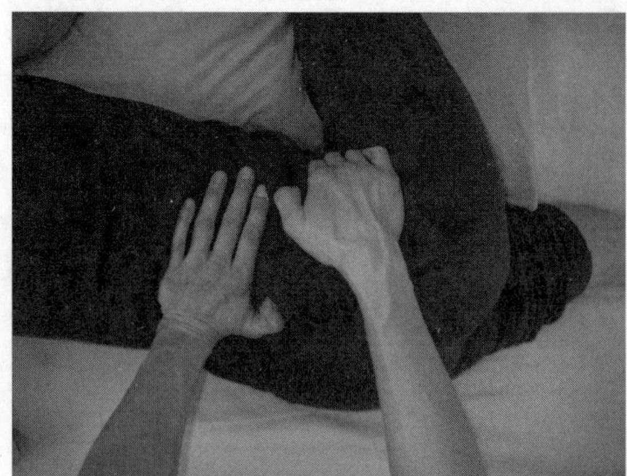

FIGURE 15-60 **Palm press, lower back.**

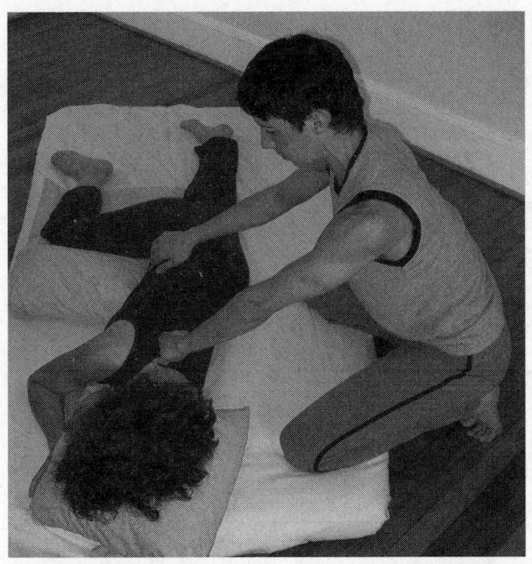

FIGURE 15-61 **Fist presses the Bladder Meridian, side view.**
Take care to avoid the spinal column when using heavy tools like the fist.

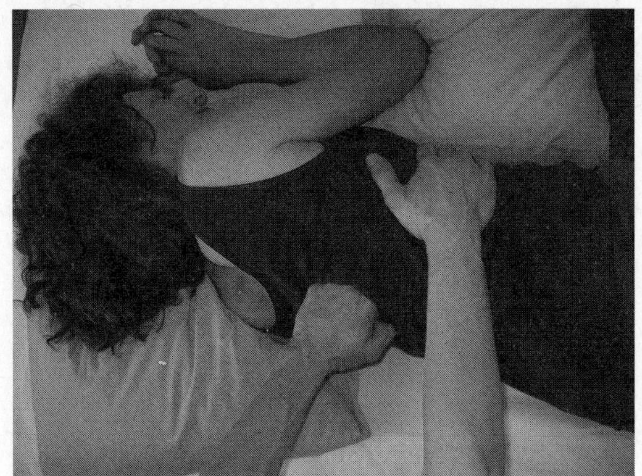

FIGURE 15-62 **Fist press, middle back.**

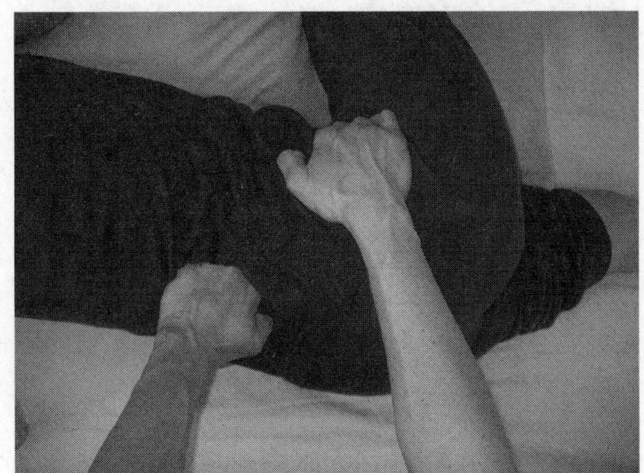

FIGURE 15-63 **Fist press, lower back.**

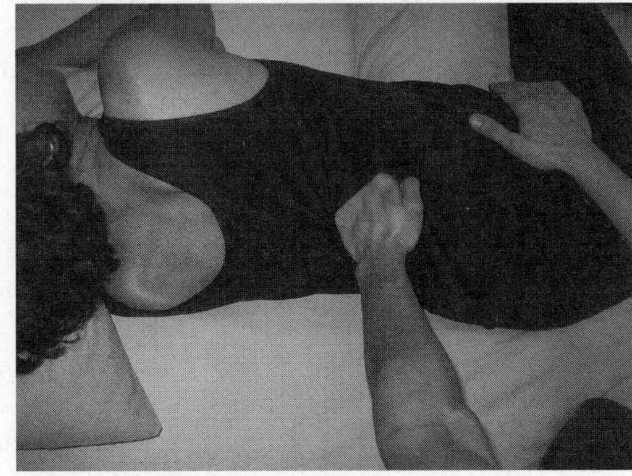

FIGURE 15-64 **Fist twist.**
Engage the deeper layer of muscle.

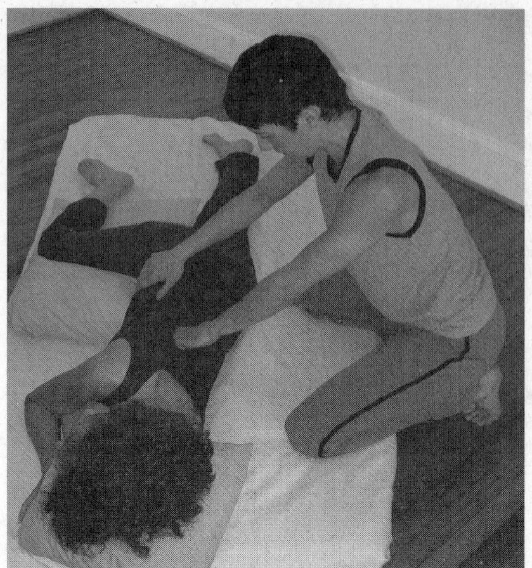

FIGURE 15-65 **Knuckles press the Bladder Meridan, side view.**
Take care to avoid the spinal column when using heavy tools like the knuckles.

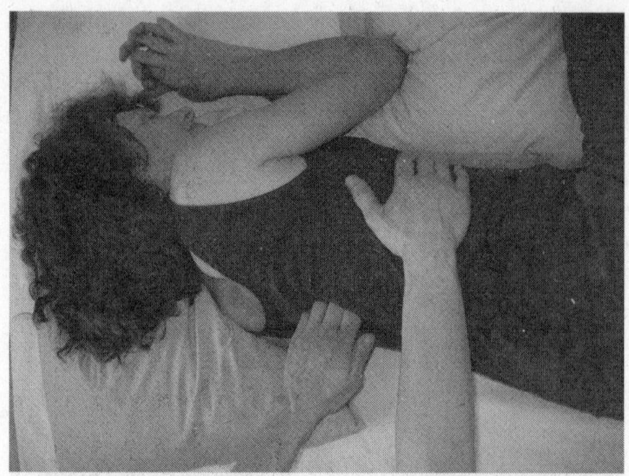

FIGURE 15-66 **Knuckle press, middle back.**

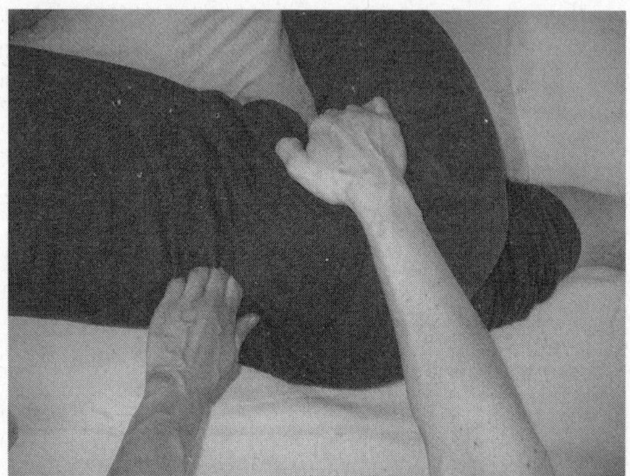

FIGURE 15-67 **Knuckle press, lower back.**

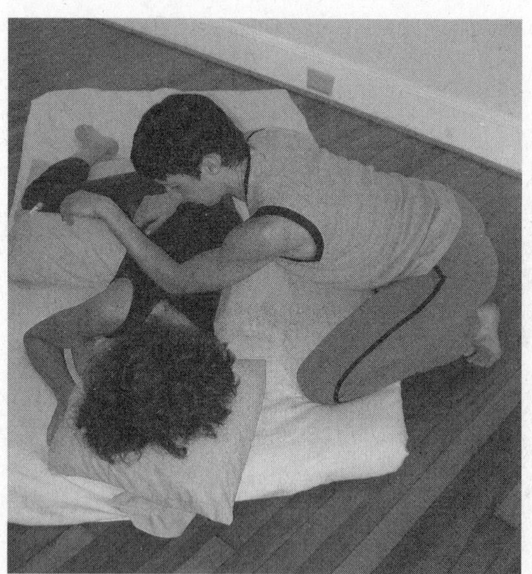

FIGURE 15-68 **Elbow presses the Bladder Meridian, side view.**
Take care to avoid the spinal column when using heavy tools like the elbow.

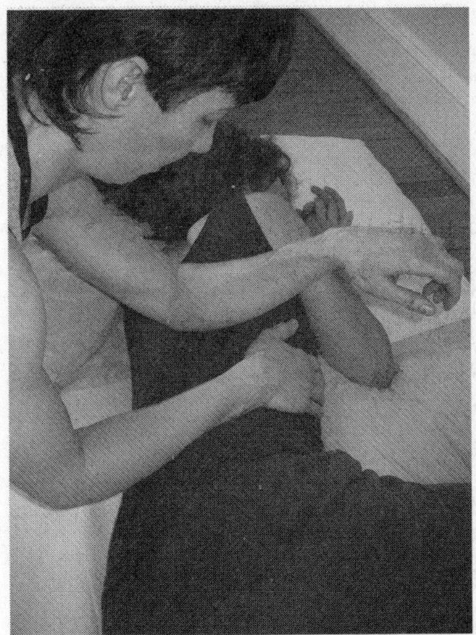

FIGURE 15-69 **Elbow press, middle back.**

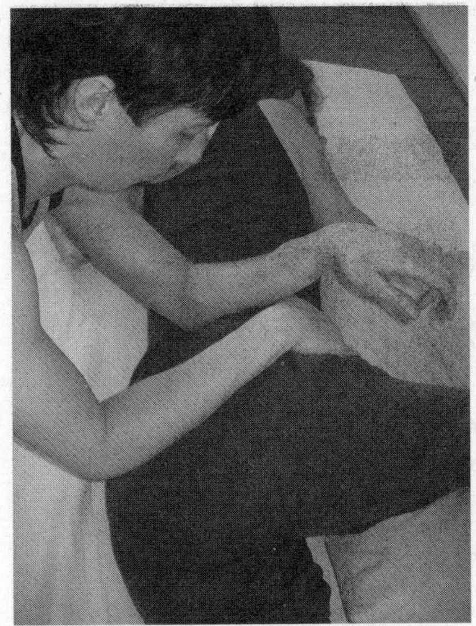

FIGURE 15-70 **Elbow press, lower back.**

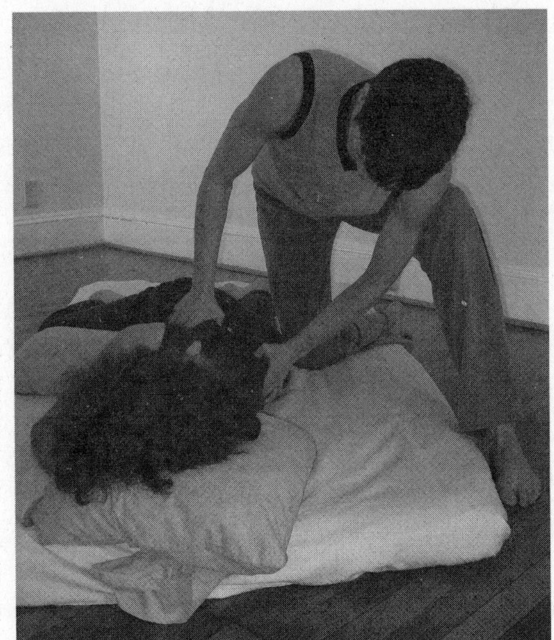

FIGURE 15-71 **Thumbs press the Bladder Meridian.**
To create leverage, brace your arm against your leg to provide firm resistance as you press along the inner and outer Bladder Meridians.

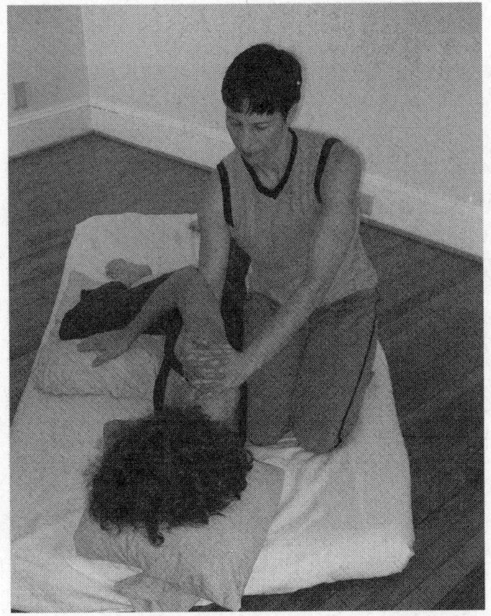

FIGURE 15-72 **Shoulder traction.**
Support the client's back with the side of your thigh. Wrap one arm under the client's arm and clasp your hands above the client's shoulder. Pull downward and release several times.

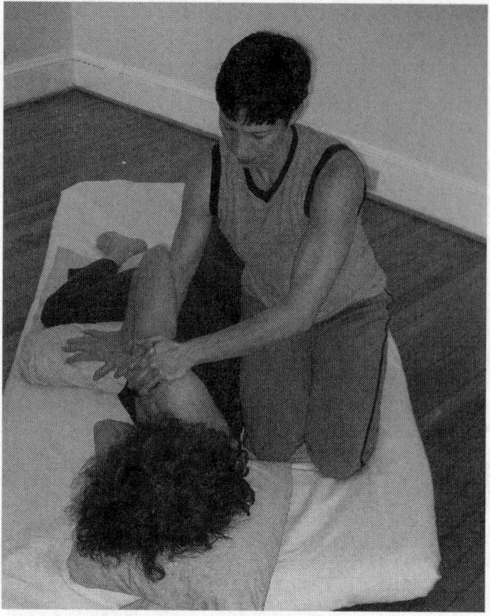

FIGURE 15-73 **Shoulder rotation, forward phase.**
Rotate the shoulder joint by first pushing forward and up, and then pulling backward and down.

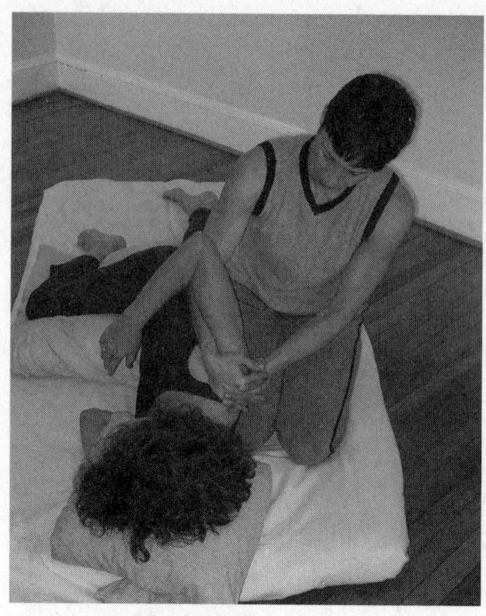

FIGURE 15-74 **Shoulder rotation, backward phase.**
Rotate several times.

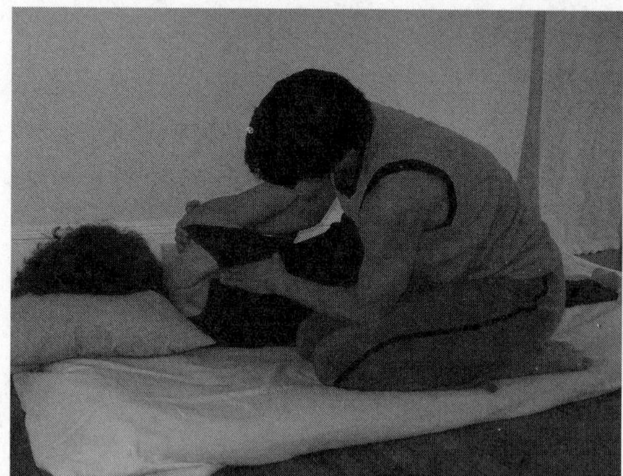

FIGURE 15-75 **Finger press under the scapula.**
With your stabilizing hand, depress and retract the shoulder by pulling it downward and backward to provide firm counterresistance. With your dynamic hand, press your fingers under the scapula (shoulderblade).

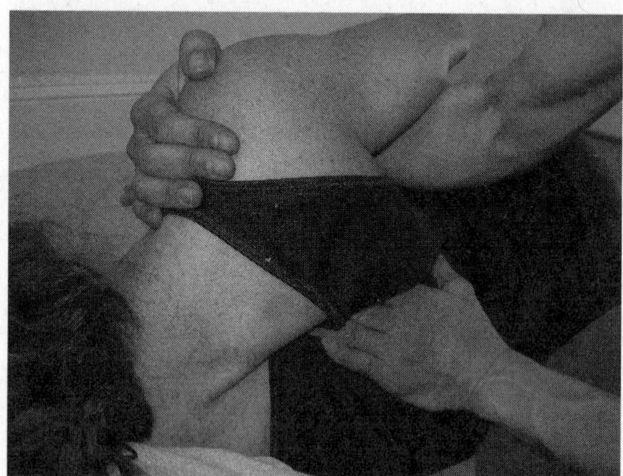

FIGURE 15-76 **Close-up of finger press.**
Repeat several times, working the entire vertebral border of the scapula (the edge of the shoulderblade next to the spine). On some clients, you will be able to insert your fingers under the scapula, as shown here.

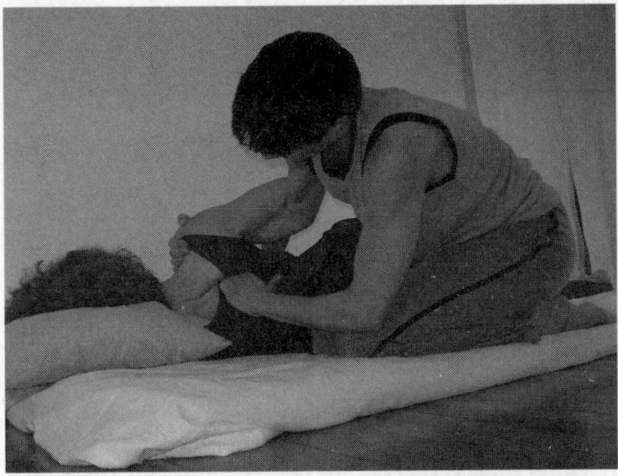

FIGURE 15-77 **Knuckles press under the scapula.**

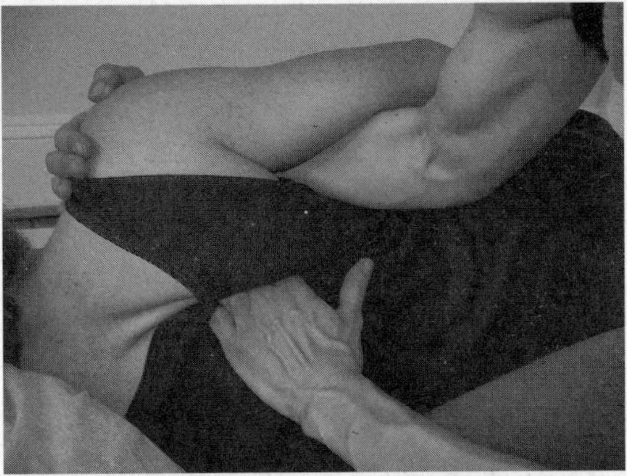

FIGURE 15-78 **Close-up of knuckle press.** As the knuckles of your dynamic hand press under the scapula, the palm of your stabilizing hand pulls the shoulder down and back.

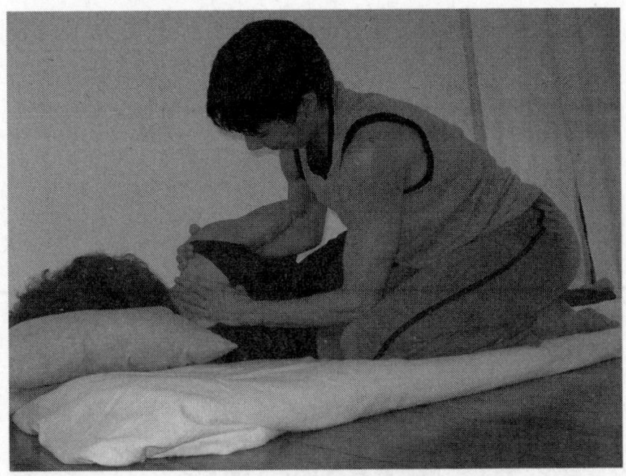

FIGURE 15-79 **Thumb presses under the scapula.**

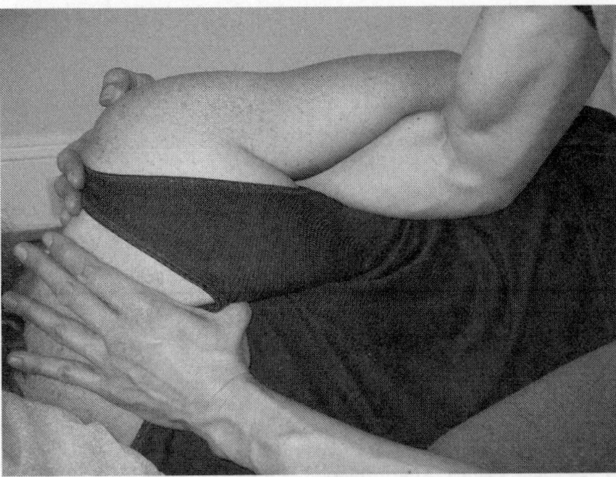

FIGURE 15-80 **Close-up of thumb press.**

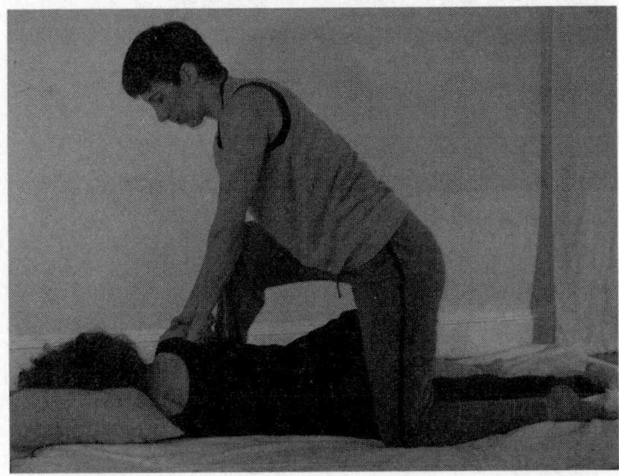

FIGURE 15-81 **Fist twist on the posterior scapula.**
Continue kneeling in seiza behind the client, or straddle the client in a kneeling lunge (as shown here). Support the front of the client's shoulder by bracing it with your stabilizing hand (as shown here) or by hooking your arm under the client's arm (see Figure 15-82).

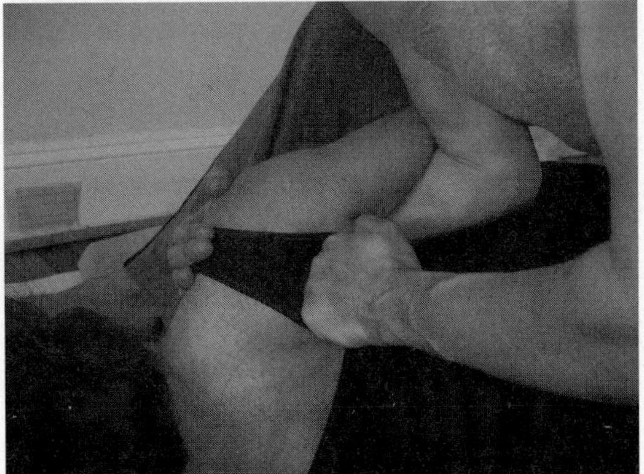

FIGURE 15-82 **Close-up of fist twist.**
Press and rotate your fist on the scapula to warm and loosen the rotator cuff.

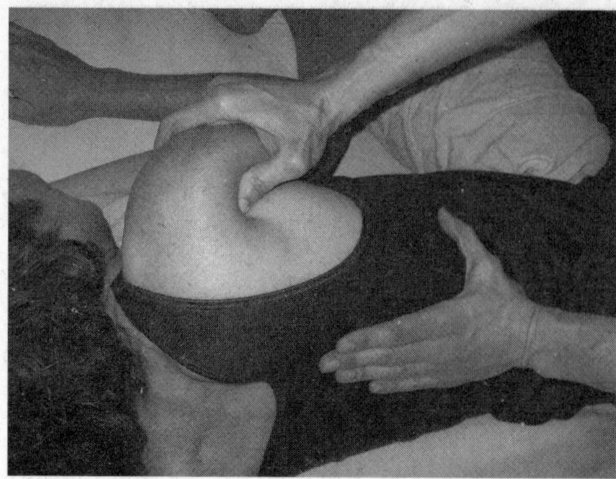

FIGURE 15-83 **SI 9.**
At the axillary (armpit) crease on the teres major.

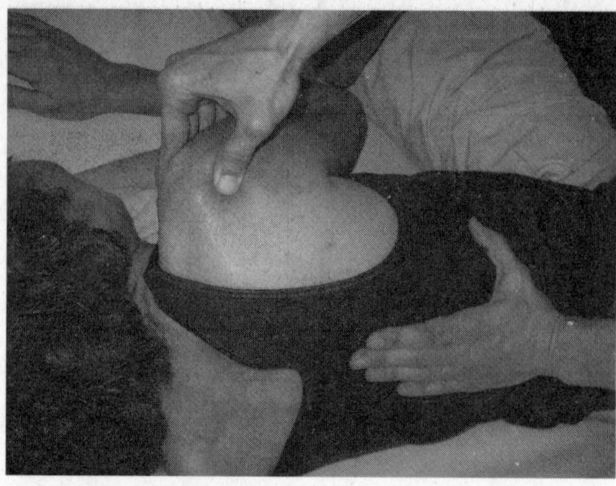

FIGURE 15-84 **SI 10.**
On the posterior deltoid.

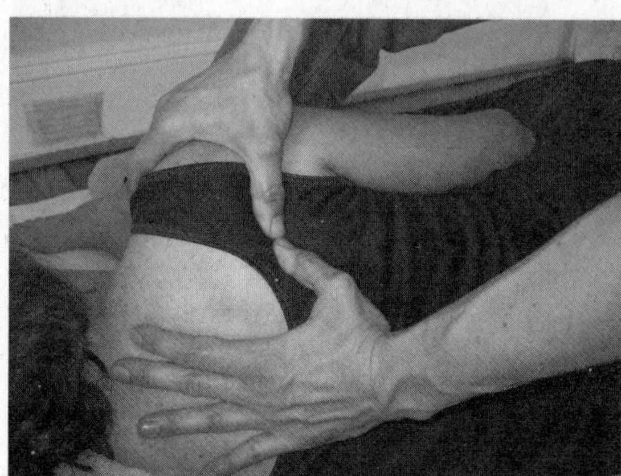

FIGURE 15-85 **SI 11.**
On the infraspinatus in the center of the scapula.

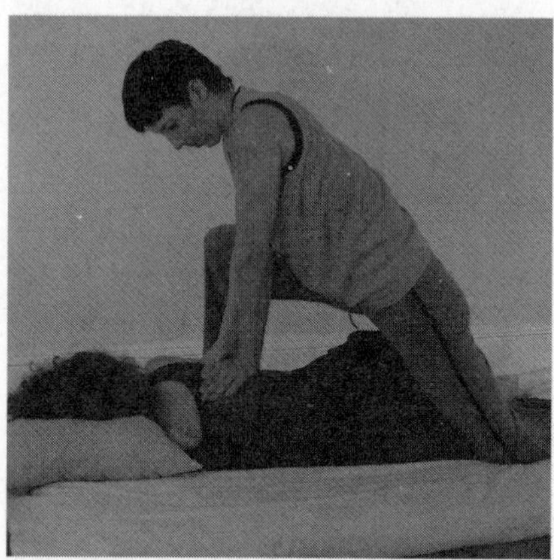

FIGURE 15-86 **Dragon's mouth on the Gallbladder Meridian.**
Continue to straddle the client's side and drape the client's arm forward to access the side of the client's torso.

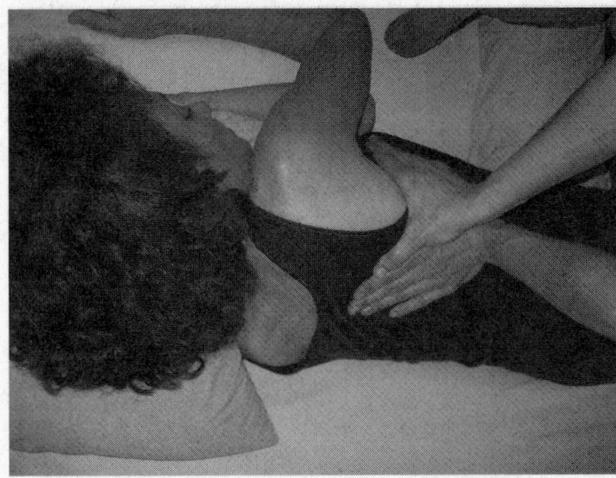

FIGURE 15-87 **Close-up of dragon's mouth on the Gallbladder Meridian.** Splay the index fingers and thumbs of both hands apart and press downward. Work down the side of the torso to the hips.

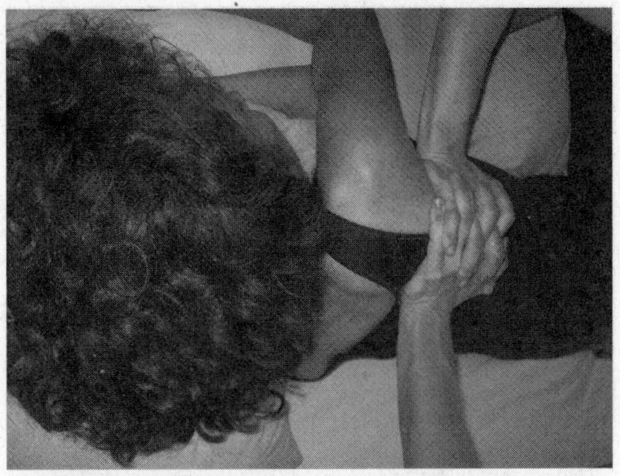

FIGURE 15-88 **Close-up of hand clasp on the Gallbladder Meridian.** Repeat with your hands clasped and your fingers interlaced, pressing the heels of your hands inward. Work down the side of the torso to the hips.

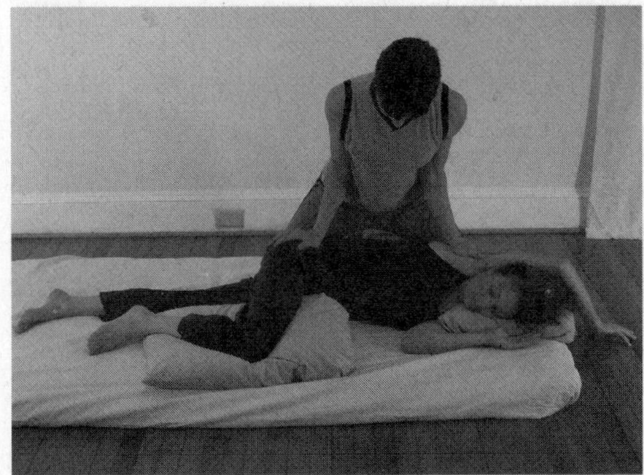

FIGURE 15-89 **Side traction.** Kneel upright, facing the client. Drape the client's arm overhead. Plant one hand below the axilla (armpit) and other on the hip. Push outward in opposite directions.

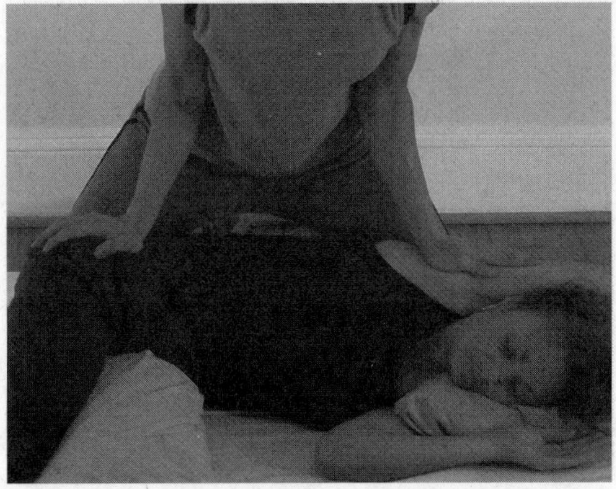

FIGURE 15-90 **Close-up of side traction.** You can also cross your arms to perform this stretch (not shown).

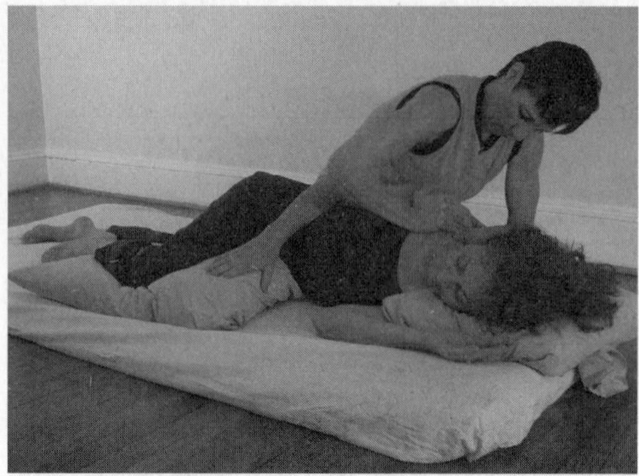

FIGURE 15-91 **Hand clasp on the chest and shoulder.**
Kneel sideways in seiza, supporting the client against your thigh. Clasp your hands around the hub of the shoulder and press and rub.

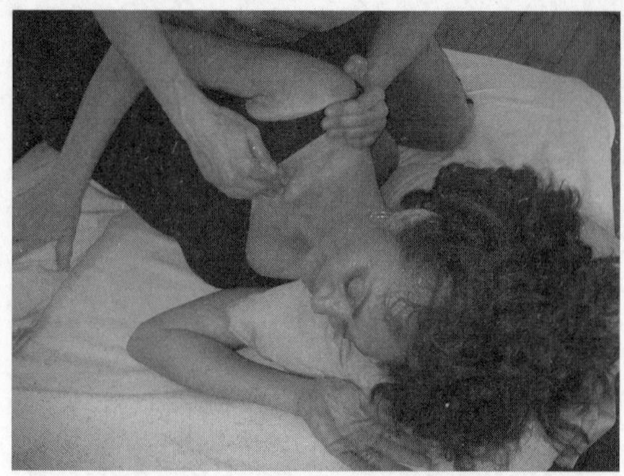

FIGURE 15-92 **Fingertip friction at Ki 27.**
At the juncture of the sternum (breastbone) and clavicle (collarbone).

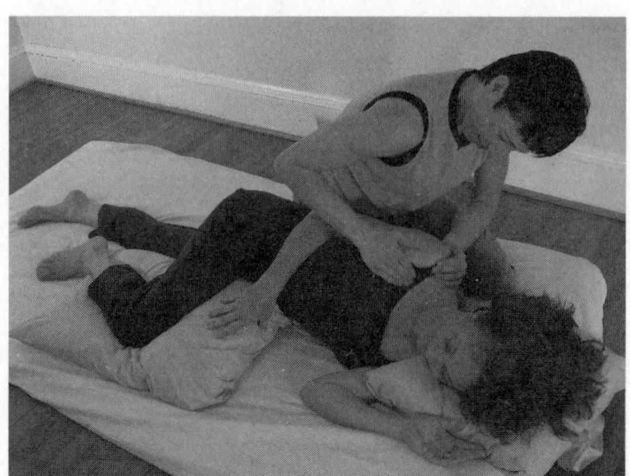

FIGURE 15-93 **Fingertip friction at Lu 1.**
Two cun down from the outer end of the clavicle (collarbone) on the pectoralis (chest muscle).

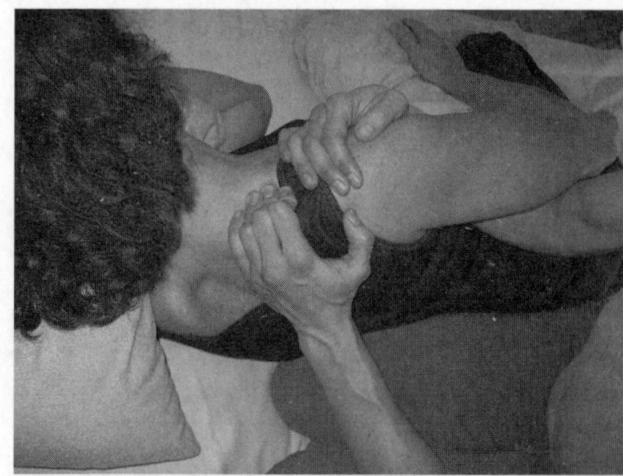

FIGURE 15-94 **Fingertips press GB 21.**
Hook your arm under the client's to stabilize the shoulder. Press and apply friction to the upper trapezius (top of the shoulder), especially GB 21.

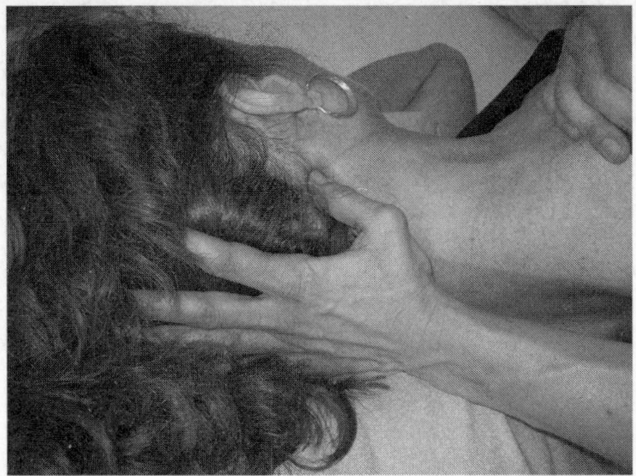

FIGURE 15-95 **Thumb presses GB 20.**
Below the occiput (bony ridge at the base of the skull) between the sternocleidomastoid and upper trapezius.

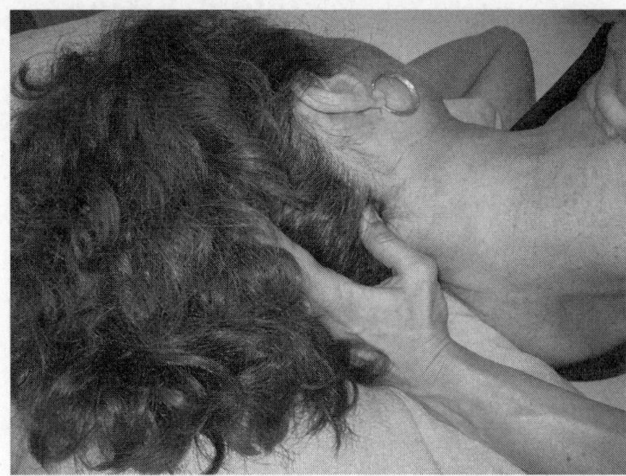

FIGURE 15-96 **Thumb presses Bl 10.**
Below the occiput on the upper trapezius, a ropey band of muscle.

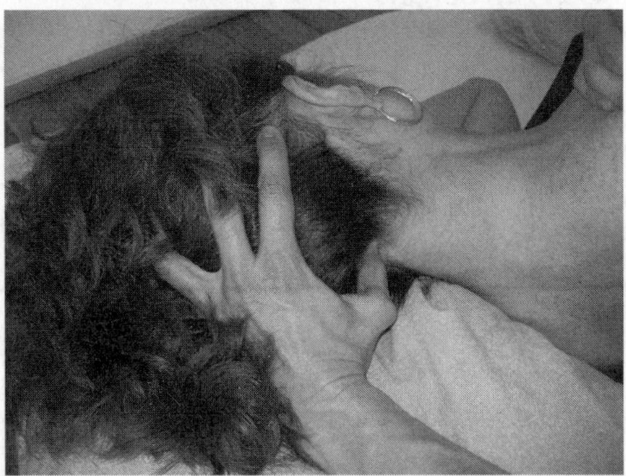

FIGURE 15-97 **Thumb presses GV 16.**
In the notch at the posterior midline of the neck.

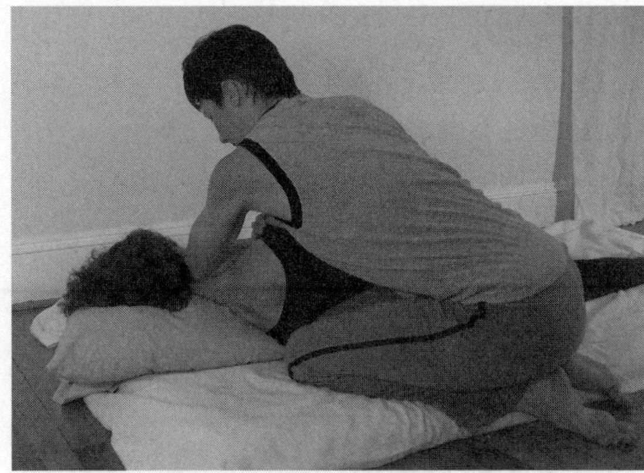

FIGURE 15-98 **Elbow tractions the neck.**
Angle your kneeling position diagonally, as shown. Press upward on the neck with the fleshy part of your forearm. Relocate your forearm and repeat, moving down to the shoulder.

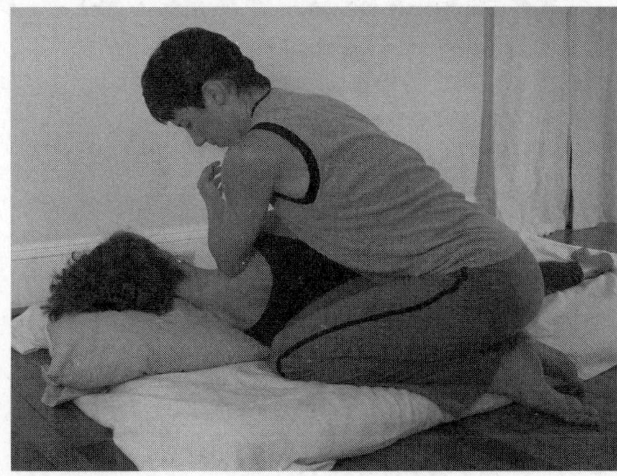

FIGURE 15-99 **Elbow depresses the shoulder.**
Press downward on the shoulder with the fleshy part of your forearm.

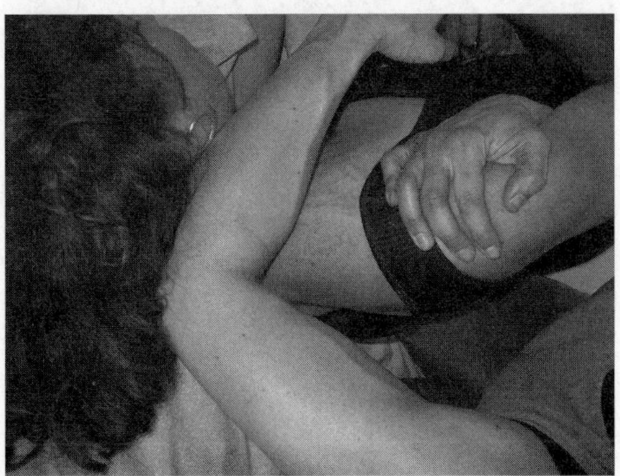

FIGURE 15-100 **Close-up of elbow tractioning the neck.**

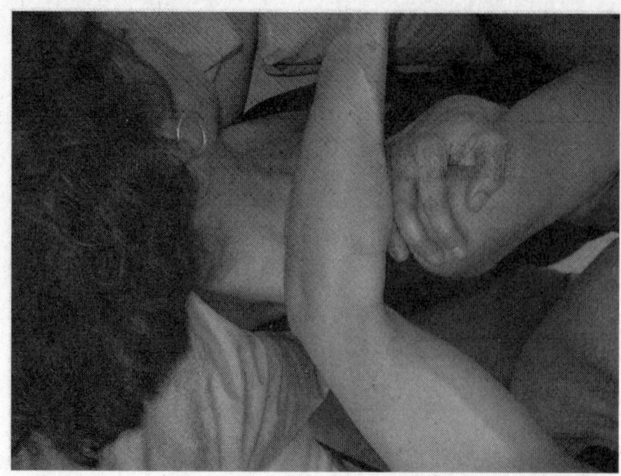

FIGURE 15-101 **Close-up of elbow depressing the shoulder.**

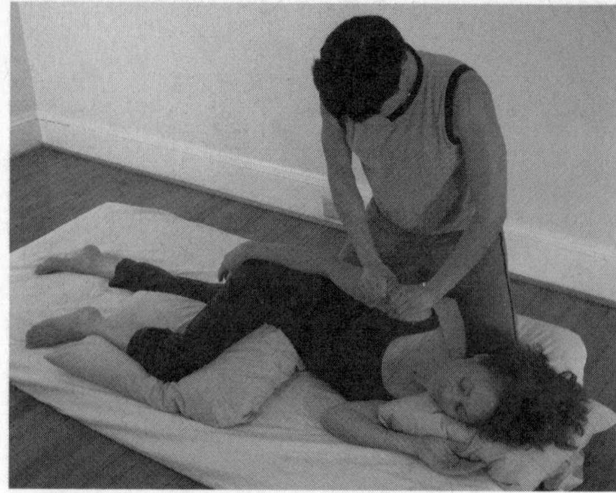

FIGURE 15-102 **Pincer grip on the Lung and Small Intestine Meridians.**
Rise to an upright kneeling position and place the client's arm alongside the client's body.

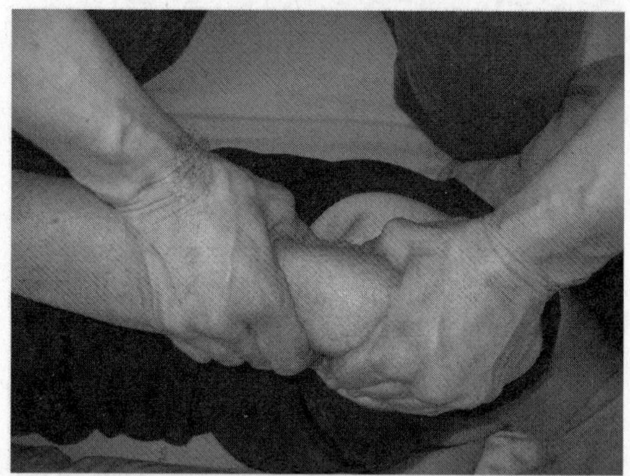

FIGURE 15-103 **Close-up of pincer grip.**
Squeeze the client's upper arm between your fingers and thumbs.

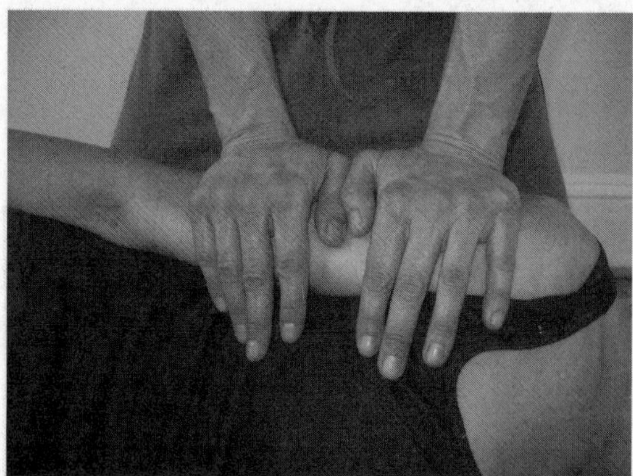

FIGURE 15-104 **Palms press the Large Intestine and Triple Heater Meridians.**
Press straight down toward the floor with both hands. Compress the length of the upper arm.

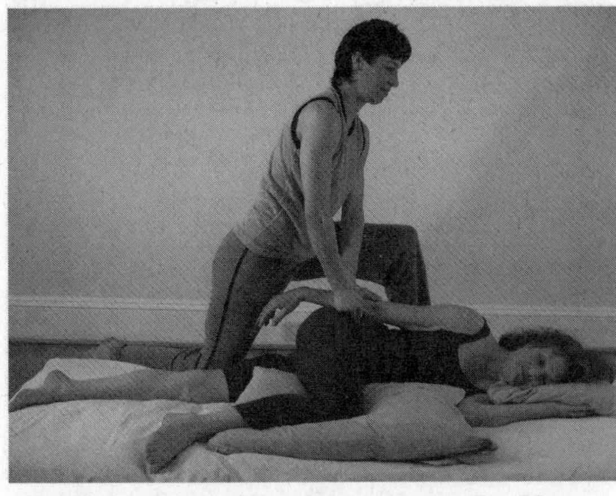

FIGURE 15-105 **Hands squeeze the Yang and Yin Meridians.**
In a kneeling lunge beside the client, wrap your fingers around the client's forearm and squeeze both sides like a torniquet.

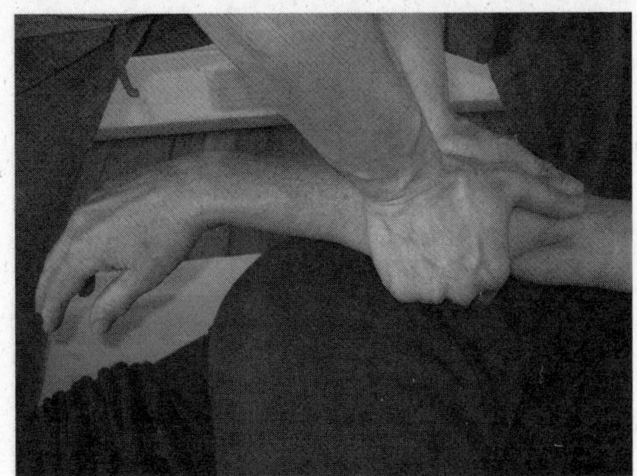

FIGURE 15-106 **Close-up of hand squeeze.**
Compress the length of the forearm.

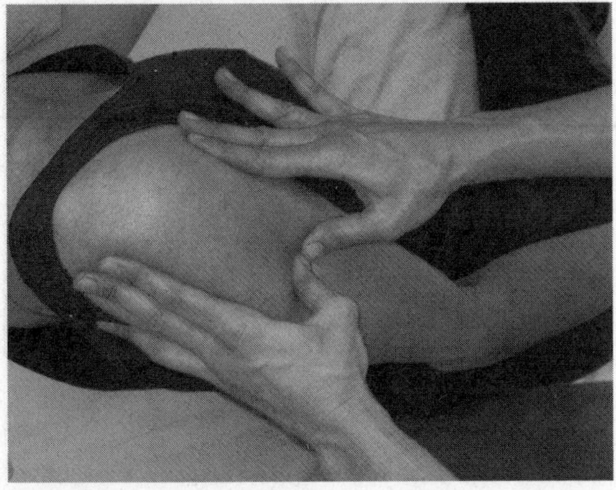

FIGURE 15-107 **LI 14.**
Just in front of and above the deltoid (shoulder muscle) insertion.

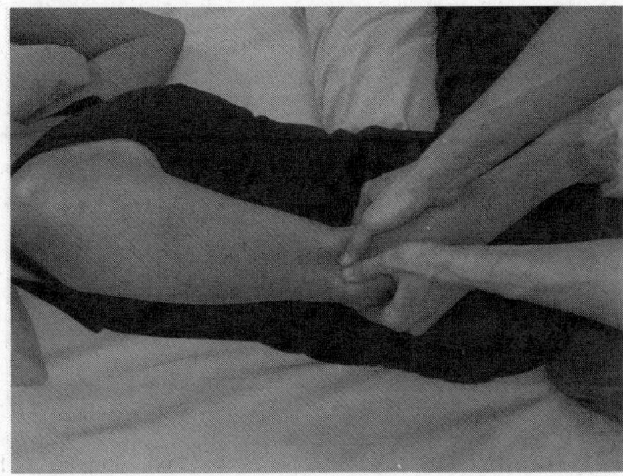

FIGURE 15-108 **LI 11.**
At the elbow on the radial (thumb) side.

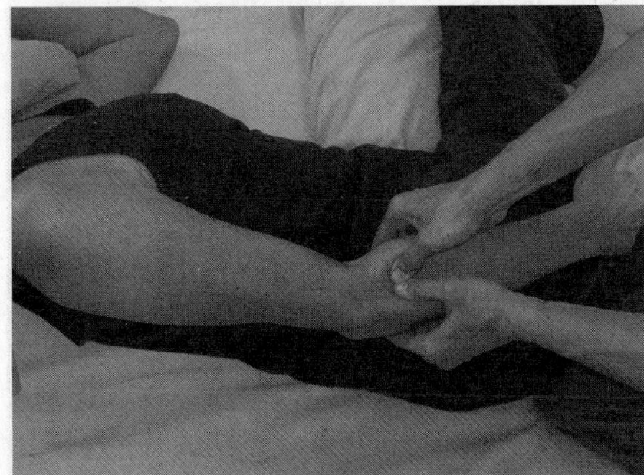

FIGURE 15-109 **LI 10.**
Two cun below the elbow on the outer forearm.

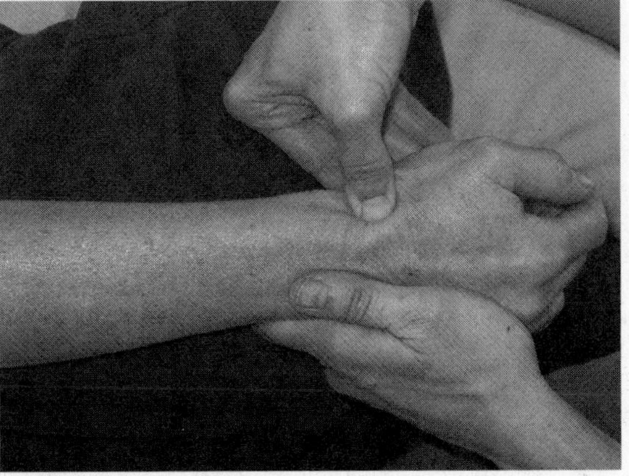

FIGURE 15-110 **LI 5.**
In the bony hollow between the two thumb tendons.

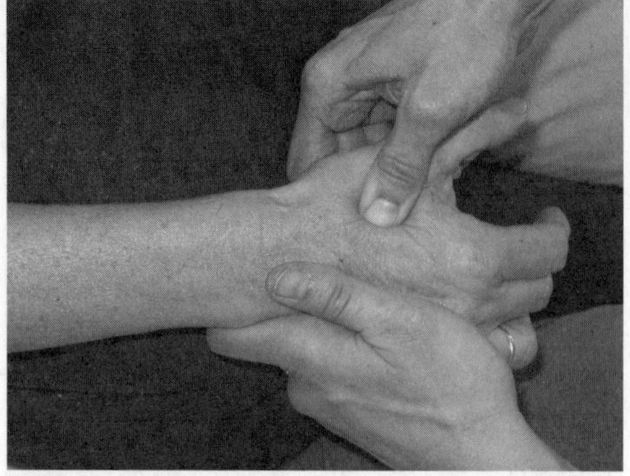

FIGURE 15-111 **LI 4.**
In the fleshy web between the index finger and thumb, pressing toward the index finger.

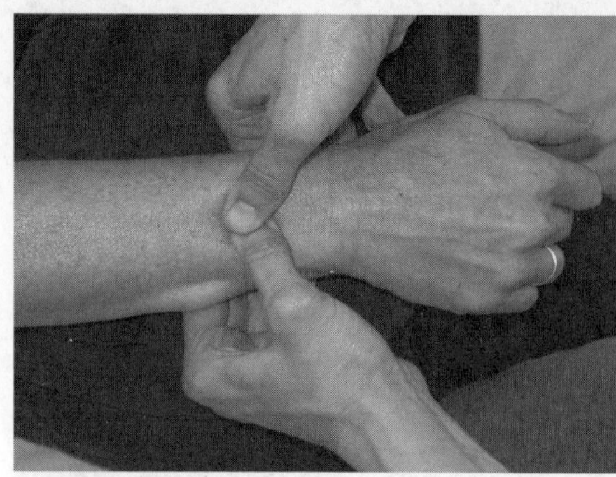

FIGURE 15-112 **TH 5.**
Two cun above the outer wrist.

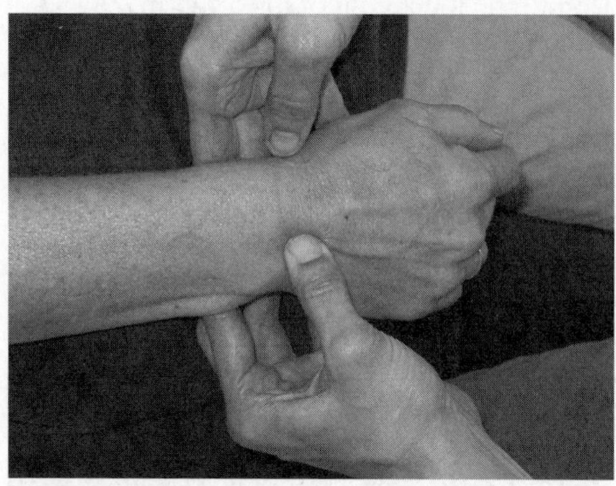

FIGURE 15-113 **TH 4.**
In the middle of the outer wrist, slightly toward the ulnar (little finger) side.

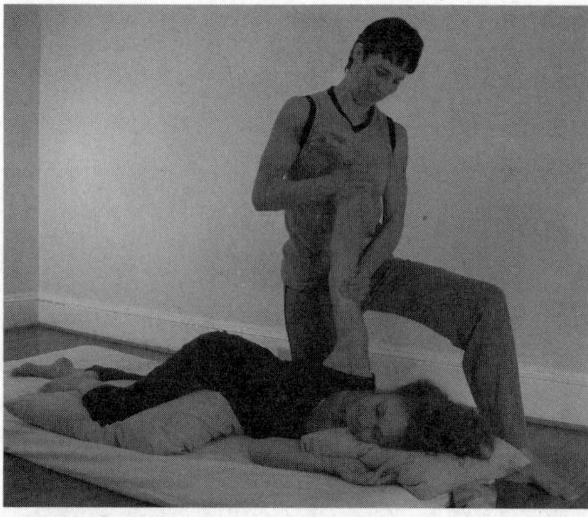

FIGURE 15-114 **Arm traction.**
Hold the client's arm above the wrist and elbow. Pull upward.

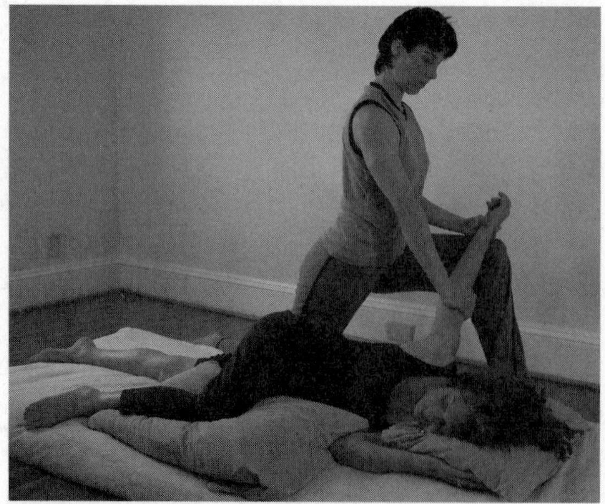

FIGURE 15-115 **Hand squeezes the Yin Meridians of the upper arm.**
In a kneeling lunge, place the client's forearm on your thigh, palm up, holding the wrist. Compress the client's upper arm.

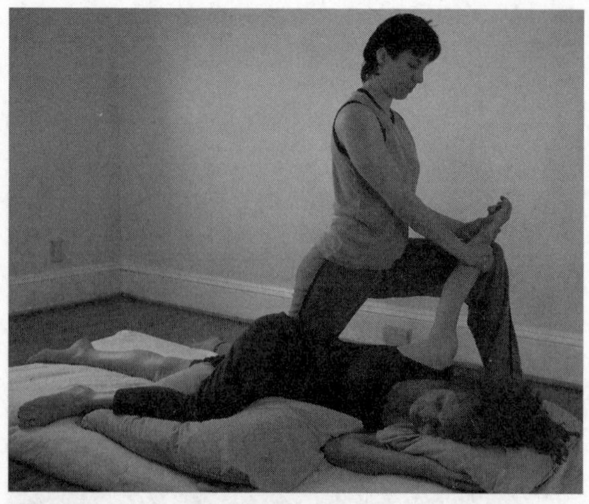

FIGURE 15-116 **Hand squeezes the Yin Meridians of the forearm.**
Continue compressing the client's forearm.

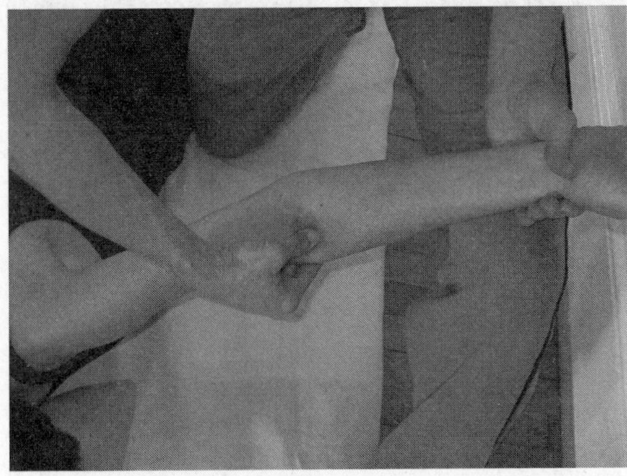

FIGURE 15-117 **Lu 5.**
On the radial (thumb) side of the inner forearm just below the elbow.

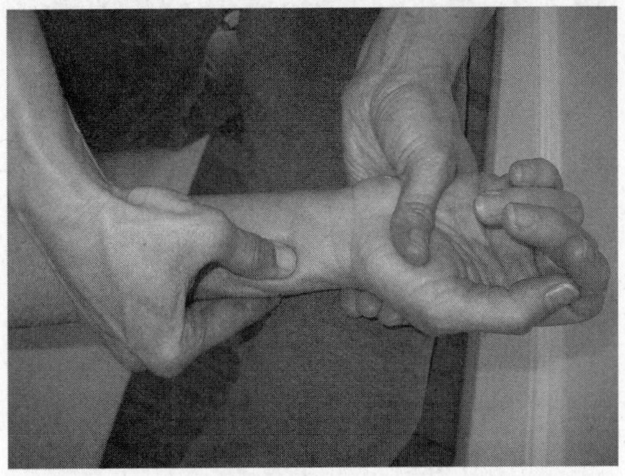

FIGURE 15-118 **Lu 7.**
One and a half cun above the radial (thumb) side of the inner wrist, just above the styloid process of the radius.

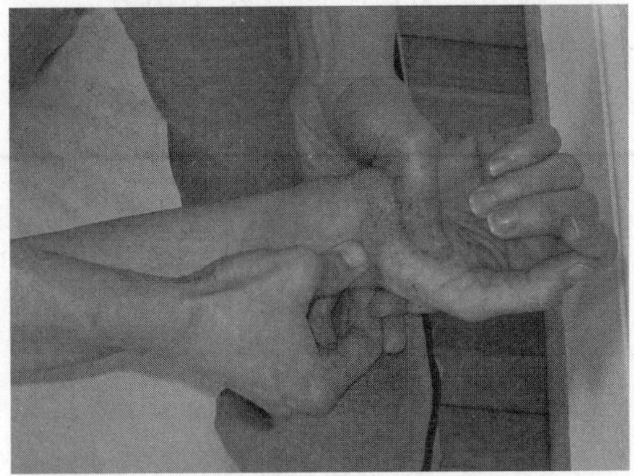

FIGURE 15-119 **Lu 9.**
On the radial (thumb) side of the inner wrist.

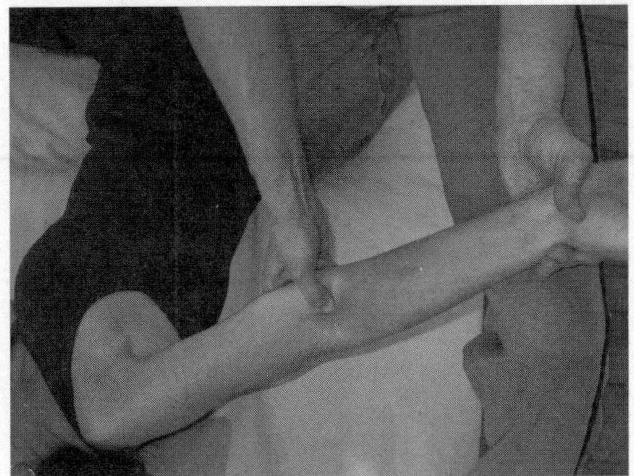

FIGURE 15-120 **PC 3.**
On the biceps tendon just above the elbow.

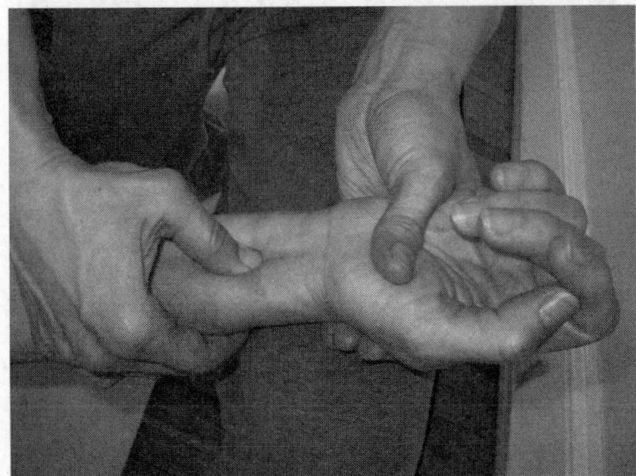

FIGURE 15-121 **PC 6.**
Two cun above the inner wrist, between the two wrist flexor tendons.

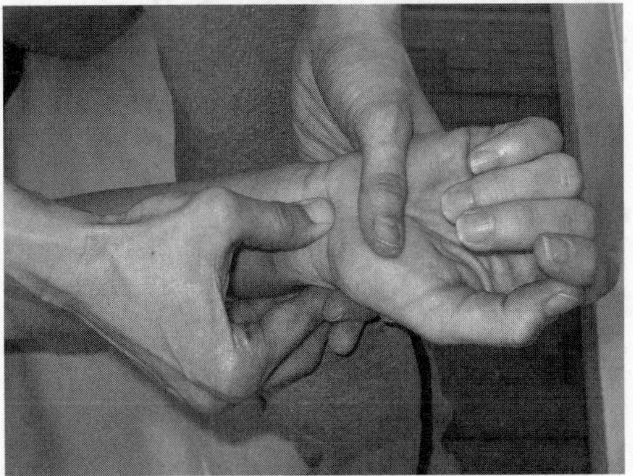

FIGURE 15-122 **PC 7.**
On the inner wrist, between the two wrist flexor tendons.

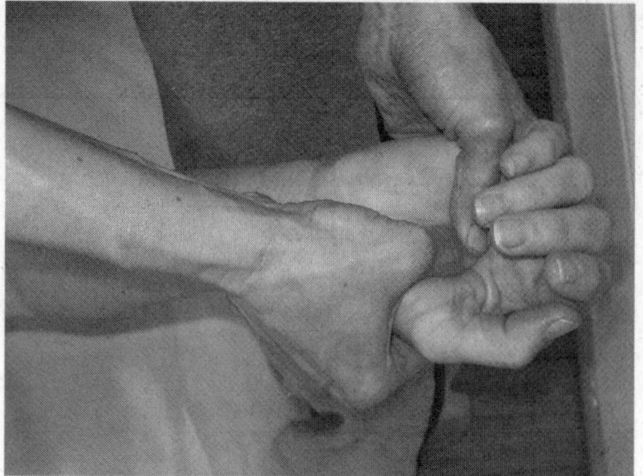

FIGURE 15-123 **PC 8.**
In the center of the palm, between the second and third metacarpals.

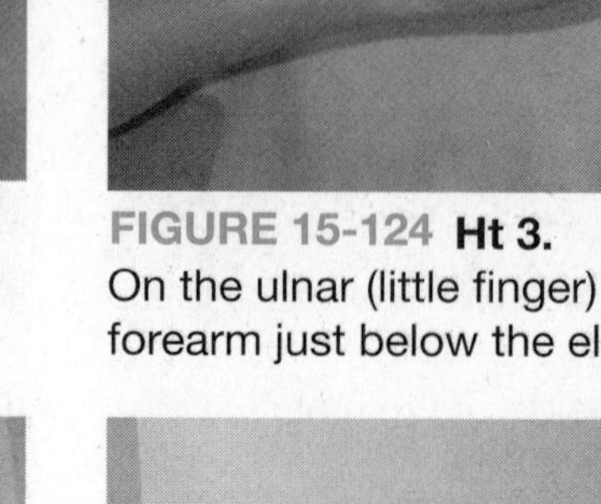

FIGURE 15-124 **Ht 3.**
On the ulnar (little finger) side of the inner forearm just below the elbow.

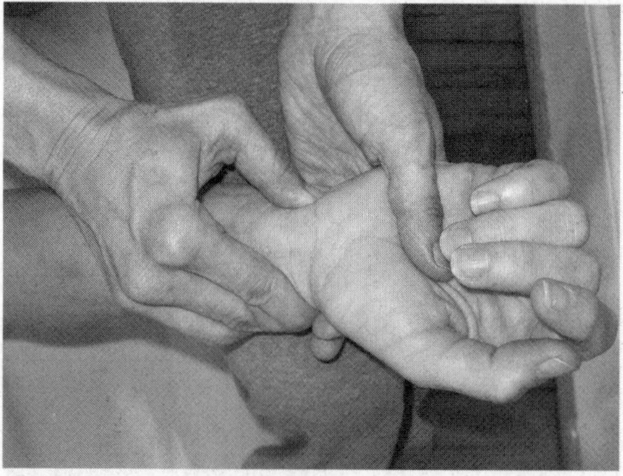

FIGURE 15-125 **Ht 7.**
In the bony hollow on the ulnar (little finger) side of the inner wrist.

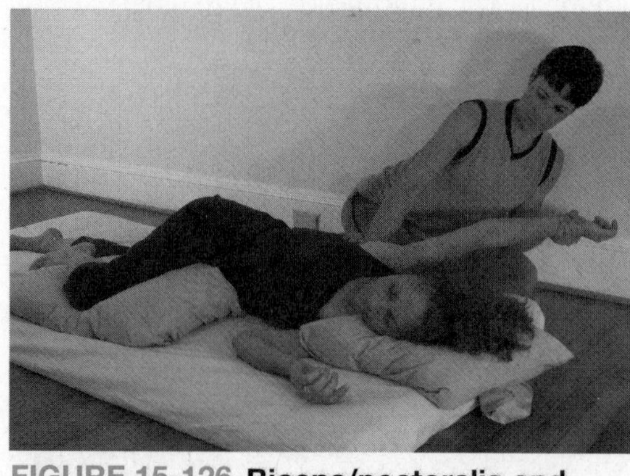

FIGURE 15-126 **Biceps/pectoralis and Lu/PC stretch.**
Hold the client's wrist, push forward at the scapula, and extend the arm up and back. Client should feel the stretch in the chest and inner upper arm.

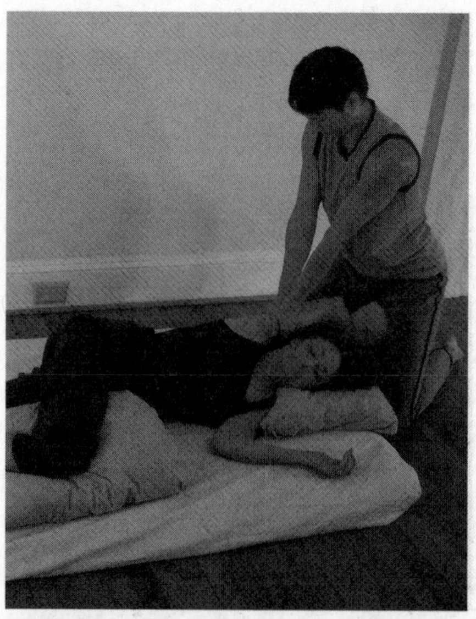

FIGURE 15-127 **Hands squeeze the Yin and Yang Meridians of the arm.**
Drape the client's arm overhead, wrap your hands around the upper arm, and squeeze.

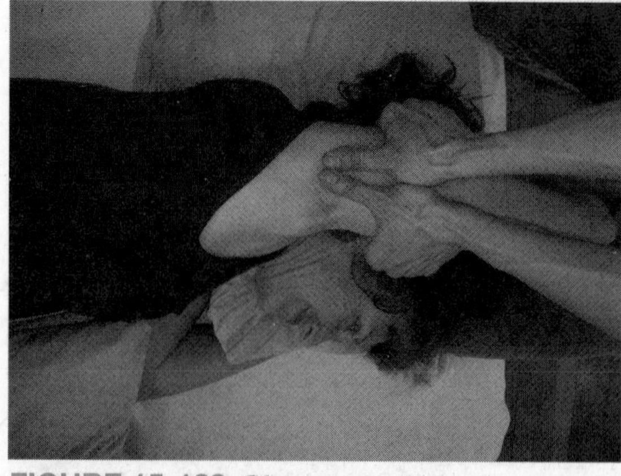

FIGURE 15-128 **Close-up of hand squeeze.**
Work down the arm toward the elbow.

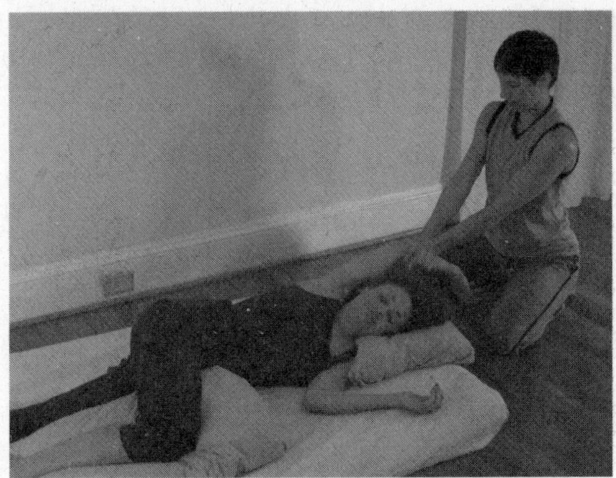

FIGURE 15-129 **Hands squeeze the Yin and Yang Meridians of the forearm.**

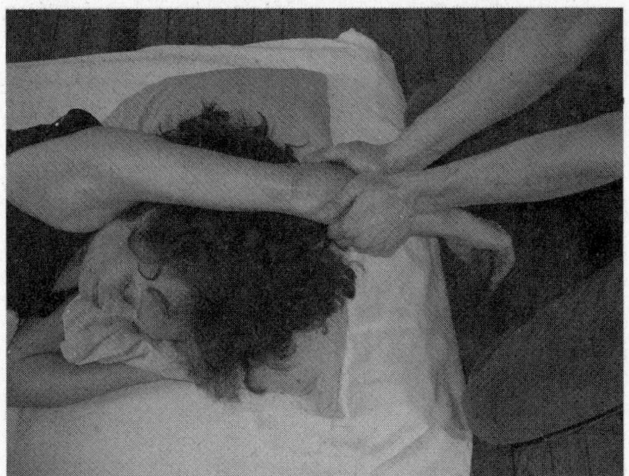

FIGURE 15-130 **Close-up of hand squeeze.**
Work down the forearm toward the wrist.

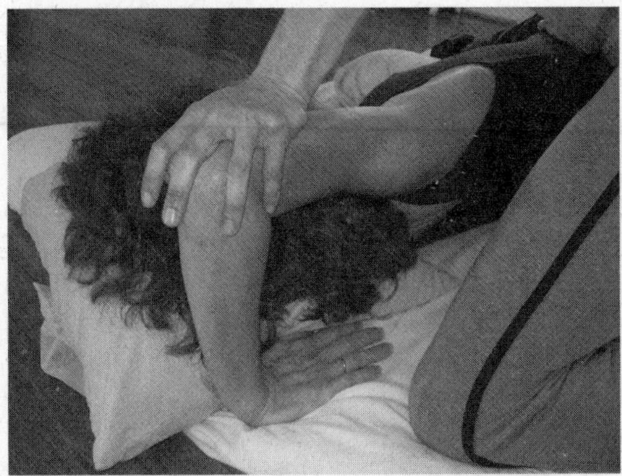

FIGURE 15-131 **Close-up of triceps/SI stretch.**
Prop the client's hand on mat with the fingers pointing toward the feet and the elbow stacked directly above the wrist.

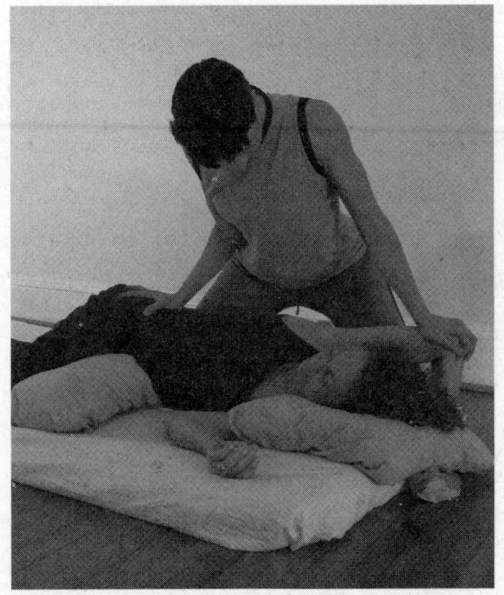

FIGURE 15-132 **Triceps/SI stretch.**
Place one hand above the elbow and the other above the pelvic crest. Push in opposite directions: upward on the client's arm and downward on the hip. Client should feel the stretch in the outer upper arm and side of the torso.

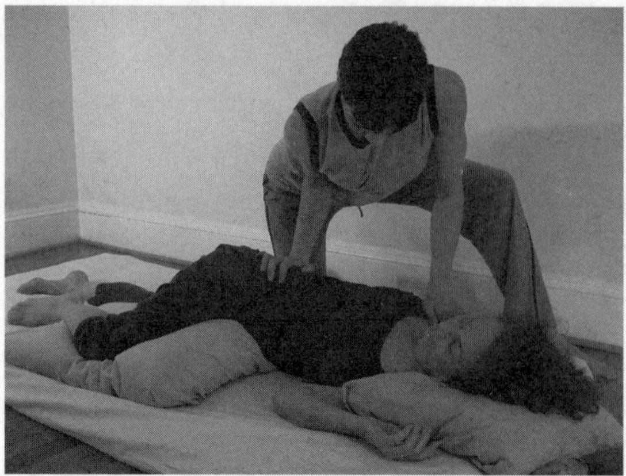

FIGURE 15-133 **Torso torque.**
In a kneeling lunge, plant one hand on the front of the client's shoulder and the other on the back of the hip. Using your body for leverage, push the shoulder down and the hip forward, twisting the torso.

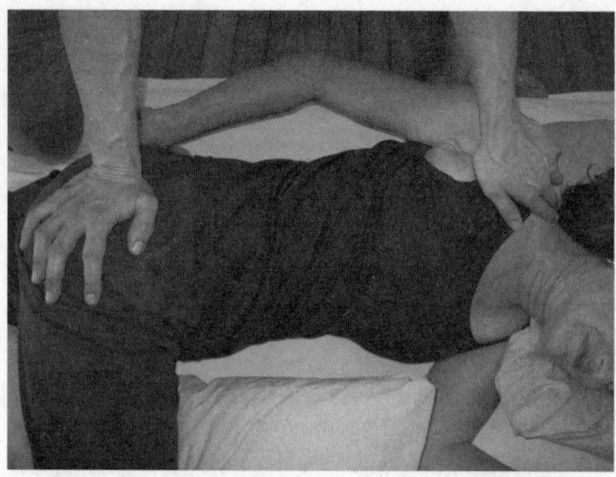

FIGURE 15-134 **Close-up of torso torque.**

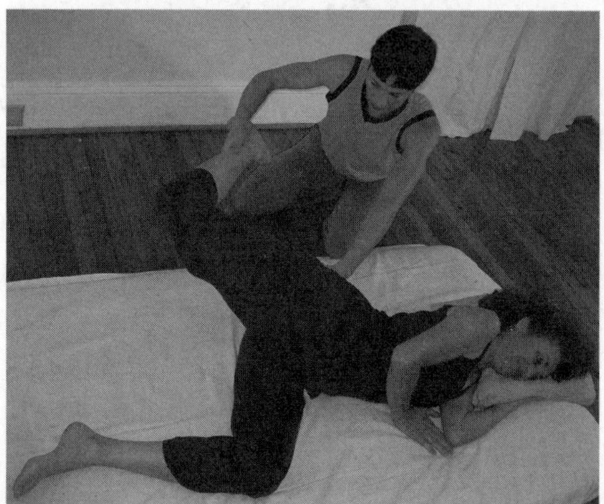

FIGURE 15-135 **Bow 1, hip flexor/ quadriceps and St/Sp stretch.**
Direct the client to rearrange the legs as shown (bottom leg bent forward; top leg extended backward). Kneel behind the client at a distance. Grab the client's ankle and firmly anchor your fist in the gluteals.

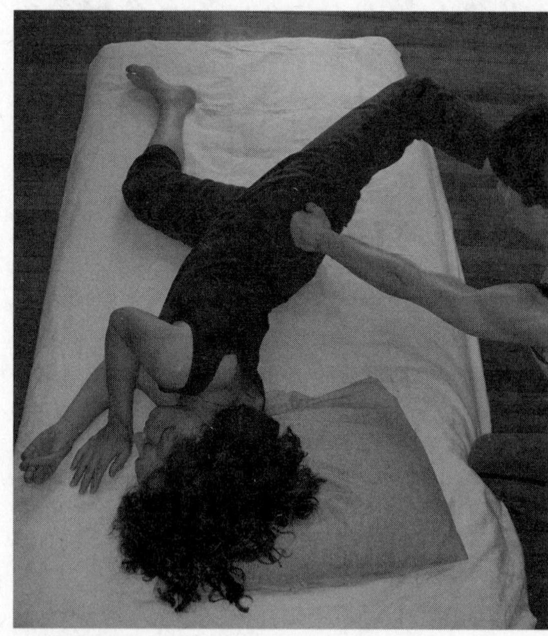

FIGURE 15-136 **Bow 1, back view.**
Push the client's hip forward with your fist and pull client's ankle back with your hand. The client should feel the stretch on the front of the hip and thigh. Release and repeat, as desired.

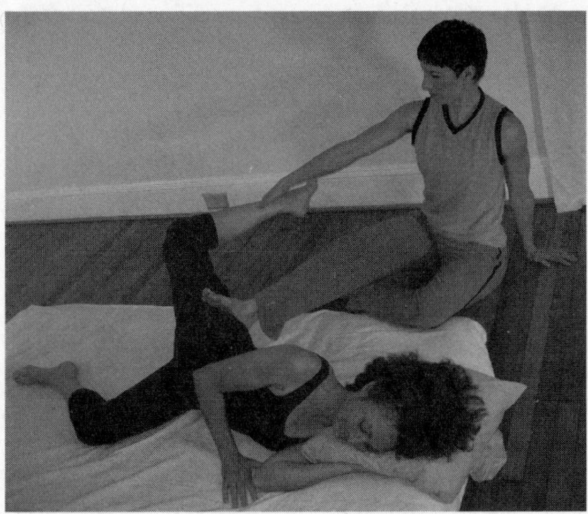

FIGURE 15-137 **Bow 1, variation and transition.**
This foot variation can be done instead of, or in addition to, the fist variation. Grab the ankle; plant your foot on the gluteals and pull the leg back.

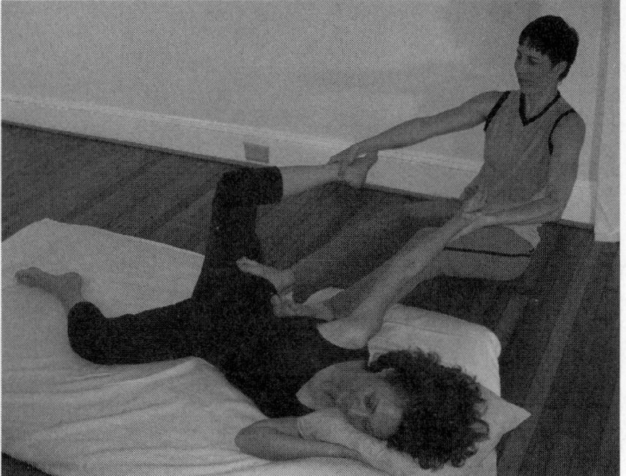

FIGURE 15-138 **Bow 2, adding pectoralis/biceps and Lu/PC stretch.**
Direct the client to extend her arm back. Grab her wrist. Plant your other foot on her middle to lower back. Press forward with your feet and pull back with your hands, more on the leg and less on the arm.

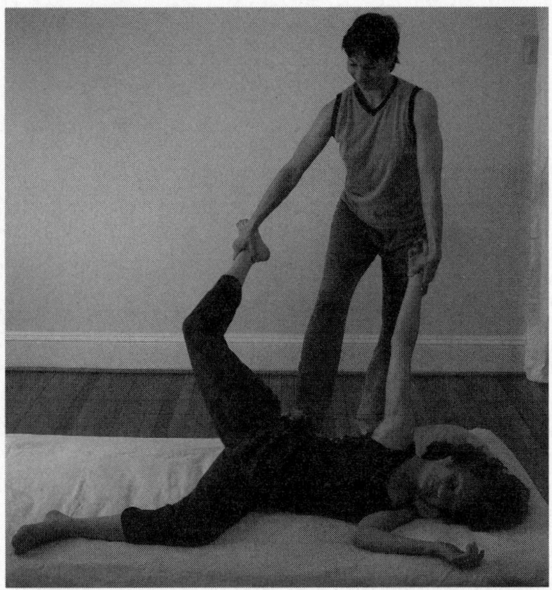

FIGURE 15-139 **Bow 3 (standing variation).**
In a standing position, grab the client's ankle and wrist. Plant one foot on the gluteals. Press forward with your foot and pull back with your hands, more on the leg and less on the arm. Direct the client to turn over, and repeat the entire protocol (Figures 15-1 through 15-139) on the other side.

16

SEATED PROTOCOL

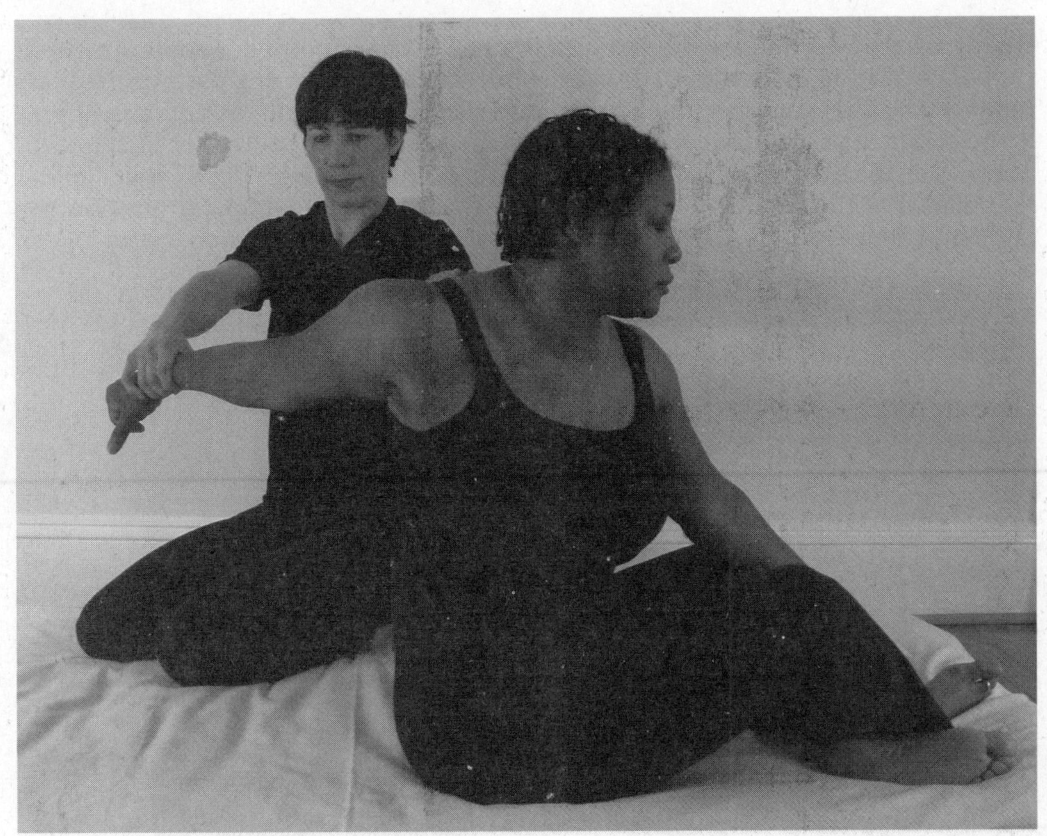

THERAPEUTIC EMPHASIS

The seated protocol is a shorter session that focuses on the neck, upper and outer shoulders, and upper back between the shoulders, areas that often become tense and fatigued from prolonged desk work (for a more detailed analysis of energetic disharmonies associated with prolonged sitting, see "Kyo Jitsu Imbalances" in Chapter 12). Typically, the head is craned forward to look at a computer screen or tilted downward to look at a keypad, mouse, or text on the table; the back is slumped; the shoulders are stooped; and the chest is collapsed. In this slouched posture, the muscles in the back of the neck and upper back are placed in a partial stretch position, and they, rather than the spinal column, must support the weight of the head and upper torso, which is why they become strained after an extended period of time. Additionally, the right hand is typically raised to operate a mouse, which can create tension in the deltoid and supraspinatus (outer shoulder muscles).

KEY ACUPRESSURE POINTS

- Neck: GV 16, Bl 10, GB 20
- Upper shoulders: GB 21, SI 12
- Between the shoulders: Bl 11–16, Bl 41–44, especially Bl 43
- Outer shoulders: LI 14, LI 15, TH 14

CLIENT COMFORT AND PRACTITIONER LOGISTICS

Giving Shiatsu without a chair requires the practitioner to provide some structural support so that the client can relax more fully. This entails using parts of the body to brace or prop the client and may require practice, especially during transitions. If the client is uncomfortable sitting cross-legged on the floor, many of the techniques can be adapted to a low-back chair. Before working down the Bladder Meridian into the lower back, give the client a voluminous pillow to support the chest and abdomen.

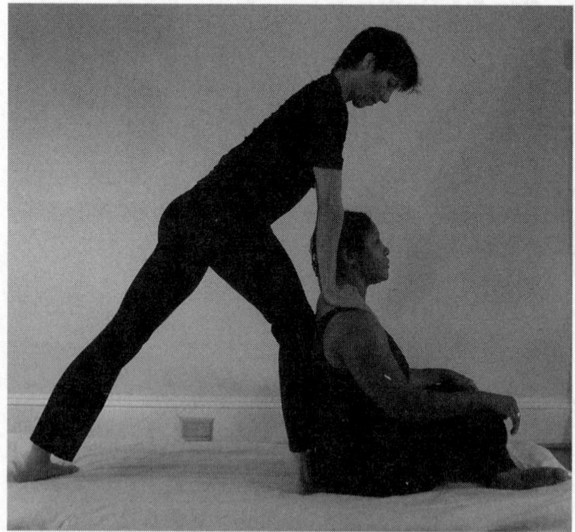

FIGURE 16-1 **Standing lunge.**
Stand in a lunge behind your client. Turn your front leg inward so that the fleshy outer part of your leg forms a backrest for your client. Lean the client back against your leg.

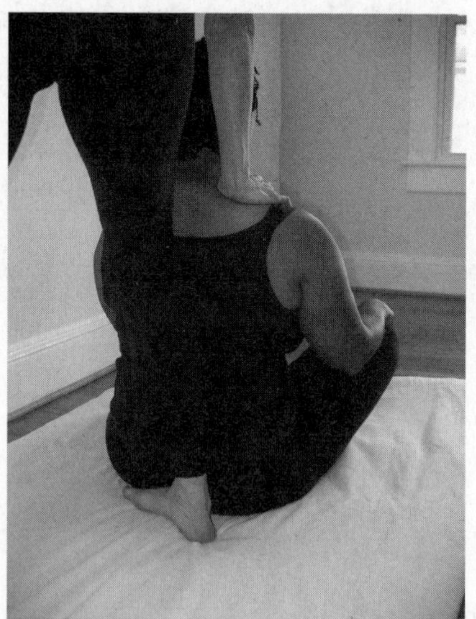

FIGURE 16-2 **Close-up of standing lunge.**
Your front leg is rotated medially so that your outer shin props and supports the client.

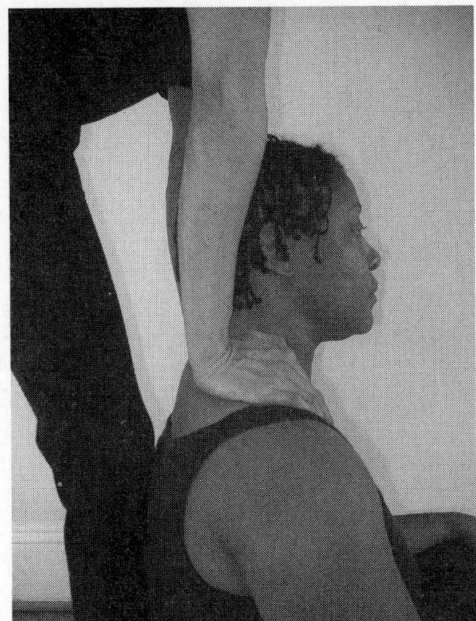

FIGURE 16-3 **Palm press, forward.** With your fingers facing forward, press down on the upper trapezius (upper shoulder). Your shoulder should be directly over your wrist.

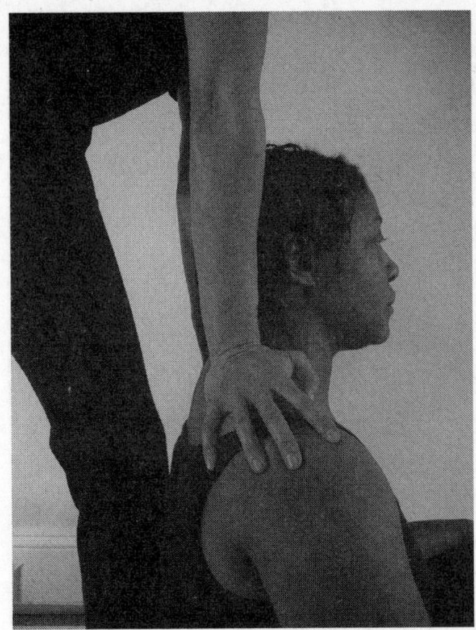

FIGURE 16-4 **Palm press, sideways.** With your fingers turned sideways, press down again on the upper shoulders.

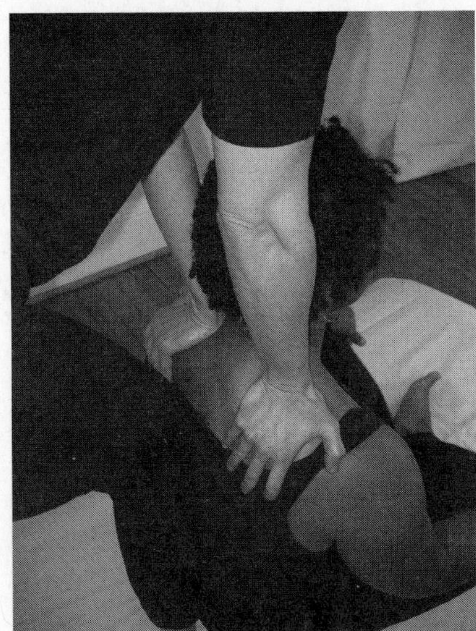

FIGURE 16-5 **Palm press, backward.** With your fingers turned backward, press down one more time on the upper shoulders. Repeat Figures 16-3 through 16-4 three times to warm up the muscles.

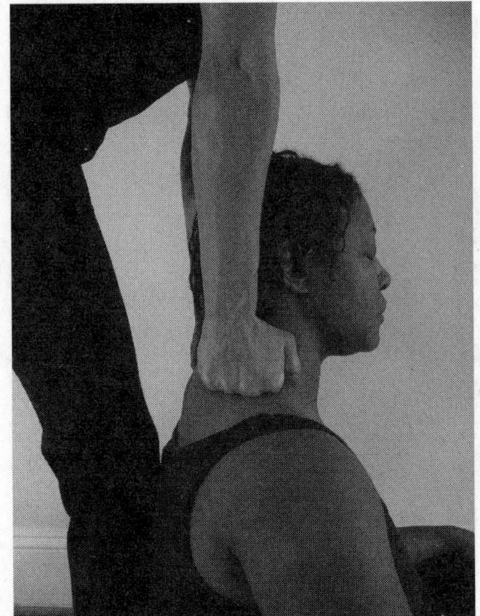

FIGURE 16-6 **Fist press.** Make a fist and press firmly down on the upper shoulders. Relocate and repeat several times. Your forearm should be in line with your knuckles: your wrist should not hyperextend backward or deviate sideways.

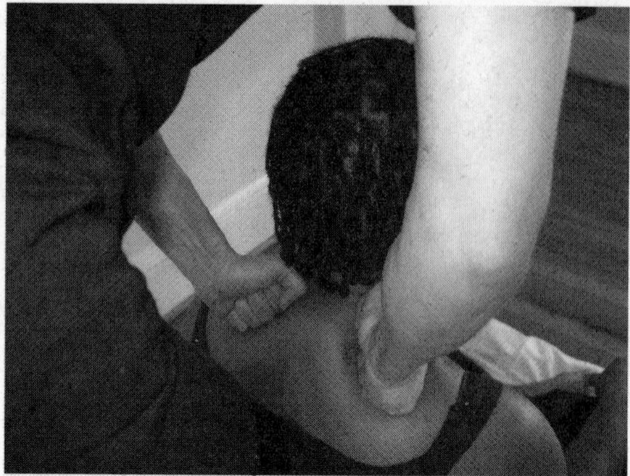

FIGURE 16-7 **Fist twist.**
Bend your elbows; anchor your fists into the muscle and torque outward. Repeat several times.

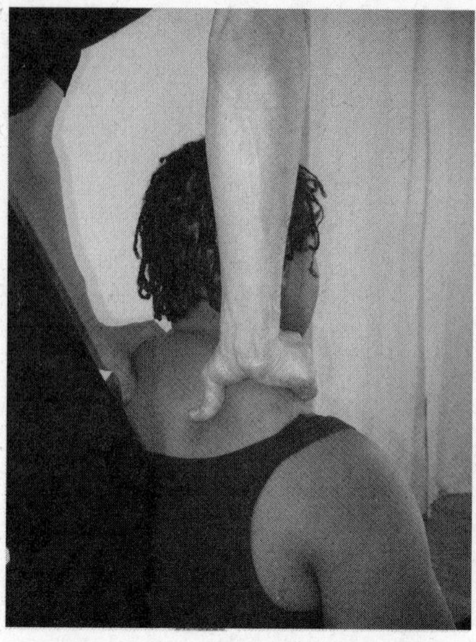

FIGURE 16-8 **Shoulder squeeze.**
Grab the upper shoulder muscles, and with a pincer grip, lift and squeeze. If the client's muscles are bulky, use both hands to lift and squeeze one side at a time.

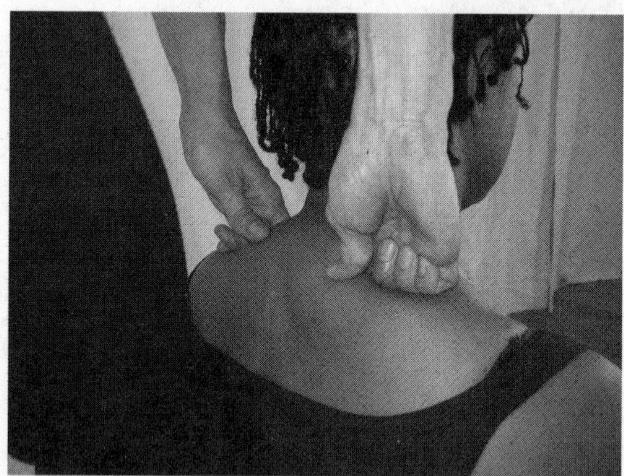

FIGURE 16-9 **Knuckle press.**
Press your knuckles into the upper shoulders. The bottom segment of your phalanges (finger bones) should be in line with your metacarpals (the bones forming the hand). Pause at GB 21 on the belly of the upper trapezius.

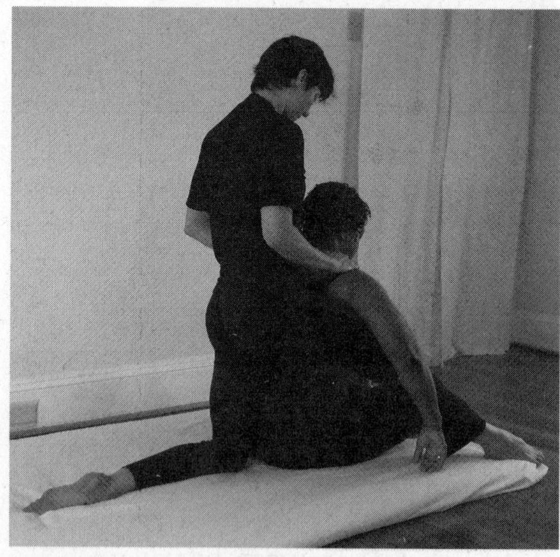

FIGURE 16-10 **Kneeling lunge.**
Descend into a kneeling lunge. Position your kneeling thigh flush against the client's back as support. Grab the client's arm above the elbow and drape it over your front leg.

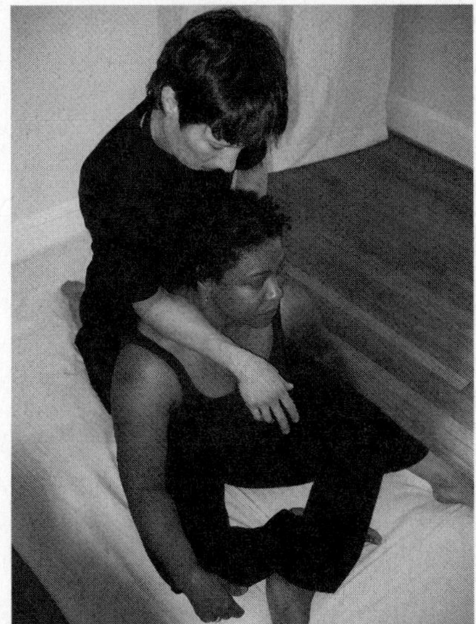

FIGURE 16-11 **Rolling pin forearm, palm down.**
Press your forearm, palm down, on the upper shoulder that is opposite the client's draped arm. Press the fleshy part of your pronated forearm into the muscle.

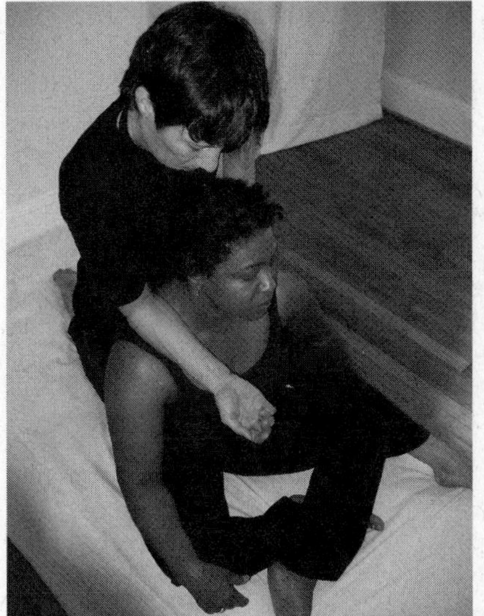

FIGURE 16-12 **Rolling pin forearm, palm up.**
Maintaining pressure, supinate your forearm by rolling it outward and turning your palm upward. Alternate pronation and supination, pressing and rolling several times. Reverse sides, repeating Figures 16-10 through 16-12.

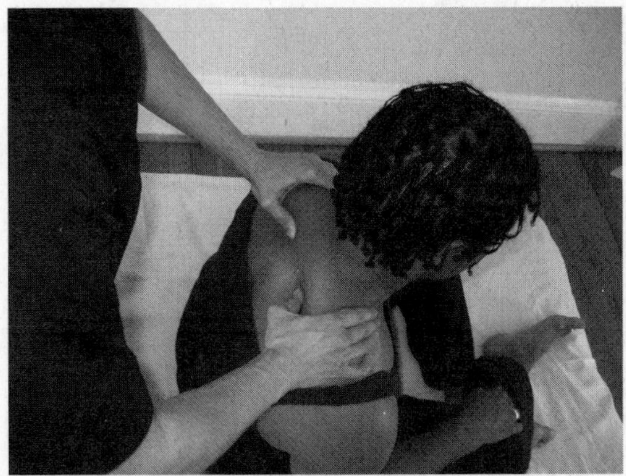

FIGURE 16-13 **Thumbs press and apply friction to the upper Bladder Meridian.**
Slip out of the kneeling lunge and into an upright kneeling position. Press your thumbs and apply friction—side to side, up and down, or in circles—to the erector spinae of the upper back on either side of the vertebral column, pausing at Bl 13, 14, and 15.

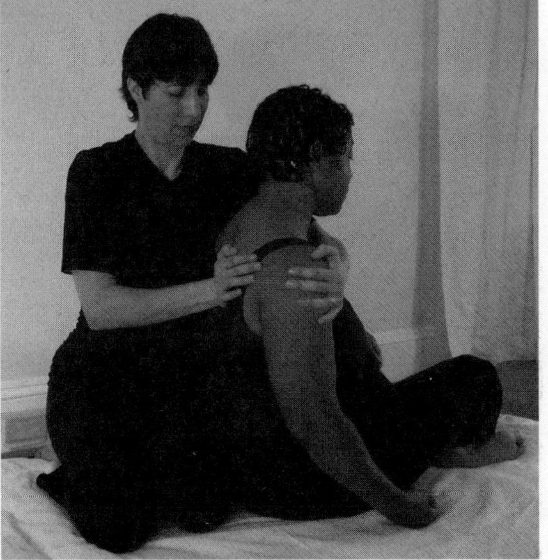

FIGURE 16-14 **Heel of the hand press.**
Kneel beside your the client, your thigh propped against the client's lower back and hip. Wrap your upper arm around and above the client's chest and hold the opposite shoulder. Press the heel of your hand along the vertebral border of the scapula (edge of the shoulderblade).

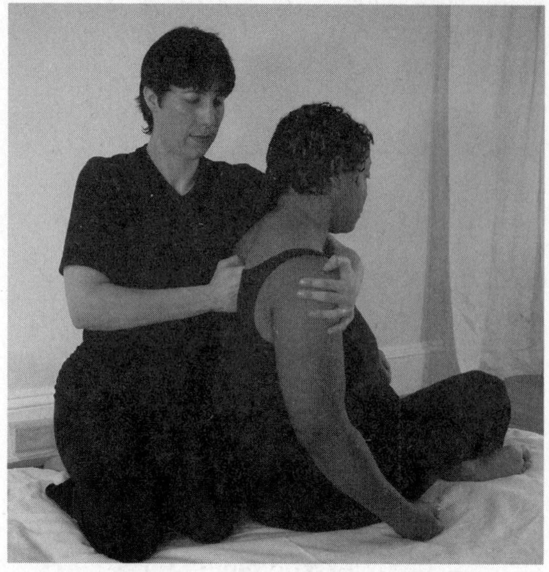

FIGURE 16-15 **Fist press or twist.**
First press, then twist your fist along the vertebral border of the scapula, taking care to avoid the spine. Accentuate the fist press by pushing the client's shoulder back into your fist with your stabilizing hand.

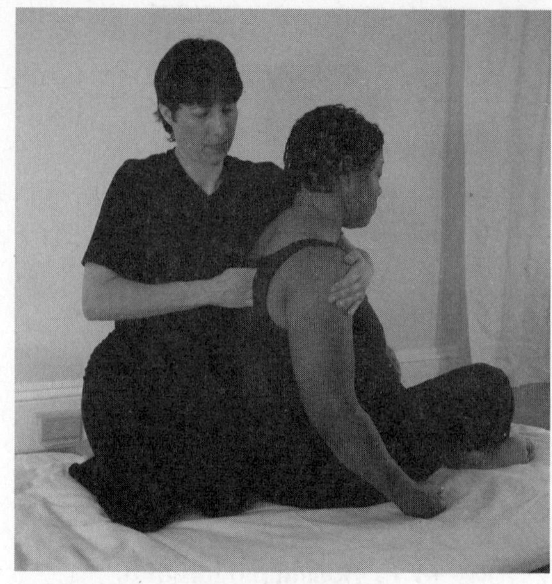

FIGURE 16-16 **Knuckle press.**
Press your knuckles along the vertebral border of the scapula. Accentuate the knuckle press by pushing the client's shoulder back into your knuckles with your stabilizing hand.

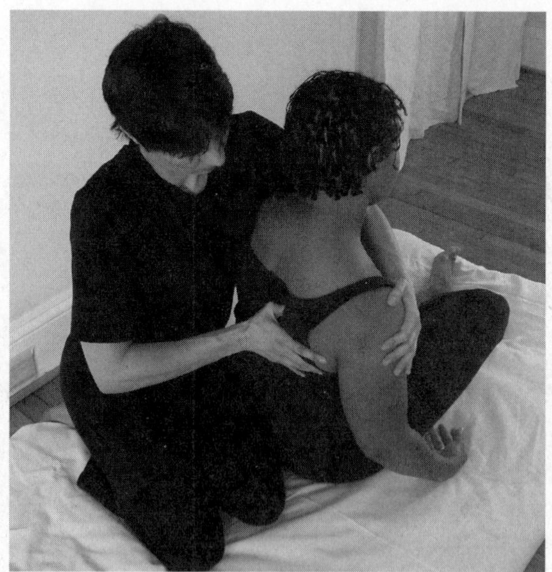

FIGURE 16-17 **Thumb press.**
Press your thumb along the vertebral border of the scapula. Accentuate the thumb press by pushing the client's shoulder back into your thumb with your stabilizing hand. Repeat Figures 16-14 through 16-17 on the other side.

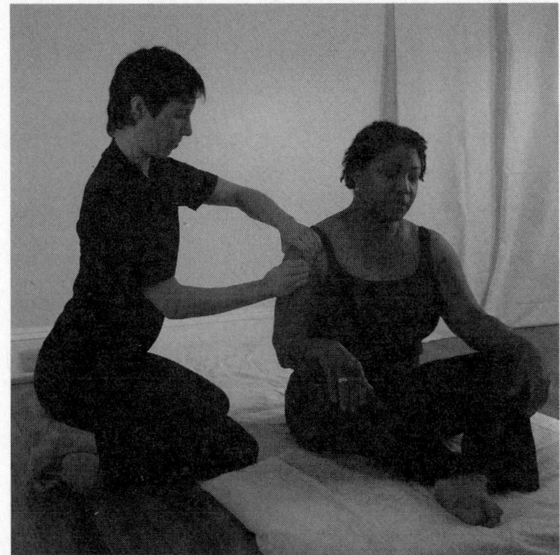

FIGURE 16-18 **Shoulder squeeze.** In a seated kneeling position or kneeling lunge beside the client, squeeze the anterior and posterior deltoid (outer shoulder muscle) with both hands, using a pincer grip.

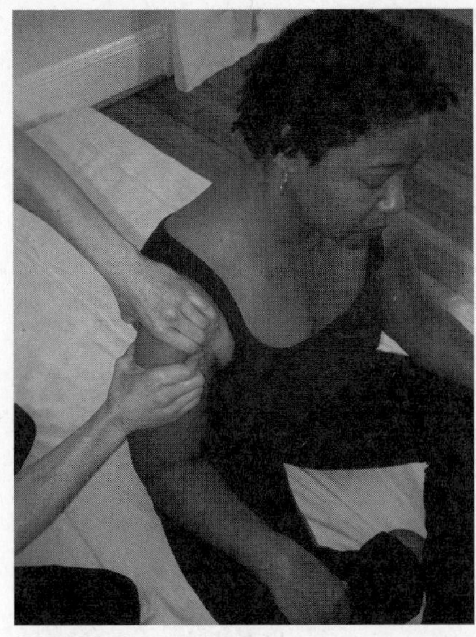

FIGURE 16-19 **Close-up of shoulder squeeze.**

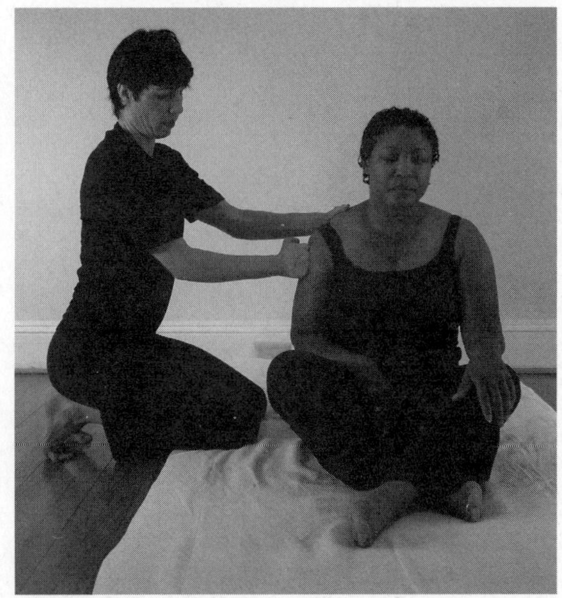

FIGURE 16-20 **Fist press or twist.** First press, then twist your fist into the medial deltoid (outer shoulder muscle).

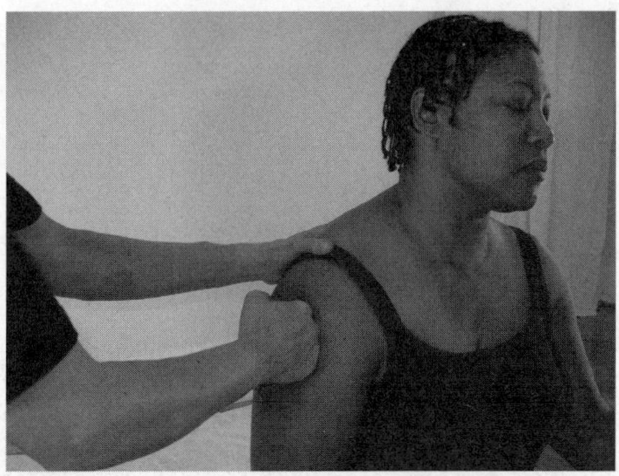

FIGURE 16-21 **Close-up of fist press or twist.**

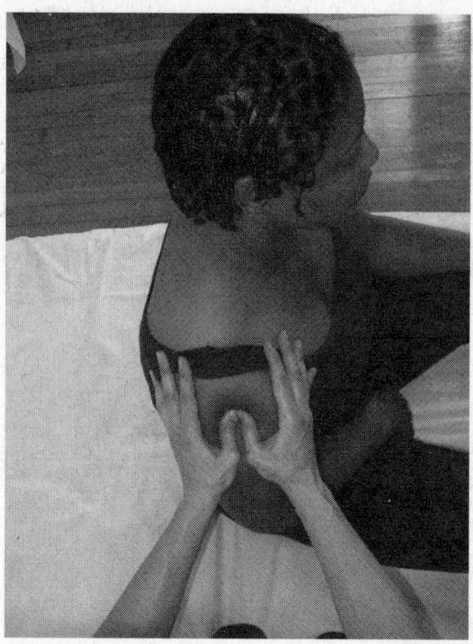

FIGURE 16-22 **Thumbs press down the outer shoulder.**
Pause at LI 14 near the deltoid insertion on the humerus. Repeat Figures 16-18 through 16-22 on the other side.

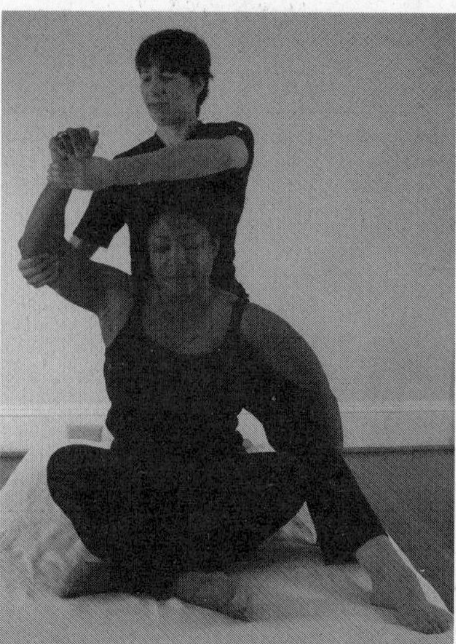

FIGURE 16-23 **Triceps/SI stretch, phase 1.**
Return to a kneeling lunge with the client's arm draped over your front leg. Grab the client's opposite arm under the elbow; lift and hold the wrist.

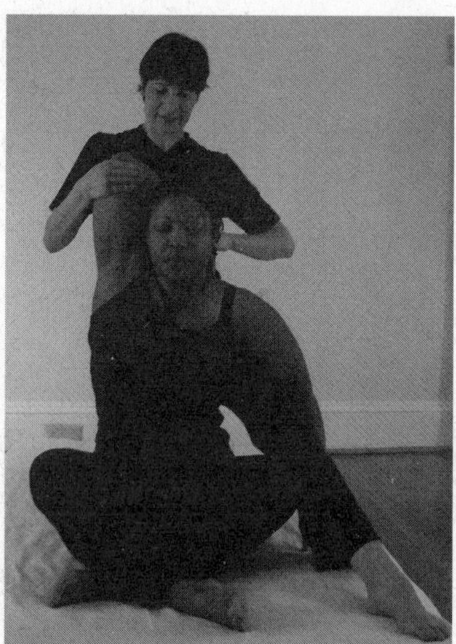

FIGURE 16-24 **Triceps/SI stretch, phase 2.**
Pull the client's arm back and down until resistance is felt. The client should feel a stretch on the upper outer arm.

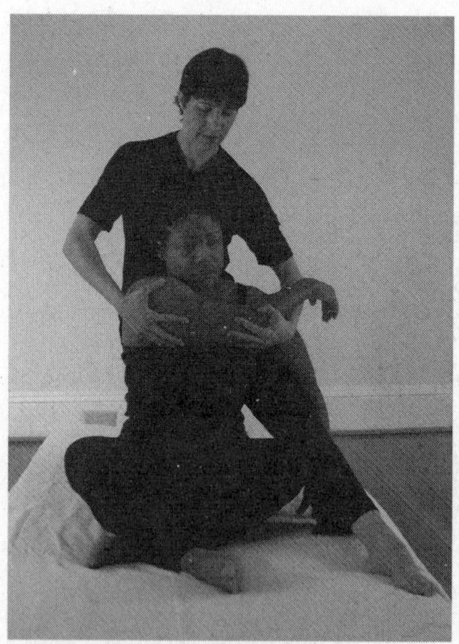

FIGURE 16-25 **Deltoid/rotator cuff/TH stretch.**
Draw and pull the client's arm down and across the chest. The client should feel a stretch in the back of the outer shoulder.

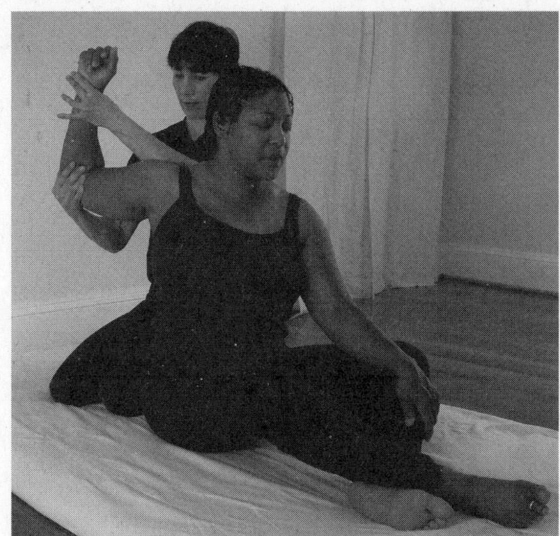

FIGURE 16-26 **Pectoralis/LU stretch.** Slip out of the kneeling lunge and into a seated kneeling position behind and beside the client. Scoop the client's arm under the elbow. Hold the wrist with your other hand and pull back. The client should feel a stretch in the chest and front of the shoulder.

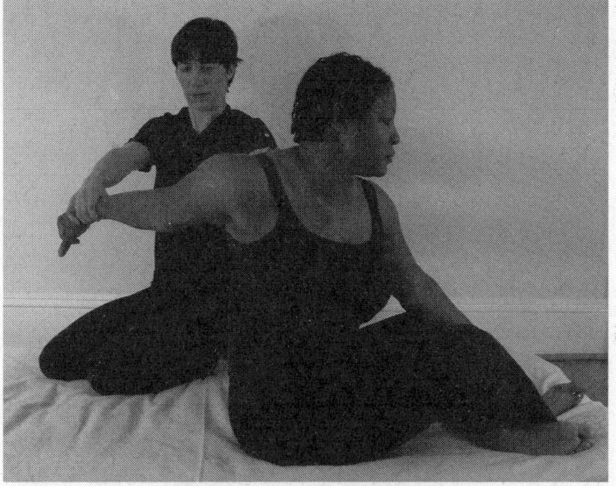

FIGURE 16-27 **Biceps/PC stretch.** Extend the client's arm, holding the wrist. Place your hand on the client's scapula (shoulder blade) and scoot farther back until the client feels stretch in the inner upper arm Repeat Figures 16-23 through 16-27 on the other side.

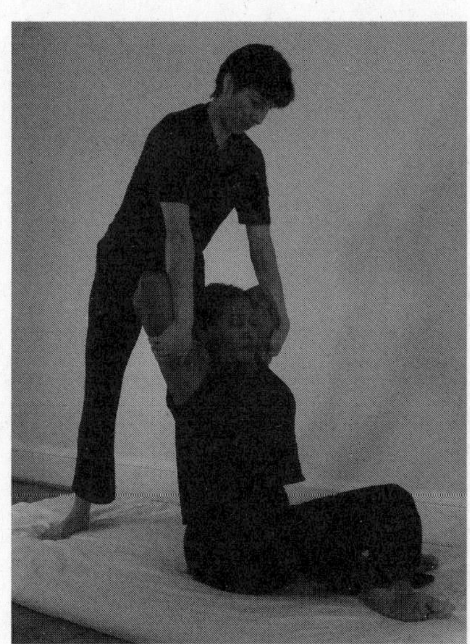

FIGURE 16-28 **Double arm chest stretch, phase 1.** Return to a standing lunge, turning your front leg inward so that the fleshy outer part of your leg forms a backrest for your client. Direct the client to clasp the hands behind the head.

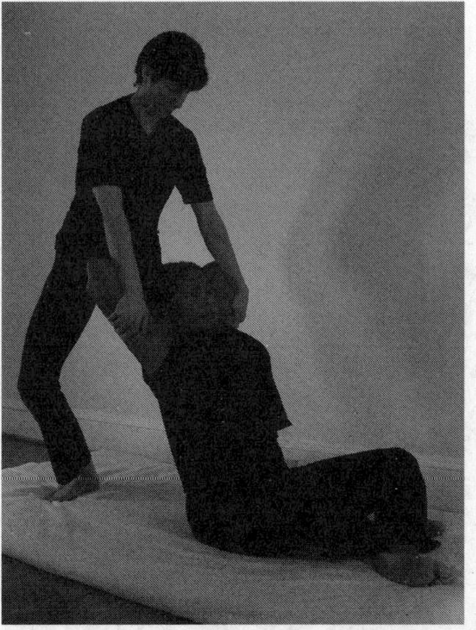

FIGURE 16-29 **Double arm chest stretch, phase 2.** Place your forearms over and your hands under the client's upper arms. Hold firmly; pull up and back, shifting your weight from your front to your back leg while leaning the client against your front leg. Repeat several times.

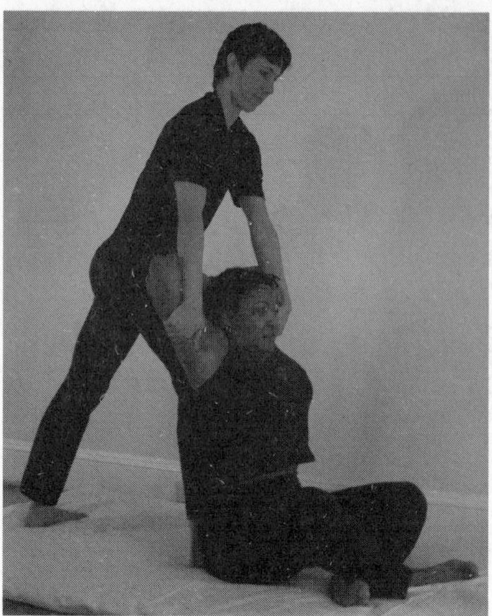

FIGURE 16-30 **Double arm chest stretch, other side, phase 1.**
Reverse sides and repeat.

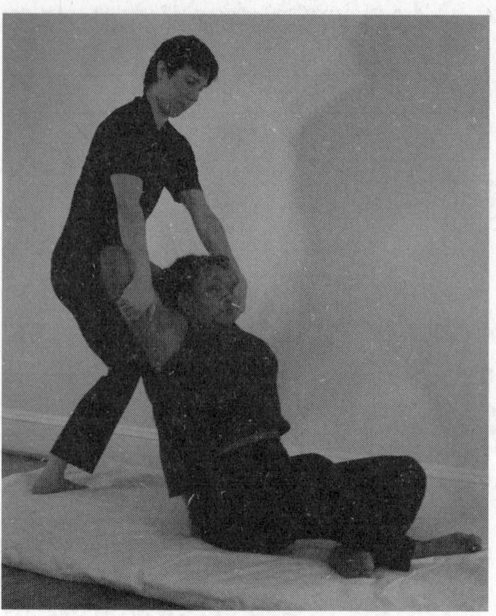

FIGURE 16-31 **Double arm chest stretch, other side, phase 2.**

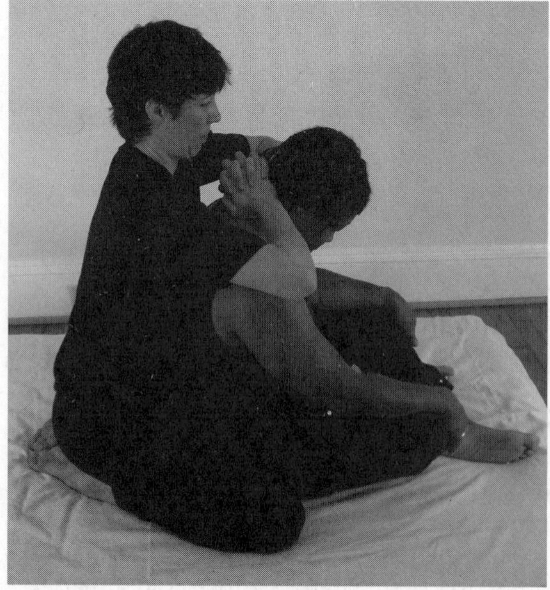

FIGURE 16-32 **Neck clasp.**
Straddle your client in a seated kneeling position. Direct the client to tilt the head forward slightly. Clasp your hands and squeeze the client's neck with the heels of your hands. Repeat several times.

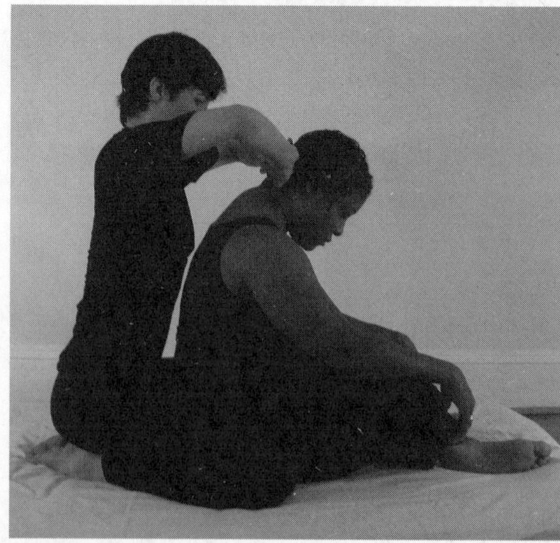

FIGURE 16-33 **Clasped-hand thumb press.**
Starting below the occiput (back of the skull), press inward with your thumbs toward Bl 10 (on the upper trapezius). Inch down the neck until you reach the shoulders.

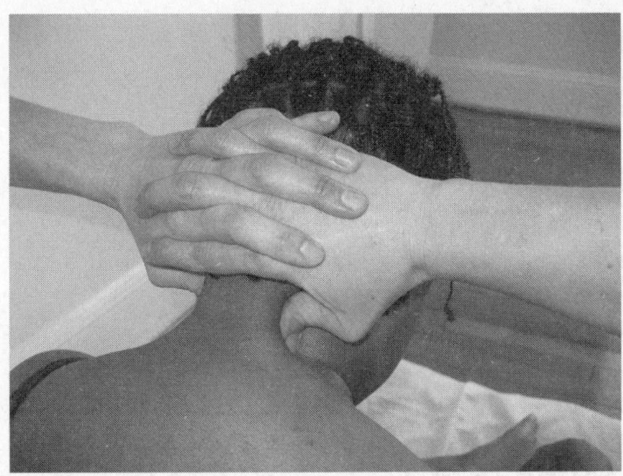
FIGURE 16-34 Close-up of clasped-hand thumb press.

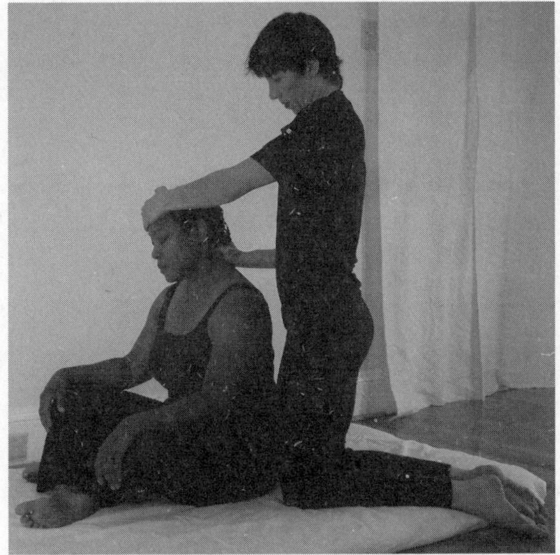
FIGURE 16-35 Hand squeeze.
Rise to an upright kneeling position. Stabilize the client's forehead and squeeze the neck with a pincer grip. Pause at GB 20, between the upper trapezius and sternocleidomastoid. Switch hands and repeat.

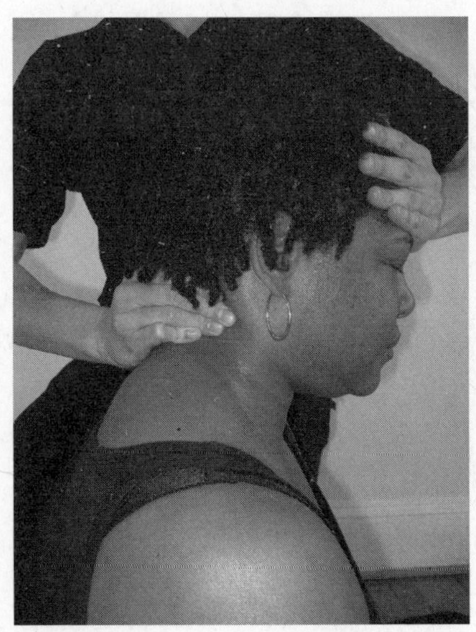
FIGURE 16-36 Close-up of hand squeeze.

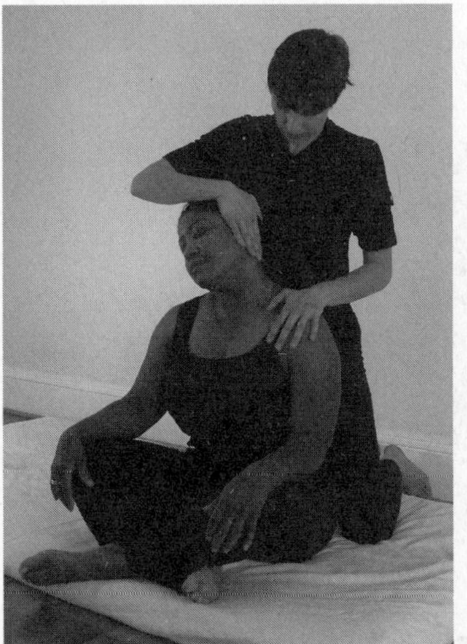
FIGURE 16-37 Lateral neck stretch.
Plant one hand on the client's shoulder and the other on the side of the client's head, covering the ear. Slowly tilt the head sideways, pressing the opposite ear toward the shoulder.

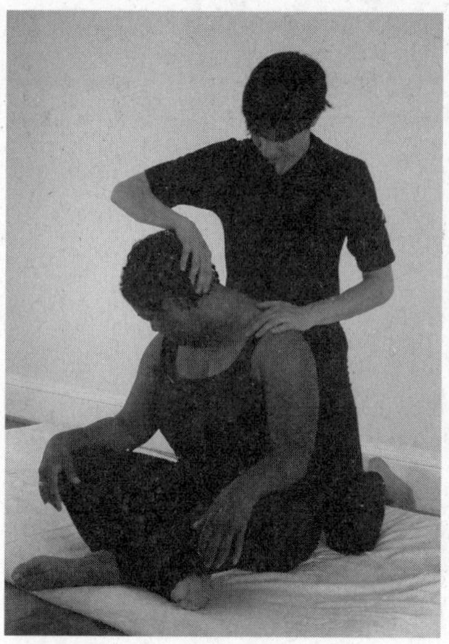

FIGURE 16-38 Forward flexion and rotation of the neck.
Plant one hand on the client's shoulder and the other on the back of the head. Slowly tilt the head forward and sideways, pressing the chin toward the opposite shoulder. Repeat the Figures 16-37 and 16-38 on the other side.

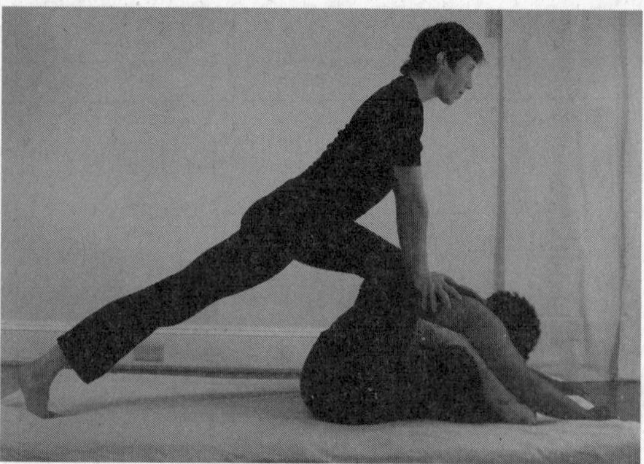

FIGURE 16-39 Palms press Bladder Meridian.
Place a big pillow between the client's legs and chest for cushion. In a standing lunge, palm press down the upper back.

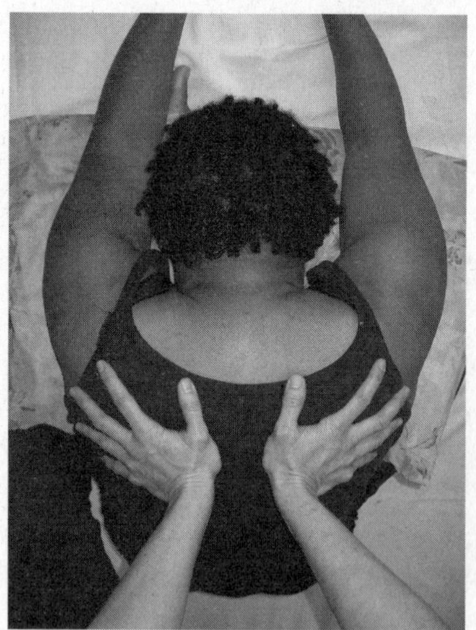

FIGURE 16-40 Close-up of palm press.

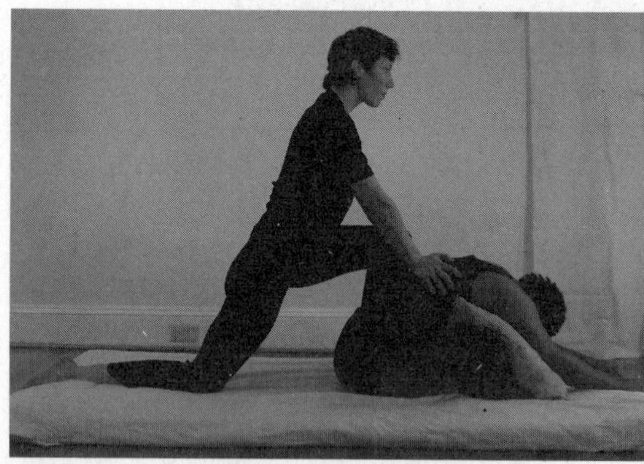

FIGURE 16-41 Palms press Bladder Meridian in middle back.
Lower to a kneeling lunge and continue pressing down the middle back.

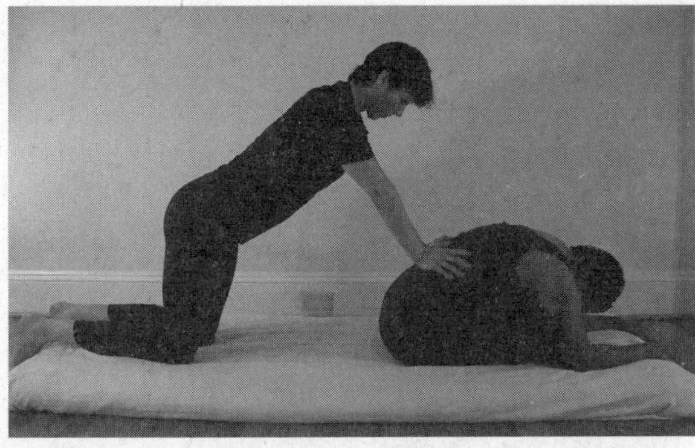

FIGURE 16-42 Palms press lower Bladder Meridian in lower back.
Reposition to an upright kneeling position and continue pressing down the lower back.

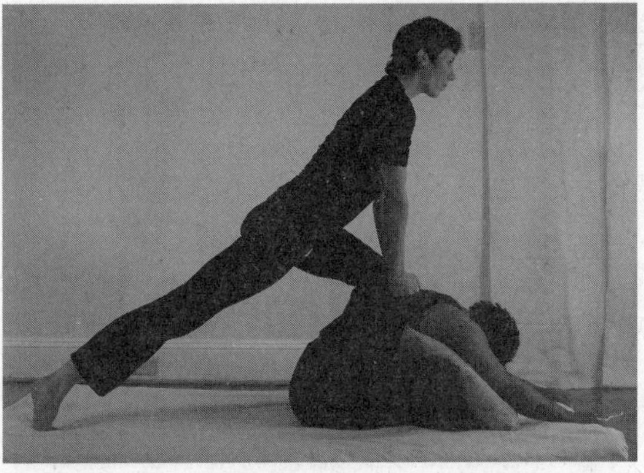

FIGURE 16-43 Fists press or twist Bladder Meridian in upper back.
Revert to a standing lunge and repeat compressions with a fist press or twist.

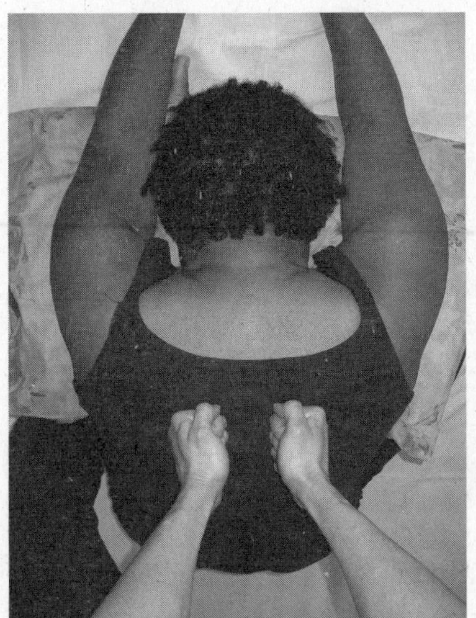

FIGURE 16-44 Close-up of fist press or twist.

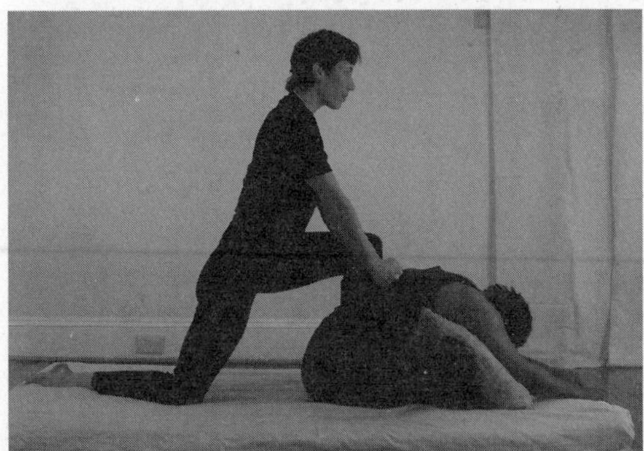

FIGURE 16-45 Fists press or twist Bladder Meridian in middle back.
Lower to a kneeling lunge and continue compressions down the middle back.

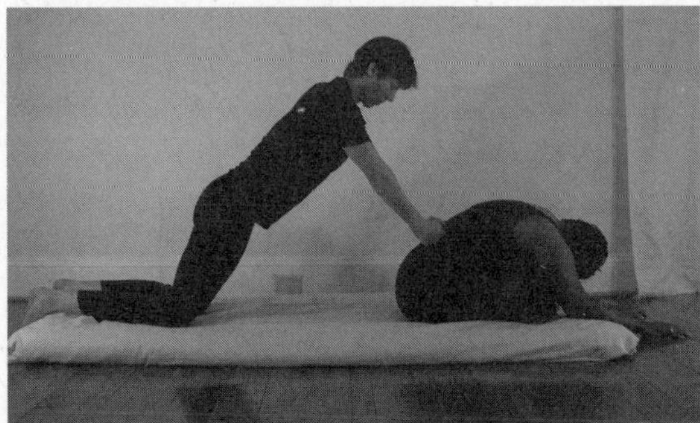

FIGURE 16-46 Fists press or twist Bladder Meridian in lower back.
Reposition to an upright kneeling position and continue pressing down the lower back.

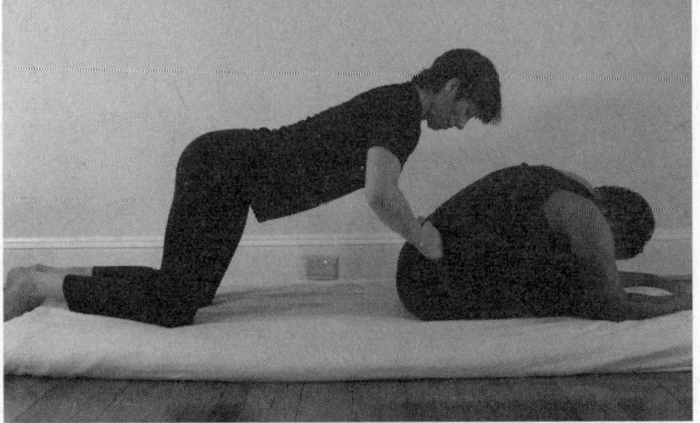

FIGURE 16-47 Fist twist in hips.
Bend your elbows; press and torque.

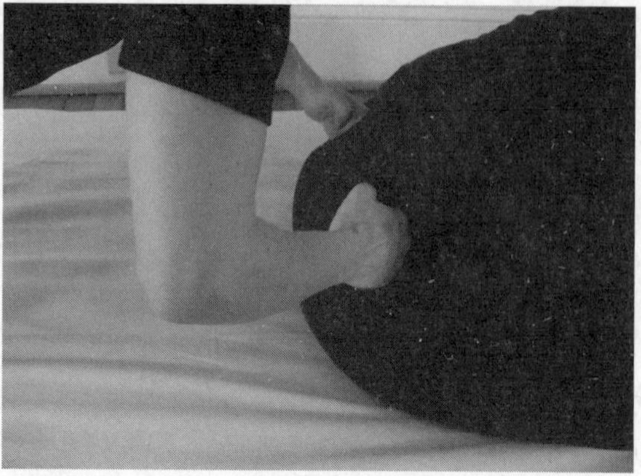

FIGURE 16-48 Close-up of fist twist in hips.
Work the gluteals along the sacrum (triangular-shaped bone at the base of the spine) and iliac crest (pelvic bone) to the greater trochanter of the femur (hipbone).

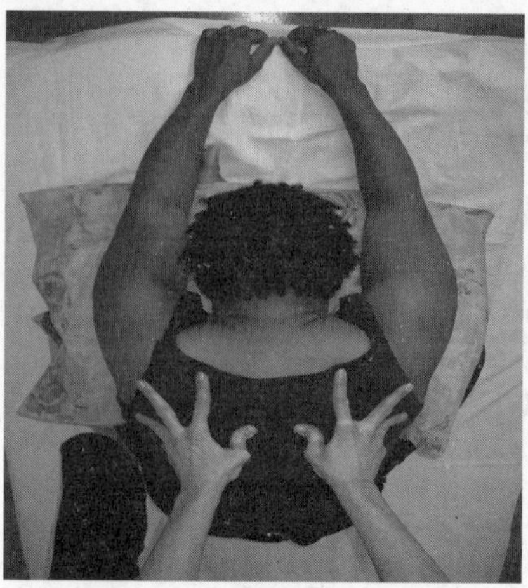

FIGURE 16-49 Thumbs press down the inner Bladder Merdian.

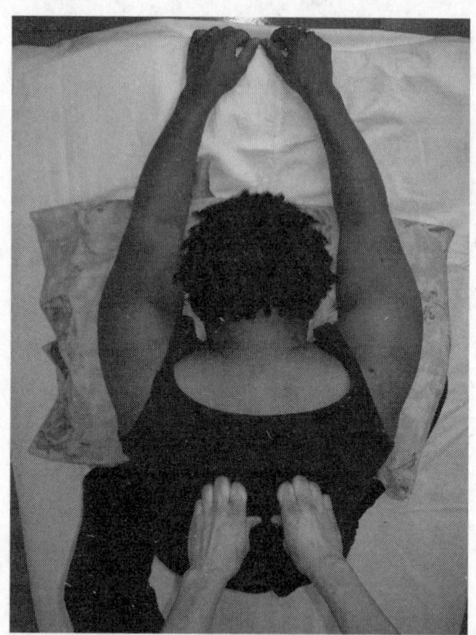

FIGURE 16-50 Knuckles press down the outer Bladder Meridian.

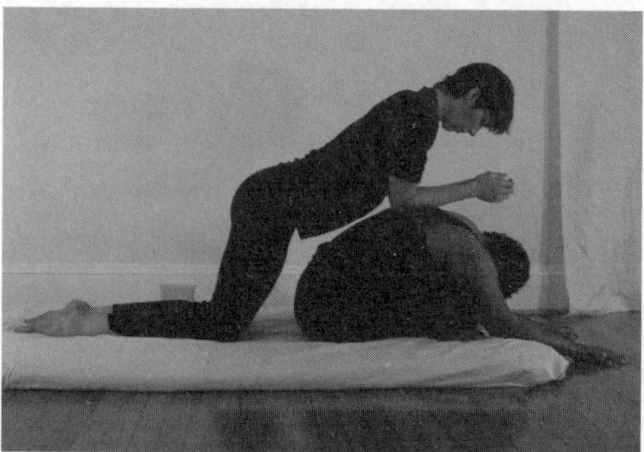

FIGURE 16-51 Elbows press down the Bladder Meridian.

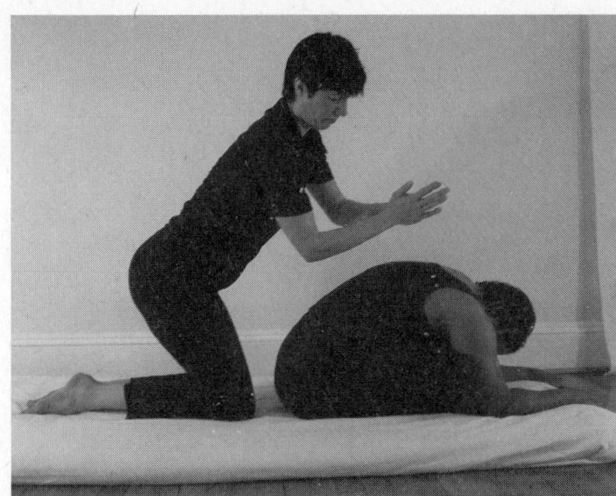

FIGURE 16-52 **Double-handed hacking, upper.**
Avoid the spine; chop lightly over the kidney area.

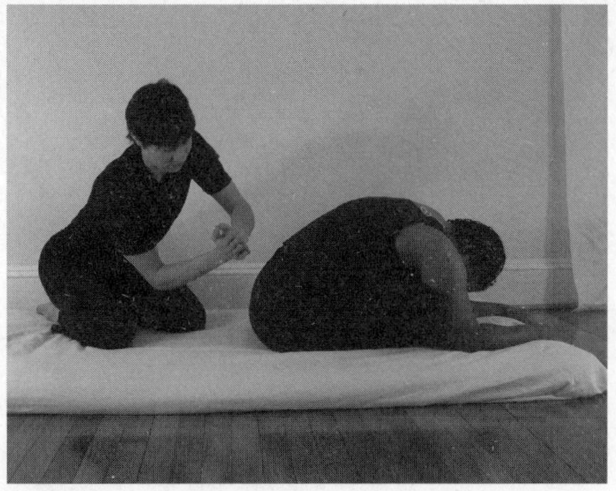

FIGURE 16-53 **Double-handed hacking, lower.**
This technique is used to disperse stagnation (tension).

REFERENCE

Chow, K.T. (2002). *Thai Yoga massage: A dynamic therapy for physical well-being and spiritual energy.* Rochester, VT: Healing Arts Press.

17

MOXA AND GUA SHA PROTOCOL

THERAPEUTIC EMPHASIS

MOXA

Moxabustion, an herbal heat therapy, is applied to acupressure points, penetrating these points with the strong Yang energy of fire. This heat therapy can reinforce a weak area, dispel Cold, clear Damp, and disperse stagnation. As a Yang therapy, it is especially helpful during the Yin seasons—autumn and winter—to counteract the tendency to develop Yin conditions like cold extremities; stiff, achy joints; weariness, lethargy, and malaise; susceptibility to illness; a foggy, muddled mental state; and a downbeat mood. Moxa specifically counteracts Yin disorders due to Cold, Damp, and sinking Qi (see "Moxa Indications and Contraindications" in Chapter 8).

GUA SHA

Gua Sha, a friction therapy and exterior releasing technique, is traditionally applied to ward off the onset of a seasonal illness or to expel it quickly after it has settled in the body. Gua Sha also neutralizes Cold/Heat and Deficiency/Excess imbalances, dispelling excess Cold or Heat and dissipating fullness. For example, Gua Sha can relieve a client who has the sensation of being uncomfortably cold or hot or who feels a disagreeable pressure inside. Finally, Gua Sha disperses the fluid and waste buildup and the stasis caused by rigorous exertion or unaccustomed activity. It can relieve tissue tenderness and stiffness due to delayed onset muscle soreness (see "Gua Sha Uses and Indications" in Chapter 8).

CAUTIONS AND CONTRAINDICATIONS

MOXA

Moxa is contraindicated for Yang conditions, such as fever and inflammation, since heat would worsen these conditions. Moxa is also contraindicated for conditions of reckless blood, such as hemorrhaging, menorrhagia (excessive menstrual flow), and hypertension (high blood pressure), as moxa stimulates blood flow. Obviously, moxa should not be applied to skin disorders or to breaches in the skin because heat could damage or destroy troubled skin or raw tissues.

Because moxa entails the burning of mugwort, a substantial amount of smoke is produced, which can irritate the lungs and mucous membranes of the eyes and nose, and leave a scorched odor that clings to textiles. Minimize this by opening windows and operating fans. If adequate ventilation cannot be provided then moxa should be performed outdoors or not at all (see "Ventilation" in Chapter 8).

Since moxa entails some risk of burning, precautions should be taken (see "Practitioner Administration Versus Client Self-Administration" in Chapter 8). Ask the client to alert you before the sensation of heat becomes too strong. Additionally, make the peace or victory sign with your nonworking hand and place it on either side of the acupressure point that is to receive moxa. When you begin to feel the heat intensify, retract the moxa before it stings. If you allow the moxa to sting, most likely a blister will form, which will be followed by a scar that gradually fades. Periodically tap the ash into a basin so that it does not aggregate and drop off onto the client. Properly extinguish the moxa to avoid a fire hazard (see "Indirect Application" in Chapter 8).

GUA SHA

Gua Sha is contraindicated when the client has any skin anomaly, skin disorder, or breach in the skin, including moles, pimples, rashes, burns, bruises, scrapes, cuts, scabs, and open wounds. The contraindication may be local or total, depending on how widespread the condition is. For example, isolated pimples or moles can be covered with a finger and worked around. However, if the entire target area is covered with pimples or moles, Gua Sha is contraindicated. Gua Sha is contraindicated on the abdomen of a pregnant woman but may be applied to her lower back, sacrum, and hips. Exercise caution with a client who is taking blood-thinning medication (prescribed for cardiovascular diseases). Spot treat a limited area to assess the client's reaction before proceeding further. If in doubt, abstain from Gua Sha. Finally, the frequency of Gua Sha sessions should be limited to once every two weeks.

The Asian custom of applying Gua Sha to avert or expel a seasonal illness contravenes the Western practice of refusing to give therapy to sick clients. This creates an interesting dilemma for the practitioner, who must choose between a conventional or unconventional approach (see "Gua Sha Uses and Indications" in Chapter 8 and "Contraindications" in Chapter 9). Certain professional imperatives, such as honoring a business policy or a local health department mandate, may militate against working on a sick client in favor of protecting the public health. However, if no professional constraints exist, the practitioner may want to consider administering Gua Sha to ward off a full-blown cold or flu or to accelerate its departure. If the practitioner decides to offer treatment, certain precautions can be taken to reduce the risk of becoming infected. Among these are working only when one feels healthy, taking immune-boosting vitamins and herbal supplements, abstaining from Gua Sha during the brief, acute, contagious phase of the illness when the client first manifests symptoms, ventilating during treatment, and disinfecting the air, contact surfaces, and hands after treatment. The ideal time to apply Gua Sha is when the client has the first inkling that she is getting ill or when the illness has matured. Aside from working on clients in a private practice, friends and family can be ideal candidates for Gua Sha.

CLIENT INFORMATION AND CONSENT

Because moxa entails a minor risk of burning, blistering, and temporary scarring and because Gua Sha leaves painless, temporary patches of reddish, millet-like speckles on the skin, informed client consent to treatment should be obtained, preferably in writing. As a professional courtesy to clients, you may want to prepare an informational handout to educate them about each therapy (see Exhibit 8-1 on self-administered moxa and Exhibit 8-2 on Gua Sha).

KEY THERAPEUTIC AREAS AND ACUPRESSURE POINTS

For acupressure point and Meridian locations, see Appendix 1, the Flow of Qi chart in Figure 2-1, and the enlarged views of the Shu/Yu and Mu/Bo points in Figures 7-6 and 7-7. For further instructions on moxa and Gua Sha treatment, see Chapter 8.

MOXA

- For colds, moxa Lu 1, Ki 27, CV 17, Bl 10, Bl 12, Bl 13, Bl 14, GV 16, GB 20, and GB 21.
- For sinking Qi disorders, such as hemorrhoids and chronic diarrhea, moxa GV 20, CV 6, CV 12, Sp 3, St 25, St 36, and LI 11.
- For lower burner disorders of a Cold, Damp nature, such as bladder infections and vaginal yeast infections, moxa CV 3, CV 4, CV 5, and CV 6.
- For lower back pain, moxa Bl 23, Bl 25, GV 4, St 25, and St 27.
- For knee aches, moxa points around the knee, such as Sp 9, Sp 10, St 34, St 35, St 36, GB 34, and Bl 40.
- For ankle aches, moxa points around the ankle, such as St 41, GB 40, Bl 60, Ki 3, Ki 4, Ki 5, and Ki 6.
- For foot aches, moxa points on the foot, such as Sp 3, Lr 3, St 41, St 42, St 43, GB 40, GB 41, Ki 1, and Bl 67, as well as the points (called Bafeng) between the metatarsals or webs between the toes (see Appendix 1: Glossary of Acupoints).
- For wrist aches, moxa points around the wrist, such as LI 5, TH 4, TH 5, SI 5, Lu 9, PC 7, Ht 4, Ht 5, Ht 6, and Ht 7.
- For hand aches, moxa points on the hand, such as LI 4, SI 3, and PC 8, as well as the points (called Shangbaxie) between the metacarpals or webs between the fingers (see Appendix 1).
- To rotate a fetus in a breech position, moxa Bl 67 around the thirtyeighth week of pregnancy.
- For delayed or difficult childbirth, moxa LI 4, Sp 6, and GB 21 to facilitate labor; also moxa Lr 3, Ki 1, and Bl 67. *Note*: LI 4, Sp 6, and GB 21 are contraindicated during pregnancy because they draw energy downward and could induce a miscarriage; vigorous stimulation of any points below the knee is contraindicated during pregnancy.

GUA SHA

- For a cold, Gua Sha downward on the midline over the breastbone, covering CV 17; Gua Sha outward under the collarbone from the breastbone to the shoulder, covering Ki 27, St 13, and Lu 2; Gua Sha outward again on a lower swath, covering Ki 26, St 14, and Lu 1; continue with another, still lower swath; Gua Sha downward on the midline from GV 16 to the middle back; Gua Sha down the inner Bladder Meridian from Bl 10 at the neck to the middle back, covering Bl 12, Bl 13, and Bl 14; repeat another swath on the outer Bladder Meridian from the neck to the middle back.
- For a sore, stiff shoulder, Gua Sha downward on the midline from GV 16 at the neck to the middle back; Gua Sha down the inner Bladder Meridian from Bl 10 at the neck to the middle back; repeat again on the outer Bladder Meridian from the neck to the middle back, covering Bl 43; Gua Sha outward from GB 20 at the neck to the shoulder crest, covering GB 21; Gua Sha outward over the shoulder blade, covering SI 12, SI 11, SI 10, and SI 9; Gua Sha downward over the side of the shoulder, covering LI 15, LI 14, TH 14, and TH 13; continue down the arm, if necessary.
- For a sore, stiff lower back, Gua Sha downward on the midline from the middle back to the tailbone, covering GV 4; Gua Sha downward from Bl 20 at the middle back to the sacrum, covering Bl 23 and Bl 25; repeat again on the outer Bladder Meridian, covering Bl 53 and Bl 54 in the buttock; Gua Sha the buttock from the edge of the sacrum to the hipbone, covering GB 30; continue down the leg, if necessary.

MOXABUSTION

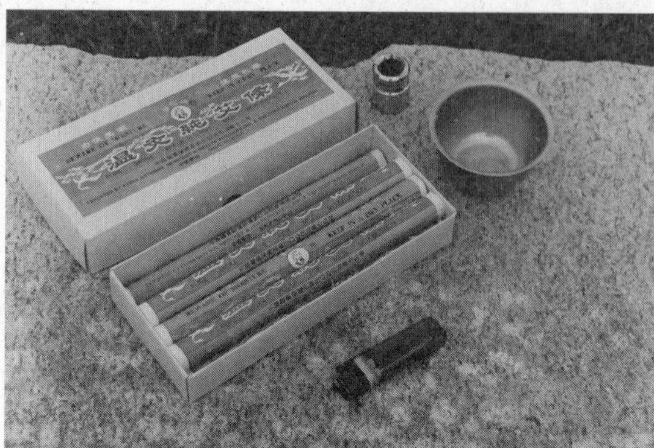

FIGURE 17-1 Indirect moxabustion supplies: box of moxa rolls, lighter, ash basin, and snuffer.
Choose a venue with good ventilation (outdoors is best).

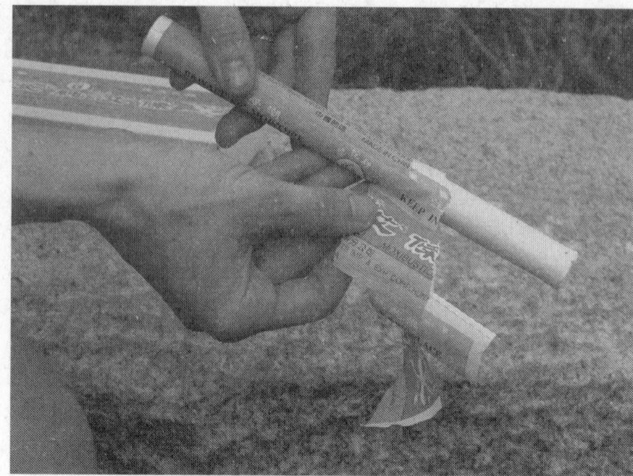

FIGURE 17-2 Peel back the paper lining.

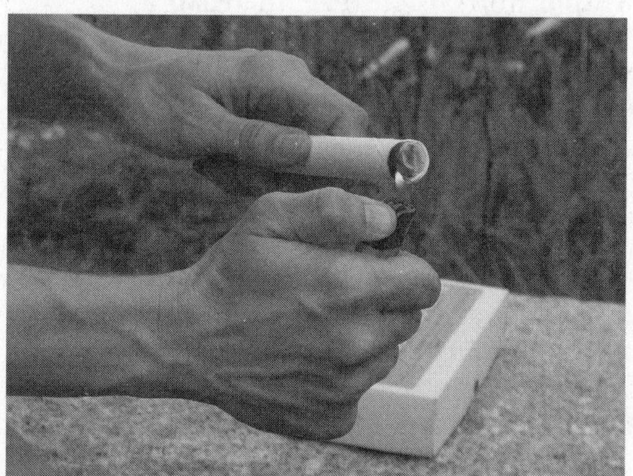

FIGURE 17-3 Light the moxa roll or "cigar."

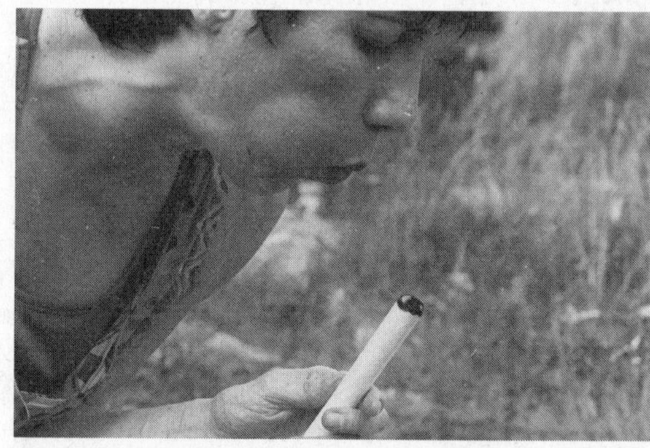

FIGURE 17-4 Oxygenate the fire.
Note: Blowing on the ignited moxa cigar to fan the flame is safe only at the beginning, before ash accumulates. Later, after ash accumulates, blowing can disperse hot ash on your person or elsewhere.

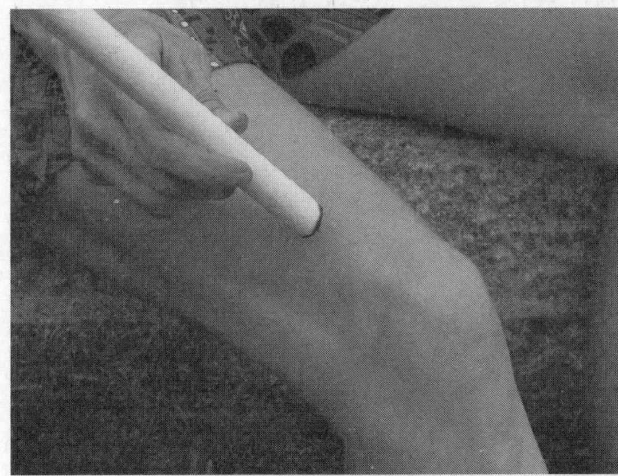

FIGURE 17-5 **St 34.**
Hold the moxa cigar over the point, or circle the cigar around the point, or peck the cigar toward and away from the point. Here a circular orbit is applied (the cigar tip is above to the point).

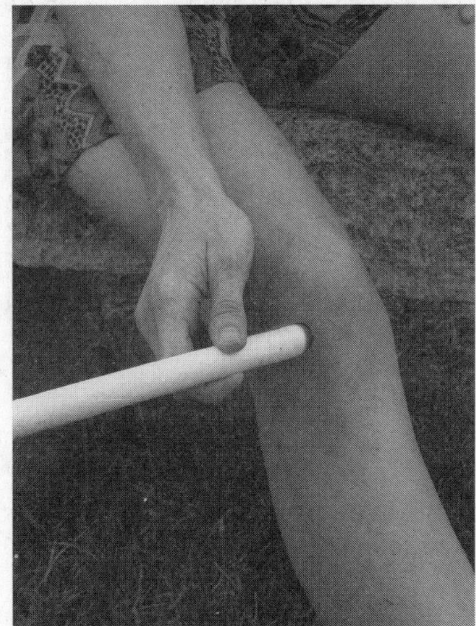

FIGURE 17-6 **St 35.**
Initially, while the cigar end is still blunt, you can hold the cigar over a point for a longer period of time before the heat sensation becomes intolerable.

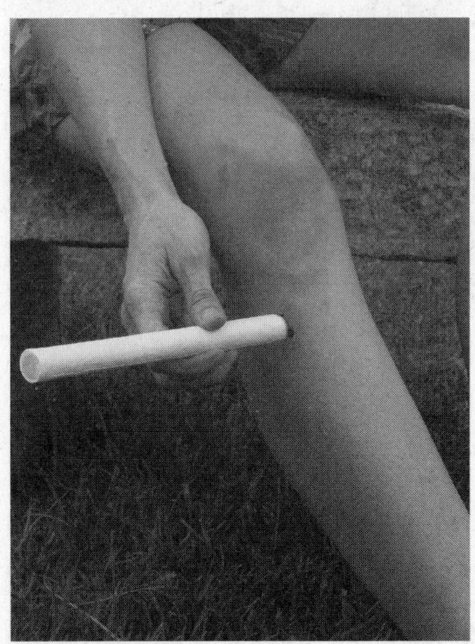

FIGURE 17-7 **St 36.**

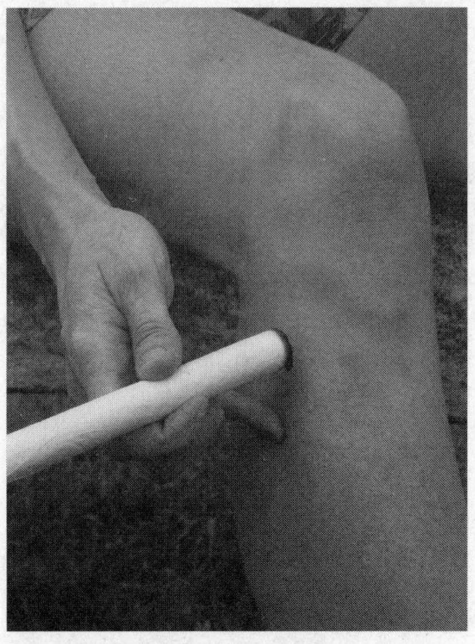

FIGURE 17-8 **GB 34.**

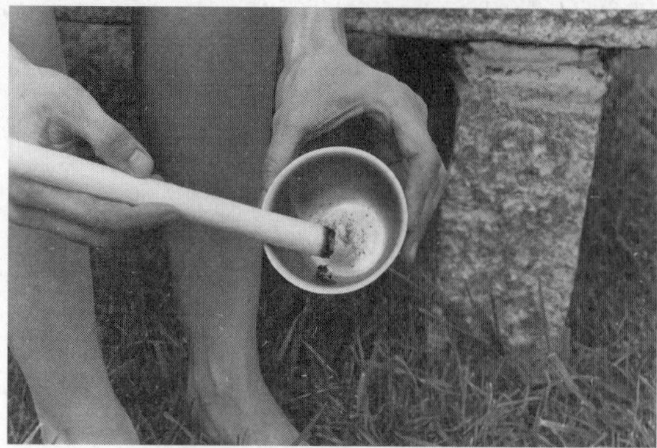

FIGURE 17-9 Tap the ash.
Periodically tap the ash to avoid dropping it on your person. Tapping loose ash becomes more important as the cigar end gets hotter and more pointed. A habit of tapping can preempt the spontaneous detachment of glowing chunks, which sometimes occurs.

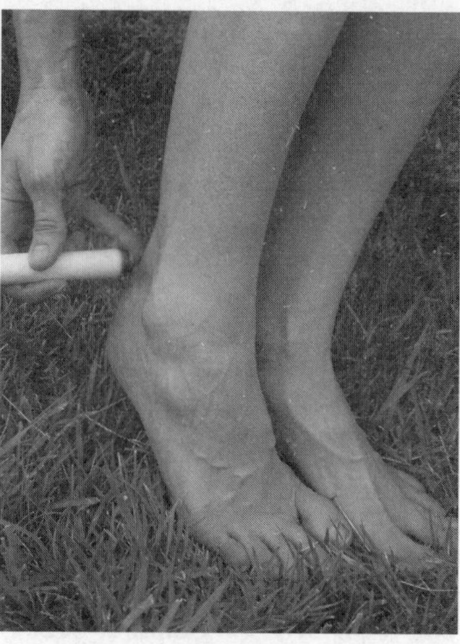

FIGURE 17-10 Bl 60.
Once the cigar end turns into a glowing red cone-shaped tip, you'll have to move it more often to prevent stinging and burning.

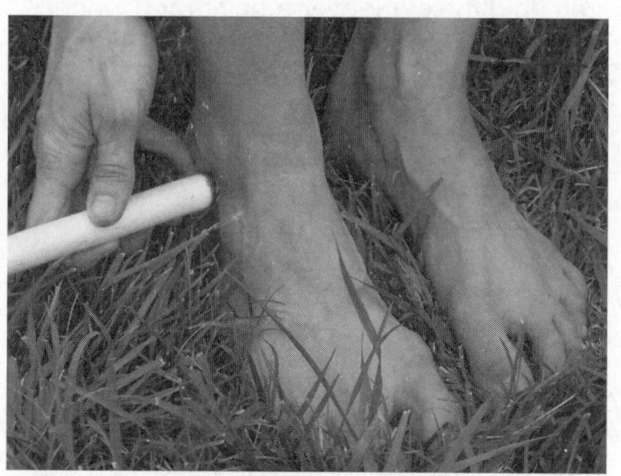

FIGURE 17-11 GB 40.
Quickly withdraw the cigar when you begin to experience a sharp, hot, stinging sensation. Move to another point, or repeat the treatment on that point three to seven times, as needed.

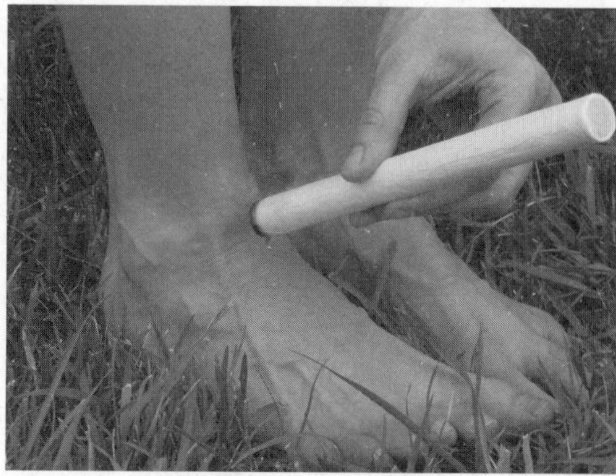

FIGURE 17-12 St 41.

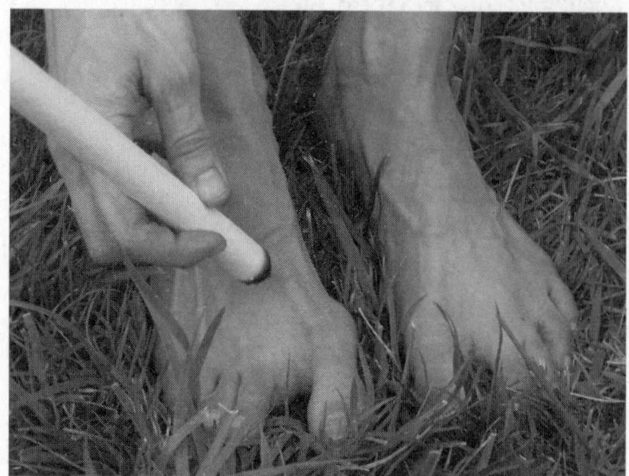

FIGURE 17-13 Lr 3.

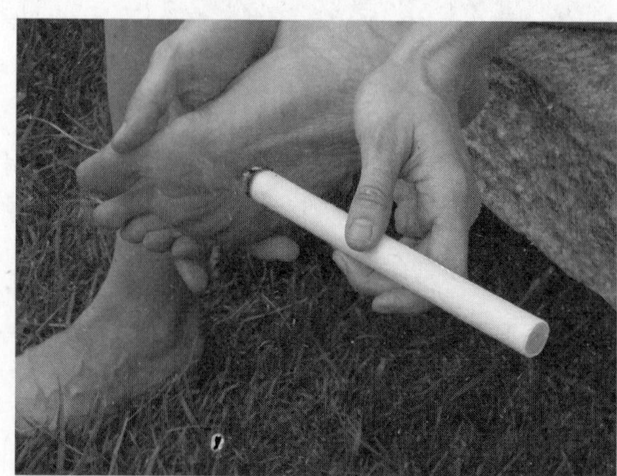

FIGURE 17-14 Ki 1.

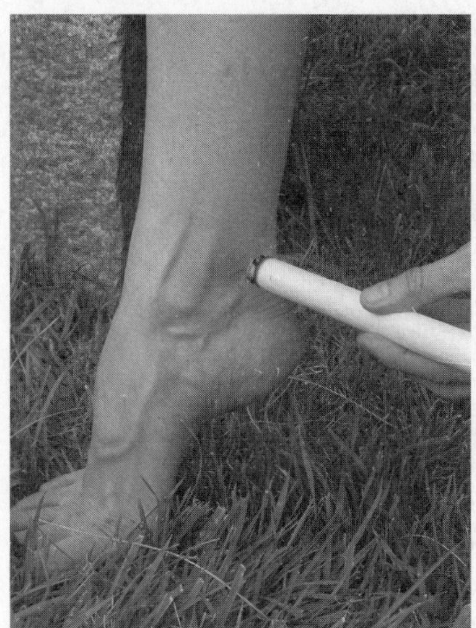
FIGURE 17-15 **Ki 3.**

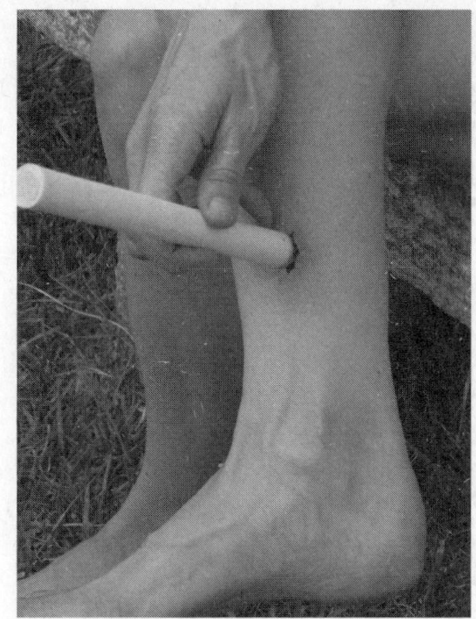
FIGURE 17-16 **Sp 6.**

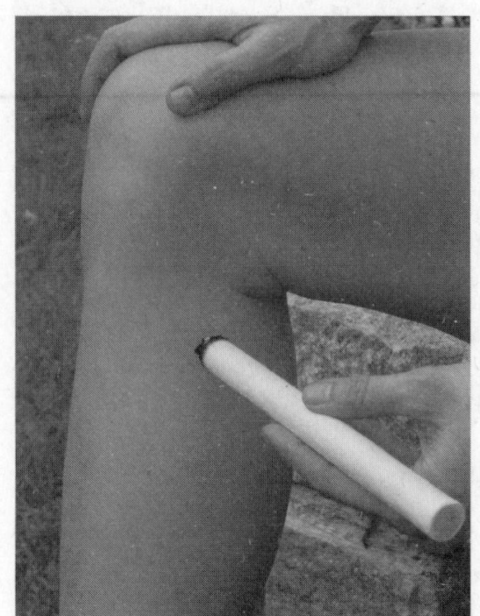
FIGURE 17-17 **Sp 9.**

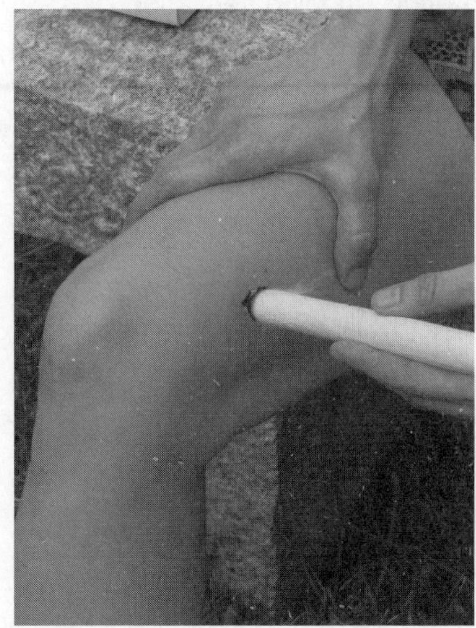
FIGURE 17-18 **Sp 10.**

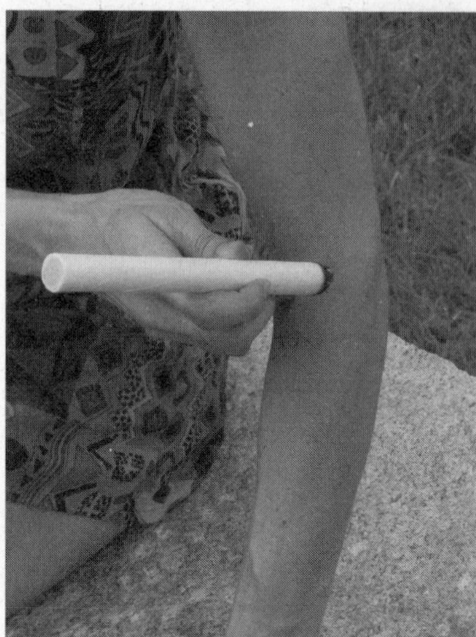

FIGURE 17-19 LI 11.
When the cigar end turns into a glowing cone shape, take care not to linger too long over a point, as you may experience a sudden, sharp, penetrating, stinging sensation.

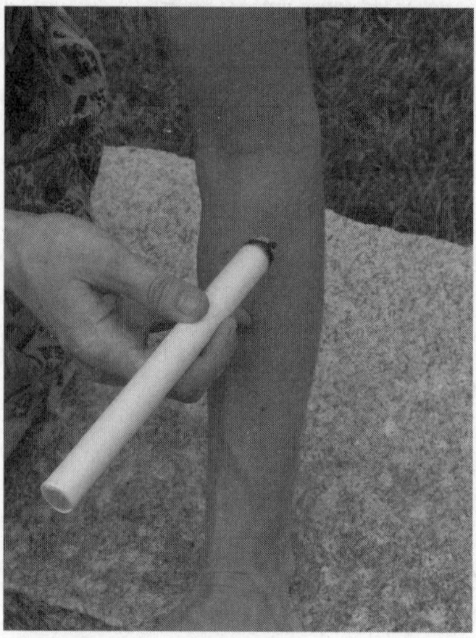

FIGURE 17-20 LI 10.
Lingering too long over a point when the heat is very intense can cause blistering and possibly scarring. The regenerated skin will be browner and rosier than the surrounding area.

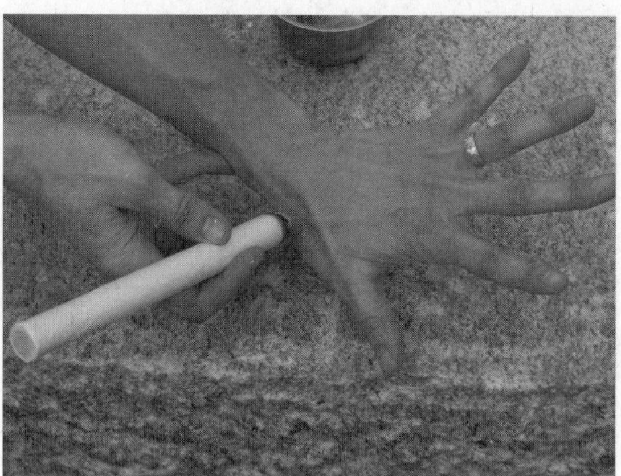

FIGURE 17-21 LI 5.

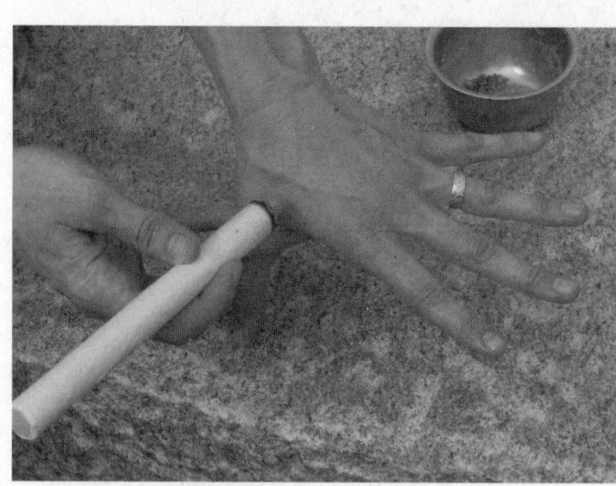

FIGURE 17-22 LI 4.

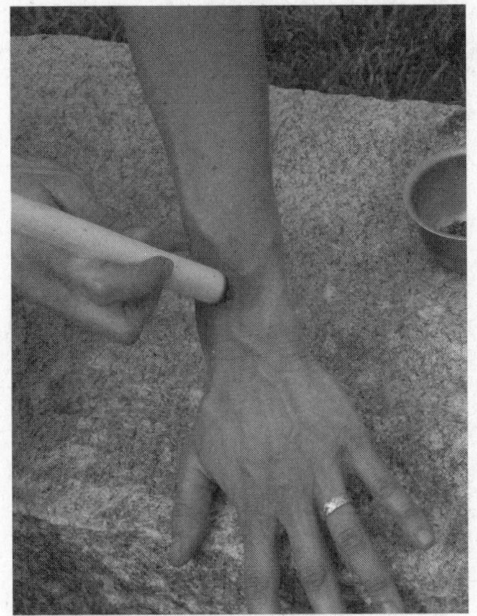
FIGURE 17-23 TH 5.

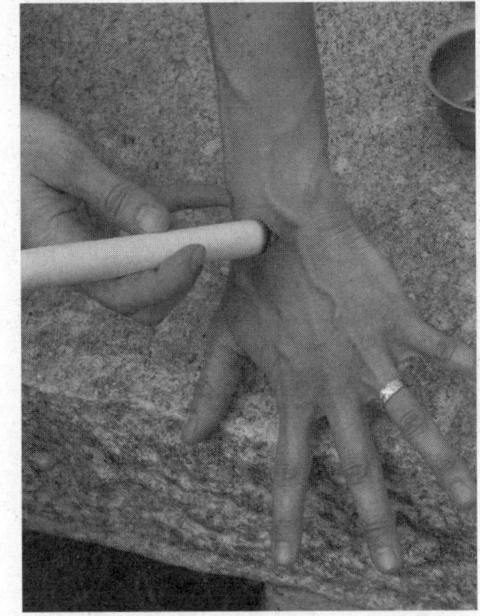
FIGURE 17-24 TH 4.

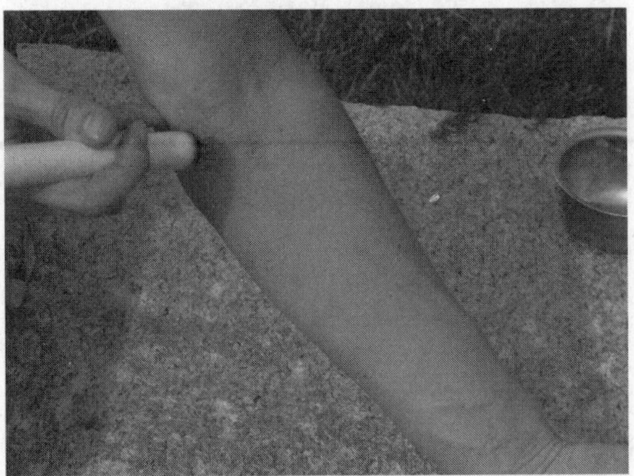
FIGURE 17-25 Ht 3.

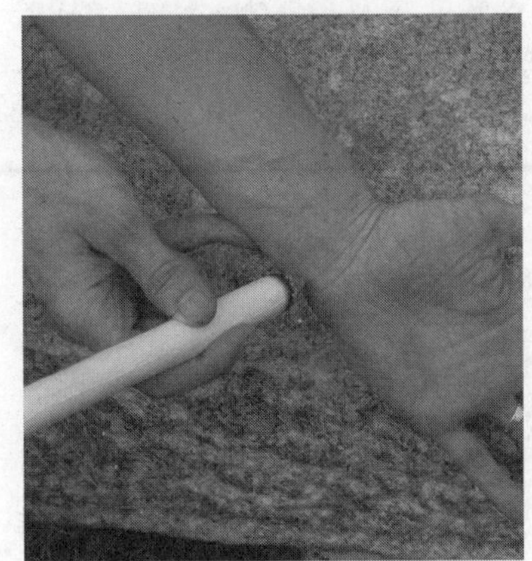
FIGURE 17-26 Ht 7.

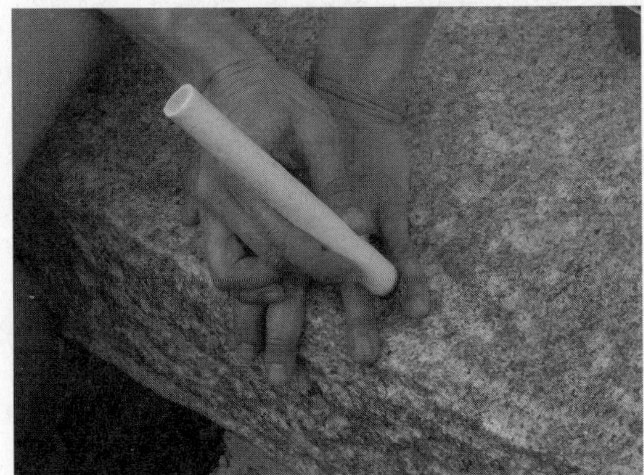
FIGURE 17-27 Ht 9.

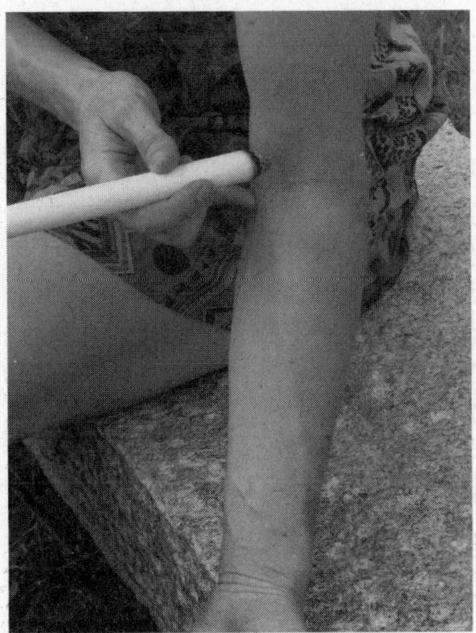
FIGURE 17-28 PC 3.

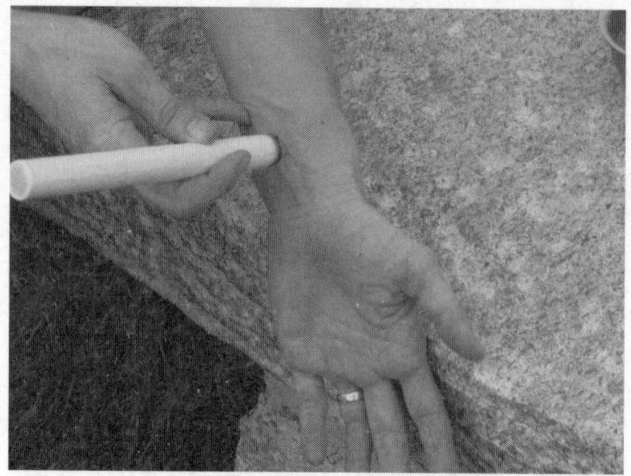

FIGURE 17-29 PC 6.

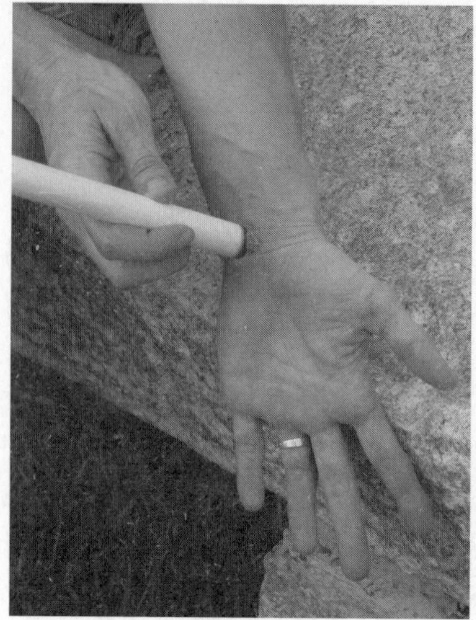

FIGURE 17-30 PC 7.

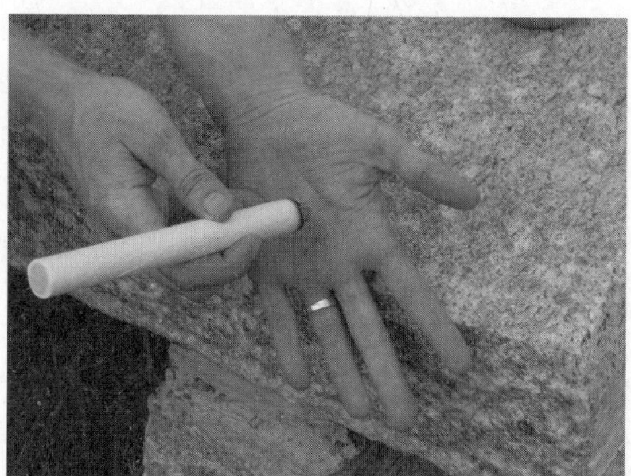

FIGURE 17-31 PC 8.

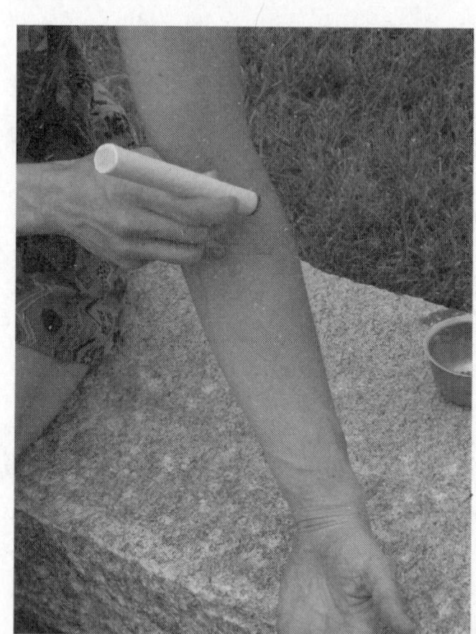

FIGURE 17-32 Lu 5.

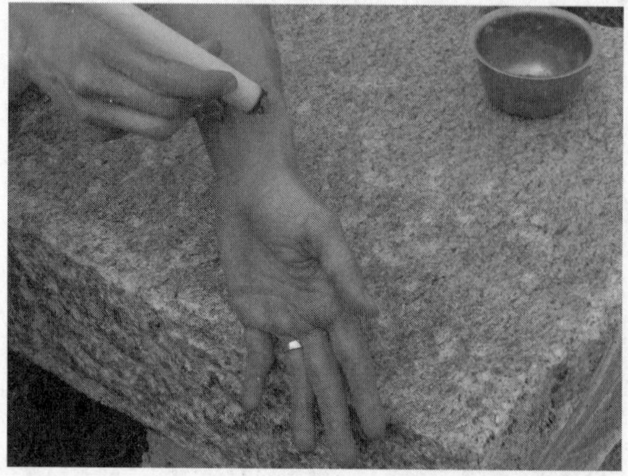

FIGURE 17-33 Lu 7.

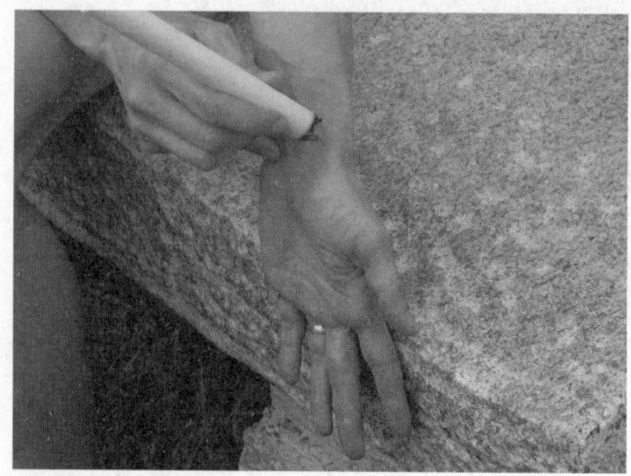

FIGURE 17-34 Lu 9.

GUA SHA

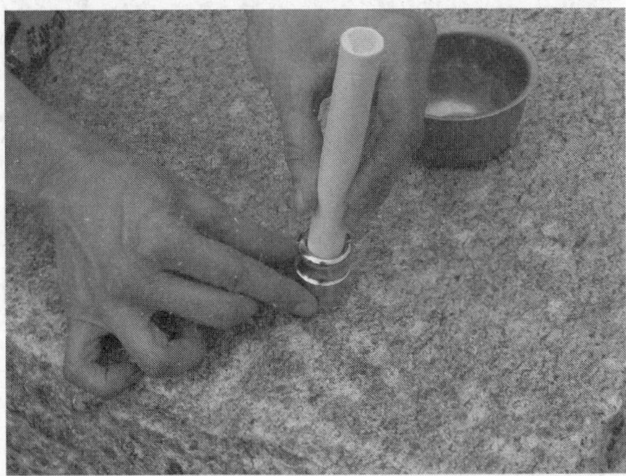

FIGURE 17-35 **Extinguish the roll.** The best way to extinguish the cigar and keep it intact for future use is to deprive it of oxygen, as this snug snuffer does.

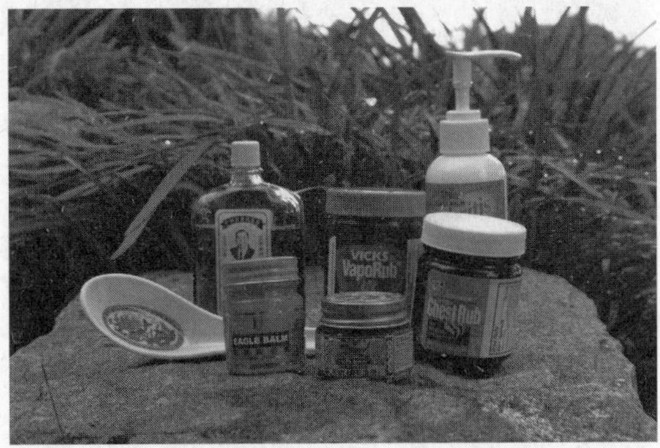

FIGURE 17-36 **Gua Sha supplies and tools.** Select a favorite balm or liniment to provide lubrication and a Chinese soup spoon or Tiger Balm lid to scrape. The best lubricants have a Vaseline base containing essential oils such as menthol, peppermint, eucalyptus, and camphor.

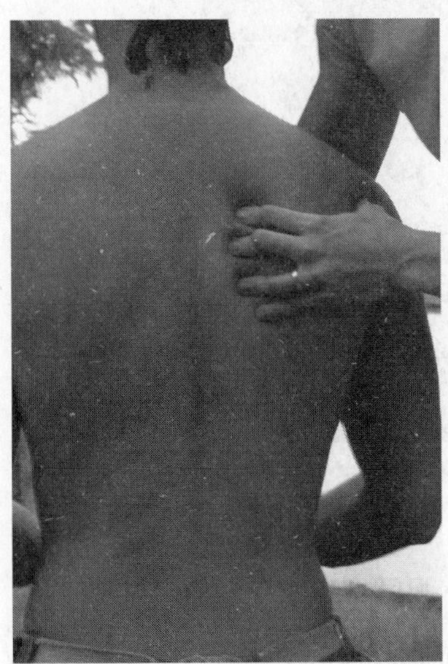

FIGURE 17-37 **Press and blanch, step 1.** Ask the client to point out any problem areas. Press your fingers into the client's tissues and remove them quickly.

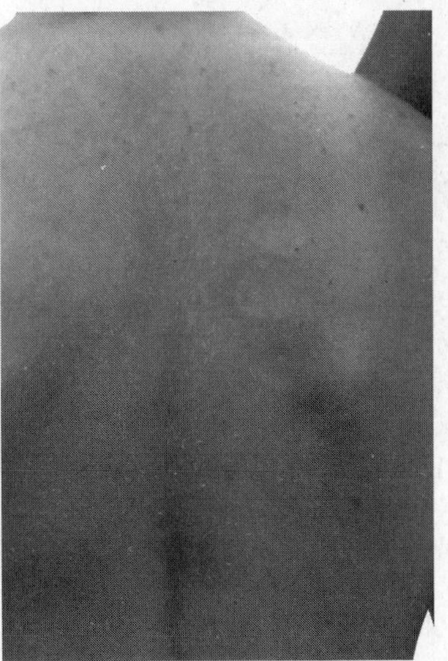

FIGURE 17-38 **Press and blanch, step 2.** Any pale, almond–shaped afterimages of your fingerprints indicate the presence of Sha and the need for Gua Sha.

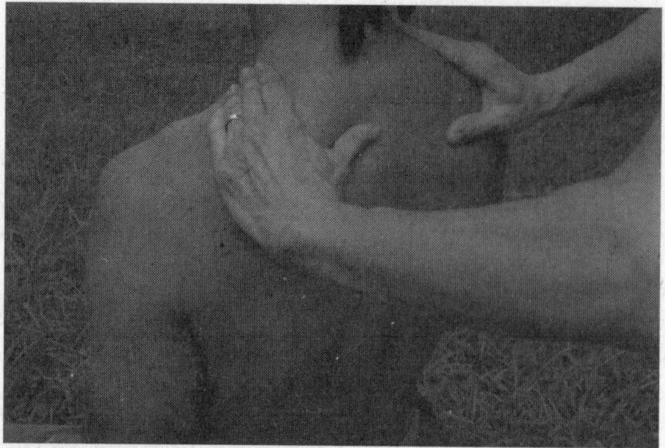

FIGURE 17-39 Spread the balm or liniment.
Vicks® VapoRub® or its generic version, Tiger Balm, and Eagle Balm all provide smooth traction for scraping.

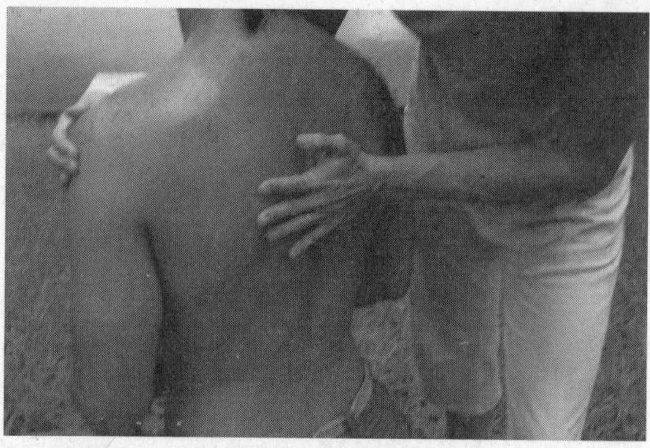

FIGURE 17-40 Spread the balm.

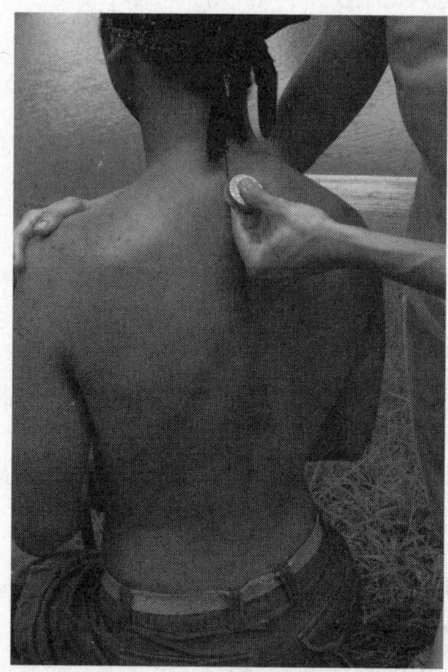

FIGURE 17-41 Gua Sha the Governing Vessel.
Begin by lightly scraping the Governing Vessel. Do not press too hard on this Meridian, as the spinous processes of the vertebrae protrude.

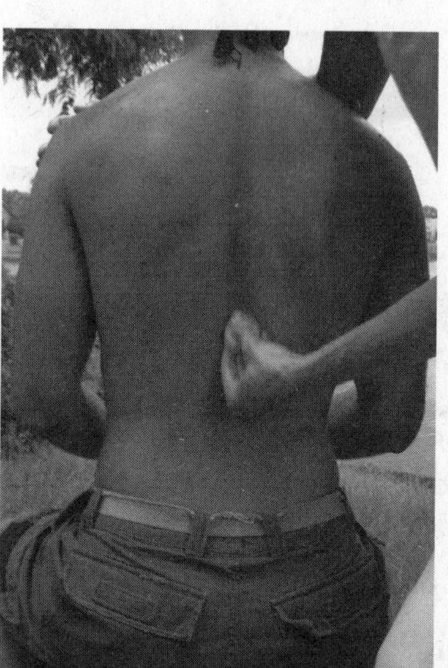

FIGURE 17-42 Direction, length, and number of strokes.
Scrape superior to inferior, from the neck downward. Swaths are from 4 to 7 inches in length, depending on the area. At the end of each stroke, lift the tool, reset it at the top, and repeat 7 to 11 times or until petechiae manifest or the client reports surface irritation (which is uncommon).

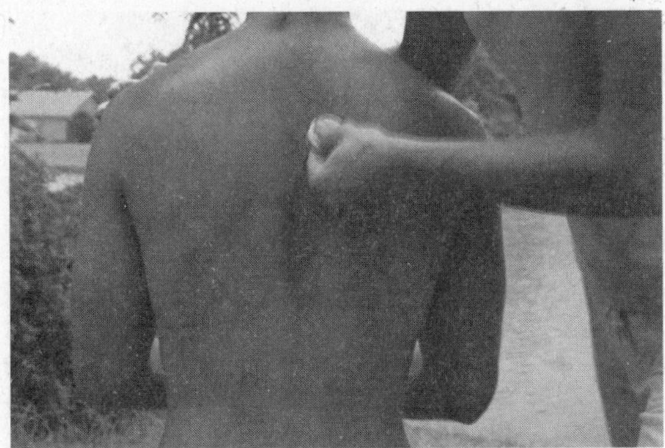

FIGURE 17-43 Gua Sha the inner Bladder Meridian.
Relocate the scraping tool about one and a half cun lateral to the midline and scrape the inner Bladder Meridian.

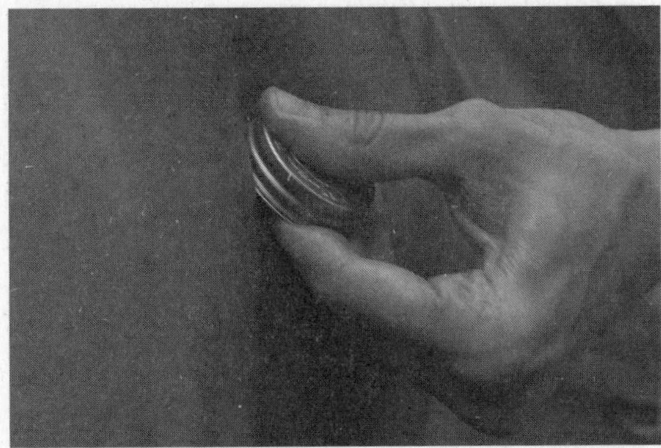

FIGURE 17-44 Angle of the scraping tool.
Hold the scraping tool at an angle close to the client's flesh—about 10 to 15 degrees—allowing enough space for your fingers to wrap underneath the tool. Your fingers should initiate and lead the stroke, maintaining contact with the client's tissues at all times.

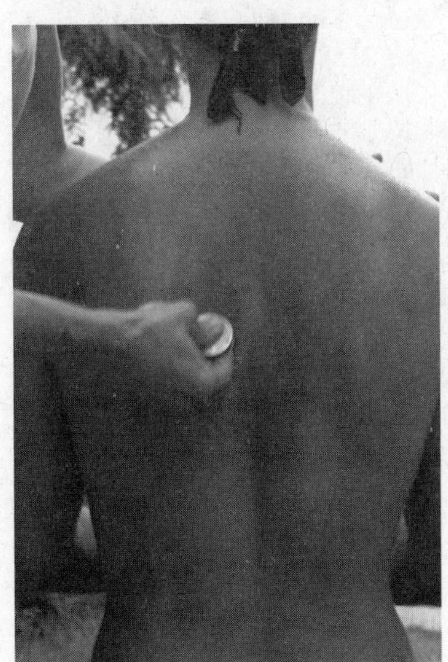

FIGURE 17-45 Gua Sha the other side of the inner Bladder Meridian.

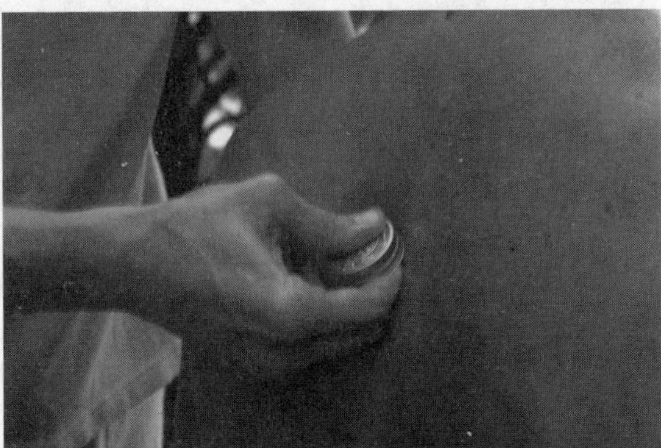

FIGURE 17-46 Press the scraping tool into the fascia.
Apply enough pressure to penetrate beyond the superficial layer of skin into the connective tissue beneath.

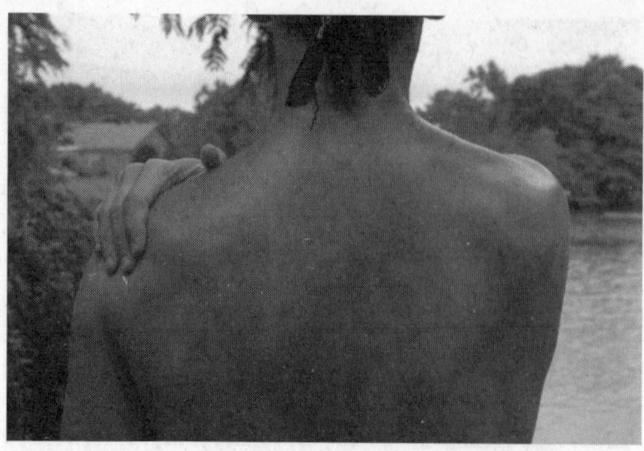

FIGURE 17-47 Wrapped arm position.
If the client is seated, direct the client to wrap his arm across his chest and drape his hand over the opposite shoulder. This protracts the vertebral border of the scapula in order to expose the area for scraping. If the client is lying prone on a table, dangle the arm over the edge of the table.

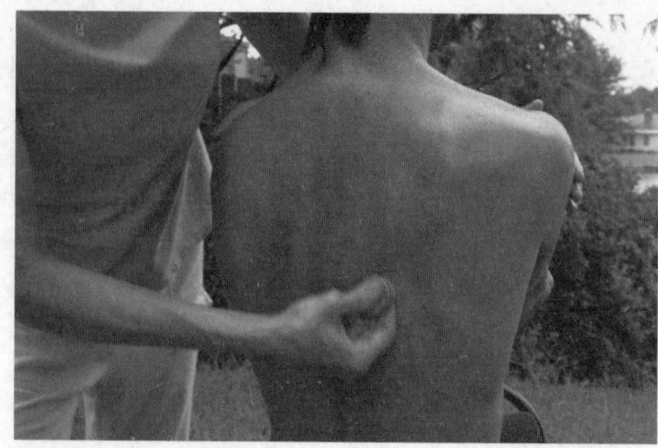

FIGURE 17-48 Gua Sha the outer Bladder Meridian.
Move laterally another $1\frac{1}{2}$ cun (3 cun from the midline) to scrape the outer Bladder Meridian. Swaths should overlap slightly so that no area is left untreated.

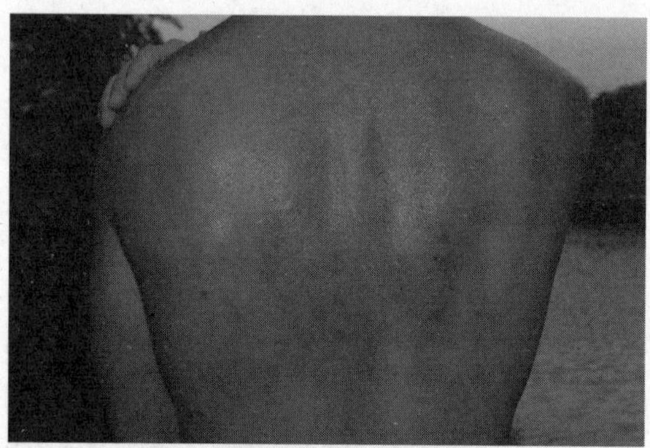

FIGURE 17-49 Examine Sha.
This young man, who is a professional modern dancer, presents red Sha, indicating Heat. Since he stays well hydrated and his vegetarian diet is fairly mild and salubrious, the Heat is probably due to the intense physical exertions and rigors of his chosen career. One could chase the dragon down his entire back; however, we will stop here.

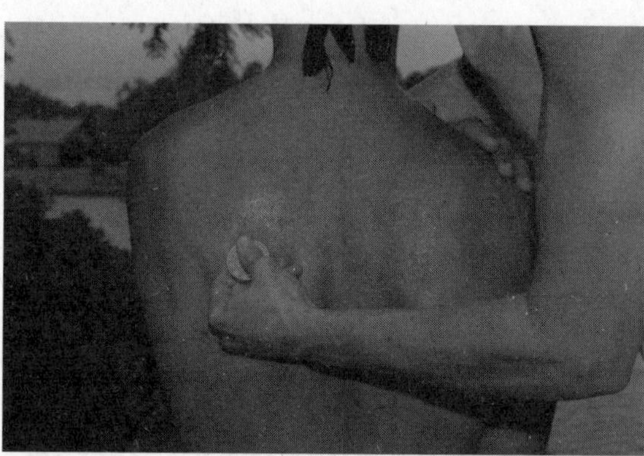

FIGURE 17-50 Gua Sha the outer Bladder Meridian, other side.

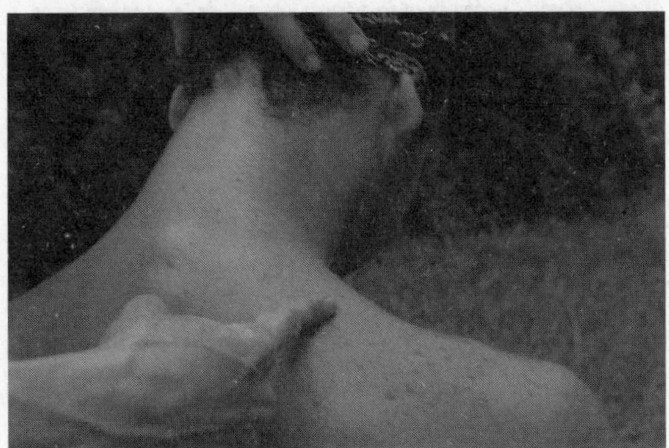

FIGURE 17-51 Forward head position. Direct the client to tilt his head forward slightly to expose the posterior surface of the neck.

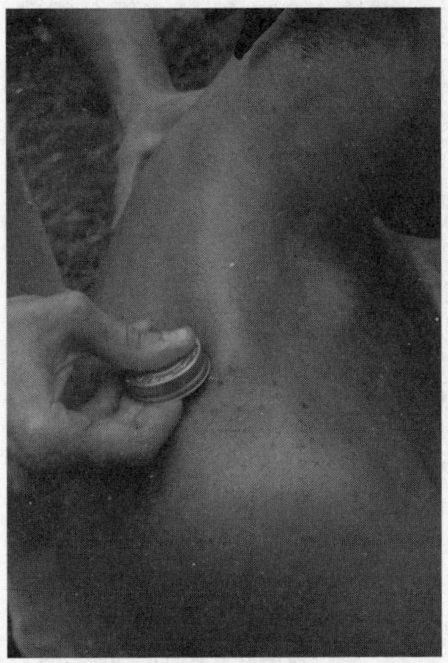

FIGURE 17-52 Gua Sha the neck and upper shoulder. Begin under the occiput at Bl 10 and scrape downward and outward, sweeping over SI 12 of the upper shoulder (shown). Move laterally to GB 20 and scrape downward and outward over GB 21, a powerful acupoint for the upper shoulder.

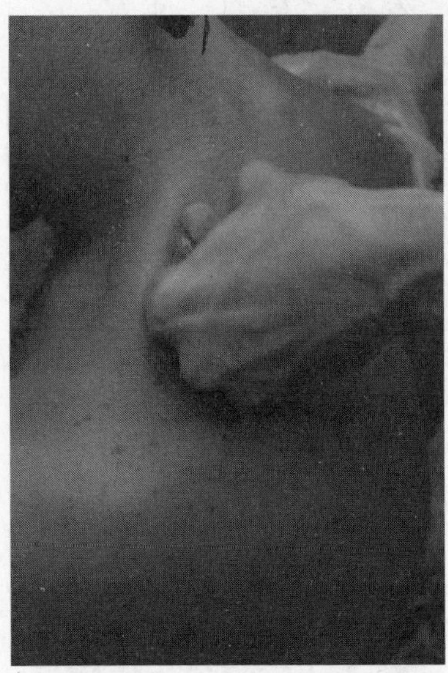

FIGURE 17-53 Neck and upper shoulder, other side. Recap: The first series of strokes begins at Bl 10 and sweeps over SI 12.

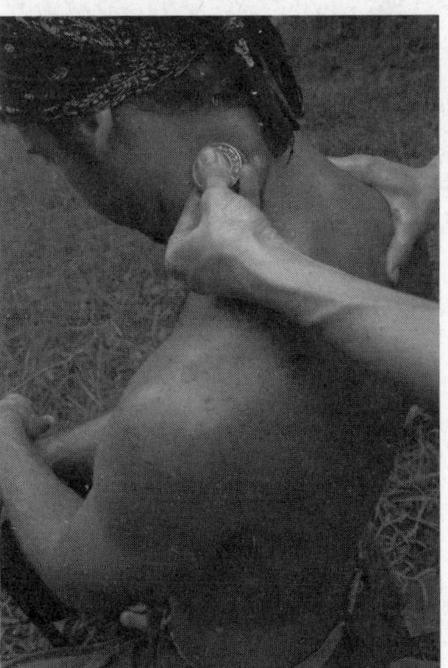

FIGURE 17-54 Neck and upper shoulder, other side. Recap: The second series of strokes begins at GB 20 and sweeps over GB 21.

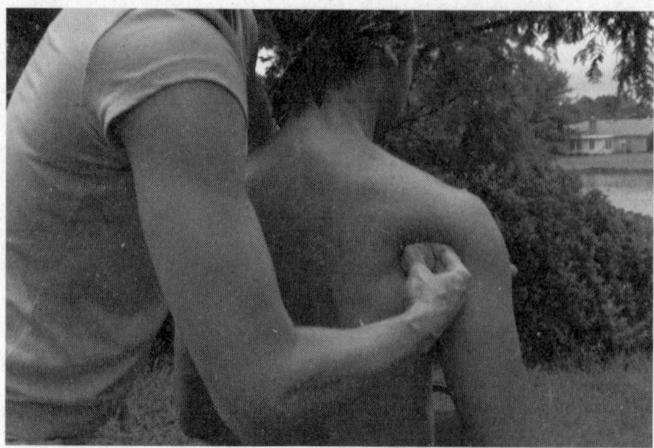

FIGURE 17-55 Gua Sha the scapula.
Scrape the shoulder blade from the vertebral border to the axilla (armpit). Begin at the superior, medial corner of the blade and move progressively lower. Here the tool is scraping over SI 11, a powerful acupoint for the rotator cuff.

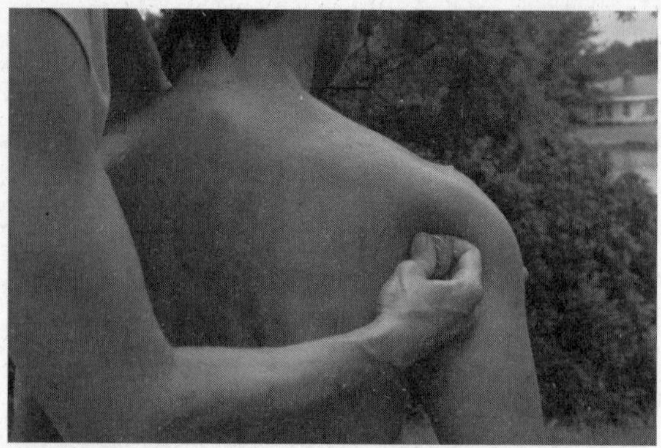

FIGURE 17-56 close-up of Gua Sha to the scapula.
Note that sufficient pressure from the scraping tool sculpts a pocket in the flesh.

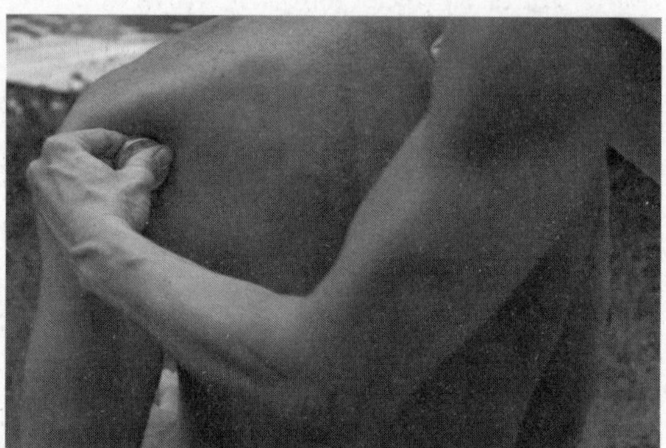

FIGURE 17-57 Gua Sha the scapula, other side.
Here the scraping tool is passing over SI 10 of the posterior deltoid.

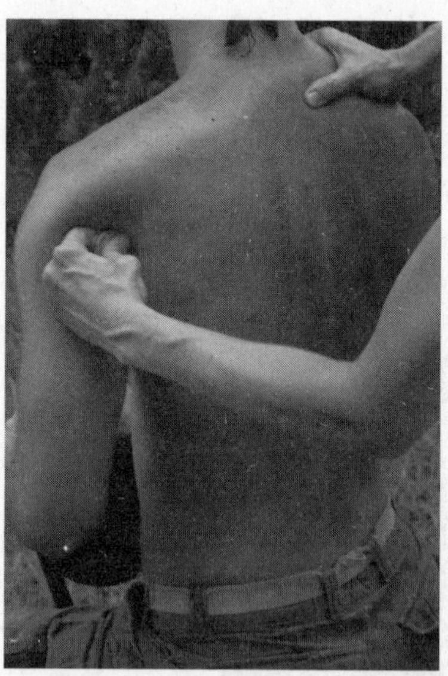

FIGURE 17-58 Further examination of Sha.
Since this model has good circulation, the Sha quickly turns from diffused red swaths to darker, crisper stripes during treatment, suggesting that the Sha will resolve and disappear fairly quickly.

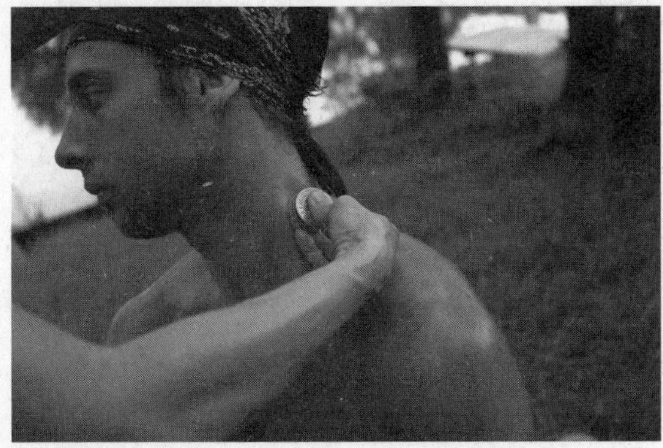

FIGURE 17-59 **Rotated head position.** Direct the client to rotate his head to the opposite shoulder to expose the anterior and lateral surfaces of the neck.

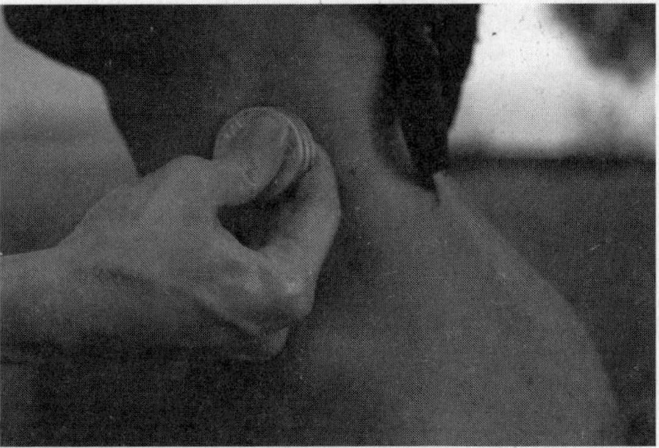

FIGURE 17-60 **Gua Sha the anterior neck.** Gua Sha the scalenes between the upper trapezius and sternocleidomastoid (SCM). The SCM may also be scraped.

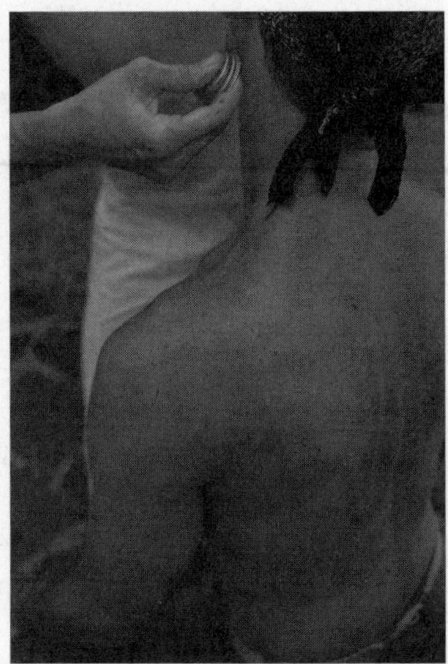

FIGURE 17-61 **Gua Sha the anterior neck.** Begin the stroke behind the ear under the mastoid process of the cranium.

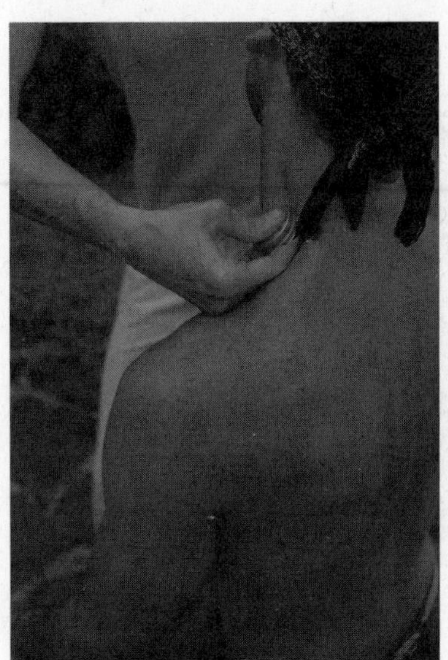

FIGURE 17-62 **Gua Sha the anterior neck.** Sweep downward and outward over the upper shoulder.

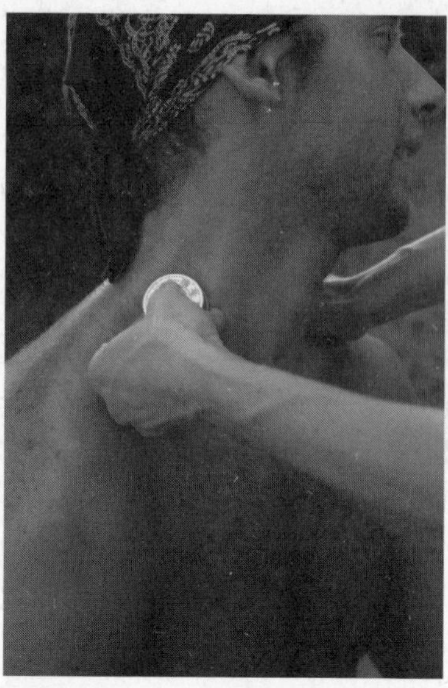

FIGURE 17-63 Gua Sha the neck, other side.

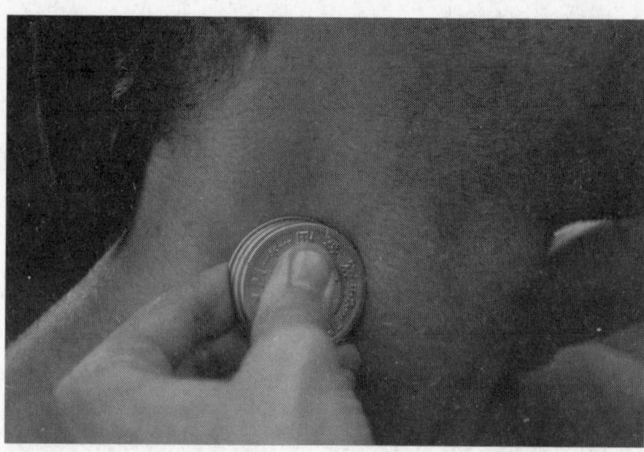

FIGURE 17-64 Close-up of Gua Sha to the neck, other side.
Note that sufficient pressure from the tool sculpts a trough between the muscles. Here the tool delineates the division between the SCM and the upper trapezius.

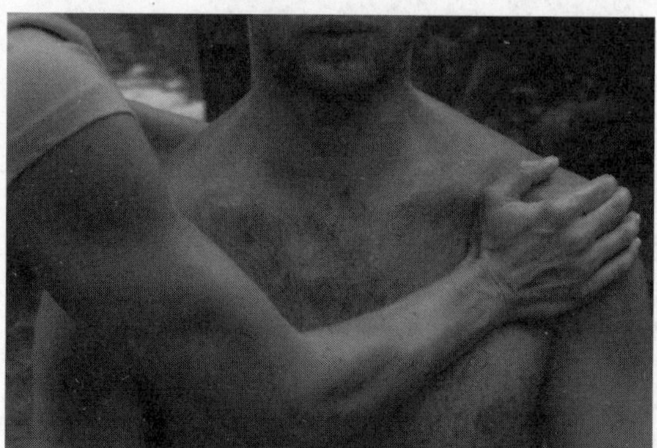

FIGURE 17-65 Spread balm on the upper chest and sternum.

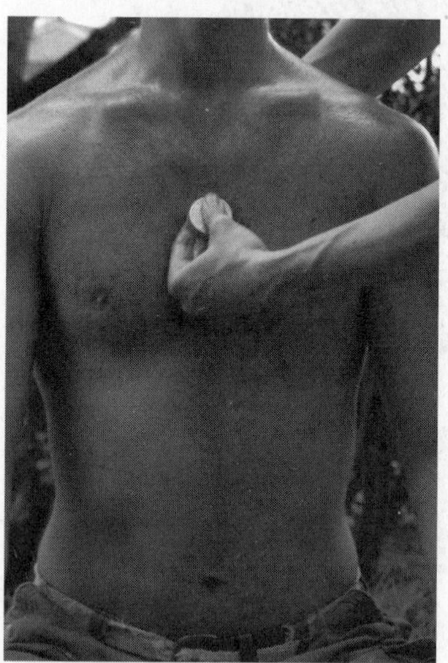

FIGURE 17-66 Gua Sha the sternum.
Apply lighter pressure on the Conception Vessel Meridian, since the sternum is a bony surface.

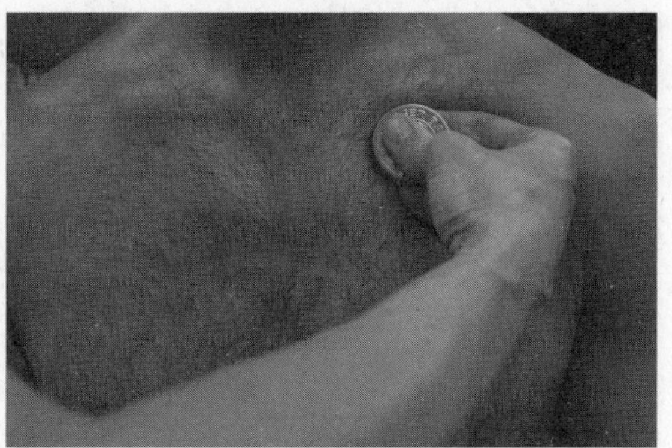

FIGURE 17-67 Gua Sha the pectoralis under the clavicle.
Start at Ki 27 and scrape laterally to Lu 2.

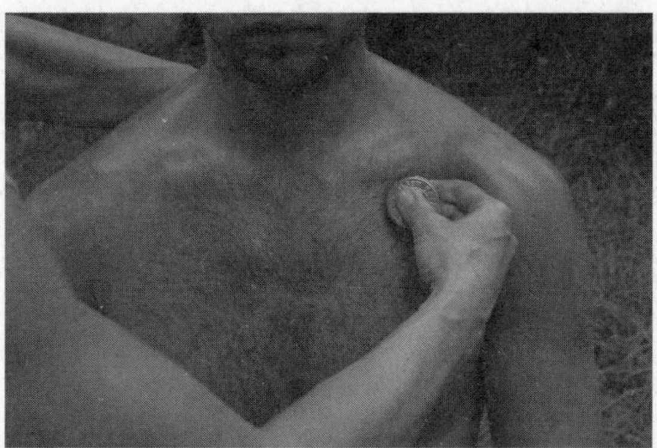

FIGURE 17-68 Gua Sha the pectoralis.

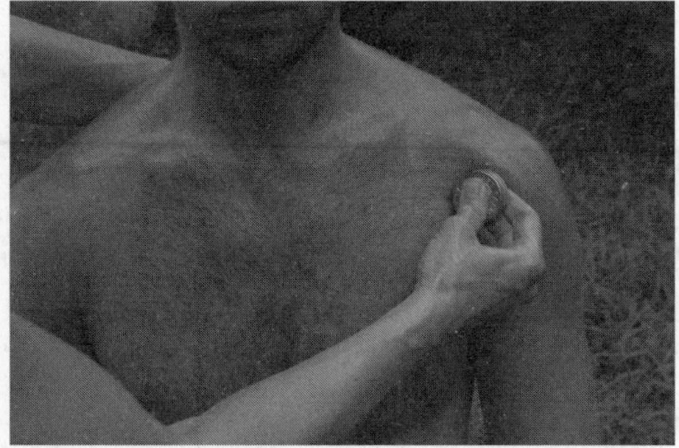

FIGURE 17-69 Extend the stroke over the anterior deltoid.
Move inferiorly and repeat the strokes, covering the upper portion of the chest.

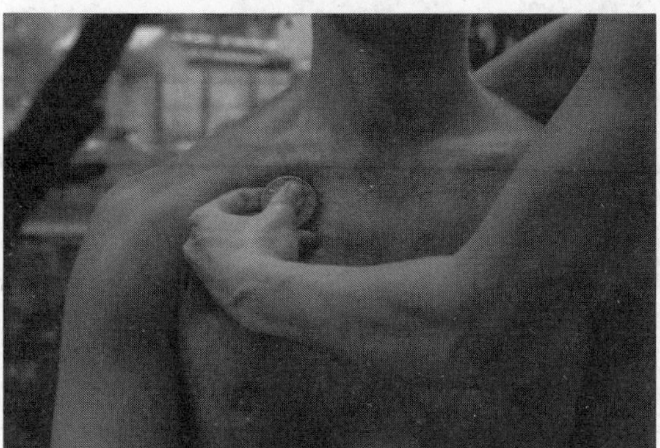

FIGURE 17-70 Gua Sha the pectoralis, other side.

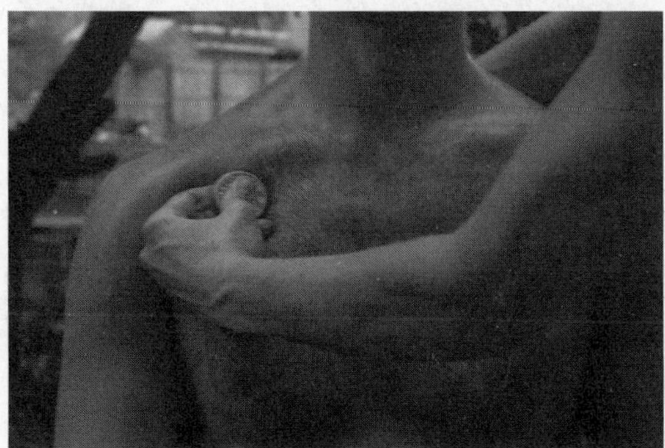

FIGURE 17-71 Gua Sha the pectoralis, other side.

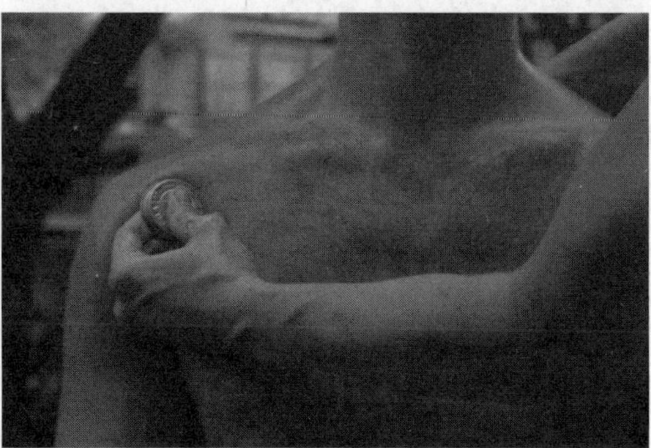

FIGURE 17-72 Gua Sha the anterior deltoid, other side.

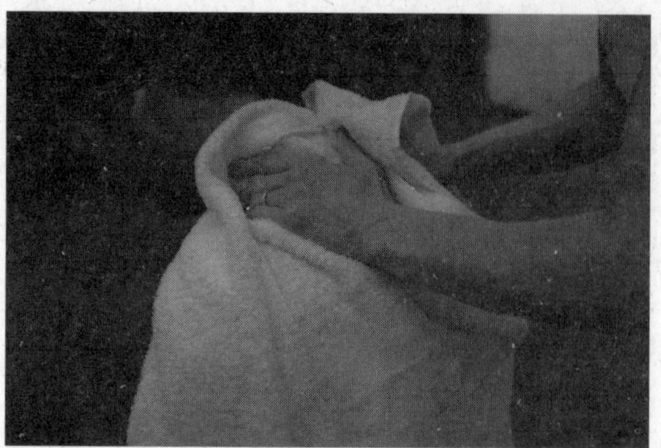

FIGURE 17-73 Wipe the balm off the client.
After treatment, remove any residual balm, which could stain the client's clothing.

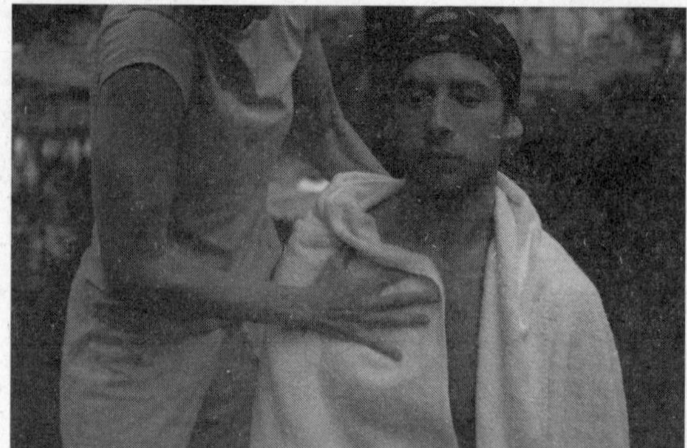

FIGURE 17-74 Wipe the balm off the client.

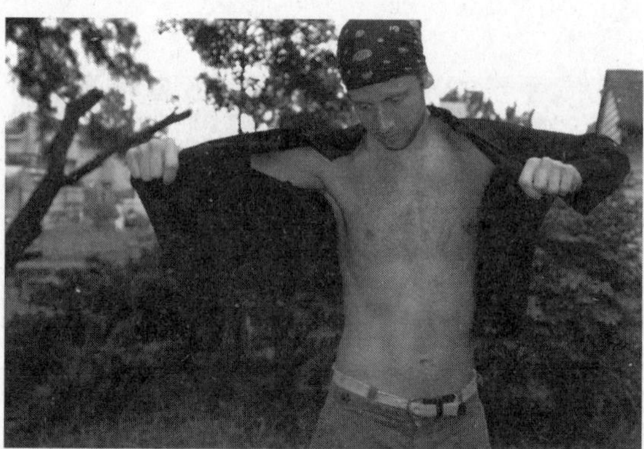

FIGURE 17-75 Instruct the client to dress.
Direct the client to dress immediately while the pores are still open and the Wei Qi or defensive armor is vulnerable.

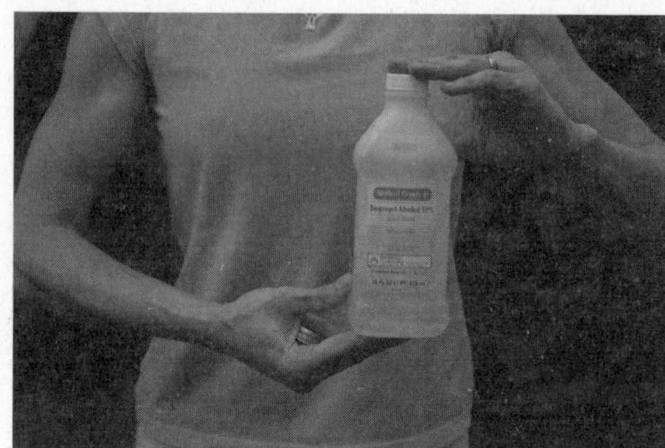

FIGURE 17-76 Sterilize tools with rubbing alcohol or other disinfectant.

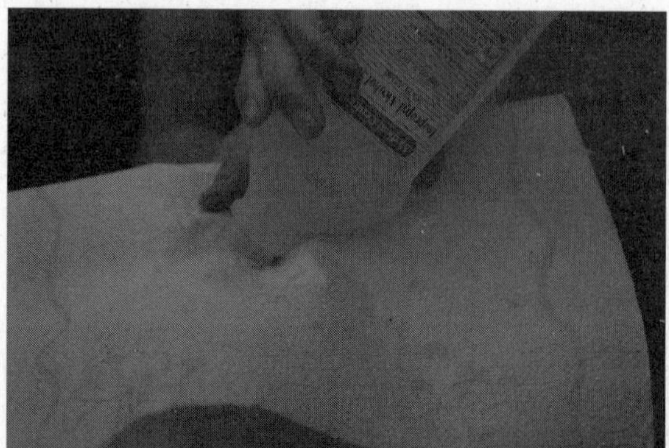

FIGURE 17-77 Soak a paper towel in rubbing alcohol.

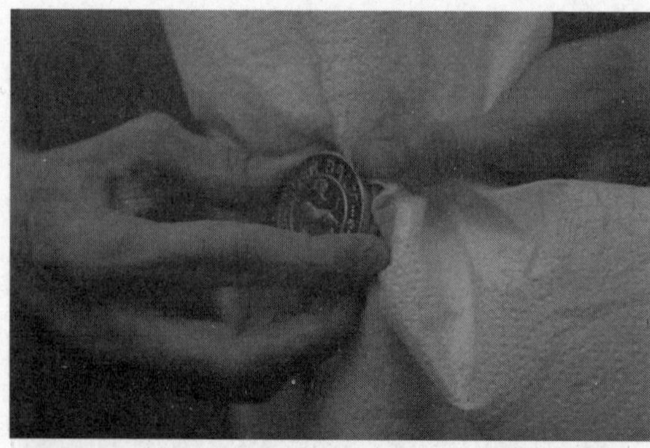

FIGURE 17-78 Sterilize the scraping tool (Tiger Balm lid).
Thoroughly wipe the tool with an alcohol-saturated paper towel, removing any bio-debris.

18

Qi Gong Exercises

Therapeutic Emphasis

The term *Qi Gong* denotes any physical discipline or exercise regimen that cultivates vital energy and develops concentration through movement of the body and regulation of the breath (see "Qi Gong" in Chapter 1). Three different cultural representations of Qi Gong are introduced in this protocol: Pal Dan Gum, Makko Ho, and Yoga. The Pal Dan Gum section is included because it is based on TCM, the theoretical and practical basis for Shiatsu. The Makko Ho section is included because it is of Japanese origin and designed for practice in a Shiatsu context. The Yoga section is included because at the time of this writing Yoga is probably the most popular form of Qi Gong in mainstream American culture. Those practitioners who are already familiar with Yoga should educate themselves about the benefits of the poses from an energetic perspective, identifying which Meridians are stimulated by a particular pose. Those who are not familiar with Yoga may want to consider developing a Yoga practice or another form of Qi Gong that is more comprehensive than either Pal Dan Gum or Makko Ho.

In any case, every practitioner should regularly do some form of Qi Gong to foster health, cultivate kinesthetic intelligence and grace, condition the body for the rigors of manual labor, prevent injury, develop concentration, and focus healing intention. Regular Qi Gong practice does all these things and is essential to a long-lasting, high-quality experience as a Shiatsu practitioner.

Pal Dan Gum are traditional Taoist (Chinese) exercises that coordinate movement with breath. Any movement that extends upward, outward, or backward is synchronized with an inhalation, and any movement that folds downward, inward, or forward is synchronized with an exhalation. These simple exercises recharge the energy of the body, cleansing the Meridians and revitalizing the organs and harmonizing their functions. They also ground and center the physical structure of the body, developing stability and balance. The whole set can be done in 5 to 10 minutes, depending on the pace and number of repetitions. Pal Dan Gum can be incorporated into a warm-up routine before a Shiatsu session and into a cool-down routine afterward. Collectively, the movements emphasize the upper body, stretching the wrist flexors (inner forearm muscles used for grasping), biceps (inner upper arm muscles used for lifting), anterior deltoids (front shoulder muscles), and pectoralis major and minor (chest muscles), all major muscles that tend to get tense and tight from giving Shiatsu.

Makko Ho are Japanese Shiatsu stretches. Each stretch expresses the nature of a particular element—a distinctive energetic state of being—and mobilizes energy in the Meridians associated with that element (see Chapter 4 on Five Element theory). Stretches are performed while regulating the breath: inhalation before the stretch; exhalation while entering the stretch, and several deep breaths while holding the stretch. Collectively, the stretches emphasize the lower body, elongating several major muscle groups in the legs, including the hamstrings (back thighs), quadriceps (front thighs), adductors (inner thighs), and, to a lesser extent, abductors (outer thighs). These stretches can be incorporated into a warm-up routine before a Shiatsu session and into a cool-down routine afterward. Additionally, the poses can be assigned to clients as a simple form of physical therapy to be practiced at home between sessions to maintain Qi flow. If a client is a classic element type who manifests physical imbalances or psychological disharmonies associated with that element, the relevant Meridian stretch can be emphasized.

Yoga poses are of Indian origin and are designed to cultivate *prana*, the Indian term for vital energy or life force, synonymous with Qi. Yoga poses are generally not performed in isolation but rather are integrated into a continuous sequence of movements, much like a dance, the core of which is the sun salutation. Depending on how the poses are performed—their number and variety, their difficulty levels, the length of time they are sustained, and the connection between them—a Yoga practice cultivates not only Qi and flexibility, but also strength, stamina, balance, mental concentration, and emotional equanimity. Most Yoga poses have several variations or modifications, each suitable for different proficiency levels. Unless a person possesses a high degree of kinesthetic awareness and conditioning, the more difficult poses should not be attempted without guidance on proper form or a thorough warm-up. With respect to breathing, any movement that extends the spine or expands the chest, such as a backbend, is performed on an inhalation, and any movement that flexes the spine or compresses the chest, such as a forward bend, is performed on an exhalation. Several breaths are taken while a holding a pose.

CLIENT INFORMATION AND CAUTIONS

When assigning a client Meridian stretch exercises or poses, provide a handout that describes the exercises, gives instructions on proper form and breathing, and, if possible, includes visual images of the poses for better recall. The handout should also include cautions about stretching. In general, the client should perform a static stretch slowly, hold the position for 10 to 30 seconds at the resistance barrier (a position of mild discomfort), ease out of it, and repeat the stretch several times. A stretch should never be ballistic (bouncing) because of the risk of pulling a muscle or initiating a defensive contraction of the muscle. Finally, a stretch should never be forced so as to elicit pain.

PAL DAN GUM

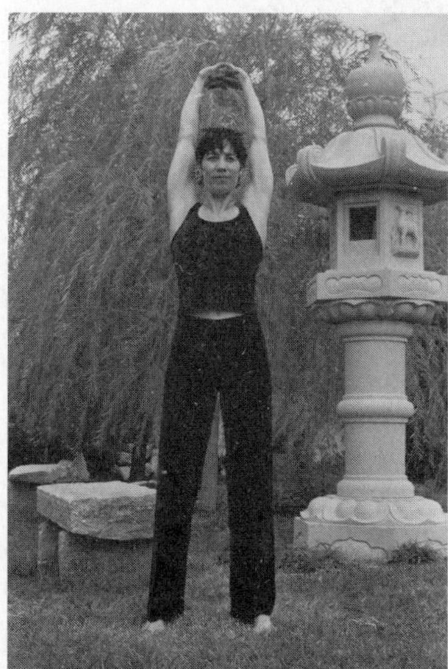

FIGURE 18-1 Upholding heaven with two hands, 1.
Inhale: Clasp the hands together; press the palms toward the sky.
Stimulates circulation and stretches the Pericardium Meridian.

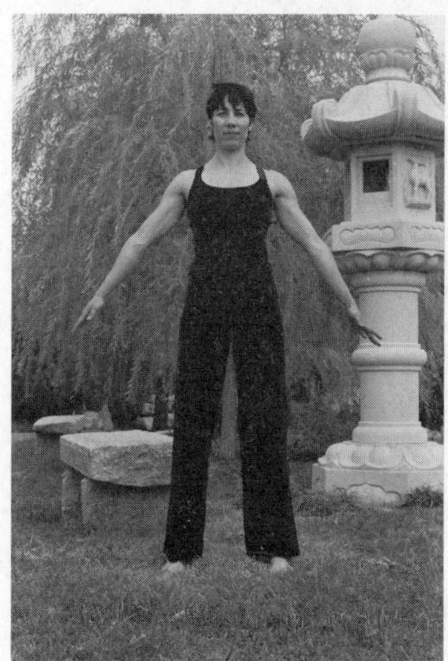

FIGURE 18-2 Upholding heaven with two hands, 2.
Exhale: Unclasp the hands; lower the arms to the sides.
Repeat several times.

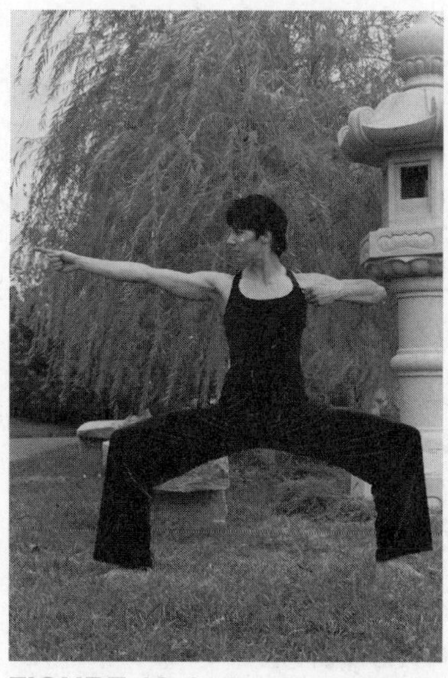

FIGURE 18-3 Opening the bow, right.
Done in a low, turned out squat
Inhale: Raise both arms to shoulder height as if drawing a bow—one arm straight, the other arm bent; fix the gaze over the index finger of the straight arm.

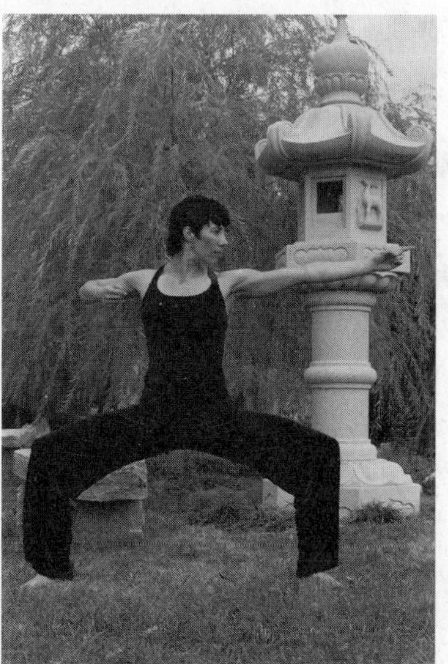

FIGURE 18-4 Opening the bow, left.
Exhale: Lower the hands to the hara (abdomen).
Inhale: Reverse sides.
Expands the chest and stretches the Lung Meridian.

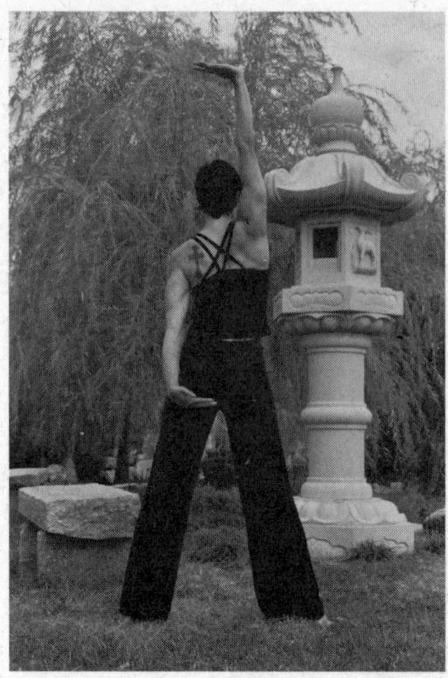

FIGURE 18-5 **Raising the hands separately, right.**
Inhale: Press one palm upward and the other downward and behind the hips, with the fingers pointing toward the midline.

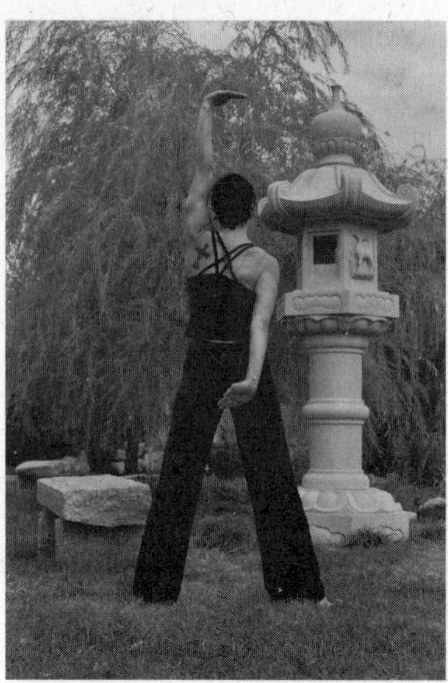

FIGURE 18-6 **Raising the hands separately, left.**
Exhale: Draw the hands together as if holding a globe in front of the hara (abdomen).
Inhale: Reverse. Repeat several times.
Stimulates the Large Intestine Meridian of the raised arm and the Small Intestine Meridian of the lowered arm.

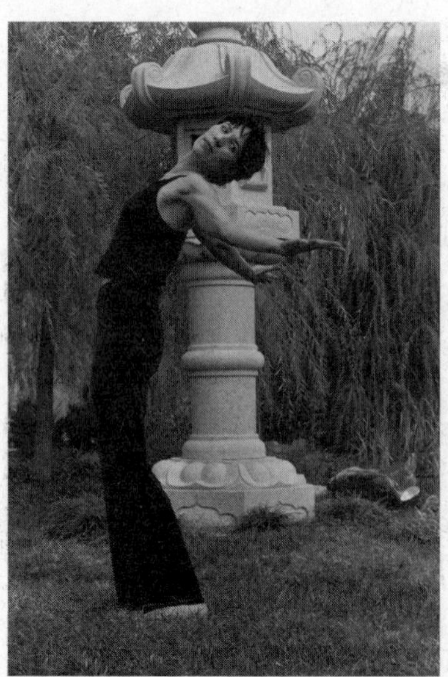

FIGURE 18-7 **Looking backwards, right.**
Inhale: With palms facing up, extend the arms sideways and bend backward; fix the gaze over one palm.

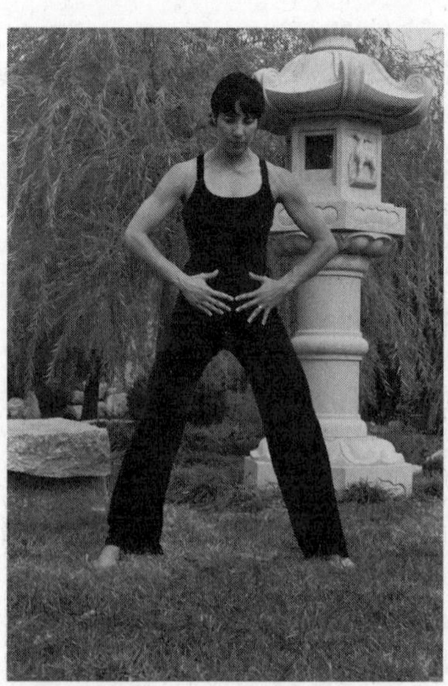

FIGURE 18-8 **Looking backwards, center.**
Exhale: Draw the hands in toward the hara.

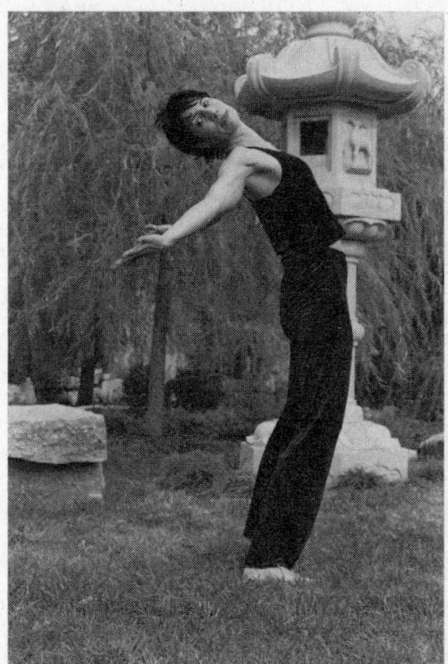

FIGURE 18-9 **Looking backwards, left.**
Inhale: Reverse the focal point.
Repeat several times.
Opens the chest and energizes the Yin organs.

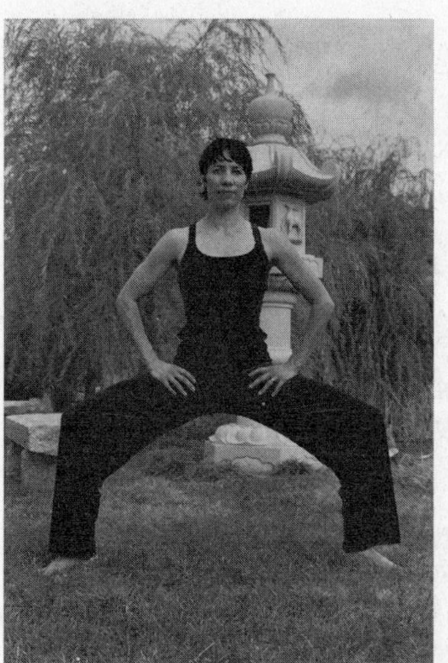

FIGURE 18-10 **Swinging trunk and head, center.**
Done in a low, turned out squat.
Inhale deeply at the center.

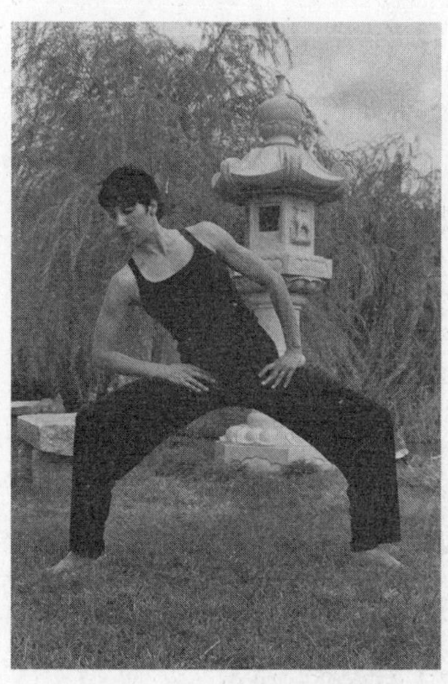

FIGURE 18-11 **Swinging trunk and head, right.**
Exhale slowly: Bend and look sideways.

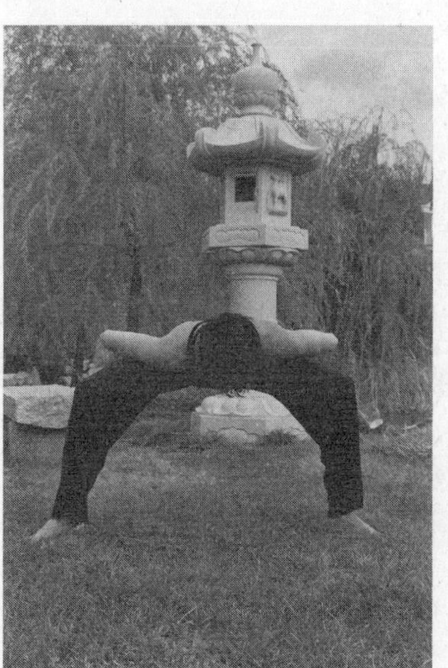

FIGURE 18-12 **Swinging trunk and head, down.**
Exhale: Bend forward and look down.

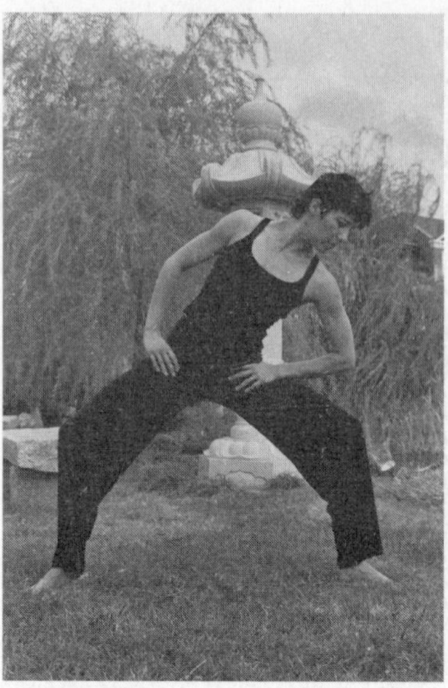

FIGURE 18-13 Swinging trunk and head, left.
Exhale: Bend and look to the other side.
Inhale: Return to center.
Repeat the torso rotation several times; then reverse. Releases Fire, limbers the lower back and waist, and soothes the Kidneys.

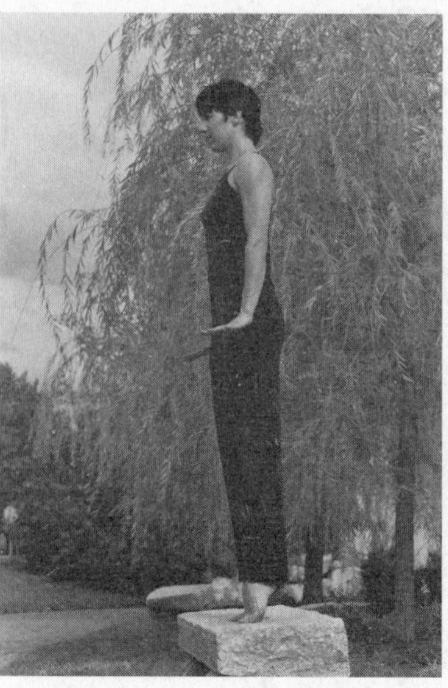

FIGURE 18-14 Standing on toes.
Inhale: Lift the heels, extend the wrists, and balance on the balls of the feet.
Exhale: Lower the heels; relax the wrists.
Repeat several times. Stimulates the Stomach and Kidney Meridians and develops balance and stability.

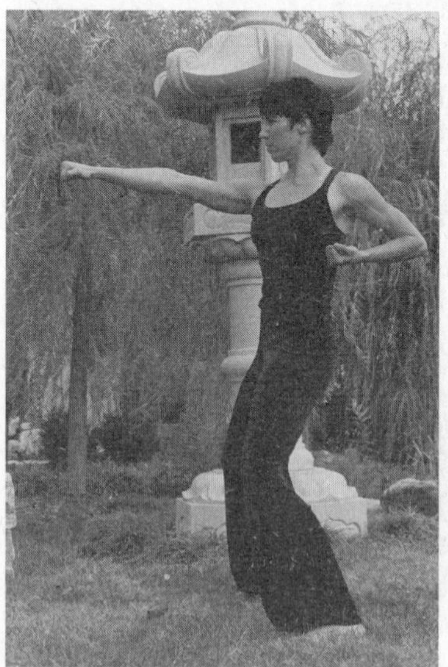

FIGURE 18-15 Punching with angry eyes, right.
Done in a bent–knee straddle.
Inhale: Draw both arms back with the elbows bent and the fists turned upward.
Exhale: Thrust one fist forward, palm down.
Inhale: Retract the arm.
Exhale: Thrust the other fist forward.

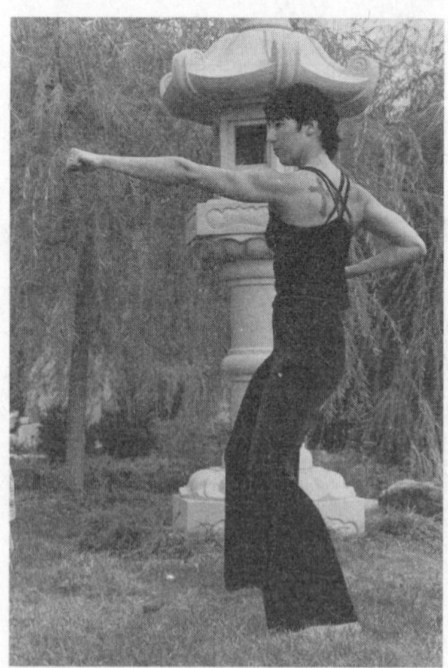

FIGURE 18-16 Punching with angry eyes, left.
Releases blocked Qi in the elbows, shoulders, and middle and upper back.
Repeat several times.

MAKKO HO

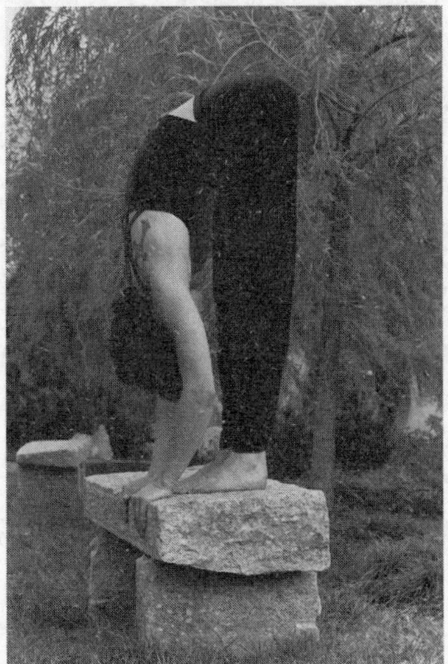

FIGURE 18-17 **Holding the toes and stretching back.**
Exhale: Bend forward, dangling the torso, neck, and head. Breathe deeply.
Inhale: Rise up; place the hands on the lower back; lift the chest and bend back.
Stretches the Bladder Meridian in the legs during the forward bend and the Stomach Meridian in the torso during the backbend.

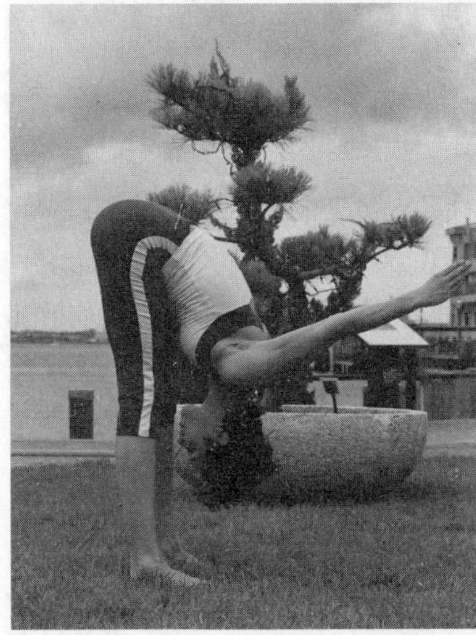

FIGURE 18-18 **Metal element stretch: Lu and LI.**
Inhale: Hook the thumbs together behind the hips and straighten the arms.
Exhale: Bend forward, extending the arms back; continue breathing.

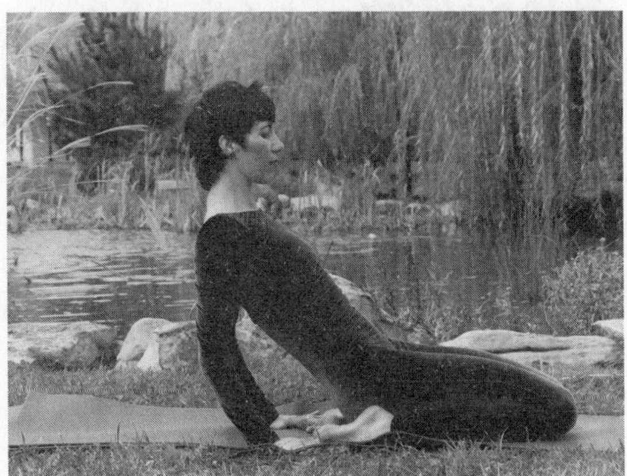

FIGURE 18-19 **Earth element stretch: Sp and St, phase 1.**
Sit on or between the heels. Place the hands behind you, fingers pointing forward. Bend the elbows and recline back until you feel a stretch in the quadriceps (front thighs). Continue breathing.

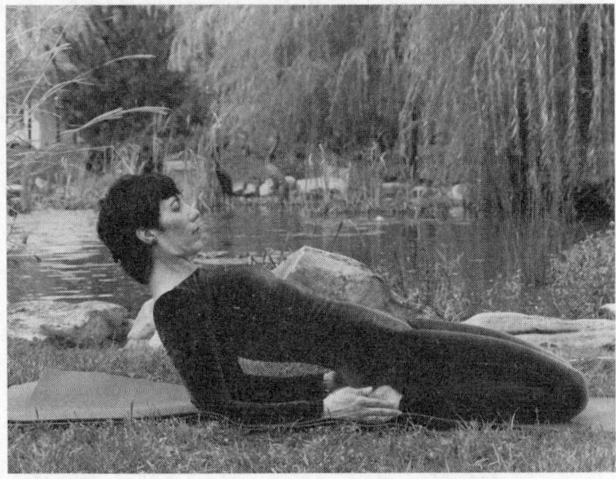

FIGURE 18-20 **Earth element stretch, phase 2.**
If flexibility permits, recline farther onto the forearms.

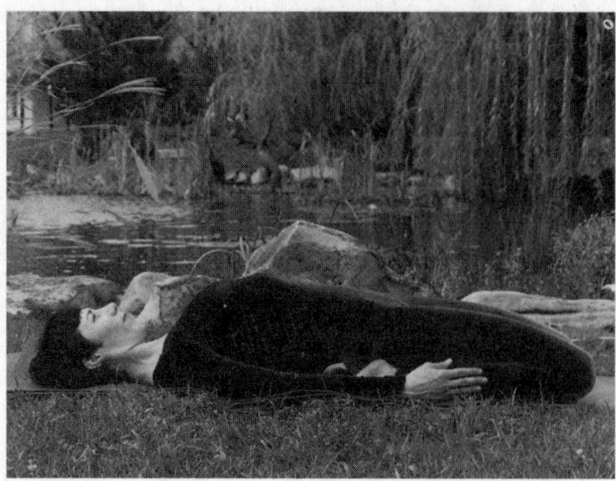

FIGURE 18-21 Earth element stretch, phase 3.
If flexibility permits, recline even farther onto the ground. To rise, bend the elbows and prop yourself up.

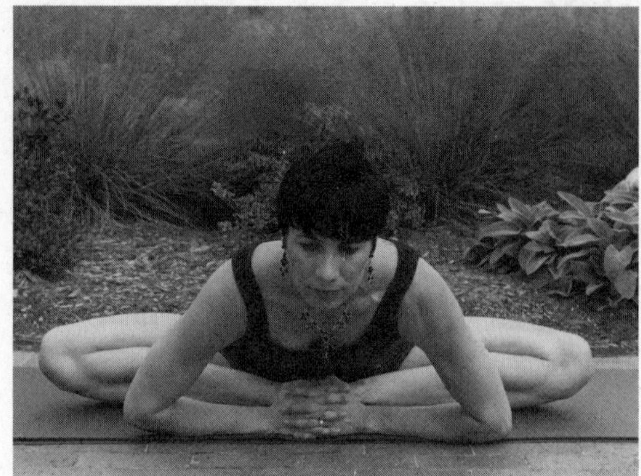

FIGURE 18-22 Primary Fire element stretch: Ht and SI.
Place the soles of the feet together; press the knees toward the ground; bend forward, lowering the torso as flexibility permits. Continue breathing.

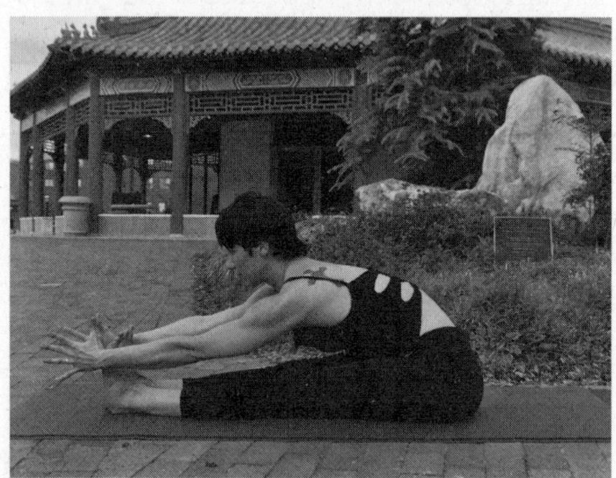

FIGURE 18-23 Water element stretch: Ki and Bl.
Extend both legs to the front; bend forward, elongating the spine (don't slump forward) and reaching toward or past the feet. Place the hands on the shins or feet and relax.

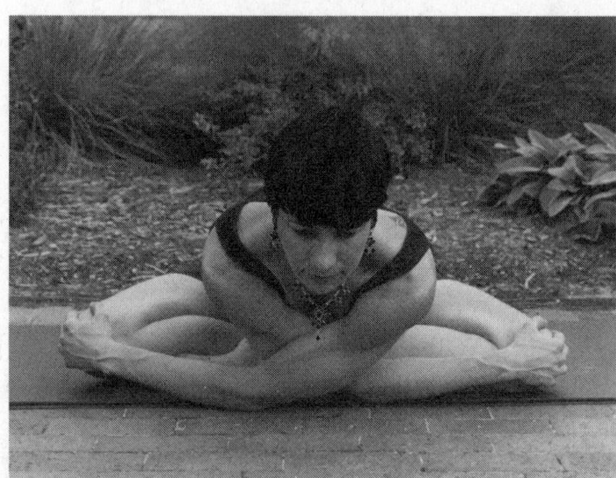

FIGURE 18-24 Secondary Fire element stretch: PC and TH.
Cross the arms; each hand holds the opposite knee. Bend forward. Reverse arms and repeat.

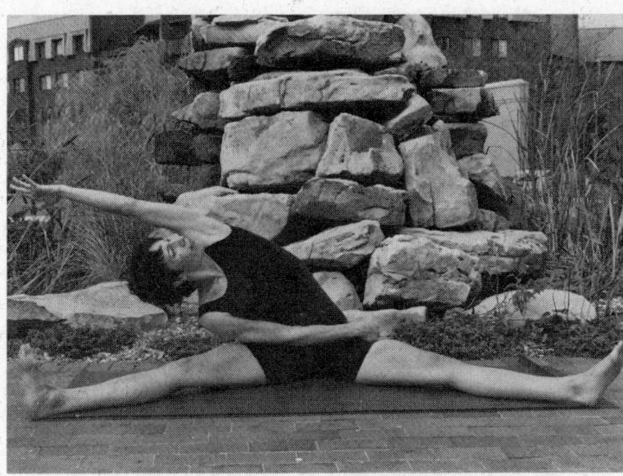

FIGURE 18-25 Wood element stretch: Lr and GB, right.
Spread the legs in a straddle split; extend the arm overhead and bend sideways.

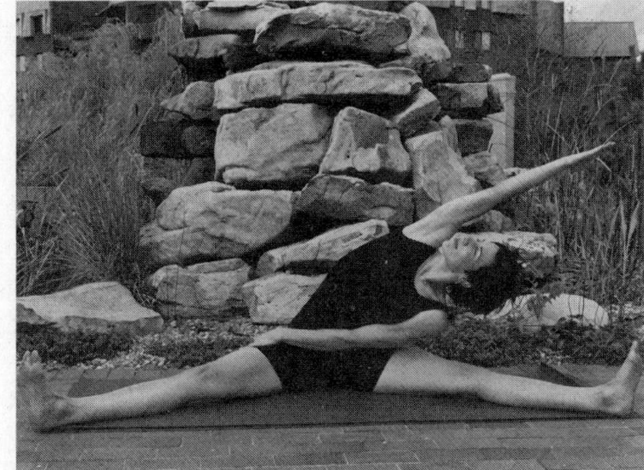

FIGURE 18-26 Wood element stretch: Lr and GB, left.
Reverse and repeat.

YOGA POSES

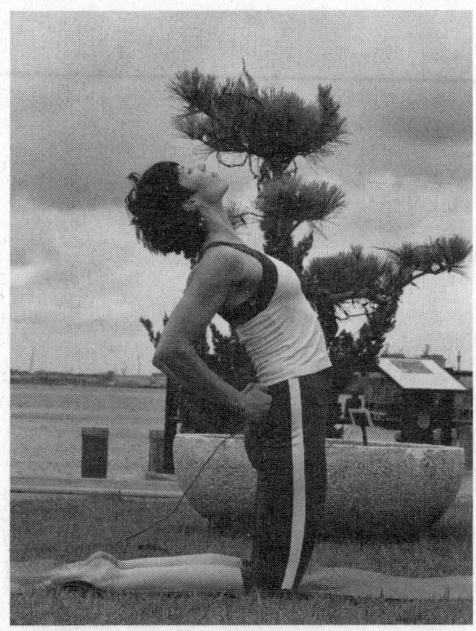

FIGURE 18-27 Metal element: beginner camel.
Place the fists on the hips; draw the elbows together; bend back.
Stretches the pectoralis (chest) and anterior deltoid (front of shoulder) and stimulates the Lung and Pericardium Meridians.

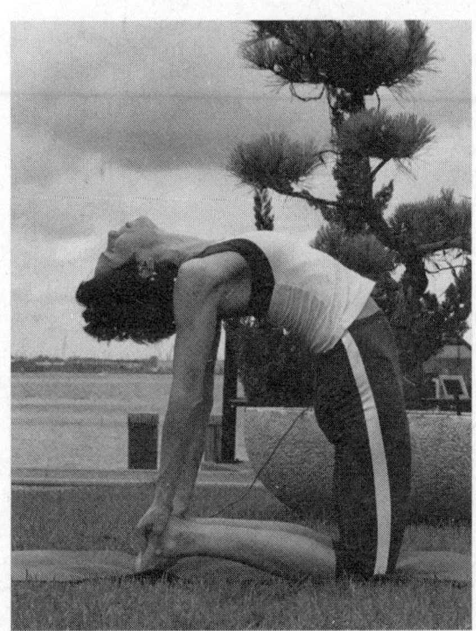

FIGURE 18-28 Metal element: intermediate camel.
Raise the heels by tucking the toes under; reach back to grab one heel with one arm and the other heel with the other arm.
Stretches the pectoralis (chest) and anterior deltoid (front of shoulder), and biceps (upper inner arms) and stimulates the Lung Pericardium, and Heart Meridians.
Contraindicated for lower back injury (bulging or herniated lumbar disk).

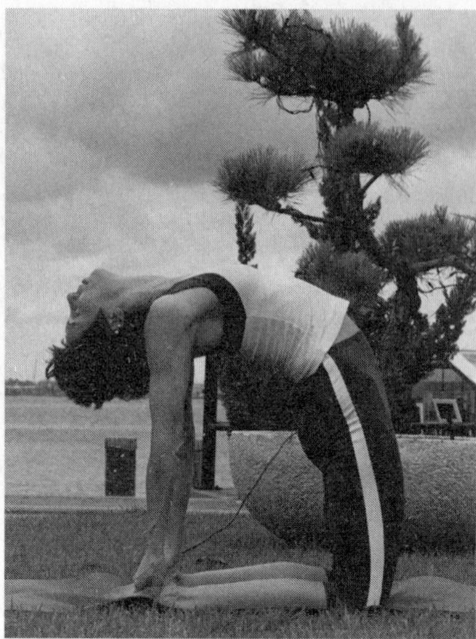

FIGURE 18-29 **Metal element: advanced camel.**
The dorsal surfaces of the feet remain on the ground. Stretches the pectoralis (chest), anterior deltoid (front of shoulder), and biceps (upper inner arms) and stimulates the Lung, Pericardium, and Heart Meridians. Contraindicated for lower back injury (bulging or herniated lumbar disk).

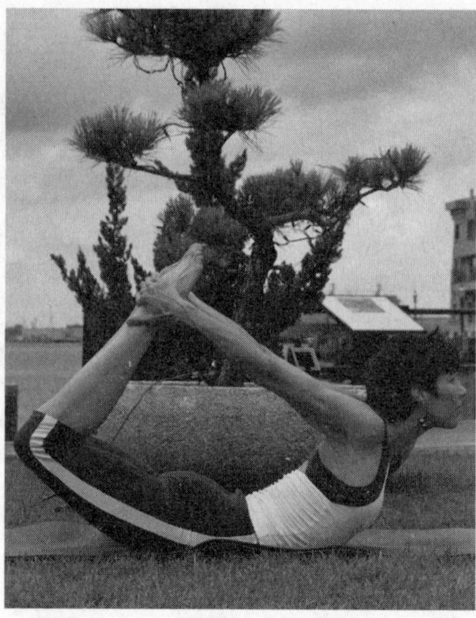

FIGURE 18-30 **Metal element: bow.**
Bend both knees and grab the ankles. Lift the thighs and chest off the ground. Stretches the pectoralis (chest), anterior deltoid (front of shoulder), and biceps (upper inner arms) and stimulates the Lung, Pericardium, and Heart Meridians. Contraindicated for lower back injury.

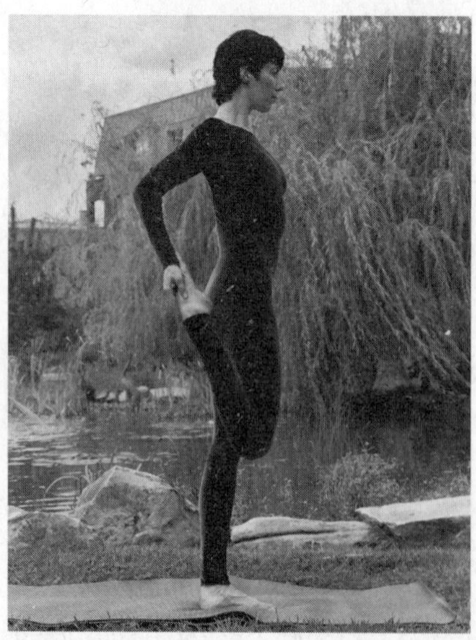

FIGURE 18-31 **Earth element: standing half frog.**
Stretches the quadriceps, especially the three vasti of the bent leg, and stimulates the Stomach and Spleen Meridians.

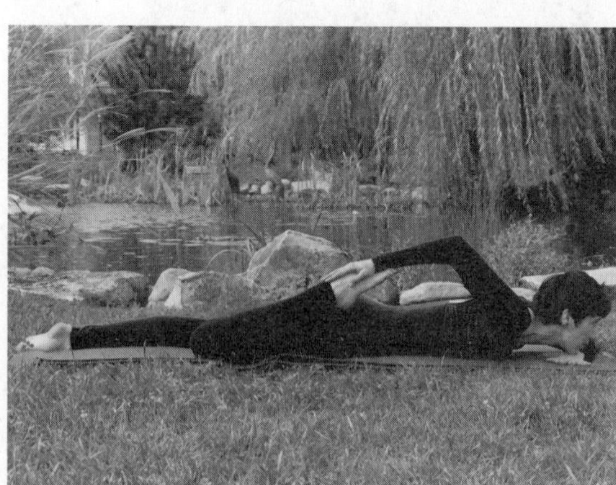

FIGURE 18-32 **Earth element: prone half frog.**
Stretches the quadriceps, especially the vasti of the bent leg, and stimulates the Stomach and Spleen Meridians.

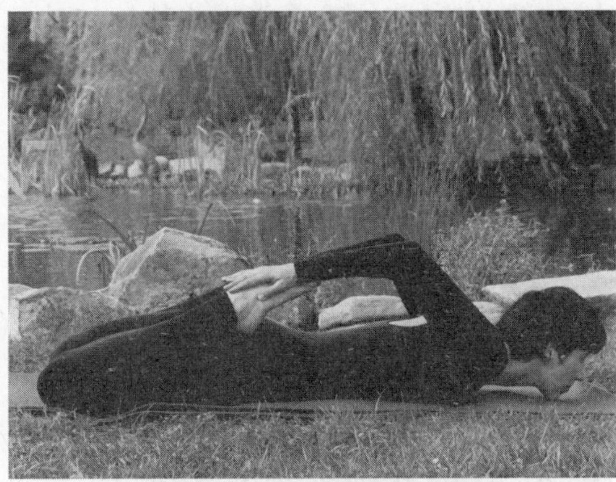

FIGURE 18-33 Earth element: frog.
Stretches the quadriceps, especially the vasti of both legs, and stimulates the Stomach Spleen Meridians.

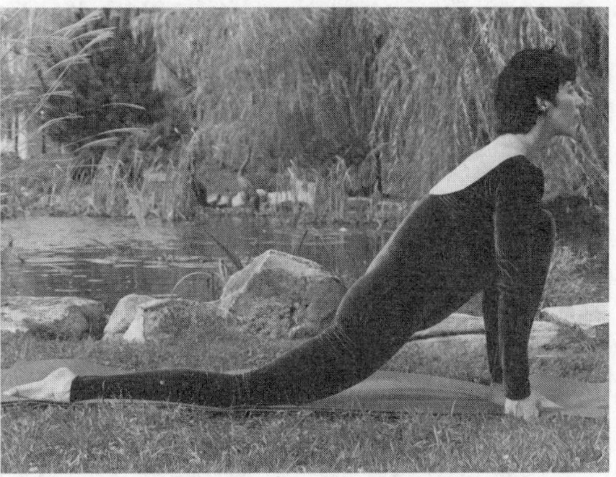

FIGURE 18-34 Earth element: beginner kneeling lunge.
Good pose to prepare for giving Shiatsu. The heel of the front foot is on the ground, and the knee of the front leg is directly over the ankle. The legs are split apart far enough to feel the stretch in the groin. Stretches the quadriceps (front thigh), especially the rectus femoris and iliopsoas (hip flexor) of the hind leg, and stimulates the Stomach and Spleen Meridians.

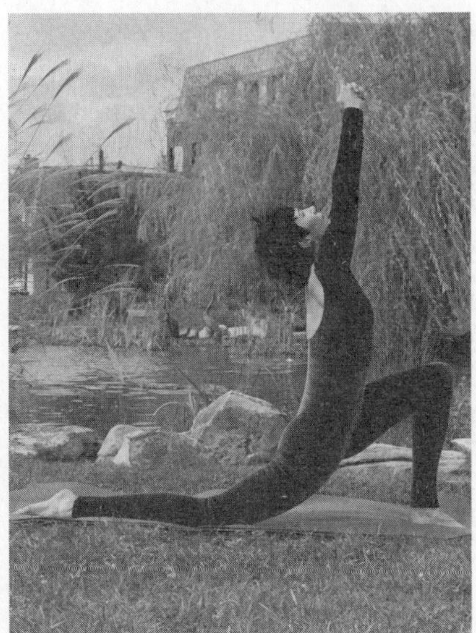

FIGURE 18-35 The Earth element: intermediate kneeling lunge.
Raise the torso and lift the arms overhead. Stretches the quadriceps (front thigh), especially the rectus femoris and iliopsoas (hip flexor) of the hind leg, as well as the rectus abdominus of the torso, and stimulates the Stomach and Spleen Meridians.

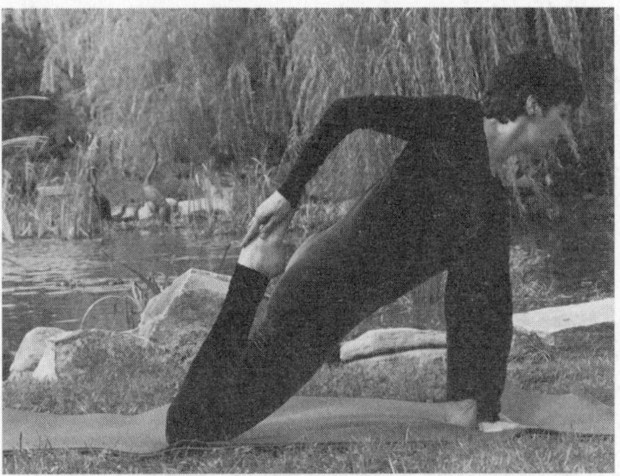

FIGURE 18-36 Earth element: advanced kneeling lunge.
Bend the knee and grab the foot of the back leg, pulling the heel toward the buttock. Strongly stretches the quadriceps (front thigh) of the hind leg, and stimulates the Stomach and Spleen Meridians.

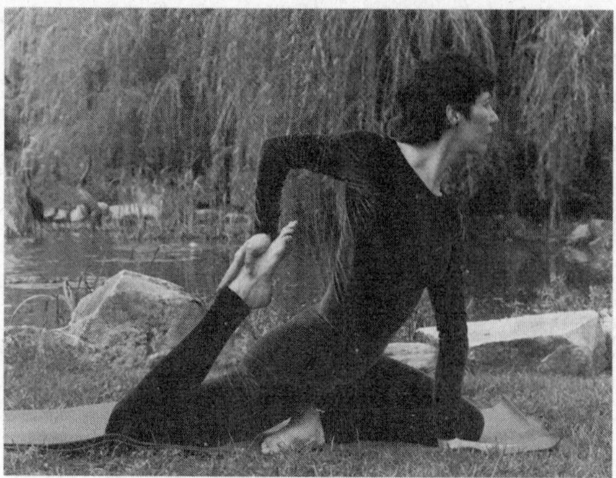

FIGURE 18-37 Earth element: advanced pigeon pose variation.
Stretches the quadriceps (front thigh) and iliopsoas (hip flexor) of the hind leg, as well as the rectus abdominus of the torso, and stimulates the Stomach and Spleen Meridians.

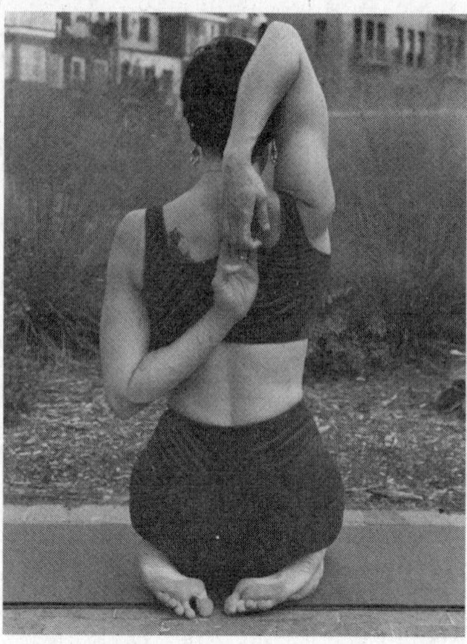

FIGURE 18-38 Primary Fire element: Archer pose.
Stretches the triceps (upper, outer muscle) of the upper arm and the teres minor and infraspinatus (rotator cuff muscles) of the lower arm, and stimulates the Small Intestine and Heart Meridians.

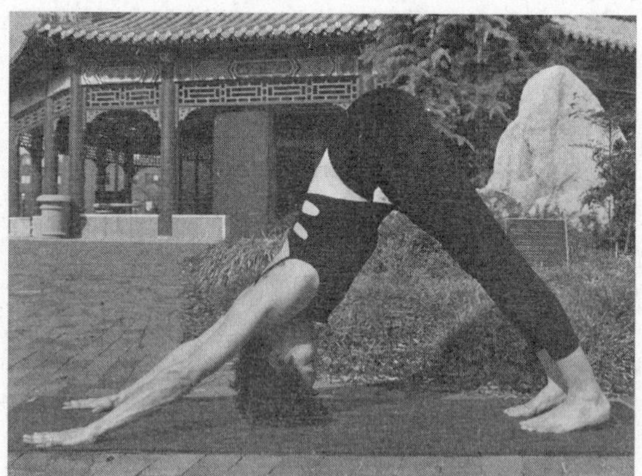

FIGURE 18-39 Water element: down dog.
The hands are parallel and shoulder width apart; the feet are parallel and hip width apart. Press the heels toward ground.
Stretches the hamstrings (back of thighs) and gastrocnemius (calf) of both legs and stimulates the Bladder Meridian.

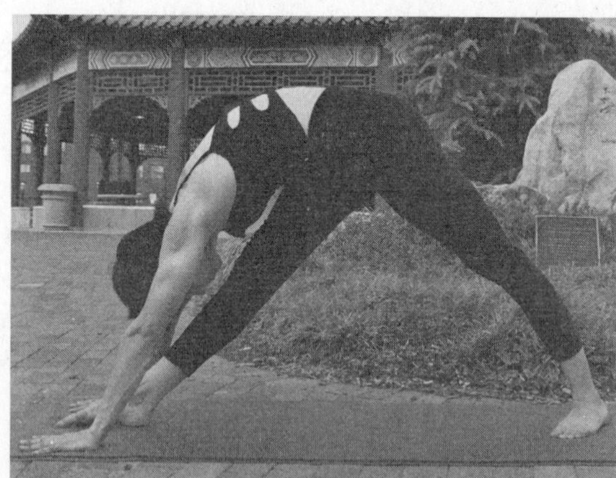

FIGURE 18-40 Water element: pyramid.
The toes of the front foot point toward the front of the mat; the toes of the back foot point toward the side of the mat. Place the hands on the front leg and slowly lower toward the ground, if possible.
Stretches the hamstrings of the front leg and stimulates the Bladder Meridian.

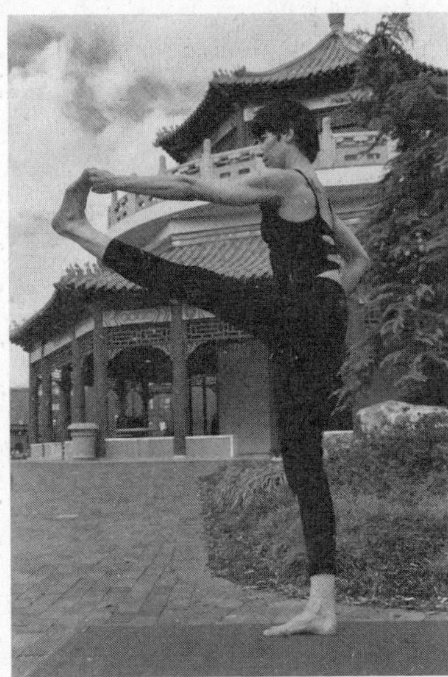

FIGURE 18-41 Water element: standing front-leg extension.
Grab the big toe with the ipsilateral (same side) hand. Extend the leg partially (modified) or fully (advanced) to the front.This pose stretches the hamstrings (back of the thigh) and gastrocnemius (calf) of the raised leg and stimulates the Bladder Meridian.

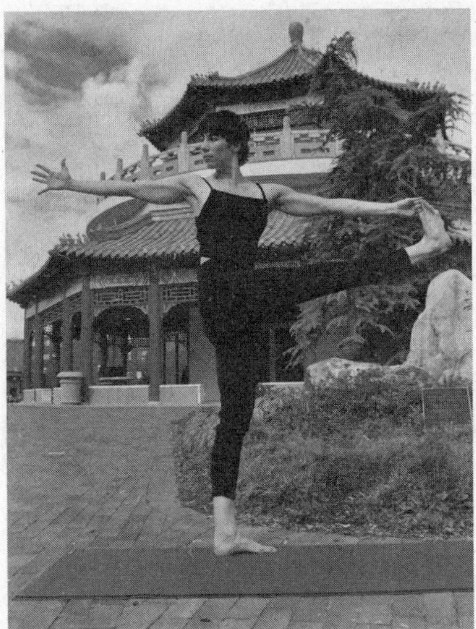

FIGURE 18-42 Water element: standing front-leg extension with twist.
Grab the big toe with the contralateral (opposite side) hand. Extend the leg partially (modified) or fully (advanced) to the front. Rotate the torso to the side. This pose stretches the hamstrings (back of the thigh), gastrocnemius (calf) of the raised leg and the Bladder Meridian.

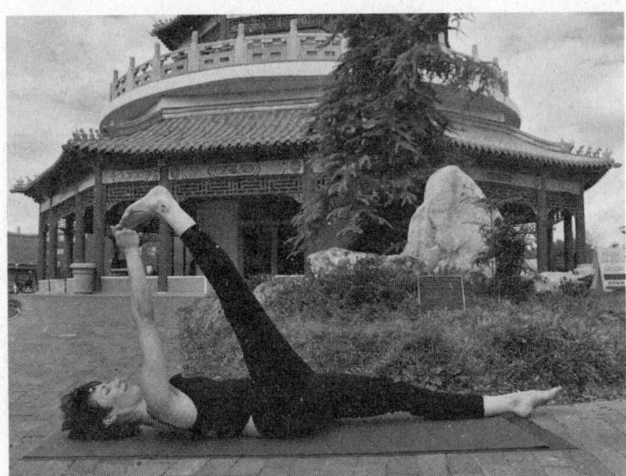

FIGURE 18-43 Water element: supine front-leg extension.
To modify this pose, grab the extended leg behind the thigh instead of the toe and bend the nonworking leg. Stretches the hamstrings (back of the thigh) and gastrocnemius (calf) of the raised leg and stimulates the Bladder Meridian.

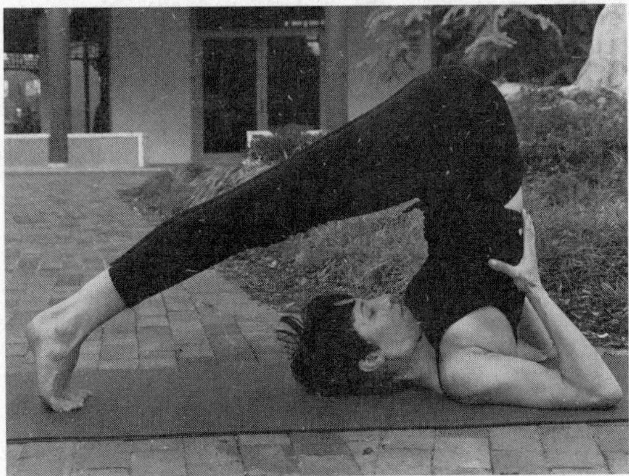

FIGURE 18-44 Water element: plough.
This advanced pose stretches the erector spinae of the back and stimulates the Bladder Meridian.

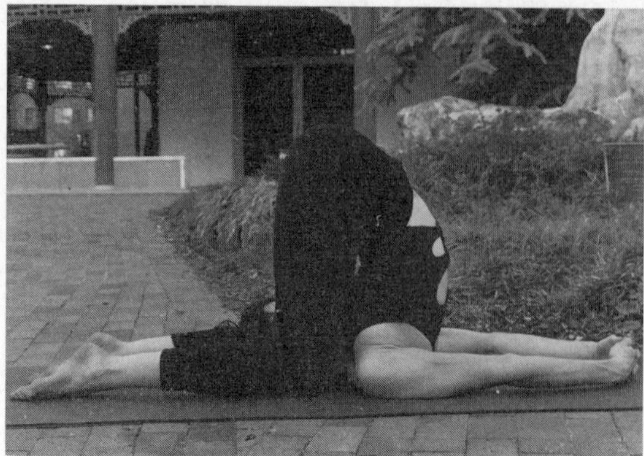

FIGURE 18-45 Water element: bent knees over ears.
This advanced pose stretches the erector spinae of the back and stimulates the Bladder Meridian.

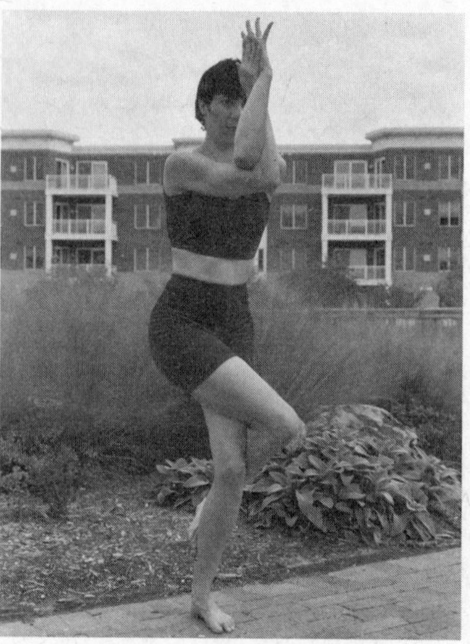

FIGURE 18-46 Secondary Fire element: eagle pose.
Cross one arm over the other at elbow level; bend the elbows; interlock the hands; raise the elbows to shoulder height. Cross one leg over the other; if possible, hook the foot behind the calf. Stretches the teres minor and infraspinatus (rotator cuff muscles) and the posterior deltoid (back shoulder) of the inner arm, and stimulates the Triple Heater and Small intestine Meridian.

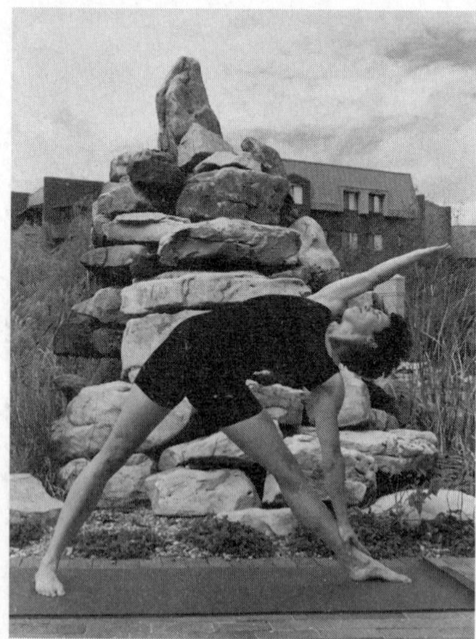

FIGURE 18-47 Wood element: extended triangle.
Separate the legs in a wide straddle split. The toes of the front foot point toward the front of the mat; the toes of the back foot point toward the side of the mat. Rotate the torso sideways. Place the front hand on the shin and slide down toward the ground, if possible. Stretches the adductors of the front leg and the latissimus dorsi, quadratus lumborum, obliques, and transverse abdominus of the torso, and stimulates the Liver and Gallbladder Meridians.

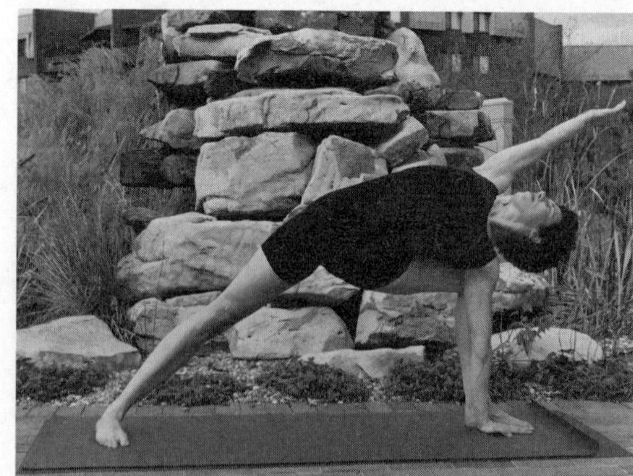

FIGURE 18-48 Wood element: extended side angle.
Bend the front leg to create a side lunge. To modify, prop the forearm on the ledge of the front thigh rather than lowering the hand to ground level, as shown. Stretches the adductors of the front leg and the latissimus dorsi, quadratus lumborum, obliques, and transverse abdominus of the torso, and stimulates the Liver and Gallbladder Meridians.

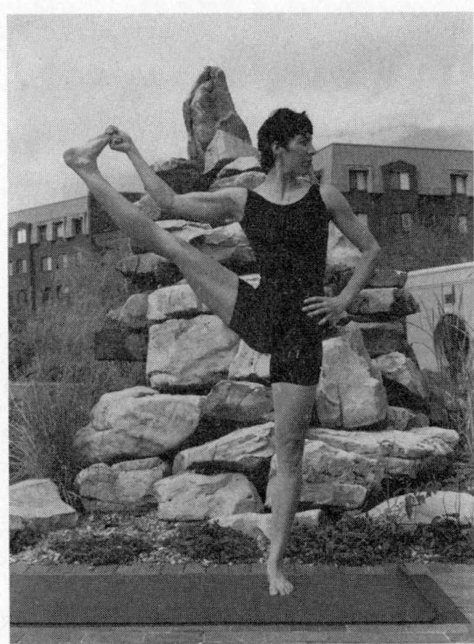

FIGURE 18-49 **Wood element: standing side-leg extension.**
Grab the big toe with the ipsilateral (same side) hand. Extend the leg partially (modified) or fully (advanced) to the side. Stretches the adductors of the raised leg and stimulates the Liver Meridian.

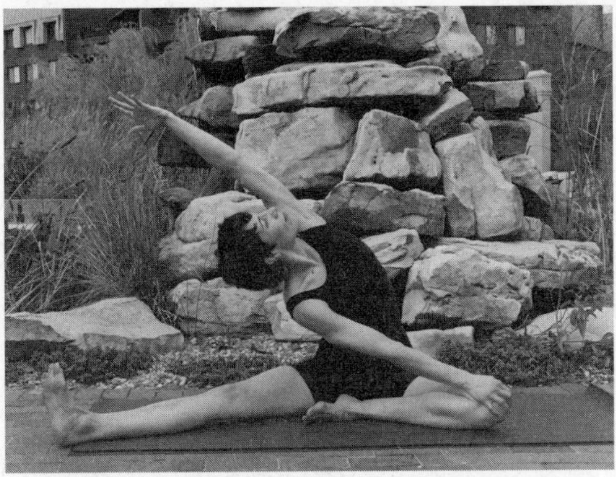

FIGURE 18-50 **Wood element pose: seated half straddle split.**
Grab the bent knee with the contralateral (opposite side) hand. Bend sideways. Stretches the adductors of the extended leg and the latissimus dorsi, quadratus lumborum, obliques, and transverses abdominus of the leaning torso, and stimulates the Liver and Gallbladder Meridians.

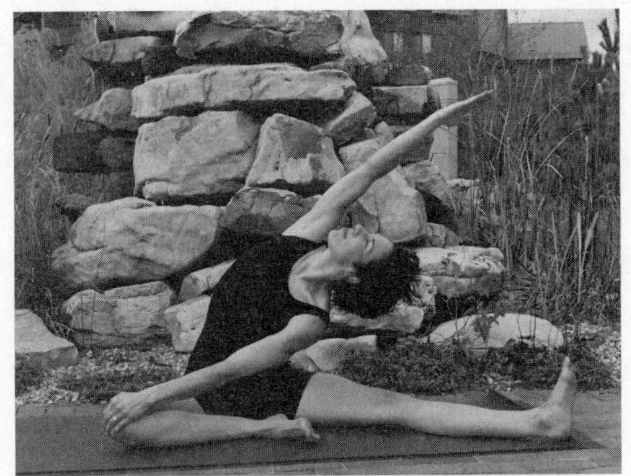

FIGURE 18-51 **Wood element pose: seated half straddle split.**

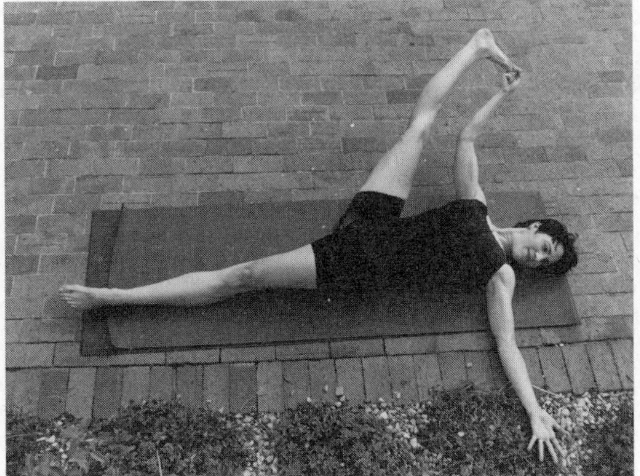

FIGURE 18-52 **Wood element pose: supine side-leg extension.**
To modify this pose, support the extended leg with the hand and the bend nonworking leg. Stretches the adductors of the extended leg and stimulates the Liver Meridian.

APPENDIX 1: GLOSSARY OF ACUPOINTS

ANATOMICAL TERMS

Anterior, ventral: Front side of the body; inner surface of a limb.
Posterior, dorsal: Back side of the body; outer surface of a limb.
Superior, cephalad: Above, higher, toward the head; in an upward direction.
Inferior, caudal: Below, lower, toward the feet; in a downward direction.
Medial: Toward the center or midline of the body; inward.
Lateral: Toward the outside or flank of the body; outward.
Proximal: Toward the torso or root of a limb; superior (refers to limbs only).
Distal: Toward the extremity or end of a limb; inferior (refers to limbs only).

MEASURING UNITS

One cun: The width of the thumb joint.
Three cun: The width of four fingers—index finger to little finger—side by side.

Abbreviations: For the sake of consistency and currency, this text uses the revised standard acupuncture abbreviations as adopted by the World Health Organization in Geneva in 1989. The Geneva abbreviations uniformly and systematically designate two letters for each Meridian, whereas the previous abbreviations adopted in Manila in 1982 designated one, two, or three letters (Institute of Acupuncture and Moxibustion, 2000). This text departs from the Geneva abbreviations only on the Triple Energizer (TE). Instead of TE, this text uses the older term Triple Heater (TH), which is a more accurate translation of the "three burning spaces" of the ancient texts and which retains the association of the Triple Heater with body heat as it transfers Source Qi to other organs to ignite their functions.

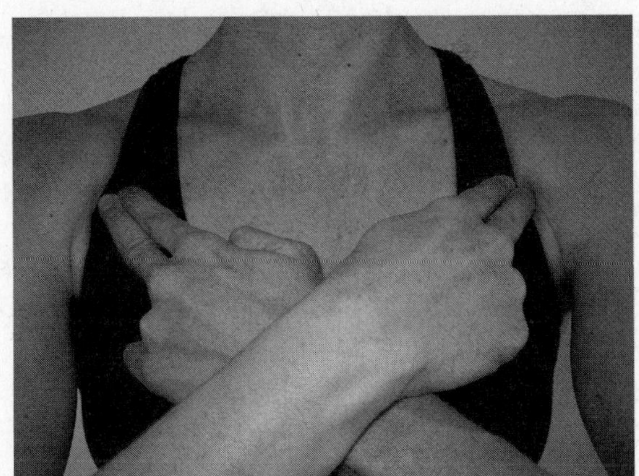

A1-1 **Lu 1.**
On the chest, 2 cun below the lateral end of the clavicle (collarbone) on the pectoralis; press down and in toward the chest. Mu/Bo point for the Lungs; promotes Lung dispersing and descending functions; good for chest pain; respiratory disorders such as asthma, labored breathing, suffocating feeling, nasal congestion, colds, flu, bronchitis; relieves anxiety, depression, sorrow, grief; releases repressed emotions.

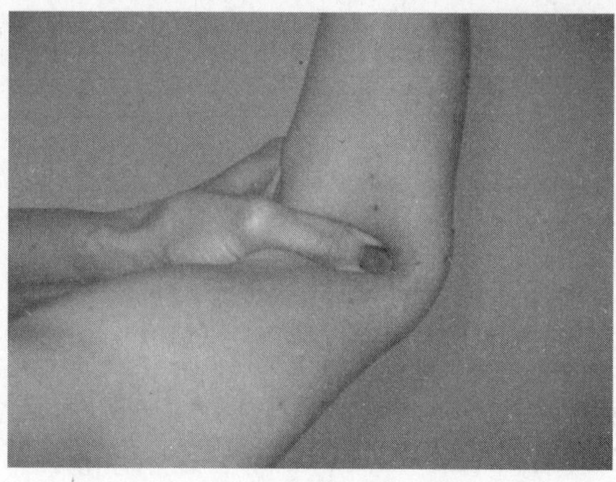

A1-2 **Lu 5.**
On the anterior forearm at the elbow crease, on the radial side of the biceps tendon; to define the biceps tendon, flex the elbow. Good for Lung Heat disorders and reversed Lung Qi such as dry cough, bloody cough, sticky and cloudy sputum, yellow phlegm, bronchitis, pneumonia; asthma, labored breathing, suffocating feeling; upper body edema.

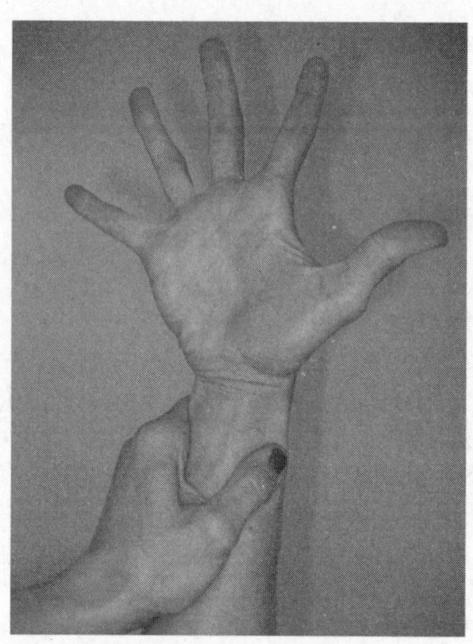

A1-3 **Lu 7.**
On the anterior forearm, 1½ cun proximal to the radial side of the wrist in a small indentation above the bony prominence of the styloid process. Expels pathogenic agents such as Cold Wind. Good for respiratory disorders such as nasal congestion, cough, dry or sore or itchy or tickly throat, colds, flu, asthma; facial edema; depression, sadness, grief.

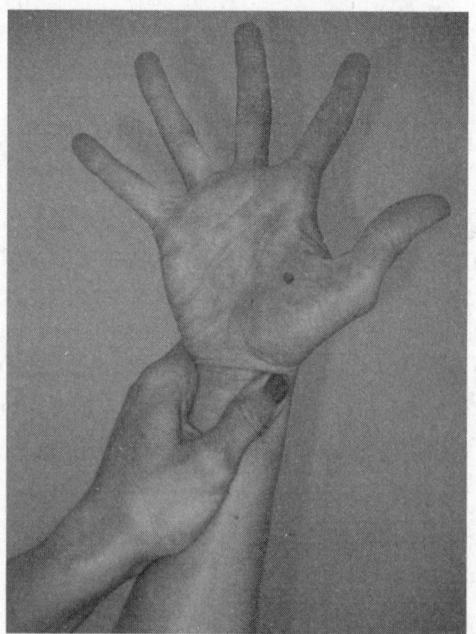

A1-4 **Lu 9.**
On the anterior wrist, on the radial side where the radial pulse is palpable. Clears Lungs; fortifies respiratory and cardiovascular systems; helps singers, public speakers, and smokers who are trying to quit. Good for chronic Lung deficiency conditions that compromise breathing and voice such as asthma, chronic cough, shallow breathing, breathlessness, hoarse or faint voice, loss of voice; cardiovascular disorders such as poor circulation, cold extremities, weak or rapid or irregular heartbeat.

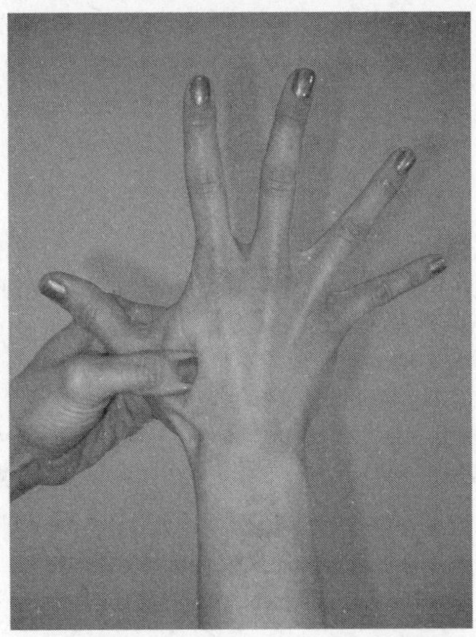

A1-5 LI 4.
On the posterior hand, in the fleshy web between the thumb and index finger; press toward the index finger. Moves energy downward and outward; expels pathogenic agents such as Wind Heat; mobilizes stagnant Qi and blood; general panacea and analgesic point; reduces physical tension and psychological stress and relaxes. Good for frontal headache, toothache, conjunctivitis, sore throat, allergy, sinusitis, colds, flu; forearm, elbow, and shoulder pain; abdominal pain or constipation; menstrual pain or delayed period. Contraindicated during pregnancy but facilitates labor.

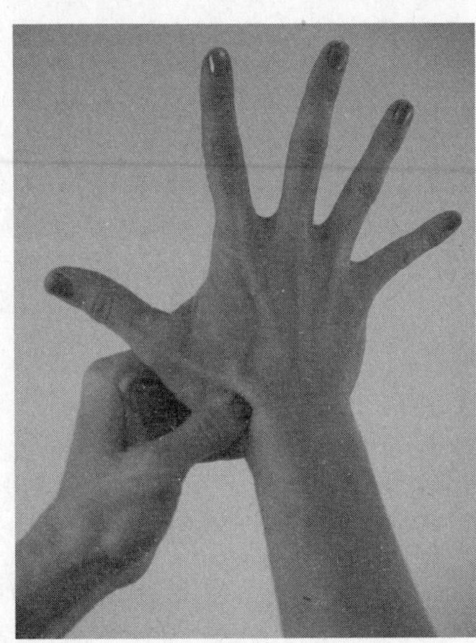

A1-6 LI 5.
On the posterior wrist, on the radial side at the base of the thumb in the anatomical snuffbox (bony hollow) between the thumb tendons; to define the tendons, extend the thumb backward. Good for wrist and thumb.

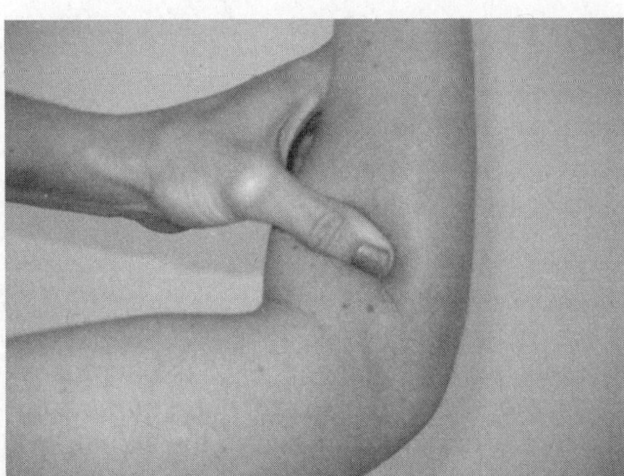

A1-7 LI 10.
On the posterior forearm, 2 cun distal to the elbow crease on the radial side on the extensor carpi radialis; to define this muscle, extend the hand backward and deviate the wrist inward. Good for painful obstruction syndrome of the hand, arm, and shoulder.

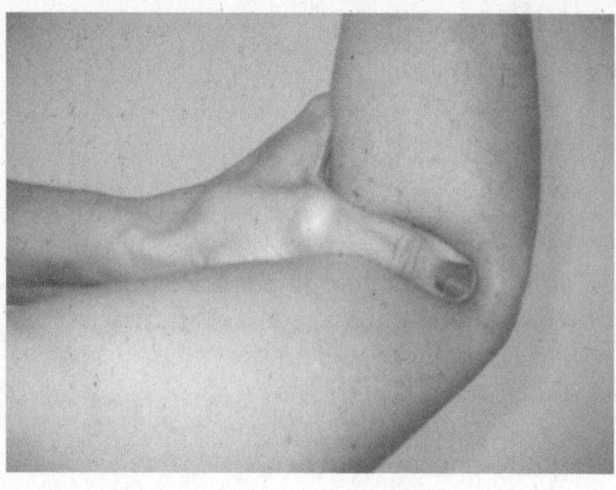

A1-8 **LI 11.**
On the posterior forearm, at the elbow crease on the radial side between the brachioradialis and extensor carpi radialis. Expels pathogenic agents such as Wind, Heat, and Damp; disperses Qi stagnation. Good for headache, hypertension, red eyes, colds, flu, swollen throat; skin disorders marked by redness and heat; abdominal pain, distention, diarrhea; painful obstruction syndrome of elbow, arm, and shoulder.

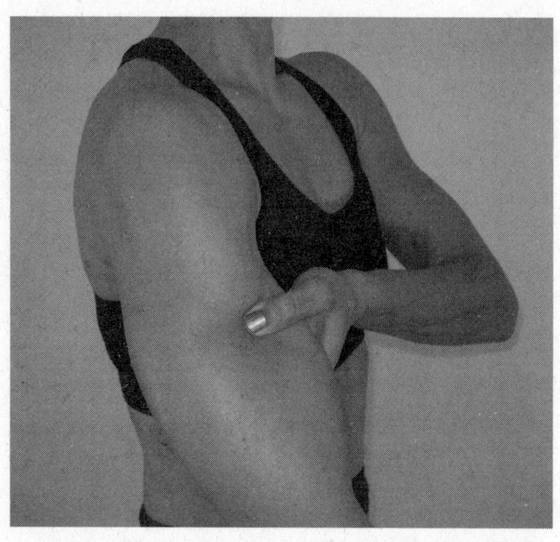

A1-9 **LI 14.**
On the arm, slightly anterior and superior to the deltoid insertion where the bulge of the shoulder muscle tapers. Good for painful obstruction syndrome of the arm and shoulder.

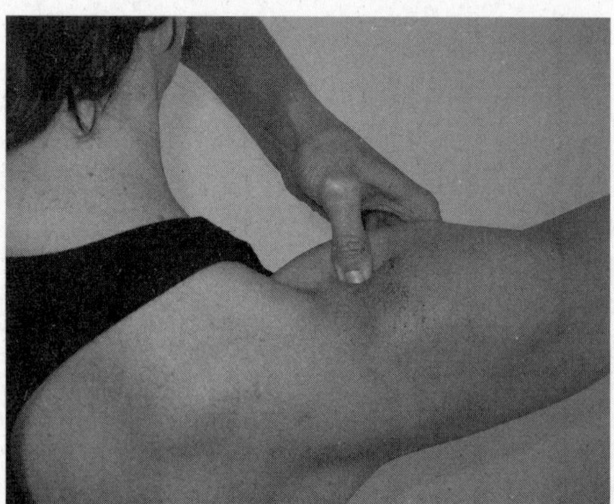

A1-10 **LI 15.**
On the upper shoulder, anterior and inferior to the acromion in the indentation formed between the anterior and medial deltoids when the arm is abducted (raised to the side). Good for painful obstruction syndrome of the shoulder and arm.

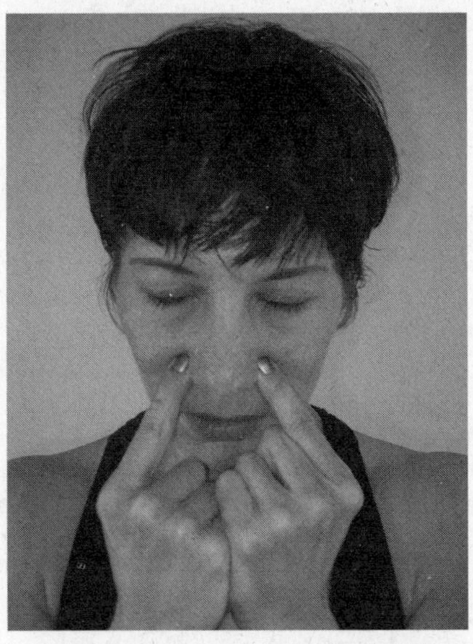

A1-11 **LI 20.**
On the face, beside each nostril. Expels pathogenic agents such as Wind and Heat; clears sinus obstructions. Good for sinus disorders, impaired breathing, impaired smell, facial paralysis.

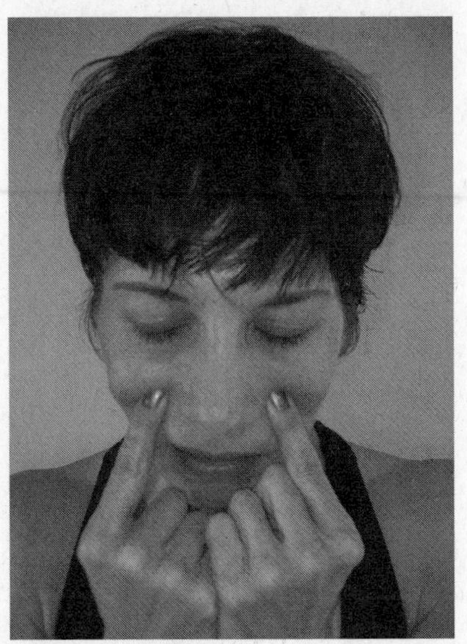

A1-12 **St 3.**
On the face, below the zygomatic arch (cheekbone) at the horizontal level of the nostrils and in vertical alignment with the pupils of the eyes. Good for facial pain and paralysis, sinus disorders, nosebleed, toothache, gum disorders, and eyes.

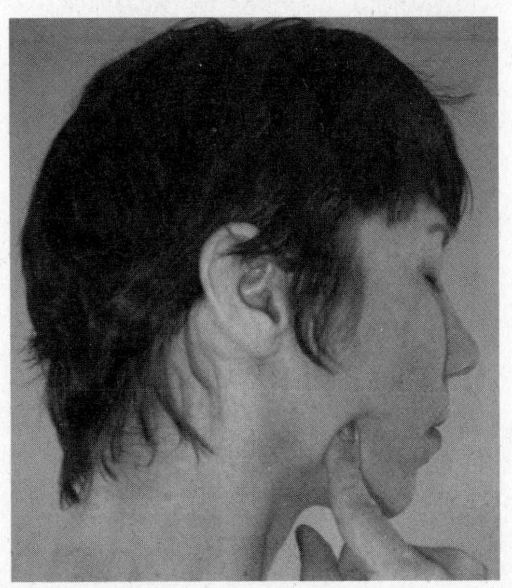

A1-13 **St 6.**
On the jaw, 1 finger width anterior and superior to the mandibular angle in a concavity formed when the masseter (jaw muscle) bulges; to define the masseter, clench the jaw. Good for jaw tension, temporomandibular joint (TMJ) syndrome (pain and difficulty in speaking, chewing, or yawning), bruxism (teeth clenching or grinding), tension headache, lower toothache, cheek swelling, facial pain and paralysis. Caution: This point is best stimulated bilaterally in the supine position, as unilateral stimulation in the sidelying position could dislocate the jaw.

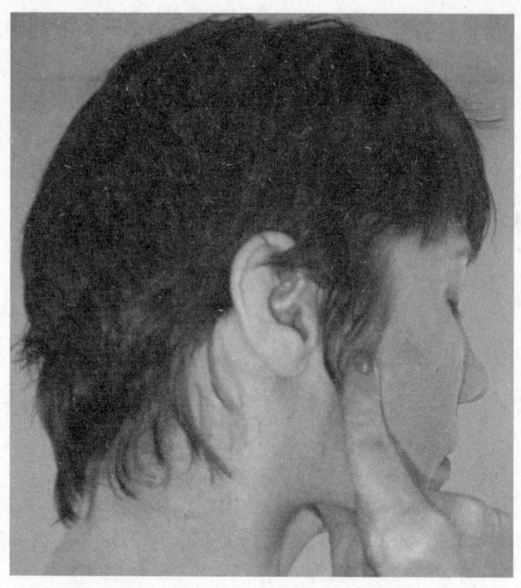

A1-14 St 7.
On the side of the face, in the hollow just below the zygomatic arch (cheekbone) and just above the mandible (jawbone). Good for TMJ (pain and difficulty in speaking, chewing, or yawning), bruxism (teeth clenching or grinding), upper toothache, facial paralysis.

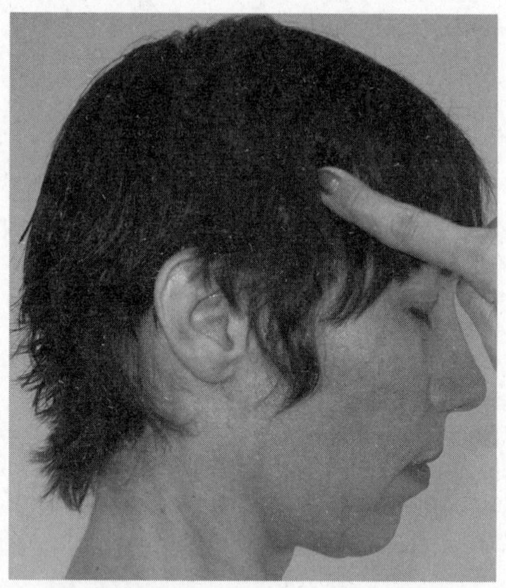

A1-15 St 8.
On the head, slightly superior to the bulge of the temporalis muscle; to define the temporalis, clench the jaw. Good for temporal tension, especially unilateral temporal headaches and migraines; dizziness, vertigo; bleary vision.

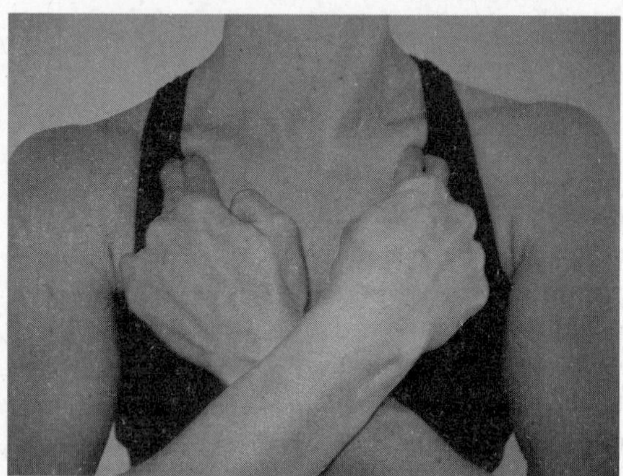

A1-16 St 13.
On the chest, below the midpoint of the clavicle or 4 cun lateral to the midline. Good for breast or chest soreness or pain, lactation difficulty, chest congestion.

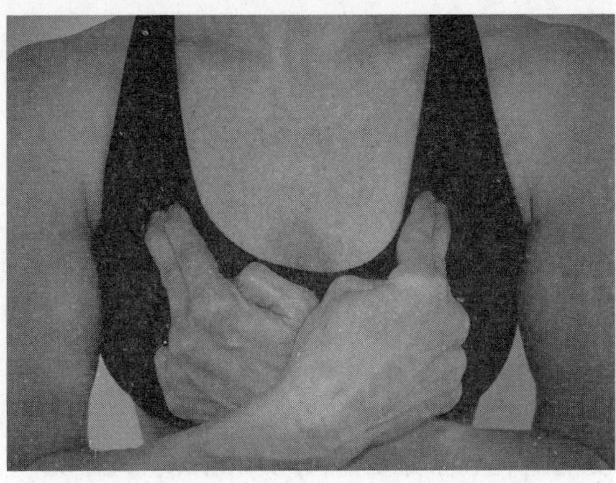

A1-17 St 16.
On the chest, in the third intercostal space (between the 3rd and 4th ribs), 4 cun lateral to the midline, on a vertical line above the nipple. Good for breast or chest soreness or pain, lactation difficulty, chest congestion.

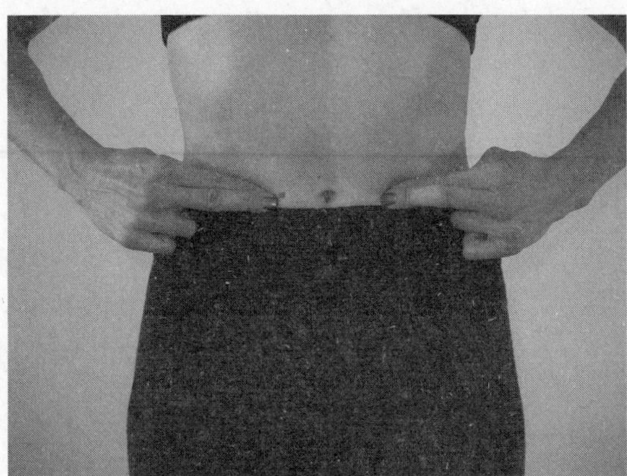

A1-18 St 25.
On the abdomen, 2 cun lateral to the navel. Mu/Bo point for the Large Intestine; cools Heat and evaporates Damp in the lower burner. Good for abdominal distention and pain, diarrhea, constipation, intestinal paralysis, irritable bowel syndrome; erratic or painful periods; excessive vaginal discharge. Place a bolster under the knees to allow the abdominal muscles to relax. *Caution:* Avoid if the abdomen is extremely painful, inflamed, or hard.

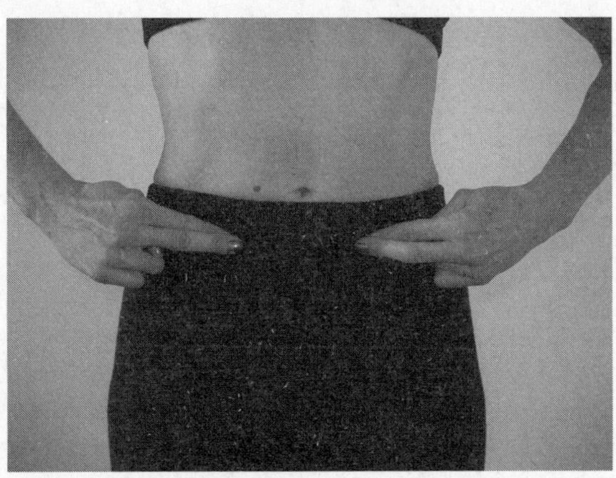

A1-19 St 27.
On the abdomen, 2 cun lateral and 2 cun inferior to the navel. Good for abdominal disorders and lumbago (lower back pain) caused by tension in the psoas muscle. Place a bolster under the knees to allow the abdominal muscles to relax.

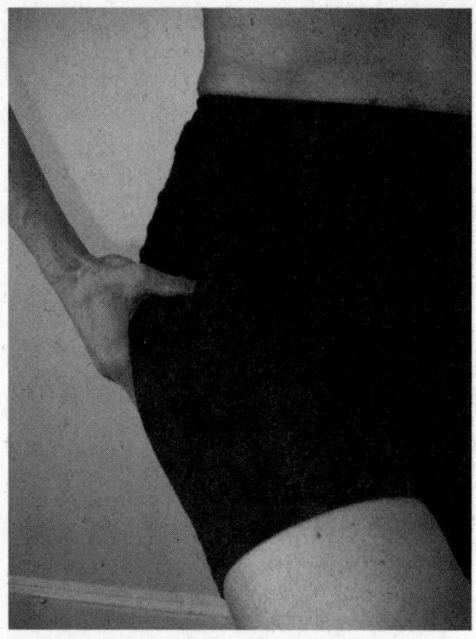

A1-20 **St 31.**
On the anterior thigh, below the ASIS (bony protrusion of the pelvic bone) between the sartorious and tensor fascia latae. Promotes blood and Qi flow to the leg. Good for painful obstruction syndrome of the hip and leg; contracture of the quadriceps; numbness, pain, and stiffness in the lower leg; atrophy or paralysis of the leg. Pressure is best applied with the hip flexed.

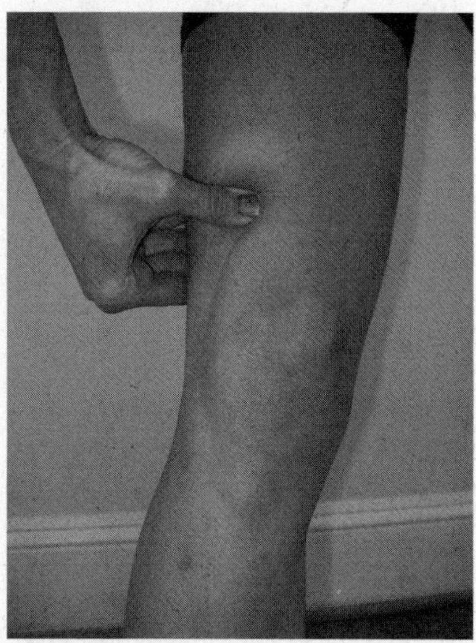

A1-21 **St 34.**
On the anterior thigh, 2 cun proximal to the superior lateral border of the patella (kneecap) between the rectus femoris and vastus lateralis (middle and outer segments of the quadriceps). Good for painful, swollen, debilitated knees; Stomach disorders such as stomachache, nausea, acid reflux.

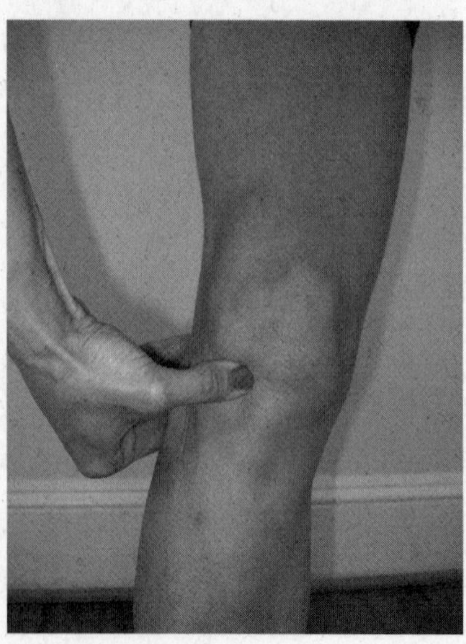

A1-22 **St 35.**
On the knee, in the hollow inferior and lateral to the patella (kneecap). Good for painful, swollen, debilitated knees.

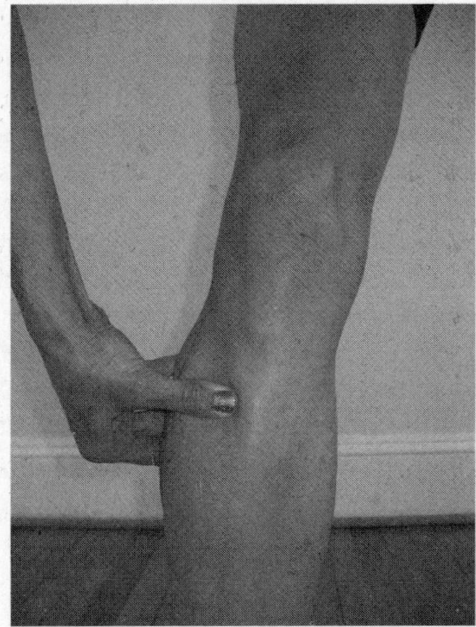

A1-23 St 36.
On the lower leg, 3 cun or 4 fingers distal to the patella (kneecap) on the anterior tibialis (shin muscle); to define the anterior tibialis, dorsiflex the foot; press inward toward the shinbone. Fortifies and nourishes the Stomach, Spleen, and entire body, especially in cases of blood or Qi deficiency. Good for digestive disorders such as poor appetite, abdominal distention and pain, indigestion, loose stools, diarrhea, constipation; knee and leg pain; fatigue, exhaustion, weakness, infirmity; scanty or absent periods.

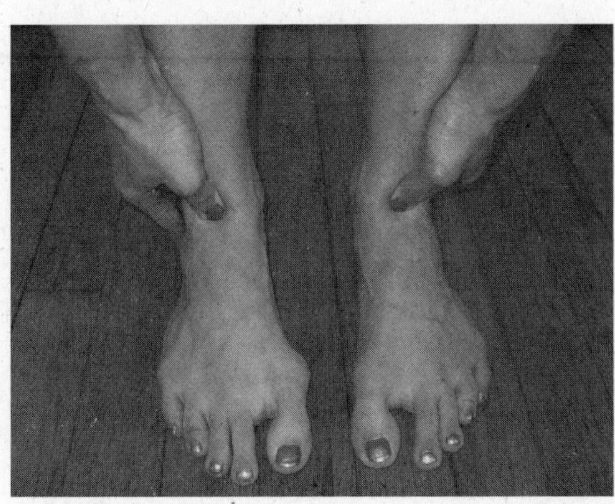

A1-24 St 41.
On the dorsal surface of the foot at the ankle, between the extensor hallucis longus (big toe tendon) and extensor digitorum longus (tendon of the other toes); to define these tendons, dorsiflex the foot and extend the toes. Good for arthritis, pain, and swelling of the ankle and foot; headache, vertigo, dizziness.

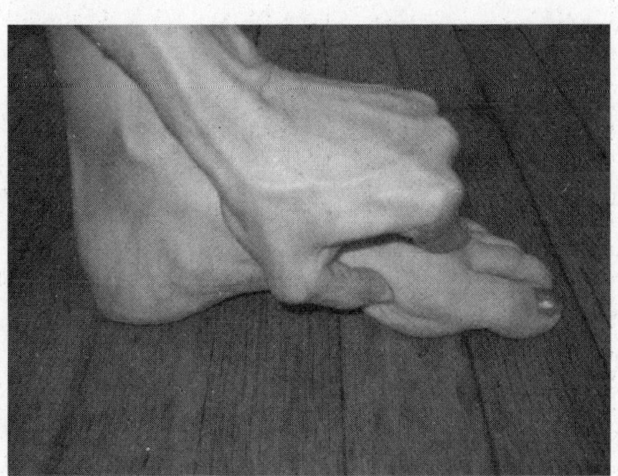

A1-25 Sp 3.
On the medial side (arch) of the foot, proximal and inferior to the head of the first metatarsal (bone at the base of the big toe, which sometimes forms a bunion) at the juncture of the red and white skin. Fortifies Spleen and evaporates Dampness. Good for weakness, tiredness, heaviness; edema in lower body; abdominal distention and pain, loose stools, diarrhea; excessive menstrual discharge; excessive urination; poor concentration, confusion, drowsiness.

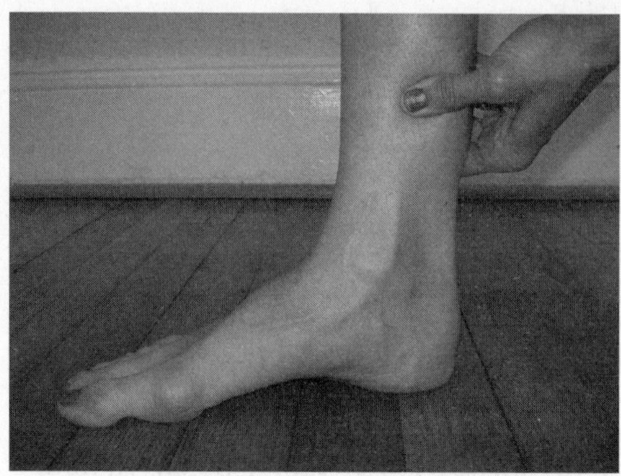

A1-26 **Sp 6.**
On the lower leg, 3 cun proximal to the medial malleolus (inner anklebone). Fortifies and nourishes the Spleen, Liver, and Kidneys, whose Meridians intersect here. Good for digestive disorders such as abdominal distention and pain, poor appetite and digestion, loose stools, diarrhea, constipation, irritable bowel syndrome, hemorrhoids; genital pain or itching; reproductive disorders such as erratic or painful or absent or copious periods, vaginal or seminal discharge, impotence or infertility; urinary disorders such as difficult or painful urination; weakness, fatigue; lower body edema; heat sensation, restlessness, insomnia, hypertension, dizziness, vertigo, tinnitus. *Contraindicated* during pregnancy but facilitates labor.

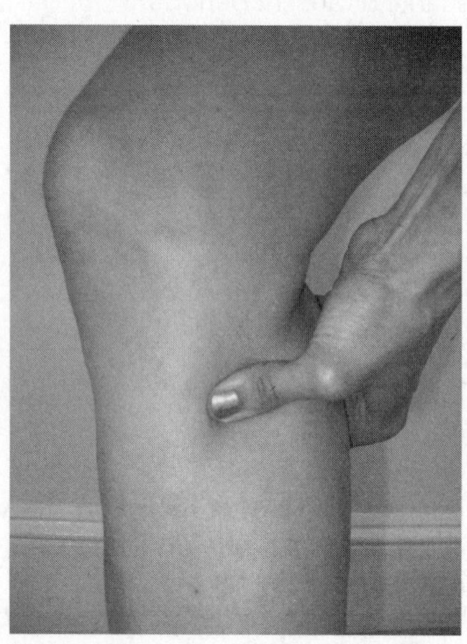

A1-27 **Sp 9.**
On the lower leg, in the depression below the medial tibial condyle (bony arch of the inner shinbone). Evaporates Dampness and cools Heat. Good for lower burner disorders such as difficult urination, retention of urine, incontinence; abdominal distention, loose stools, diarrhea, mucus in stools; vaginal discharge, erratic periods, seminal emission, impotence; edema of the lower body; leg and knee pain and swelling.

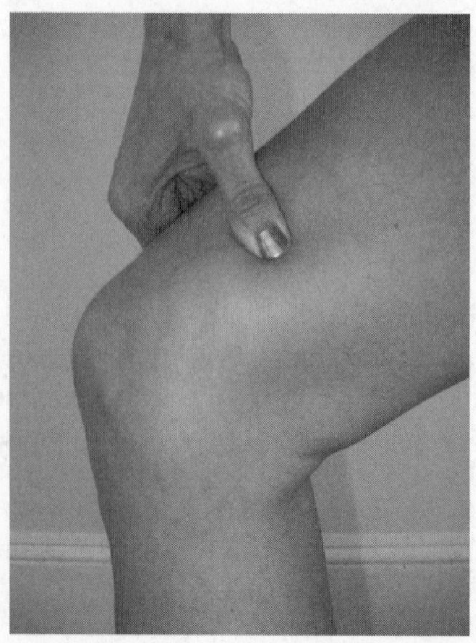

A1-28 **Sp 10.**
On the anterior thigh, 2 cun proximal to the superior medial border of the patella (inner kneecap) on the vastus medialis (inner segment of the quadriceps). Cools Heat and regulates blood flow. Good for menstrual disorders such as erratic, painful, or copious periods; inner thigh and knee pain; transient, itching, inflammatory skin disorders such as rashes, hives, herpes, eczema, psoriasis.

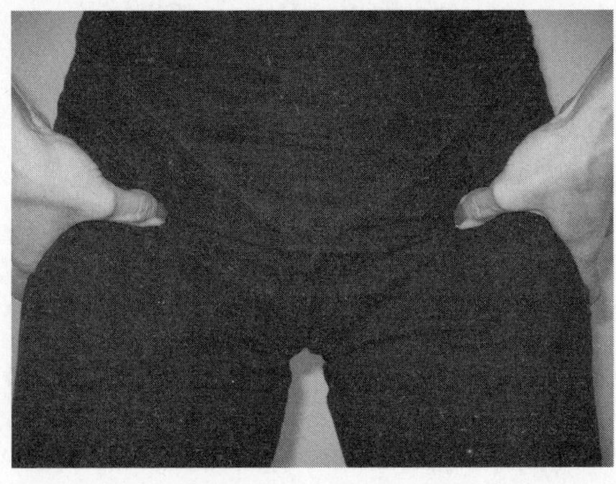

A1-29 Sp 12.
On the groin, in horizontal alignment with the upper ridge of the pubic bone just lateral to the arterial pulse. Good for abdominal pain, bloating, menstrual cramps, impotence, hip pain.

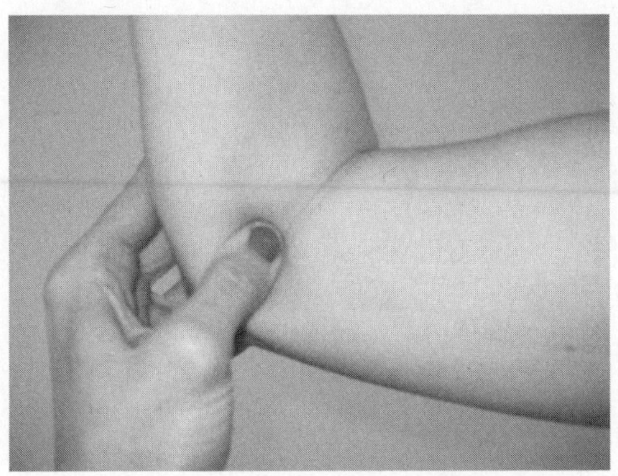

A1-30 Ht 3.
On the anterior forearm, on the ulnar side just distal to the medial epicondyle of the humerus (bony protuberance of the inner elbow) on the flexor carpi ulnaris tendon. Cools Heat, dispels Phlegm, calms Shen. Good for elbow pain, arm debility, forearm numbness, hand tremors; chest pain; forgetfulness or absentmindedness, depression, mental disorders, insomnia.

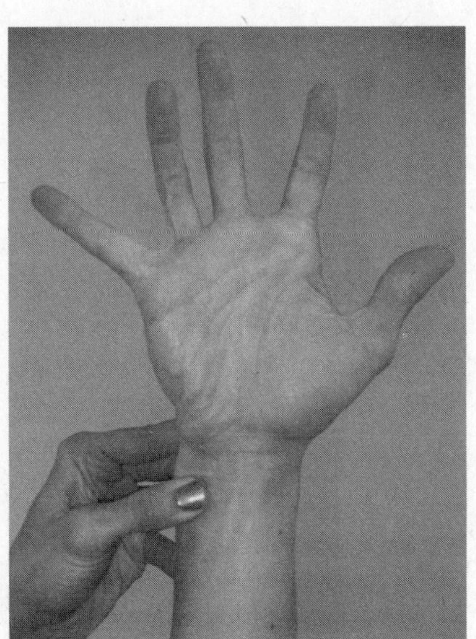

A1-31 Ht 5.
On the anterior forearm, 1 cun proximal to the wrist on the ulnar side on the tendon of the flexor carpi ulnaris. Calms Shen. Good for chest pain, palpitations, arrhythmia; stuttering, muteness; fright, shock.

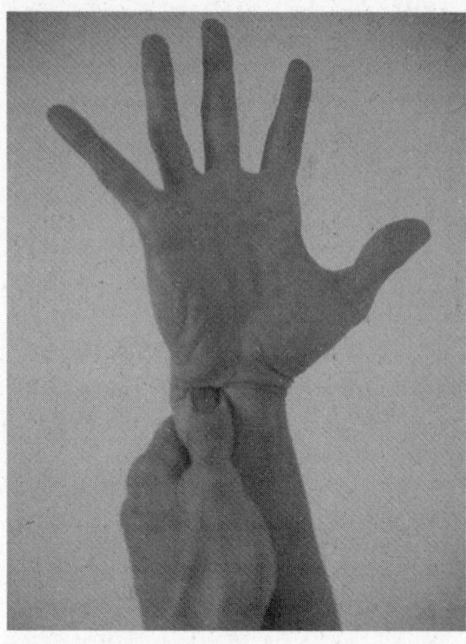

A1-32 Ht 7.
On the anterior wrist, in a small hollow on the ulnar side on the tendon of the flexor carpi ulnaris. Calms Shen. Good for Heart palpitations, chest pain; forgetfulness or absentmindedness, nervousness, emotional distress, anxiety, mental disorders, insomnia.

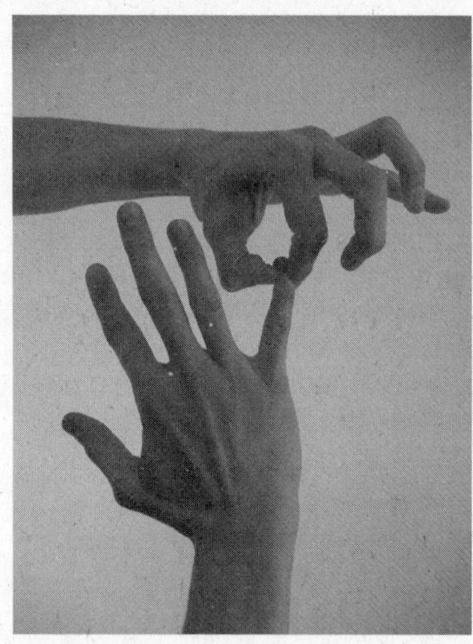

A1-33 Ht 9.
On the little finger, at the inner corner of the nailbed. Calms Shen; restores consciousness. Good for Heart palpitations, chest pain; fever, heatstroke; extreme anxiety, emotional upset, hysteria, shock.

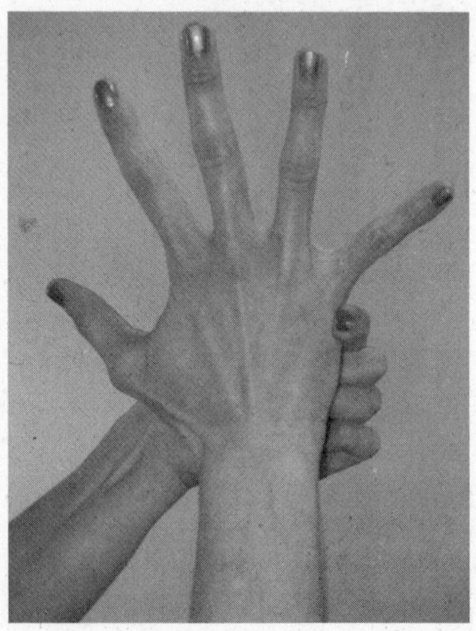

A1-34 SI 3.
On the ulnar side of the hand, proximal to the fifth metacarpal-phalangeal joint in the slight dip or fold when a lax fist is made. Dispels Wind; dissipates Heat; tonifies Yang energy; calms the mind. Good for neck, upper back, and shoulder pain and stiffness; wrist and elbow pain; occipital headache; flu; inflamed eyes; tinnitus; dizziness, hypertension, insomnia.

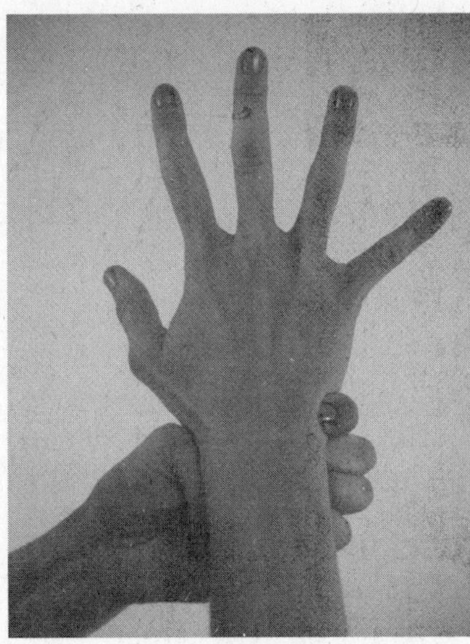

A1-35 **SI 5.**
On the ulnar side of the wrist, in the dent between the styloid process (bony prominence) of the ulna and the carpals. Good for neck, upper back, and shoulder pain and stiffness.

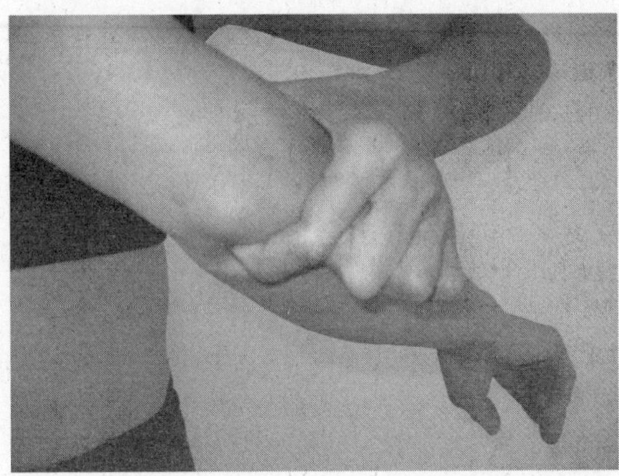

A1-36 **SI 8.**
On the inner elbow, in the nook between the oleocranon of the ulna (elbow) and the medial epicondyle of the humerus. Good for the ulnar nerve, elbow, forearm, and shoulder.

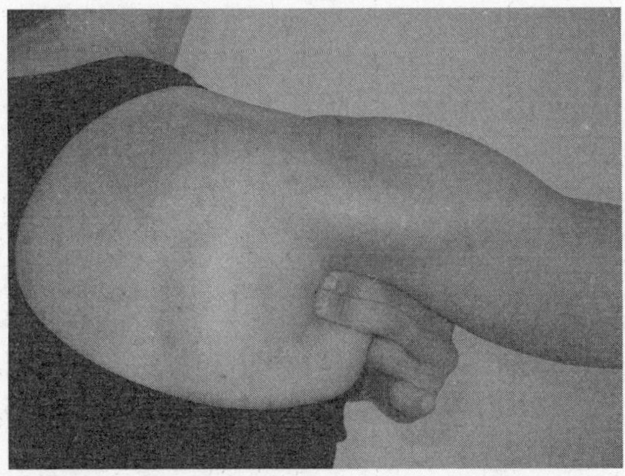

A1-37 **SI 9.**
On the posterior shoulder, 1 cun above the axillary fold (armpit crease) on the teres major. Good for inflammation, paralysis, painful obstruction syndrome of the shoulder and arm.

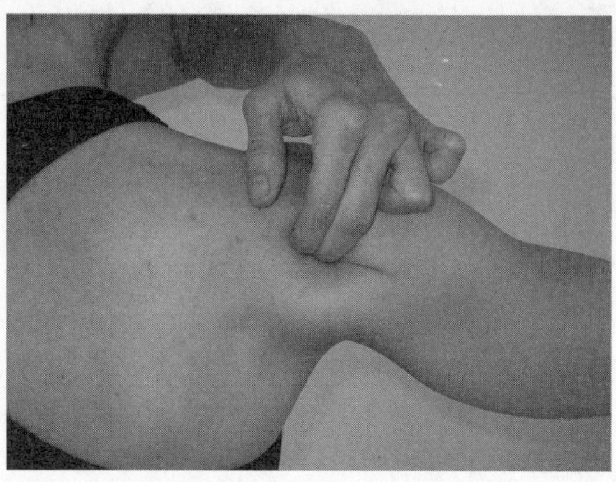

A1-38 SI 10.
On the posterior shoulder, just below the scapular spine on the posterior deltoid. Good for inflammation, paralysis, painful obstruction syndrome of the shoulder and arm.

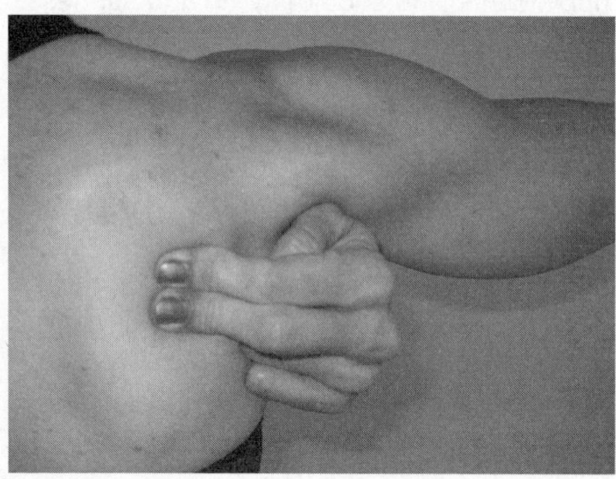

A1-39 SI 11.
On the posterior shoulder, in the center of the scapula (shoulder blade) on the infraspinatus. Powerfully relaxes the entire shoulder; good for inflammation, paralysis, painful obstruction syndrome of the shoulder and arm; calms and relaxes the alimentary tract; good for abdominal pain, indigestion, irritable bowel syndrome, diarrhea, acid reflux.

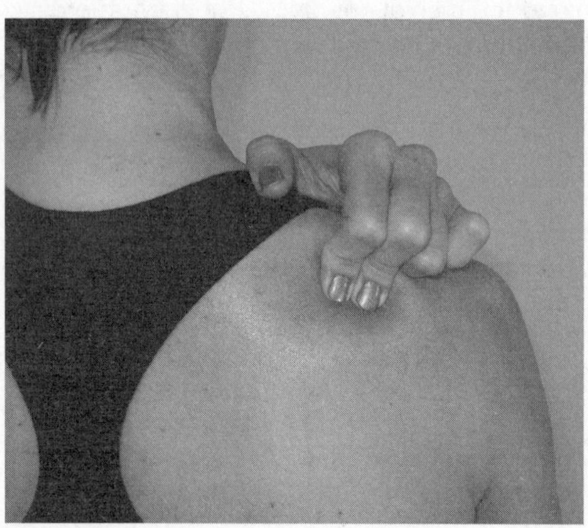

A1-40 SI 12.
On the posterior shoulder, in the center of the suprascapular fossa (bony basin above the scapular spine) on the supraspinatus; good for inflammation, paralysis, painful obstruction syndrome of the shoulder and arm; upper back and neck pain and stiffness; calms and relaxes the alimentary tract; good for abdominal pain, indigestion, irritable bowel syndrome, diarrhea, acid reflux.

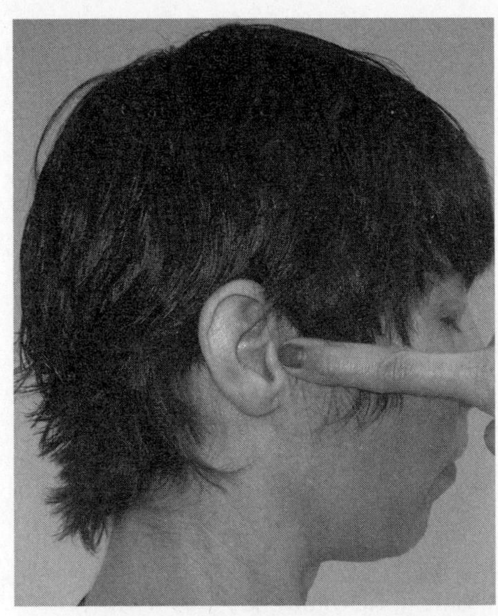

A1-41 **SI 19.**
On the side of the face, in the hollow formed in front of the tragus (ear flap); to define the hollow, open the jaw. Good for ear disorders such as ear infections, tinnitus (ringing in the ears), deafness.

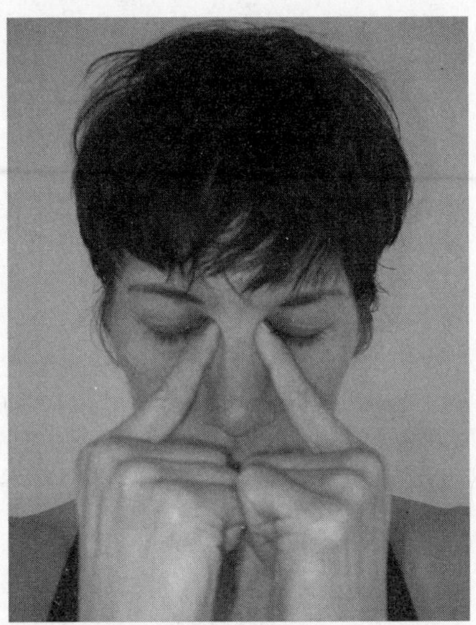

A1-42 **Bl 1.**
On the face, close to the inner corner of the eyes. Good for eye disorders such as dry eyes, tired and strained eyes, sore and red and swollen eyes, poor night vision, inflammation or atrophy of the optic nerve, glaucoma, cataract; migraine; nosebleeds.

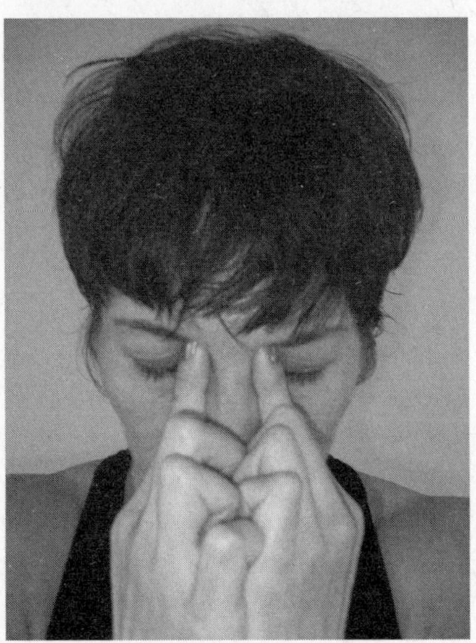

A1-43 **Bl 2.**
On the face, at the inner corners of the eyebrows; press upward against the bony ridge of the eye orbit. Good for eye disorders such as conjunctivitis, sore and strained and red eyes; frontal headache, migraine; facial paralysis.

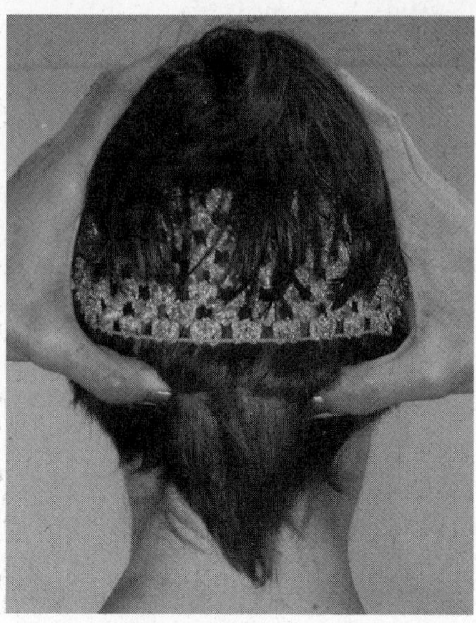

A1-44 **Bl 10.**
On the neck, below the occipital ridge (base of the skull) on the lateral aspect of the upper trapezius. Good for neck and shoulder tension and stiffness; occipital headache; dizziness; sore, strained, red eyes; emotional distress.

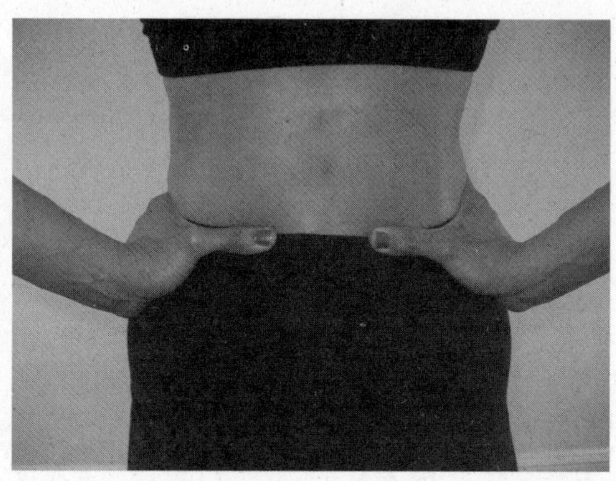

A1-45 **Bl 23.**
On the lower back at waist level, below L2, 1½ cun lateral to the spine. Shu/Yu point for the Kidneys; use moxa to fortify against general infirmity and to increase vitality. Good for lumbago (lower back pain); reproductive disorders such as low libido, infertility, seminal discharge, impotence, premature ejaculation; ear disorders such as deafness, tinnitus.

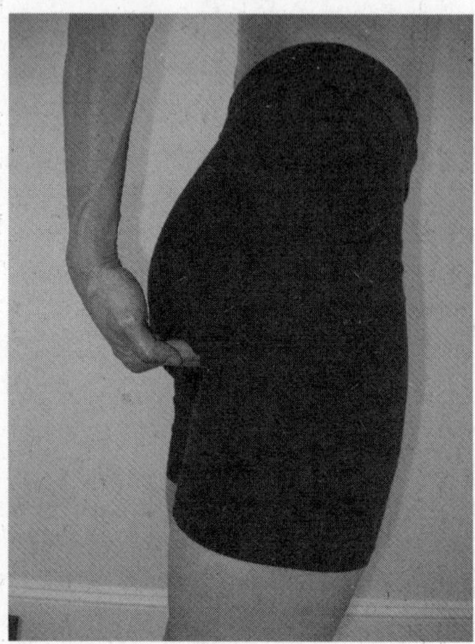

A1-46 **Bl 36.**
On the posterior thigh, directly below the cleft of the buttock just lateral to the biceps femoris (hamstring) attachment at the ischial tuberosity (sit bone). Good for lumbago (lower back pain), sciatica.

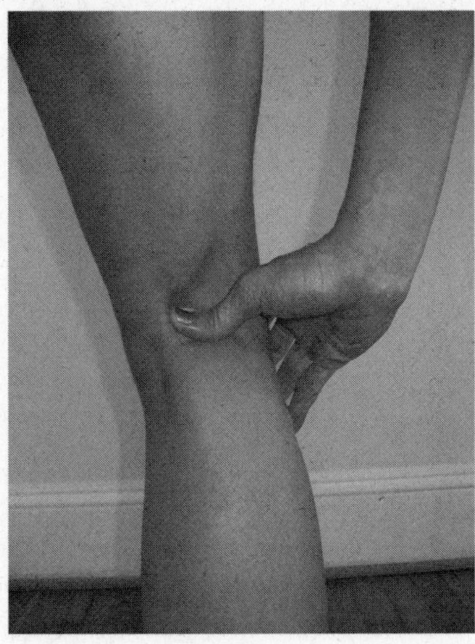

A1-47 **Bl 40.**
On the posterior knee, in the center of the popliteal crease between the biceps femoris and semitendinosus (hamstring) tendons. Good for acute and chronic back pain, leg pain, knee pain. *Caution:* Do not apply excessive pressure.

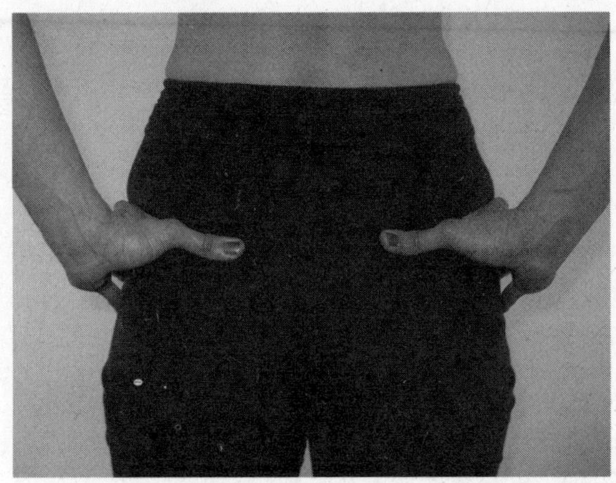

A1-48 **Bl 53.**
On the buttock, in horizontal alignment with the second sacral foramen; good for lumbago, hip tension or pain, sciatica; PMS, menstrual cramps; urinary disorders; constipation; hemorrhoids; relieves irritation, frustration.

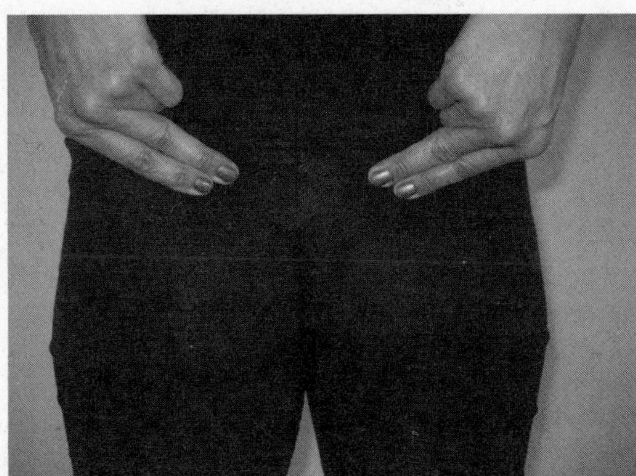

A1-49 **Bl 54.**
On the buttock, at the apex of the gluteus maximus (buttock muscle) in horizontal alignment with the fourth sacral foramen; good for lumbago, hip tension or pain, sciatica; PMS, menstrual cramps; urinary disorders; constipation; hemorrhoids; relieves irritation, frustration.

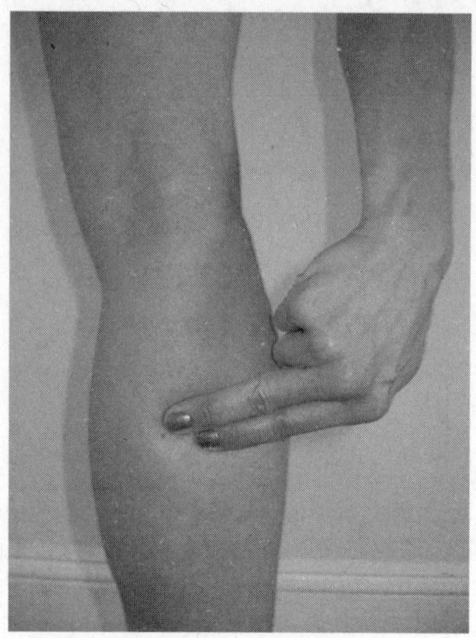

A1-50 Bl 56.
On the calf, about 5 cun below the popliteal crease on the plumpest part of the belly of the gastrocnemius (upper calf muscle). Good for lumbago, sciatica; calf cramp; leg weakness; painful period; hemorrhoids; pain in the pelvic floor or anus.

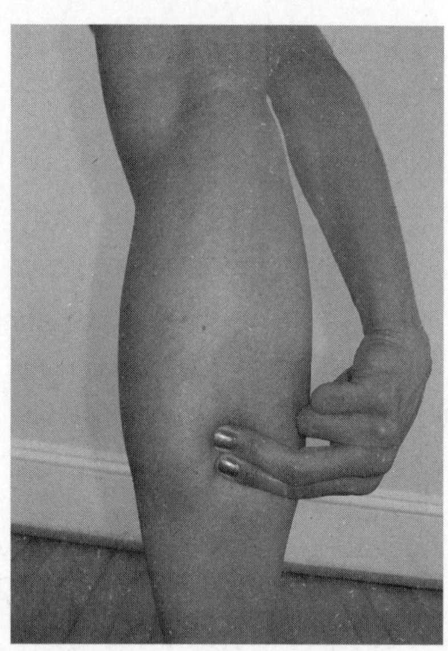

A1-51 Bl 57.
On the calf, where the calf muscle tapers in an arrowhead-shaped depression at the junction of the gastrocnemius (superficial calf muscle) and soleus (deeper calf muscle); to locate, raise the heels. Good for lumbago, sciatica; calf cramp; leg weakness; painful period; hemorrhoids; pain in the pelvic floor or anus.

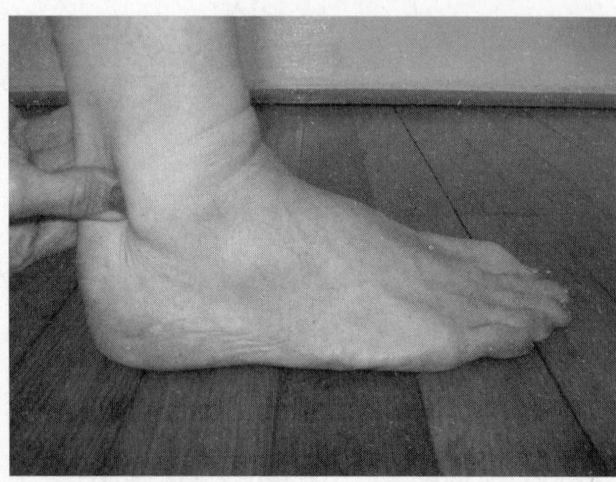

A1-52 Bl 60.
Behind the outer ankle, between the Achilles tendon and lateral malleolus (outer anklebone). Good for back pain; heel pain; headache; childbirth pain; difficult labor.

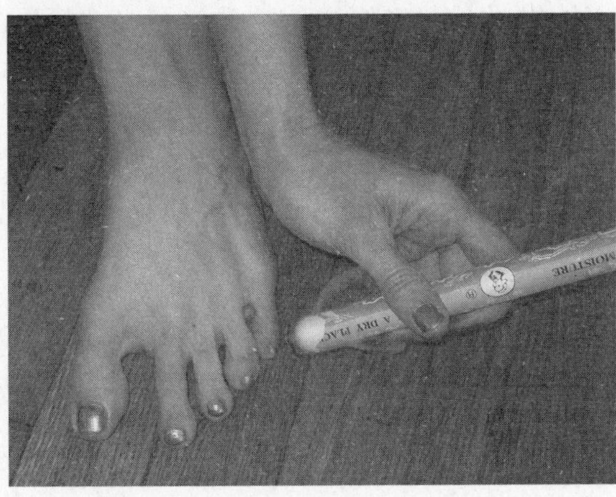

A1-53 Bl 67.
On the little toe, at the outer corner of the nailbed; resolves certain obstetric complications, including a malpositioned fetus and difficult labor; apply moxa during the 38th week of gestation to rotate a fetus in the breech position; apply moxa or vigorously stimulate to facilitate labor.

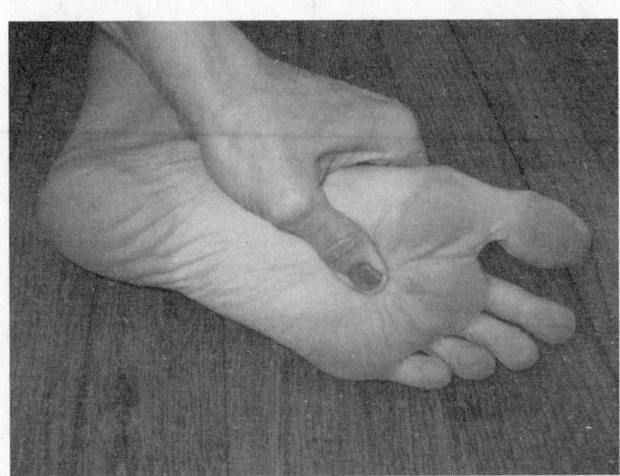

A1-54 Ki 1.
On the sole of the foot, proximal to the calloused ball of the foot between the second and third metatarsal bones in the depression formed when the foot points. Cools Heat; draws down excessive Yang energy, especially from the head. Good for vertex headache, dizziness, vertigo, hypertension, hot flashes, heatstroke; shock, mental disorder, agitation, anxiety, irritability, insomnia; seizure, convulsion; pain or spasm in the sole of the foot.

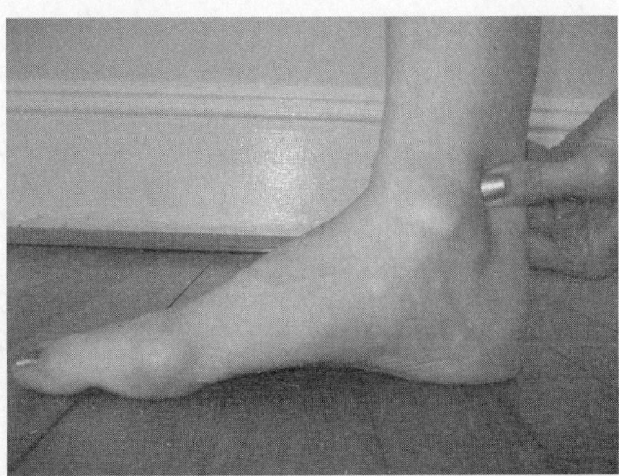

A1-55 Ki 3.
Behind the inner ankle, between the Achilles tendon and medial malleolus (inner anklebone). Fortifies and nourishes Source Qi. Good for erratic or absent periods, menopausal complaints, infertility, premature ejaculation, impotence; frequent urination, incontinence; exhaustion; lower body edema; coldness and weakness of the abdomen, lower back, legs, and knees; headache, dizziness, hypertension, poor hearing, tinnitus.

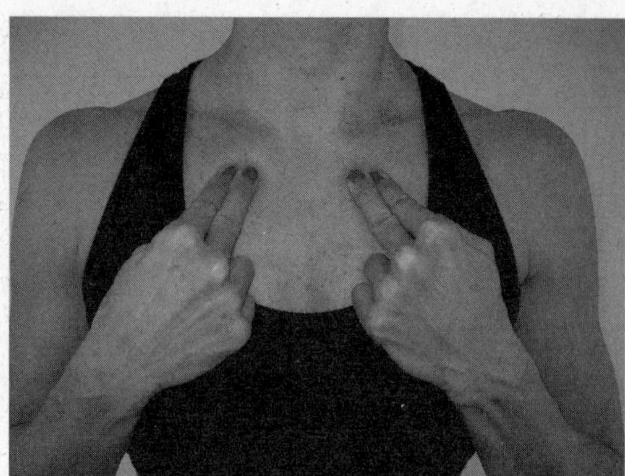

A1-56 Ki 27.
On the chest, at the juncture of the clavicle (collarbone) and sternum (breastbone) on the pectoralis. Good for respiratory disorders, chest pain, tension and constriction, palpitations; anxiety, depression.

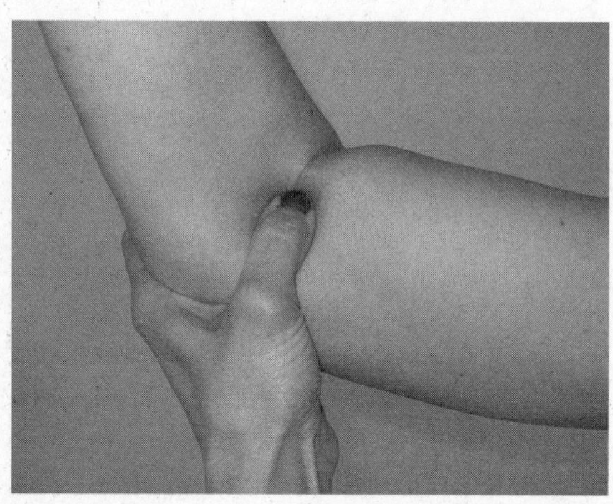

A1-57 PC 3.
On the anterior forearm at the elbow, on the ulnar side of the biceps tendon. Cools Heat; disperses stagnation; calms Shen. Good for chest pain, palpitations, rapid or racing heartbeat; labored breathing, cough; vomiting; insomnia; hyperthermia, fever; anxiety.

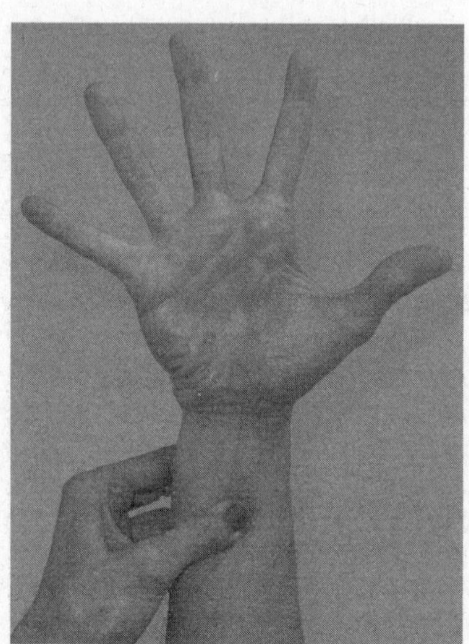

A1-58 PC 6.
On the anterior forearm, 2 cun proximal to the wrist between the two wrist flexor tendons. Cools Heat; disperses stagnation; calms Shen. Good for chest pain, distention or constriction, palpitations, cough; stomachache, rebellious Stomach Qi: hiccups, nausea, acid reflux, vomiting; PMS, breast pain; emotional distress, anxiety, irritability, insomnia.

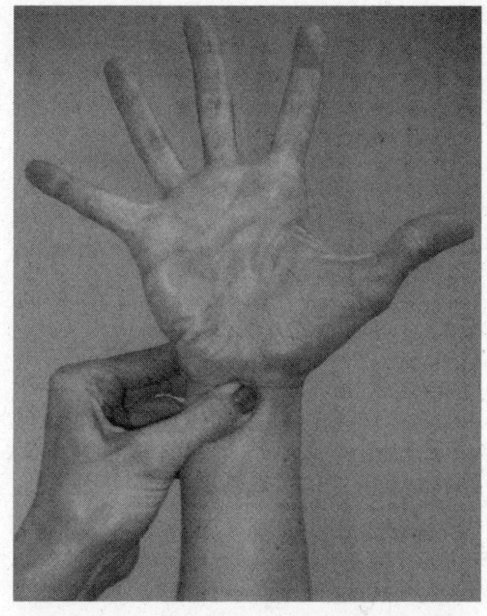

A1-59 **PC 7.**
On the anterior wrist, between the two wrist flexor tendons.
Good for nausea; emotional distress or upset, anxiety, irritability.

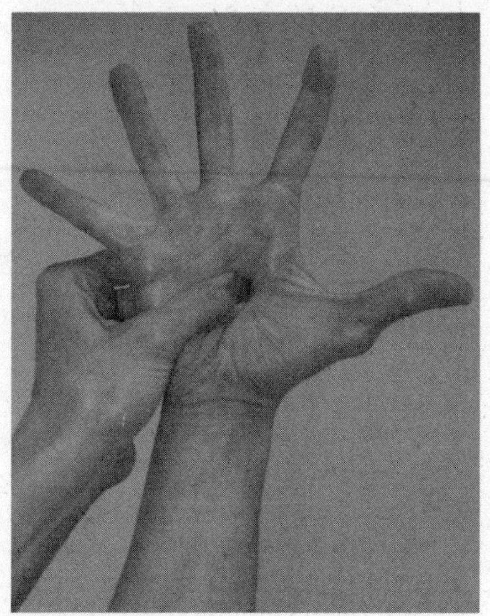

A1-60 **PC 8.**
In the center of the palm, between the second and third metacarpal bones. Cools Heat; quenches Fire; dispels Wind; calms Shen. Good for chest pain, palpitations; mouth and tongue ulcers; profuse sweating, fever, delirium, unconsciousness; hand tremors, convulsions; anxiety, nervous agitation, emotional upset, hysteria.

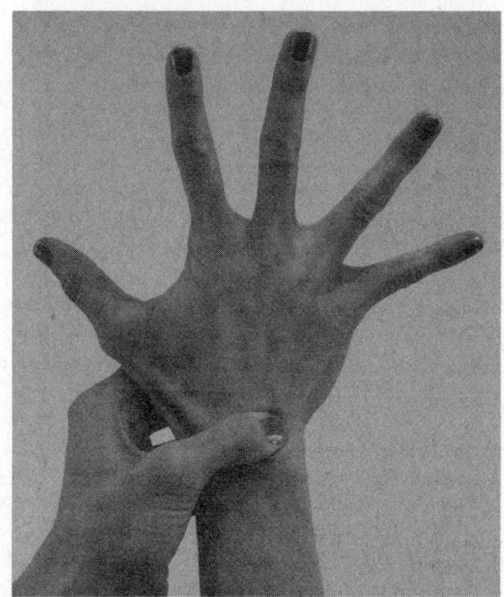

A1-61 **TH 4.**
On the posterior wrist, in a tiny depression lateral to the extensor digitorum communis tendon. Cools Heat; dispels Wind; evaporates Damp. Good for painful obstruction syndrome and swelling or inflammation of the hand, wrist, arm, and shoulder; headache, sore throat, tonsillitis, fever, inflamed eyes and ears; edema; Raynaud's disease (cold extremities).

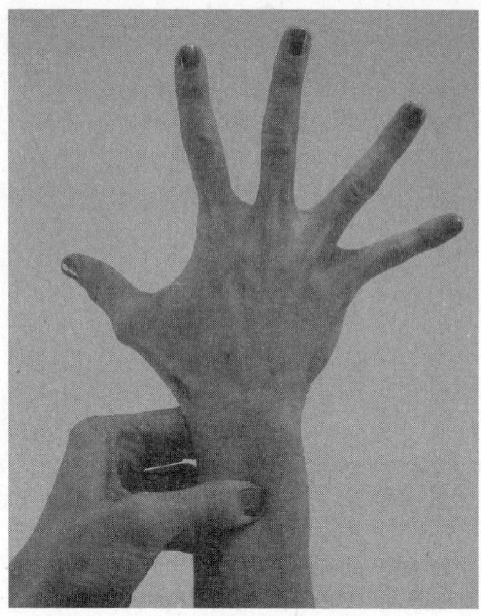

A1-62 TH 5.
On the posterior forearm, 2 cun proximal to the midpoint of the wrist between the radius and ulna. Cools Heat; dispels Wind. Good for painful obstruction syndrome of the arm, shoulder, and neck; headache, sore throat, colds, flu; inflamed eyes, ears, salivary glands; tinnitus, deafness.

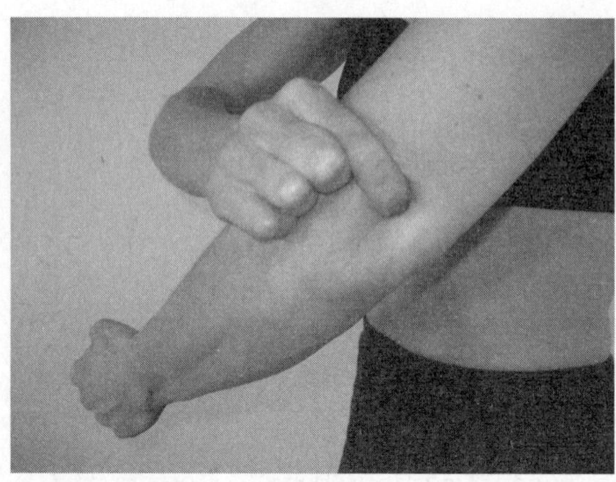

A1-63 TH 10.
On the posterior arm near the elbow, in the indentation proximal to the oleocranon of the humerus (elbow) when the arm is bent; to locate, flex the elbow. Good for elbow problems.

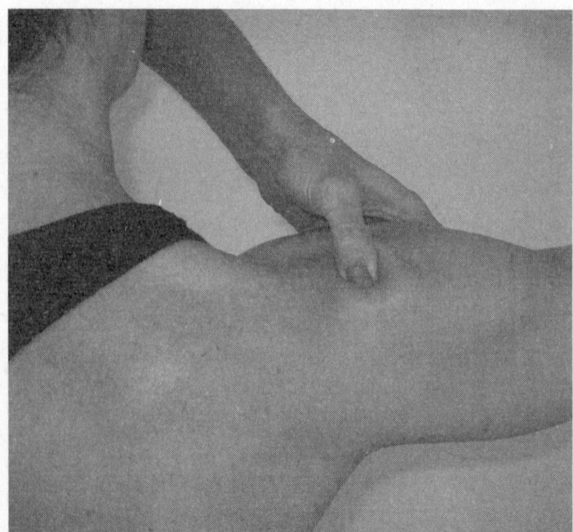

A1 -64 TH 14.
On the upper shoulder, posterior and inferior to the acromion in the indentation formed between the medial and posterior deltoids when the arm is abducted (raised to the side). Good for painful obstruction syndrome of the shoulder and arm.

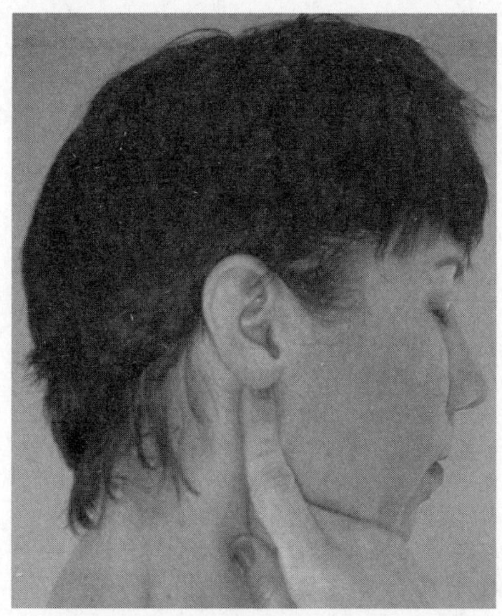

A1 -65 TH 17.
In the notch behind the earlobe and jaw. Cools Heat; dispels Wind. Good for ear disorders such as earache, pain, itching, inflammation, discharge, infection; tinnitus, impaired hearing, deafness; Meniere's disease (balance disorder, dizziness, vertigo); sore throat, inflamed salivary glands; TMJ, jaw and facial tension, pain, or paralysis.

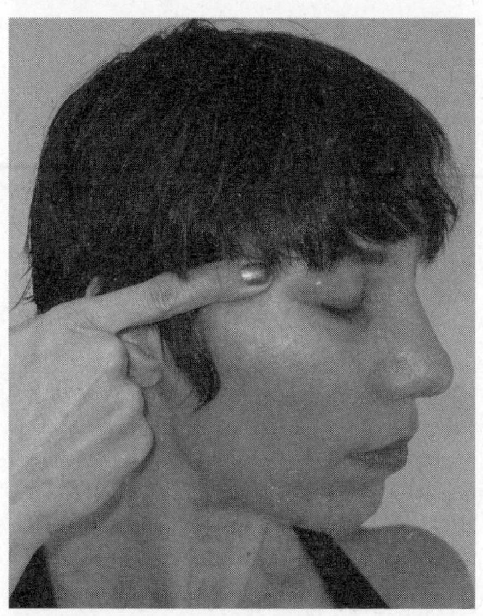

A1-66 GB 1.
On the side of the face, in the depression at the outer corners of the eyes. Good for vision.

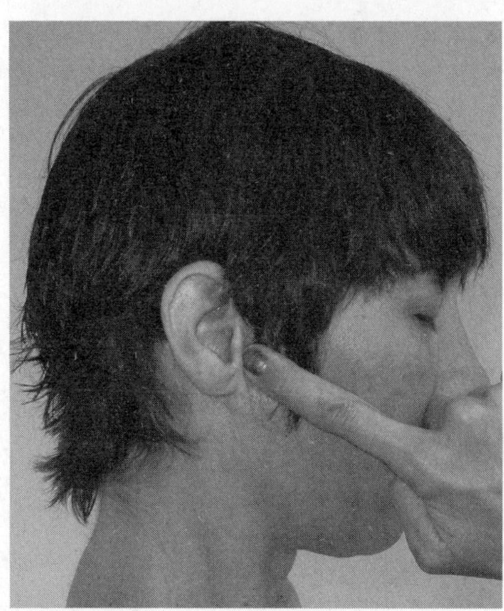

A1-67 GB 2.
On the jaw, between the tragus (ear flap) and earlobe (this point is inferior to SI 19). Good for ear disorders such as earache, pain, itching, or infection; tinnitus, temporary loss of hearing, deafness; mandibular arthritis.

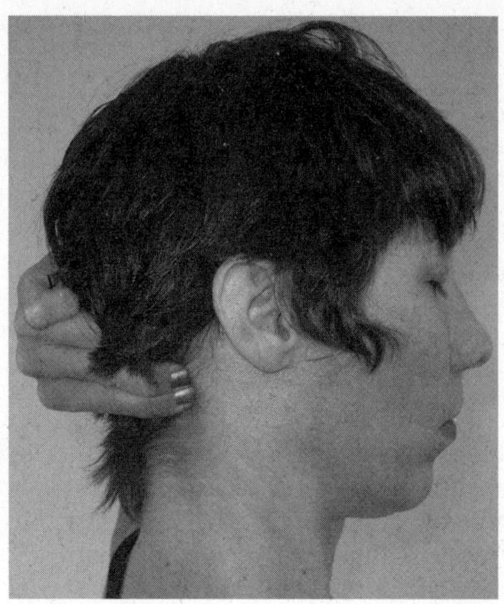

A1-68 GB 20.
On the neck, below the occiput (bony ridge at the nape of the neck) between the upper trapezius and sternocleidomastoid. Expels pathogenic agents; mobilizes stagnant Qi and blood. Good for neck and shoulder tension, stiffness, and pain; headache, migraine; dizziness, vertigo; colds, flu; inflamed eyes or ears, impaired vision or hearing; TMJ; irritation.

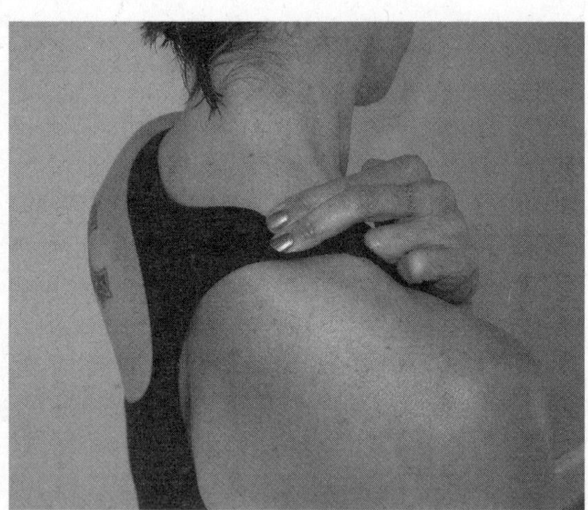

A1-69 GB 21.
On the upper shoulder, on the belly of the upper trapezius. Good for shoulder tension and stiffness; headache, migraine; painful or inflamed eyes or ears; TMJ; fatigue; frustration, irritation, nervous agitation. *Contraindicated* during pregnancy but facilitates labor.

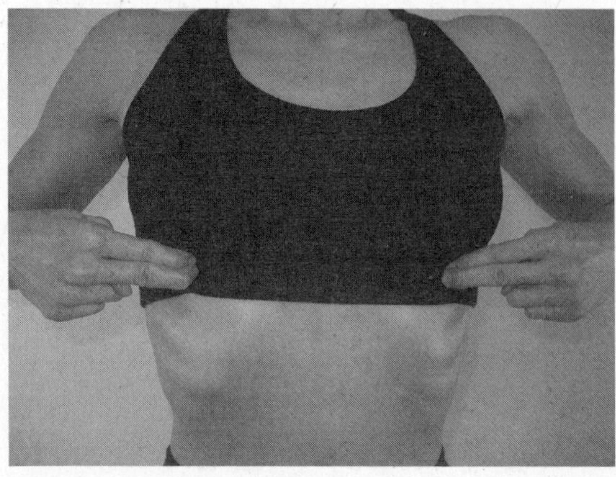

A1-70 GB 24.
On the anterior rib cage, in the seventh intercostal space (between the seventh and eighth ribs) in vertical alignment with the nipple. Mu/Bo point for the Gallbladder; good for Gallbladder and Liver disorders; pain and distention in hypochondrium (upper, lateral abdomen on either side of the Stomach); jaundice.

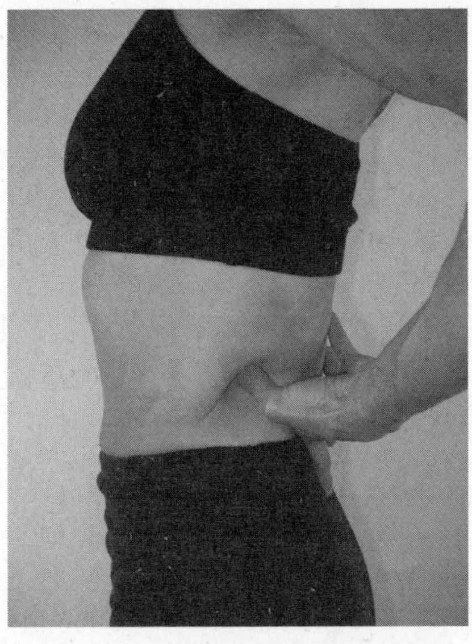

A1-71 GB 25.
On the lateral waist, inferior to the end of the twelfth floating rib. Mu/Bo point for the Kidneys; this point has properties similar to Lr 13; fortifies and harmonizes middle and lower burners; good for digestive disorders caused by Liver invading Spleen such as rebellious Stomach Qi, abdominal distention, indigestion, flatulence, diarrhea, constipation; good for distention and constriction of the chest, labored breathing, coughing; good for middle and lower back stiffness and pain that limits twisting and side bending movements. *Caution*: carefully apply mild to moderate pressure, as floating ribs may fracture.

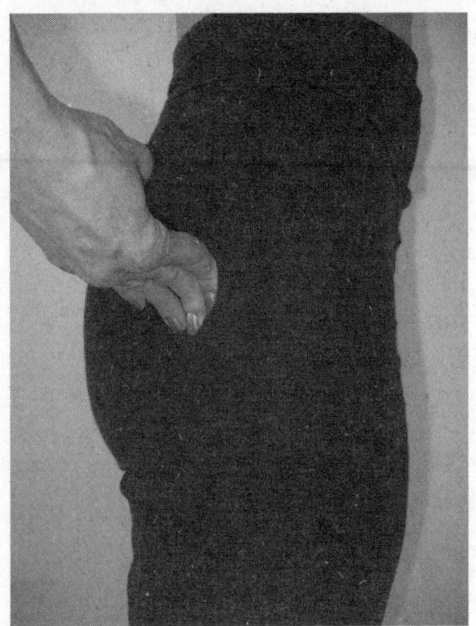

A1-72 GB 30.
On the outer buttock, one-third of the way between the greater trochanter of the femur (thighbone) and sacrum (triangular bone at the base of the spine); when standing, the buttock forms a bowl-shaped hollow at this point. Good for lumbago, sciatica, hip and lower leg pain; paralysis; frustration, irritation.

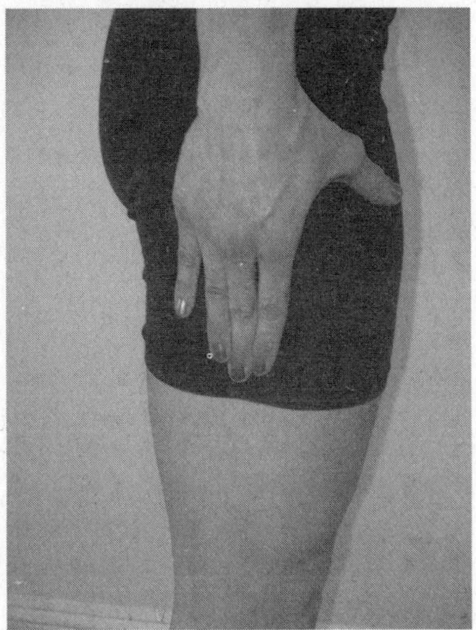

A1-73 GB 31.
At the point where the middle finger touches the lateral thigh when the arm hangs down. Good for sciatica, iliotibial band syndrome (pain or neural sensations down the side of the thigh); weakness, pain, and wasting of the lower leg; one-sided paralysis.

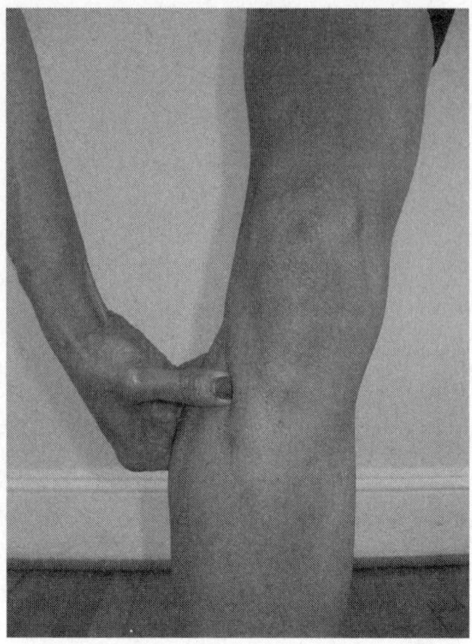

A1-74 **GB 34.**
On the lateral lower leg, anterior and inferior to the head of the fibula. Promotes the free flow of Qi and blood. Good for sinew disorders such as muscular tension, stiffness, rigidity, cramps, spasms, numbness, twitching or tremors, tendinosis, arthritis; knee pain, leg pain, lumbago; paralysis; irritability, PMS.

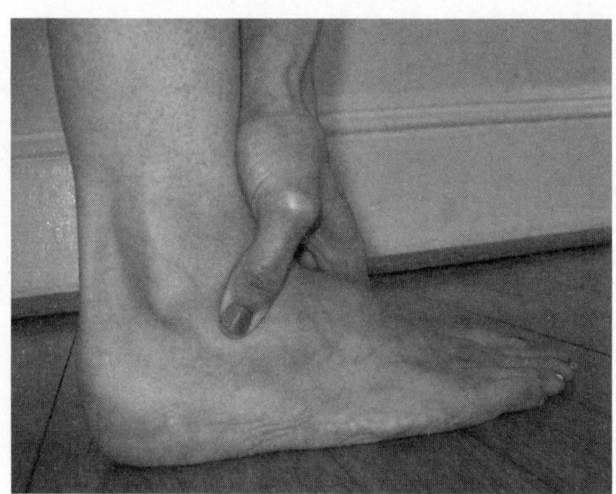

A1-75 **GB 40.**
On the dorsal surface of the foot, anterior and inferior to the lateral malleolus (outer anklebone). Good for sinew disorders such as muscular tension, stiffness, cramps, spasms; indecisiveness, timidity.

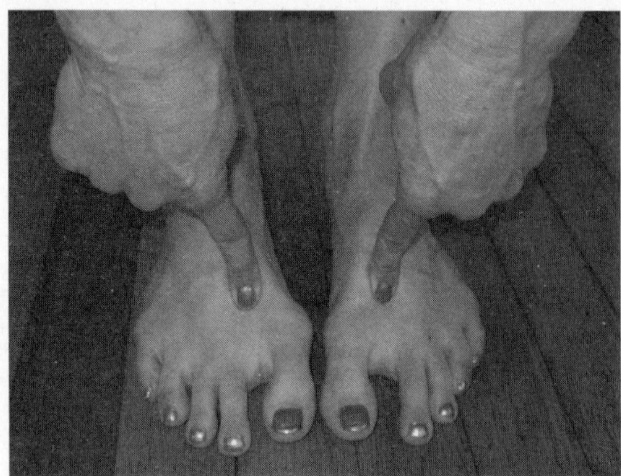

A1-76 **Lr 3.**
On the posterior foot, in the web of flesh between the first and second metatarsal bones. Quenches Liver Fire; draws excessive Yang energy down; like LI 4, this point is a general panacea and antidote for many disorders. Good for hypertension, headache, migraine, dizziness, vertigo, insomnia; strained, tired, inflamed eyes; impaired vision; rebellious Stomach Qi, abdominal distention and pain, irritable bowel syndrome; PMS, absent or erratic or painful or copious periods; irritation, frustration, agitation. Caution: do not vigorously stimulate during pregnancy, but use to facilitate labor.

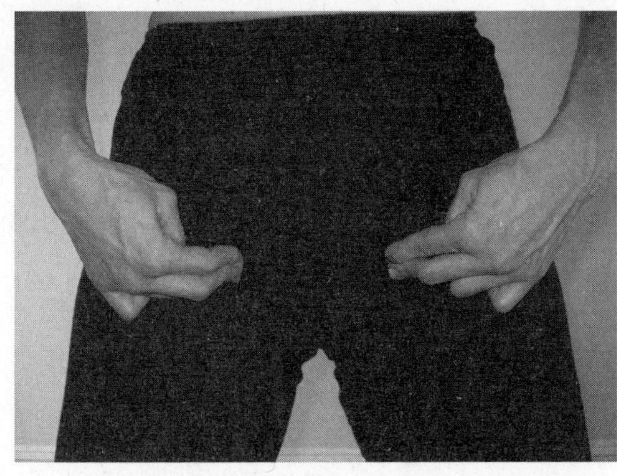

A1-77 **Lr 12.**
At the groin, lateral to the pubic tubercle (prominent corner of the pubic bone) just medial to the femoral artery. Good for hernia, prolapse of uterus; pain in lower abdomen, medial thigh, or genitals.

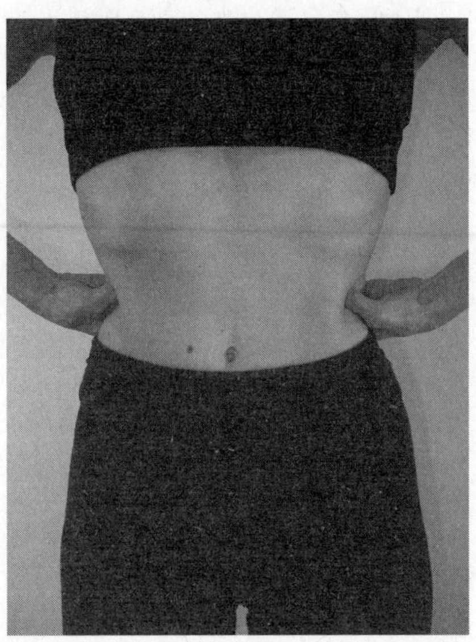

A1-78 **Lr 13.**
On the lateral waist, inferior to the end of the eleventh floating rib: Mu/Bo point for the Spleen; fortifies the Spleen; regulates Liver Qi. Good for symptoms of Liver invading Spleen such as abdominal distention and pain, indigestion, borborygmus (abdominal churning, rumbling, gurgling), nausea, belching, vomiting, flatulence, loose stools, diarrhea, constipation; distention or constriction of the chest, labored breathing, coughing; good for middle and lower back stiffness and pain that limits twisting and sidebending movements. *Caution*: carefully apply mild to moderate pressure, as floating ribs may fracture.

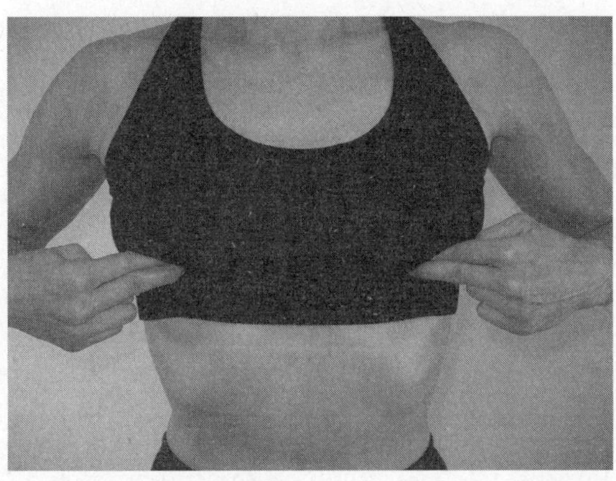

A1-79 **Lr 14.**
On the anterior rib cage, in the sixth intercostal space (between the sixth and seventh ribs) in vertical alignment with the nipple. Mu/Bo point for the Liver; promotes circulation of stagnant Qi and blood. Good for chest and abdominal pain and distention; borborygmus (abdominal churning, rumbling, gurgling), hiccupping, vomiting; hepatitis.

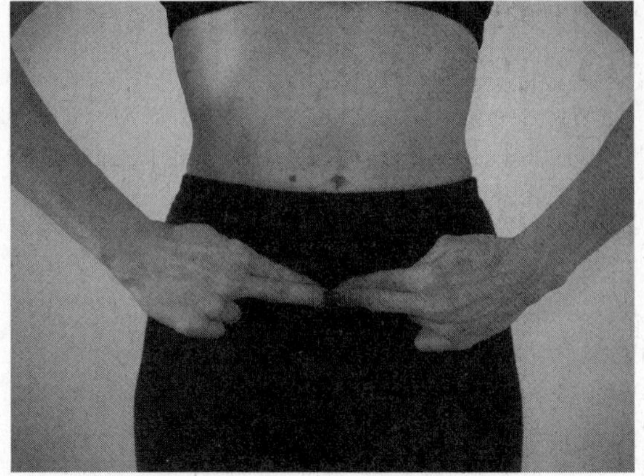

A1-80 **CV 3.**
On the lower abdomen, 4 cun below the navel. Mu/Bo point for the Bladder; use moxa with symptoms of Cold Damp. Good for lower burner disorders such as abdominal pain and distention; urinary tract infections, painful or frequent urination; erratic or painful or copious periods, vaginal discharge, seminal discharge; premature ejaculation, impotence, prostate inflammation, genital itching and pain.

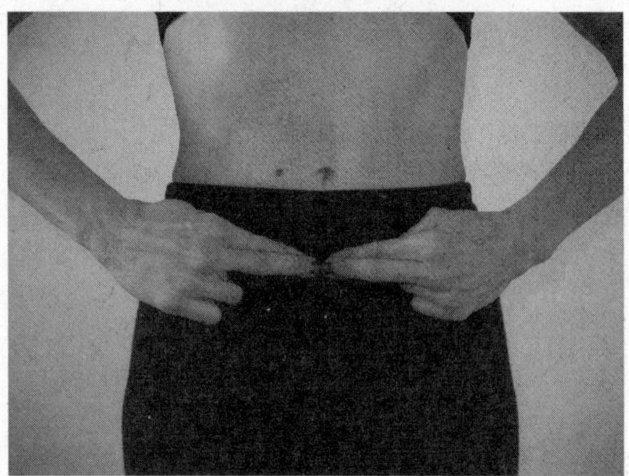

A1-81 **CV 4.**
On the lower abdomen, 3 cun below the navel. Mu/Bo point for the Small Intestine; fortifies the body in chronic illness and fatigue; use moxa with symptoms of Cold Damp. Good for lower burner disorders such as abdominal distention and pain, irritable bowel syndrome, diarrhea; retention of urine, painful or frequent urination, incontinence, bedwetting; vaginal discharge, erratic or painful or scanty or absent periods, infertility, ovarian or uterine cysts; seminal discharge, premature ejaculation, impotence; nervous agitation, anxiety, insomnia.

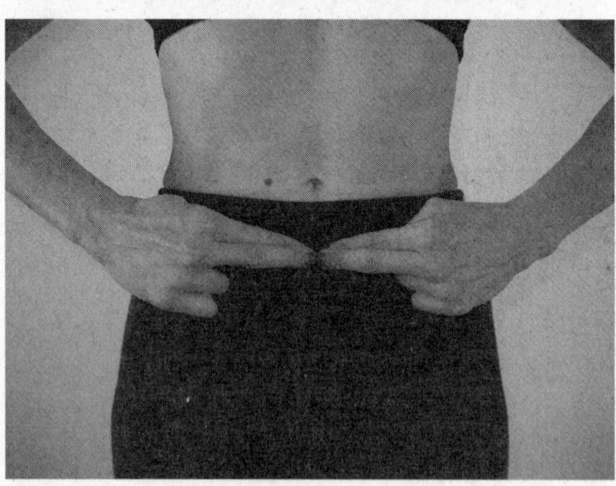

A1-82 **CV 5.**
On the lower abdomen, 2 cun below the navel. Mu/Bo point for the Triple Heater. Good for lower burner disorders, especially those involving the transformation and excretion of fluids such as fluid retention, painful urination, vaginal discharge.

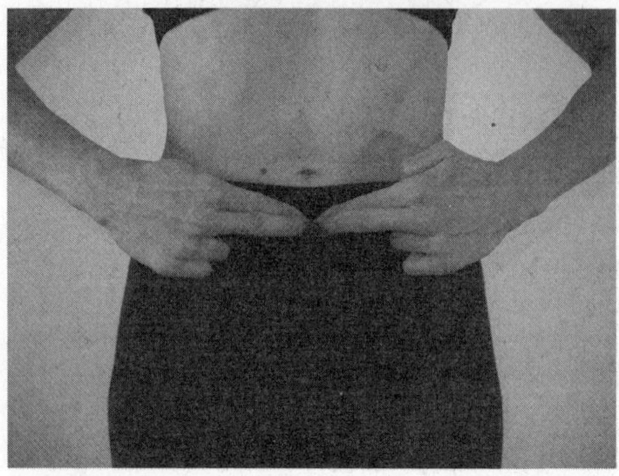

A1-83 **CV 6.**
On the lower abdomen, $1\frac{1}{2}$ cun below the navel. Fortifies Yang energy; evaporates Dampness; use moxa for symptoms of Cold Damp. Good for lower burner disorders such as abdominal distention and pain, diarrhea, constipation; incontinence, bedwetting; erratic or painful periods, vaginal discharge; whole-body malaise, infirmity, emaciation; sinking Qi; mental exhaustion, depression, lack of self-assertion or self-control.

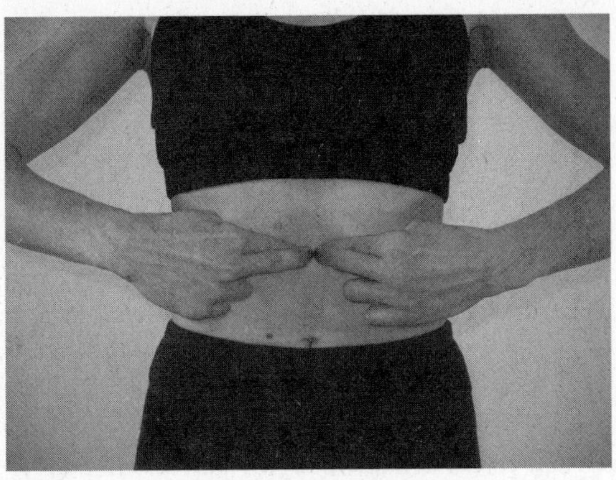

A1-84 **CV 12.**
On the upper abdomen, halfway between the navel and xiphoid process of the sternum (notch of the breastbone) or 4 cun above the navel. Mu/Bo point for the Stomach; use moxa with symptoms of Cold Damp. Good for digestive disorders, especially deficiency disorders such as lack of appetite, abdominal distention and pain, borborygmus (abdominal churning, rumbling, gurgling), poor digestion, loose stools or diarrhea; rebellious Stomach Qi—hiccups, belching, nausea, vomiting; restlessness, fatigue, inability to concentrate.

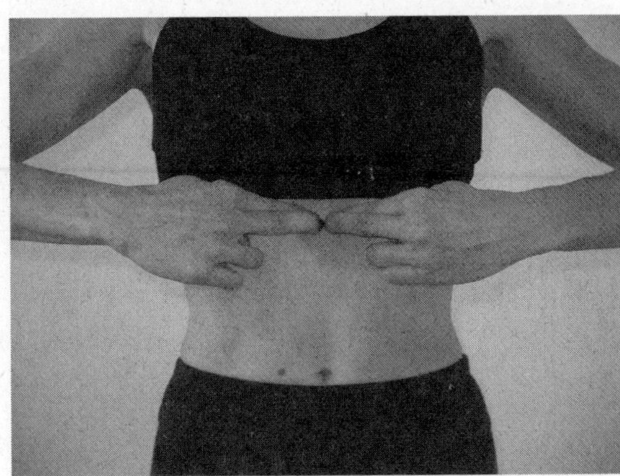

A1-85 **CV 14.**
On the upper abdomen, 6 cun above the navel. Mu/Bo point for the Heart; dissipates Heat; disperses stagnation in the chest. Good for chest pain and constriction, palpitations, labored breathing, coughing; rebellious Stomach Qi; anxiety, emotional upset, insomnia.

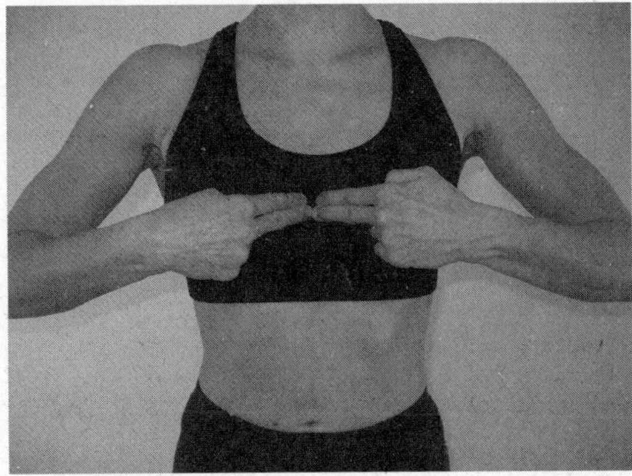

A1-86 **CV 17.**
On the chest, in the middle of the sternum (breastbone) at nipple level. Mu/Bo point for the Pericardium. Good for chest pain and constriction; asthma, labored breathing, coughing, hiccupping, lump in throat, difficulty swallowing; difficult lactation, breast pain; insomnia, nervousness, anxiety, emotional distress, anguish, depression, sorrow, grief, hysteria.

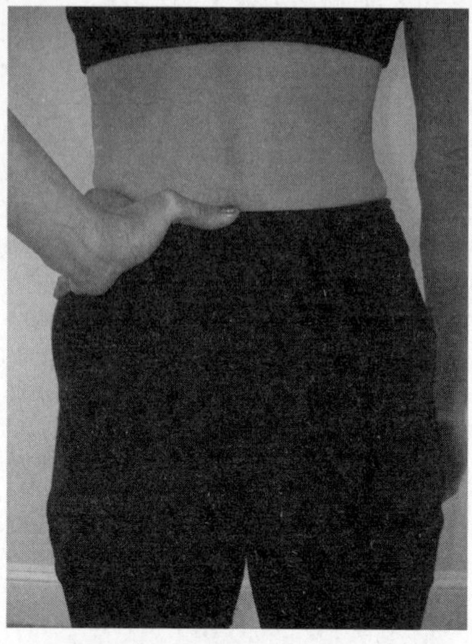

A1-87 **GV 4.**
On the lower back, below the spinous process of L2. Fortifies and nourishes Source Qi; use moxa to fortify against general infirmity and to increase vitality. Good for lumbago, weak back and knees; copious urination, incontinence; vaginal discharge; impotence; lack of vitality; chilliness.

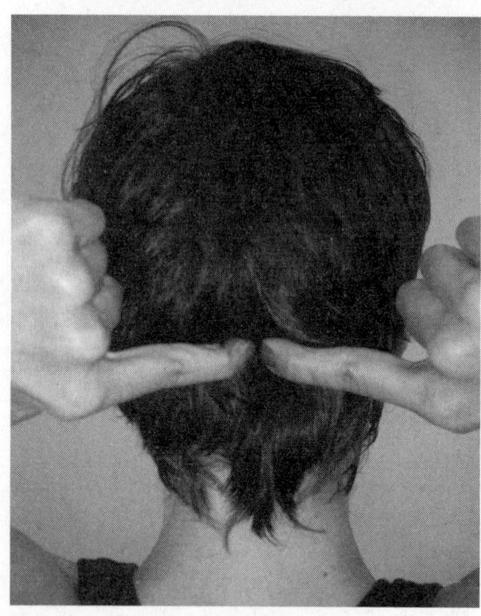

A1-88 **GV 16.**
On the posterior neck, on the midline below the occiput between the bilateral sections of the upper trapezius: good for neck tension, headache.

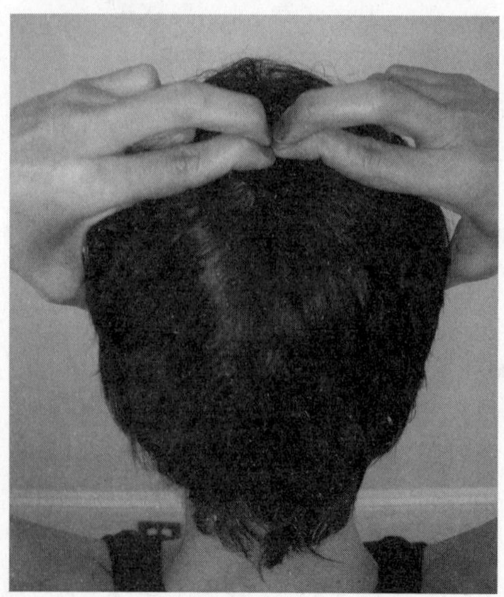

A1-89 **GV 20.**
On the crown of the head, at the midpoint of a line connecting the apex of both ears; subdues excess Yang energy in the head; calms Wind; raises sinking Qi; clears the mind; uplifts emotions; good for vertex headache, dizziness, vertigo, mental agitation; apply moxa in cases of chronic diarrhea, hemorrhoids, hernia, organ prolapse.

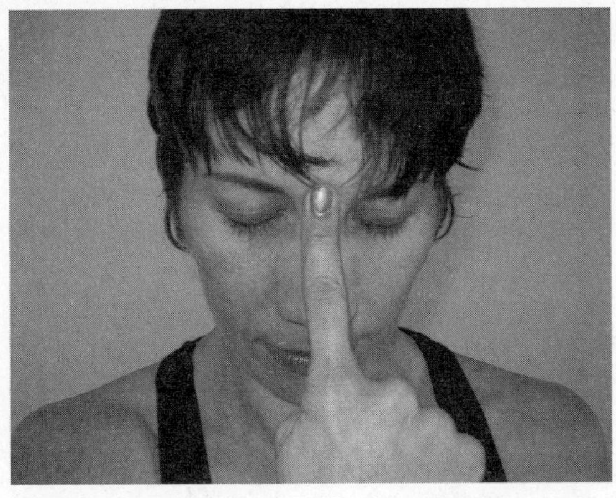

A1-90 GV 24.5 Yintang.
On the forehead, between the eyebrows (at the third eye). Calms Shen. Good for headache, dizziness, insomnia, sore eyes.

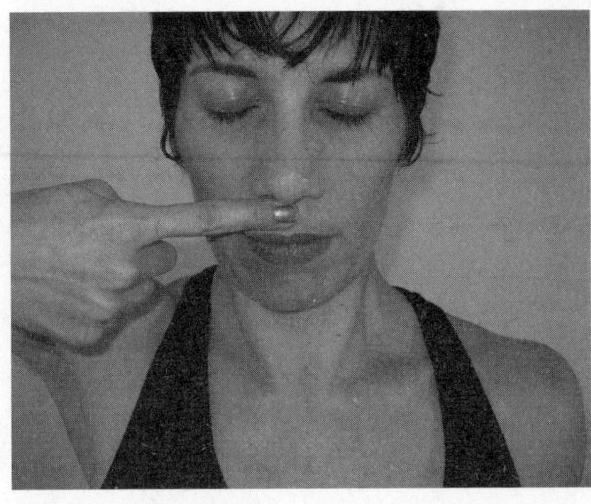

A1-91 GV 26.
On the face, between the nose and upper lip. Good for shock, restoring consciousness.

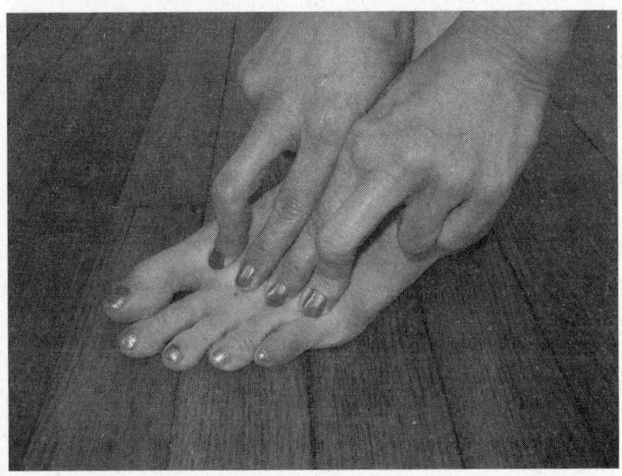

A1-92 Bafeng.
On the webs between the toes. Use moxa with symptoms of Cold Damp. Good for pain, swelling, or arthritis of toes and foot.

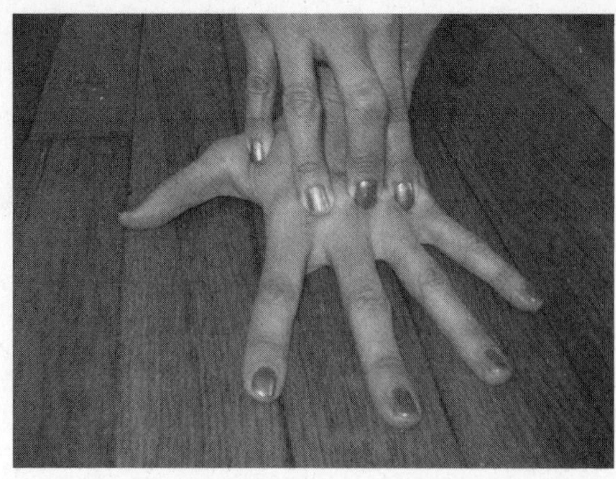

A1-93 Shangbaxie.
On the webs between the fingers. Use moxa with symptoms of Cold Damp. Good for pain, swelling, or arthritis of fingers and hands.

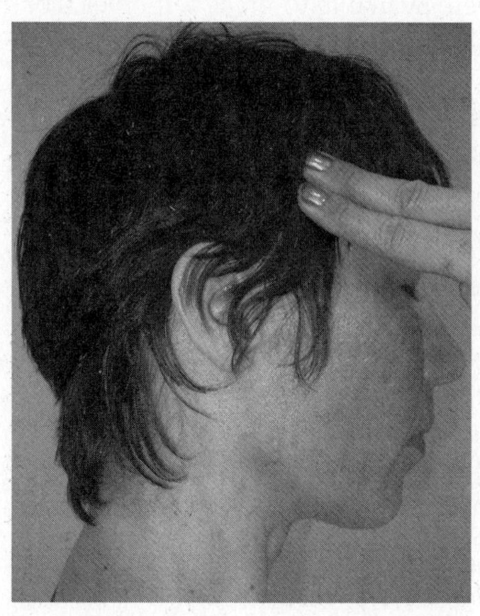

A1-94 Tai Yang.
On the temple. Good for temporal headaches, migraine, eye pain.

REFERENCES

Gach, M. R. (1990). *Acupressure's potent points: A guide to self-care for common ailments.* New York: Bantam.

Institute of Acupuncture and Moxibustion of the China Academy of Traditional Chinese Medicine & Kelin Technology Development Co. (2000). *Charts of Chinese standard location of acupoints.* Beijing: Morning Glory.

Jarmey, C., & Mojay, G. (1999). *Shiatsu: The complete guide.* (1st Rev. ed.). London: Thorsons.

Junying, G., & Zhihong, S. (1997). *Practical Traditional Chinese Medicine and Pharmacology: Acupuncture and moxibustion.* Beijing: New World Press. (Original work published 1991).

Liechti, E. (1998). *The complete illustrated guide to Shiatsu: The Japanese healing art of touch for health and fitness.* New York: Barnes and Noble.

Appendix 2: Answers to Study Questions

Chapter 1 History of Shiatsu

1. Shiatsu originated in China and was further developed in Japan.
2. TCM stands for Traditional Chinese Medicine.
3. TCM is at least 4,000 years old (it predates 2000 B.C.).
4. The *Nei Jing* is *The Yellow Emperor's Classic of Internal Medicine*, the oldest extant medical text.
5. The development of TCM was influenced by the kinds of disorders that were prevalent in a particular region of China and the kinds of natural resources that were available to make remedies. For example, in northern China, where cold disorders and mugwort (an herb) were prevalent, moxabustion (a heat therapy) was developed.
6. The four main healing modalities are acupuncture, herbalism, moxabustion, and Qi Gong. Qi Gong includes breathing and movement exercises (Tao-Yin) and massage therapy (An Mo or "press rub" and Tui Na or "push grab").
7. Like Tui Na and An Mo, Shiatsu is a type of massage therapy; like Tao-Yin, Shiatsu incorporates passive BMTs and stretches and, to some extent, coordinates breathing and movement through the application of pressure; like acupuncture, Shiatsu stimulates the body's vital energy by manipulating acupoints; some practitioners also incorporate moxabustion and herbalism into their practice, though these are considered supplementary.
8. Tui Na and An Mo are Chinese forms of massage therapy. The literal translations are "push grab" for Tui Na and "press rub" for An Mo.
9. Martial artists practice Tui Na to rehabilitate themselves after incurring injuries during practice.
10. Medical doctors practice Tui Na to heal patients.
11. Dian Xue is "cavity press" massage, the precursor to modern acupressure.
12. Martial artists strike acupressure points to disable, incapacitate, or kill.
13. The amount of force applied to a pressure point determines whether it is beneficial or harmful.
14. There is no manual contact or manipulation in Qi massage, just the transmission of energy.
15. TCM was introduced to Japan in the late sixth or early seventh century A.D., a time when China and Japan exchanged diplomatic and trading missions.
16. In seventeenth-century Japan, the study of Amma (massage) and Do-In (breathing and movement exercises) was a prerequisite to the study of medicine.
17. The Shogun used his authority to express his gratitude for being healed by a blind acupuncturist. Some sources also suggest that blind practitioners of bodywork were preferred because they ostensibly have an acute sense of touch, which is naturally suited to massage, and their blindness ensures the client's privacy.
18. In the zeal to adopt Western medicine, the Japanese aristocracy of the nineteenth century banned traditional medicine, and Amma lost its medical stature. By the early twentieth century, Amma had declined to a form of pleasure associated with bath services.
19. Ampuku is a Japanese form of abdominal massage. It is used to diagnose internal organ maladies and has special application to obstetric/gynecological concerns.
20. Amma was renamed Shiatsu to reestablish the credibility of the profession by disassociating it from mere relaxation or pleasure massage and also to evade the restrictive governmental regulations imposed on pleasure massage.

21. In Japan, Shiatsu is considered a form of medicine, used to diagnose and treat diseases (this is not so in the West).
22. Tempaku is regarded as the founder of Shiatsu and was the first person to integrate Asian healing arts with Western anatomy and physiology.
23. Namikoshi's main contribution was gaining official recognition of Shiatsu as a medical modality.
24. Namikoshi eliminated all references to TCM and based Shiatsu on Western anatomy and physiology, much like Trigger Point Therapy or forms of neuromuscular therapy.
25. Masunaga's main contribution was reconnecting Shiatsu to its ancient Chinese heritage, which views health as dependent on the free flow of Qi through Meridians and illness as the result of energetic imbalances and which emphasizes psychological factors in diagnosis and treatment. Some also regard his extension of the classical Meridian system as a major contribution.
26. Masunaga's style is distinguished by the addition of industrial-strength body tools (knuckles, elbows, and knees) to apply pressure, tonification and sedation techniques, the Mother/Son hand technique, and the energetic connection between client and practitioner.
27. Serizawa's main contribution was his scientific research verifying the location and electrical properties of acupressure points.
28. Acupressure is based on Serizawa's Tsubo Therapy.
29. Acupressure stimulates isolated points or combinations of points to treat particular disorders, whereas Shiatsu is a whole-body therapy that stimulates entire sequences of points (Meridians).
30. In general, Qi Gong includes any discipline that cultivates the flow of vital energy. Specifically, Qi Gong may refer to a particular type of movement and breathing exercise regimen.
31. A massage practitioner should practice some form of Qi Gong regularly to increase cardiovascular fitness, muscular strength and flexibility, mental focus, and healing power. Qi Gong reduces the likelihood of illness and the risk of injury and enhances performance.

CHAPTER 2 QI AND MERIDIANS

1. Shiatsu is based on TCM.
2. The concept of vital energy informs TCM; vital energy can manifest as substance (matter) or activity (energy).
3. Ki is the Japanese word for vital energy.
4. Chi or Qi is the Chinese word for vital energy.
5. Qi/Ki can manifest as matter.
6. No; Qi has no beginning or end.
7. In humans, Qi manifests as flesh (cells, tissues, and organs), physiological and psychological functions, and physical activities.
8. When the smooth flow of energy is disrupted, dis-ease or disease ensues.
9. Yes; the body responds to electromagnetic therapy because it is itself electromagnetic in nature.
10. Yes; the practitioner's body is an electromagnetic instrument that transmits electromagnetic energy and facilitates the client's own healing power.

11. The ancient Chinese ideogram for energy means "no fire"; it indicates a state of balance or optimal health where there is neither excess (fire) nor deficiency.
12. The modern Chinese ideogram for energy means "space rice," referring to the two postnatal sources of energy in the body: air and food.
13. The three primary sources of Qi in humans are one's parents (prenatal ancestral inheritance), air (postnatal), and food (postnatal).
14. The five basic functions of Qi in humans are movement (voluntary and involuntary), protection (defense against External Pernicious Influences), transformation (the conversion of air and food into bodily substances and activities), stabilization or retention (the preservation of structural integrity), and warmth (the regulation of body temperature).
15. The four disharmonies of Qi are deficient Qi (insufficient energy to make tissues and fluids or to propel organ functions), sinking or collapsed Qi (insufficient energy to support and uphold structures or retain substances), stagnant or excessive Qi (congested or blocked energy), and rebellious Qi (energy that moves in the wrong direction, usually a reversal of the normal energy flow).
16. Diarrhea, hernia, hemorrhoids, hemorrhaging, varicose veins, and organ prolapse are examples of sinking Qi.
17. Nausea, belching, hiccupping, acid reflux, and regurgitation are examples of rebellious Stomach Qi; coughing and sneezing are examples of rebellious Lung Qi.
18. Jing is essence; Jing is roughly equivalent to one's inherited constitution.
19. Jing determines the quality and rate of development and aging, procreative ability, and physical robustness.
20. Jing dysfunctions include developmental disorders, constitutional infirmities, sexual dysfunctions and procreative disorders, and premature aging.
21. An abusive lifestyle exhausts Jing, while a healthy lifestyle conserves it.
22. The literal translation for Shen is "spirit" or "mind"; Shen refers to the human psyche.
23. Shen encompasses consciousness, psychological characteristics, and social tendencies.
24. Mental and emotional states affect physical health, and vice versa.
25. Meridians are invisible channels, pathways, or routes of Qi flow. Collectively, they form an energy network or system that transmits energy to all parts of the body.
26. No; Meridians do not correspond to a physical structure in the body.
27. Slow, weak, or blocked Qi flow can lead to slow, weak, or blocked blood flow and nerve conduction, and vice versa.
28. Meridians do not exist in a corpse because moving, flowing Qi is an aspect and sign of life, just as circulating blood is a sign of life.
29. There are 12 main Meridians and 2 extra Meridians.
30. Except for the Conception and Governing Vessels, which run along the midline of the torso, the 12 main Meridians are structured in bilateral pairs that are mirror images of one another.
31. In addition to particular organs, organ systems, or functions, Meridians are also associated with psychological capacities.
32. In general, the posterior and lateral aspects of the body (back and outer sides) correspond to Yang Meridians.

33. Yang Meridians flow from superior to inferior (from the head down to the feet) and from lateral to medial (from the fingertips in toward the midline).
34. In general, the anterior and medial aspects of the body (front and inside) correspond to Yin Meridians.
35. Yin Meridians flow from inferior to superior (from the feet up to the head) and from medial to lateral (from the torso out toward the fingertips).
36. When Qi reaches the end of one Meridian, it flows into the next (its Meridian pair) in one continuous circuit during a 24-hour period.
37. Qi flow peaks for 2 hours in each Meridian.
38. Symptoms of distress, illness, or irregularity that occur at approximately the same time every day indicate an energetic imbalance in the corresponding Meridian.
39. A pattern of disharmony in a Meridian should be treated with Shiatsu.
40. The Conception Vessel influences all Yin Meridians; it acts as an energy reservoir that drains off excess Qi, supplies Qi where there is deficiency, and holds in Qi reserve; it is associated with reproduction.
41. The Governing Vessel influences all Yang Meridians; it acts as an energy reservoir that drains off excess Qi, supplies Qi where there is deficiency, and holds Qi in reserve; it is associated with the brain and spinal cord.

CHAPTER 3 YIN YANG

1. The Yin Yang paradigm is derived from Taoism. *Note*: It is inadequate to say that Yin Yang is based on Chinese philosophy, since Chinese philosophy could refer to Taoism, Buddhism, or Confucianism.
2. The dark half represents Yin, and the light half represents Yang.
3. The dark dot represents the seed of Yin within Yang and the potential of Yang to turn into Yin. The light dot represents the seed of Yang within Yin and the potential of Yin to turn into Yang.
4. The curved line dividing the two halves represents change and indicates that Yin and Yang are not constant entities or static qualities but rather are in dynamic flux.
5. The Chinese ideogram for Yin means the shady slope of the hill; it represents quiescence. The ideogram for Yang means the sunny slope of the hill; it represents activity.
6. The temporal correspondences for Yin are night and winter; the spatial correspondences for Yin are inside and earthward.
7. The temporal correspondences for Yang are day and summer; the spatial correspondences for Yang are outside and heavenward.
8. Yin forms are soft and concave; Yin substances are solid.
9. Yang forms are hard and convex; Yang substances are immaterial.
10. Yin movement is contracting, centripetal, descending, and heavy.
11. Yang movement is expanding, centrifugal, ascending, and light.
12. The Yin zones of the body are anterior (front), interior, and inferior (bottom).
13. The Yang zones of the body are posterior (back), exterior, and superior (top).
14. Yin symptoms of illness are pale, cold, weak, tired, and chronic.
15. Yang symptoms of illness are red, hot, strong, agitated, and acute.

16. Western thought tends to be individualistic and compartmentalized in perspective; Chinese thought tends to be relational and holistic or global in perspective.
17. Newton's third law of motion ("To every action, there is an equal and opposite reaction") emphasizes the synchronous nature of opposing forces. Opposing forces that arise together exactly describes Yin Yang dynamics.
18. Yes; everything contains both Yin and Yang.
19. The human personality contains Yin qualities like the desire for solitude and contemplation and Yang qualities like the desire to socialize and do something.
20. Nothing is exclusively or absolutely Yin or Yang.
21. Tepid (warm) water is Yang compared to cool water, but it is Yin compared to hot water.
22. Yin and Yang are relative rather than absolute entities; whether something is Yin or Yang can be determined only by comparing it to other things in a larger context.
23. The ocean floor is generally considered Yin (Cold and Damp), but where molten magma erupts from rifts in the earth's crust, the ocean floor is Yang (Hot), with temperatures far exceeding the boiling point.
24. Yin and Yang keep each other in check (they control or limit one another).
25. A balance of Yin and Yang in the body corresponds to good health.
26. An imbalance of Yin and Yang in the body corresponds to illness.
27. When Yin has reached its maximum fullness or is too dominant, Yin turns into Yang; likewise, when Yang has reached its maximum fullness or is too dominant, Yang turns into Yin.
28. No; a change from Yin to Yang is not necessarily a sign of disorder; it could be a natural change, as in a rotational cycle of reversals.
29. Mundane examples of transformation are the desire to move after sitting a long while and the desire to sit after moving a long while.

CHAPTER 4 THE FIVE ELEMENTS

1. The Five Elements are not fixed entities or stable constituents of matter; rather, they represent the quality of energy embodied by a particular form.
2. A more accurate translation is five Processes, Stages, Phases, Transitions, Transformations, or Metamorphoses.
3. The Five Elements are emblems for Qi in different conditions or states of existence.
4. The Water element is greater Yin (utmost Yin); its energy has stored potential; it is associated with winter, old age, and the Kidney and Bladder Meridians.
5. The Wood element is lesser Yang (increasing, growing Yang); its energy expands upward and outward; it is associated with spring, childhood, and the Liver and Gallbladder Meridians.
6. The Fire element is greater Yang (utmost Yang); its energy peaks; it is associated with summer, adolescence, the Heart and Small Intestine Meridians (primary pair), and the Pericardium and Triple Heater Meridians (secondary pair).
7. The Earth element is between Yin and Yang; its energy is centered, balanced, and poised; it is associated with Indian summer or the end of each season, adulthood, and the Spleen and Stomach Meridians.
8. The Metal element is lesser Yin (increasing, growing Yin); its energy contracts downward and inward; it is associated with autumn, middle age, and the Lung and Large Intestine Meridians.

9. Shen refers to the Creative Cycle.
10. Wood fuels Fire; Fire's ashes furnish Earth; Earth condenses and consolidates into Metal; Metal melts into or condenses Water; Water irrigates Wood.
11. No; each stage is not equal in duration.
12. The Mother is the element that nourishes or produces the Child element.
13. "Problem child, problem parent" refers to the relational nature of imbalances or dysfunctions. If an element is deficient, most likely the Mother is deficient, too, and has transmitted her deficiency to the Child. Conversely, if an element is excessive, most likely the Mother is excessive, too, and has transferred her excess to the Child.
14. Treat the element and its Mother.
15. If an element is deficient, tonify (nourish) the Child and its Mother (if indicated).
16. If an element is excessive, sedate (calm) the Child and its Mother (if indicated).
17. Ko refers to the Control Cycle.
18. Ko is necessary to limit the generative power of the Shen Cycle; otherwise, there will be unbridled production.
19. Wood penetrates, pries apart, or holds together Earth; Earth channels, blocks, or dams Water; Water extinguishes Fire; Fire melts Metal; Metal chops or cuts Wood.
20. Insult occurs when an overregulated element rebels and "insults" its controller, disabling the controller.
21. Sedate (calm) the rebellious element, and tonify (nourish) the controller.
22. Humiliation occurs when an overregulated element is "humiliated" or disabled by its controller.
23. Sedate (calm) the controlling element, and tonify (nourish) the controlled element.
24. The Cosmological sequence emphasizes the importance of the Water element to our physical well-being through prenatal Qi (because the Water element is our ancestral inheritance), the importance of the Earth element to our physical well-being through postnatal Qi (because the Earth is associated with food), and the importance of the Fire element to our psychological well-being (because the Fire element is associated with the Heart, which houses Shen).
25. An individual response is required.
26. Knowledge of the element types gives the practitioner convenient assessment profiles; each element type tends to manifest certain physical and psychological imbalances that can be treated through the associated Meridians.
27. Irritability; anger.
28. Joy; agitation.
29. Overthinking; worry.
30. Sadness; grief.
31. Angst; fear.
32. Knowledge of the element correspondences gives the practitioner convenient assessment patterns. Each element has characteristic qualities such as skin hue, tone of voice, preferred flavor, preferred climate, issues with an associated sense organ and tissue, and a habitual emotional or mental state. A constellation of qualities belonging to a certain element suggests Shiatsu on the associated Meridians.

33. Yin Yang theory was developed first.
34. Five Element theory and Yin Yang theory were both developed by the naturalist school and view the body as a landscape. Both theories are premised on the concept of Qi.
35. No; Five Element theory does not always yield the same diagnostic results as Yin Yang theory.
36. Five Element theory tends to be very formulaic in its approach to assessment. While this may be convenient and expedient, it is not as accurate or precise as Yin Yang theory.

CHAPTER 5 THE ZANG FU ORGAN SYSTEM

1. Zang organs are Yin organs.
2. Zang organs are solid (except for the Heart); they produce, store, and distribute the body's vital substances.
3. Fu organs are Yang organs.
4. Fu organs are hollow; they digest and assimilate nutrients and eliminate wastes.
5. All organs and their Meridians are important to the Shiatsu practitioner, since their functions affect the body-mind.
6. Bone is the tissue associated with the Water element. Bone includes teeth, considered an outgrowth of bone, as well as the TCM concept of Marrow, which consists of the brain, spinal cord, and nerves.
7. The Water element influences the autonomic nervous system in several ways. First, the associated tissue, Marrow, includes the brain, spinal cord, and nerves, which are all involved in our relative state of excitation or calm; second, the energy flow in the Bladder Meridian, which runs parallel to the spine, affects the spinal cord; third, the Kidney organ complex includes the adrenal glands, which release the stress hormone adrenaline.
8. Physiological effects of the sympathetic mode include increased heartbeat and respiration, increased blood flow to the skeletal muscles, and decreased digestive and reproductive functions.
9. Psychological characteristics of the sympathetic mode include a heightened awareness or perception of environmental threats, motivation, ambition, and drivenness.
10. Physiological effects of the parasympathetic mode include decreased heartbeat and respiration, decreased blood flow to the skeletal muscles, and increased digestive and reproductive functions.
11. Psychological characteristics of the parasympathetic mode include a dulled awareness or perception, lack of motivation, lack of ambition, and inertia.
12. The Water element is considered the foundation of the other elements because it is the basis of Yin and Yang in the body. The Kidneys house Jing, which creates and sustains the Yin form of the body, and they house Ming-Men, which provides the impetus for the Yang activities of the body.
13. Ming-Men, also known as Life Gate Fire, Gate of Vitality, Original Qi, and Source Qi, is the root of Yang, or energy, in the body and the source of Fire, or heat, in the body.
14. Ming-Men provides the impetus for all physiological processes and transformations—all active, dynamic, heating, and converting functions in

the body. It has been compared to a pilot light that ignites the fire of the other organs in the body.

15. Jing, translated as Essence, is the root of Yin, or form and substance, in the body and the source of Water in the body.
16. Jing is roughly equivalent to our inherited constitution: It governs the development and decline of our physical form over time, our basic vitality, and our ability to procreate.
17. Although other organs are involved in processing Water, the Kidneys "rule" or control Water—that is, all bodily fluids, including sweat and urine. This is because Kidney Jing is the basis for all fluids and bodily substances and for all supportive, nourishing, and moistening functions. Additionally, Kidney Fire regulates Water.
18. Kidney Ming-Men is the source of the body's Fire, or Yang energy and animating power. Ming-Men is the starter for all physiological processes and transformations—in short, all active, dynamic, heating, and converting functions. Ming-Men empowers all organ functions via the Triple Heater, which transmits Ming-Men to each organ, igniting its activity. A byproduct of organ activity is Heat.
19. Kidney dysfunctions usually entail a disproportion of Fire to Water.
20. The main signs of Kidney Fire deficiency are Water and Cold symptoms. When Kidney Fire is deficient, Kidney Water overflows, and Water and Cold symptoms arise not only in the Kidneys, but also in other organs, especially the Spleen.
21. Disorders due to Kidney Fire deficiency include frequent, pale, copious urine; nighttime urination; urinary incontinence; genital discharges; low sex drive; lower body edema; cold back and knees; and apathy.
22. The Spleen may be adversely affected by a deficiency of Kidney Fire; symptoms include poor appetite, loose stools or diarrhea, and listlessness.
23. The main sign of Kidney Water deficiency is Heat. When Kidney Water is deficient, Kidney Fire burns, and Heat symptoms arise not only in the Kidneys, but also in other organs, especially the Heart and Liver.
24. Disorders due to Kidney Water deficiency include thirst; abnormal body heat; dark, scanty urine; dry stools or constipation; dizziness; vertigo; amnesia; tinnitus; deafness; sore lower back; and achy bones.
25. The Liver and Heart may be adversely affected by a deficiency of Kidney Water. Liver symptoms include headaches, inflamed eyes, and visual impairment. Heart symptoms include mental restlessness, insomnia, and palpitations.
26. The ears are the sense organ associated with the Water element.
27. In disharmony, hearing disorders such as tinnitus, tone deafness, and deafness can arise.
28. The psychological capacity of the Water element is will; the Yang aspect is volition, motivation, and drive, and the Yin aspect is yielding.
29. Fear and fearlessness are the emotions associated with Water. An emotional imbalance exists when a person has no reason to fear but does (insecurities and phobias) or has reason to fear but doesn't.
30. Creativity, direction, purpose, planning, control, and industriousness are all psychological qualities associated with the Wood element.
31. Anger is the main emotion associated with Wood. Variations on anger include impatience, frustration, irritability, resentment, rigidity, recklessness, hostility, fury, and rage.

32. Headaches, inflamed eyes, and hypertension are examples of disorders due to Liver Yang rising.
33. Deficient Wood energy manifests as lack of creativity, lack of direction and purpose, irresoluteness, and timidity.
34. The Liver's main physiological functions are the detoxification and distribution of blood and the distribution of free-flowing Qi.
35. Disturbances in Liver function may manifest in excess patterns, such as stagnant Qi (characterized by distention, migrating pain, and transient abdominal masses) or congealed blood (characterized by fixed, stabbing or boring pain, permanent abdominal masses, and purple discoloration of various tissues). PMS is an example of stagnant Qi due to Liver excess, and dysmenorrhea (painful period) is an example of congealed blood due to Liver excess. Additionally, Liver dysfunction can manifest as deficiency conditions, such as Liver blood deficiency. Amenorrhea (no periods) and oligomenorrhea (infrequent periods with scanty blood flow) are examples.
36. A disharmony in the Wood element can disrupt Earth element functions. Various digestive problems arise, according to the pattern of Liver invading Spleen (poor appetite, abdominal distention and pain, intestinal rumblings, flatulence, alternating diarrhea and constipation, and tiredness) or Liver invading Stomach (abdominal distention and pain, nausea, belching, acid reflux, and vomiting).
37. The Gallbladder's main function is to produce bile, a bitter yellow fluid that digests fats.
38. The nails and sinews are the tissues associated with Wood.
39. Deficient Liver blood can make the nails pale, thin, brittle, and indented, and stagnant Liver Qi can make the sinews stiff and rigid or cause painful obstruction syndrome.
40. The eyes are the sense organ associated with Wood.
41. Liver disharmonies can cause inflammatory eye disorders and visual impairment.
42. The Fire element is the only element that has two pairs of Meridians—a primary pair (Heart and Small Intestine) and a secondary pair (Pericardium and Triple Heater). Additionally, two Meridians do not correspond to actual organs. The Pericardium is a protective sheath that encloses the Heart, and the Triple Heater refers to a complex or system of organs.
43. The Heart influences the psychosocial aspect of one's being.
44. Joy is the main emotion of Fire.
45. In excess, the disposition of Fire is overstimulated, hyperactive, agitated, and manic.
46. In deficiency, the disposition of Fire is apathetic, impassive, or emotionally vapid.
47. The main physiological function of the Heart is the circulation of blood.
48. The associated tissue of Fire is the blood vessels, which are considered an extension of the Heart.
49. Heart disorders are cardiovascular in nature; examples include hypertension, arteriosclerosis, aneurysm, varicose veins, phlebitis, thrombosis, heart attack, and stroke.
50. The Heart enshrines Shen, variously translated as consciousness, awareness, mind, and spirit.
51. Shen governs psychosocial aspects of being, memory, and sleep.

52. Signs of a disturbed Shen include frenzied thoughts, agitation, nervous excitability, hysteria, shock, delirium, unconsciousness, inappropriate or exaggerated emotional responses, maladjusted social interactions, amnesia, disrupted sleep, and troubling dreams.
53. The Heart influences psychosocial dynamics, including the appropriateness of behavior in terms of time, place, and manner. When Shen is disturbed, a person will say or do something at the wrong time, in the wrong place, or in the wrong manner, making the person's behavior socially maladaptive, awkward, eccentric, or offensive.
54. The sense organ associated with the Heart is the tongue.
55. Pathological conditions of the tongue include speech impediments, stuttering, stammering, and muteness.
56. The abilities to communicate well, to connect with others, to articulate meaning, and to respond appropriately are qualities associated with a healthy Fire element. Often Fire element types talk speedily and at length.
57. The Small Intestine's main physiological function is to "separate the pure from the impure"—that is, to absorb nutrients and water and to pass wastes on to the organs of elimination.
58. The Spleen is often implicated in Small Intestine disorders, since the Spleen directs the Small Intestine's functions.
59. The Small Intestine's main psychological function is to "separate the pure from the impure"—that is, to accept what is healthy for the psyche and to reject what is harmful.
60. Other names for the Pericardium are Heart Constrictor, Heart Master, and Heart Governor.
61. The Pericardium assists, shares, and reinforces Heart functions in several ways. As a connective tissue sheath enclosing the Heart, the Pericardium assists the Heart in pumping blood (hence, the name Heart Constrictor) and defends the Heart against invasion by External Pernicious Influences (Heart Protector). It also acts on behalf of the Heart and supplements its functions (Heart Master/Heart Governor).
62. Like the Heart, the Pericardium influences the quality of social interactions and relationship dynamics.
63. Psychological imbalances of the Pericardium manifest as social defensiveness or social insecurity (shyness, social vulnerability).
64. The Triple Heater shares influence over social interactions and relationship dynamics with the Pericardium.
65. Other names for the Triple Heater are Triple Warmer, Triple Burner, and Sanjaio.
66. The *Nei Jing* likens the Upper Burner to a mist, with the Lungs dispersing Water throughout the body to moisten its tissues; the Middle Burner to a foam or bubbling cauldron, with the Spleen and Stomach churning food in digestion; and the Lower Burner to a swamp or drainage ditch that dredges bodily sewage for evacuation via the Large Intestine and Bladder.
67. The zone of the Upper Burner extends from the chest to the diaphragm, encompassing the Heart and Lungs; the zone of the Middle Burner extends from the diaphragm to the navel, encompassing the digestive organs; and the Lower Burner extends from the navel to the pubis, encompassing the organs of elimination.
68. The Triple Heater's main physiological functions are regulating body temperature, transmitting vital energy from the Kidneys to the other organs, and defending against External Pernicious Influences.

69. Triple Heater disorders include thermal disorders (especially lack of warmth), poor resistance to infections, poor immunity against External Pernicious Influences, and allergies.
70. The psychological capacity of the Earth element is cognition, analytical reasoning, rumination, and reflective thought.
71. An imbalance in Earth distorts this psychological capacity, turning cognition into mulling, brooding, worrying, obsession, and the paralysis of analysis, what the Chinese refer to as overthinking.
72. Other psychological disharmonies associated with Earth include confused, irrational thinking; boredom; disinterest; mental lethargy; and mental apathy.
73. The psychological capacity of Earth is the ability to give and receive in mutually supportive relationships.
74. When the Earth capacity for giving and receiving is imbalanced, dysfunctional, co-dependent relationships arise.
75. The giving Earth element type is a caretaker in both private and public life. This type feels secure and affirmed in giving but has difficulty receiving.
76. The receiving Earth element type enjoys being taken care of and gravitates toward a dependent role.
77. The Earth element produces Post-Heaven/Postnatal Qi.
78. The Stomach's main physiological function is "rotting and ripening" food—that is, decomposing and fermenting it for further processing by the Spleen.
79. Rebellious Stomach Qi is a reversal of the normal descending direction that manifests as nausea, hiccups, belching, acid reflux, and vomiting.
80. According to TCM, the Spleen is the primary digestive organ, and the Stomach is the secondary digestive organ, preparing food for the Spleen.
81. The Spleen's main physiological function is "transformation and transportation"—that is, converting Grain Qi into a substance compatible with and usable by the body.
82. Spleen Qi normally flows upward, sending processed Grain Qi upward for integration with Air Qi of the Lungs. Because of this lifting movement, Spleen Qi also plays a role in retention, stabilization, and structural integrity (upholding body parts in their proper place).
83. Examples of sinking Spleen Qi (a reversal of Spleen Qi flow) include diarrhea, hernia, hemorrhoids, and organ prolapse.
84. In conjunction with the Lungs, the Spleen is credited with producing Postnatal Qi, which makes the flesh of the body and provides energy for the body.
85. Examples of Spleen disorders include deficient blood (anemia); deficient Qi (low energy, lethargy, and fatigue); and malnourished, emaciated, or wasted flesh.
86. The flesh, especially muscle tissue, is associated with the Earth element. Good muscle tone and abundant physical energy indicate a healthy Spleen, whereas flaccid or atrophied muscles, weakness, enervation, or exhaustion indicate a deficient Spleen.
87. In TCM, Phlegm is a type of Dampness that manifests in both tangible and intangible forms. The tangible forms of Phlegm include lumpy masses like lipomas, cysts, and tumors, and the intangible forms of Phlegm include numbness or paralysis along a Meridian.
88. Reckless blood is a disorder in which blood is not properly contained in vessels; examples include varicose veins, hemorrhoids, and hemorrhaging (nosebleeds; blood in stools, sputum, or urine).

89. Many Earth element disorders center on the theme of eating, including appetite disorders, digestive disorders, sweet cravings, sugar addiction, and weight disorders (anorexia nervosa, bulimia, and overindulgence in food).
90. The Earth element is associated with female reproductive functions such as the menstrual cycle and female reproductive organs such as the uterus and breasts.
91. The Metal element is associated with a sense of self because its organs and tissues constitute the boundaries of our discrete physical being: The skin is our border; the nose and Lungs are an entry into the body; and the Large Intestine is an exit from the body.
92. The Lungs engage in exchange by inhaling Air Qi and exhaling carbon dioxide.
93. The Lungs are called the "tender organ" because they interface directly with the environment and are particularly susceptible to invasion by External Pernicious Influences.
94. Examples of Lung disorders include colds and flus.
95. The nose is the sense organ associated with the Metal element.
96. The Lungs affect the energy level of the body by virtue of their role in producing Postnatal Qi through the intake of Air Qi.
97. Lung Qi normally flows downward, dispersing Qi throughout the body.
98. Sneezing and coughing indicate a reversal of Lung Qi flow.
99. The Lungs moisten the periphery: the skin.
100. Examples of Lung disorders that adversely affect water metabolism are irregular sweating patterns and edema in the upper body.
101. The Spleen can cause edema in the lower half of the body, while the Lungs can cause edema in the upper half.
102. The skin and its accessories—sebaceous (oil) glands, and suderiforous (sweat) glands, and body hair—are the tissues associated with the Metal element.
103. The skin engages in exchange by absorbing emollient nutrients and air, dissipating Heat, and excreting pus.
104. The Large Intestine engages in exchange by absorbing water and expelling feces.
105. As the main organ of digestion, the Spleen is implicated in Large Intestine disorders, and the Small Intestine may also be involved.
106. The psychological associations of Metal are self-esteem (a sense of individual value), accepting and taking in, and rejecting and letting go.
107. A Metal element type might suffer from a lack of self-worth or an inability to receive something of value or to discard something of little or no value.
108. A Metal element imbalance could render a person disinclined to pursue a worthy relationship or career or to relinquish an unworthy relationship or career.
109. Sadness and grief are the emotions associated with Metal. Although sadness and grief are natural responses to loss, disproportionate or prolonged sadness and grief indicate a Metal element disharmony; so, too, does the inability to grieve when appropriate.
110. A negative outlook is associated with a Metal element imbalance; this could manifest as depression, pessimism, or cynicism.
111. Although Metal element types tend to be private, solitary types, a Metal element disharmony could render a person isolated, alienated, and estranged to an extreme degree.

CHAPTER 6 THE EIGHT PRINCIPLE PATTERNS AND KYO JITSU

1. The four classical examinations of TCM are looking, listening and smelling, asking, and touching.
2. Oriental medical doctors and acupuncturists primarily rely on tongue (looking) and pulse (touching) diagnosis, whereas Shiatsu practitioners primarily rely on observation of the body (looking, listening, and smelling) and palpation (touching).
3. Interior/Exterior refers to the location of the disorder, whether affecting the inner organs or the external tissues.
4. An internal disorder is chronic in nature, slow to develop, and difficult to resolve.
5. Internal disorders are usually caused by constitutional infirmities or prolonged emotional disturbances.
6. An external disorder is acute in nature, abrupt in onset, severe in symptom, and brief in duration.
7. External disorders are usually caused by External Pernicious Influences (climatic factors), pathogenic agents, or mechanical injuries; they correspond to Western infectious illnesses and trauma.
8. External disorders can be treated with dispersal techniques, which help the body expel invading pathogens and which stimulate blood, lymph, and Qi flow where they have become stagnant.
9. Deficiency/Excess refers to the quantity of Qi, blood, or other bodily substance (whether too little or too much) and the quality of organ function (whether sluggish or hyperactive).
10. Physical symptoms of a Deficiency disorder are a low supply of bodily substances and substandard organ function, as well as a pale complexion, a faint voice, feeble movement, and lethargy or exhaustion.
11. Psychological characteristics of a Deficiency disorder are emotional listlessness and apathy.
12. Physical symptoms of an Excess disorder are a superabundance of bodily substances and supercharged organ function, as well as a red complexion, a loud voice, forceful movement, and agitation.
13. Psychological characteristics of an Excess disorder are emotional tension and intensity.
14. Rigorous exercise or manual labor, habitually unhealthy postural and movement patterns, a sedentary lifestyle, and poor stress-management skills can all contribute to Excess disorders.
15. Painful obstruction syndrome is a type of Excess disorder caused by a block that retards or disrupts Qi flow, which leads to the accumulation and stagnation of Qi and the hyperirritability of the tissues involved.
16. Dispersal techniques clear stagnation.
17. Cold/Heat refers to temperature imbalances.
18. Cold symptoms include a white complexion, dislike of cold, a chilly feeling in the body or body parts, relief with heat, slow movement, and a reserved, inwardly drawn temperament.
19. Cold conditions can be caused by invasion of Cold, excess Yin, or deficient Yang.

20. Heat symptoms include a red complexion, dislike of heat, a hot feeling in the body or body parts, relief with cold, fast or frenzied movement, and an outward-bound temperament.
21. Heat conditions can be caused by invasion of Heat, excess Yang, or deficient Yin.
22. True Cold is too much Yin (Cold), while the appearance of Cold is not enough Yang (Heat).
23. True Fire is too much Yang (Heat), while the appearance of Fire is not enough Yin (Cold).
24. Most clients present mixed symptoms.
25. Jitsu means "full".
26. Kyo means "empty".
27. Kyo corresponds to a state of hunger or condition of need.
28. Jitsu corresponds to energy expenditure—a compensatory drive to satisfy a need.
29. Kyo arises first.
30. Kyo is the cause of the energy imbalance.
31. Once Kyo is resolved, Jitsu naturally dissipates.
32. A Kyo Jitsu energy imbalance could reflect a normal fluctuation in energy level due to biological cycles.
33. A Kyo Jitsu energy imbalance could reflect a mood.
34. A prolonged Kyo Jitsu imbalance could lead to disease.
35. Jitsu most often arises because of an underlying Kyo condition (unmet need), but it can arise from an obstruction or blockage that leads to the congestion and stagnation of Qi.
36. Kyo most often arises because of an unmet need, but it can arise from a hereditary infirmity, trauma, or prolonged illness that depletes Qi.
37. Jitsu manifests as convex protrusions.
38. Kyo manifests as concave depressions.
39. Symptoms of Jitsu include hyperactivity, excitability, heat, sharp pain, and hard distended surfaces.
40. Symptoms of Kyo include hypoactivity, inertia, cold, dull pain, and soft, flabby or hollow surfaces.
41. Jitsu hardness is reactive; it has a springy, trampoline quality; it yields to pressure and bounces back. Kyo hardness is unresponsive; it has a stiff, rigid, wooden quality; it resists pressure.
42. Pressure on Jitsu feels painful to the client and may elicit a negative reaction ("Ouch" or "That hurts").
43. Pressure on Kyo is a welcome relief to the client and may elicit a positive reaction ("Ohhh" or "That feels good").
44. Jitsu is easier to detect.
45. Jitsu is easier to detect because it is physically conspicuous.
46. Focus on Kyo.
47. By satisfying Kyo, Jitsu compensatory activity becomes unnecessary and disappears of its own accord.
48. When the client's lifestyle is causing a perpetual Kyo Jitsu imbalance, the most one can expect is temporary relief for a condition that will return or damage control (rather than abatement).

49. Begin a session by sedating Jitsu when the client is a Jitsu type (energetic, strong, productive or hyperactive, wired, or high-strung), has specifically requested relief for a Jitsu condition (tension), or is new and the practitioner is uncertain how to begin (Jitsu is easier to detect and treat than Kyo).
50. Begin a session by tonifying Kyo when the client is a Kyo type (sluggish, weak, underactive, low-key), has specifically requested relief for a Kyo condition (tired, depleted, exhausted), or is a return client whose Kyo energy pattern is familiar to the practitioner.
51. A client's facial expression and voice, body type (physique or figure), movement style, and temperament are all assessed.
52. A Kyo client may have pale skin; a skinny or flabby body; a soft voice or few words; hesitant, sluggish, or weak movements; and a retiring or bland personality.
53. A Jitsu client may have red skin; a fat or muscular body; a loud voice or many words; decisive, vigorous, or bold movements; and a forward or sharp personality.
54. Kyo clients prefer gentle therapy.
55. Jitsu clients prefer vigorous therapy.
56. The Yin Yang principle of transformation explains these client preferences. Applying gentle techniques to a Kyo client is like adding Yin to Yin, which transforms into Yang (energizes the client). Applying vigorous techniques to a Jitsu client is like adding Yang to Yang, which transforms into Yin (relaxes the client).
57. Tonify the weak side or half of the body (especially the most Kyo Meridian) and sedate the strong side or half of the body (especially the most Jitsu Meridian).
58. The Stomach and Spleen Meridians are implicated in pear-shaped, bottom-heavy body types.
59. The Gallbladder and Liver Meridians are implicated in right/left discrepancies.
60. Place the limbs in Meridian stretch positions and feel the quality of the tissues.
61. A Meridian is predominantly, but not exclusively, Kyo or Jitsu.
62. A Jitsu Meridian feels firm yet buoyant in the stretch position.
63. A Kyo Meridian feels flaccid or inflexibly hard and inert in the stretch position.
64. Light fingertip pressure is used for hara diagnosis.
65. A Jitsu area on the hara feels obvious in some way—in its form (bulging), movement (active), or reaction (shift or pain).
66. A Kyo area on the hara feels hollow, empty, static (resists change), or stiff.
67. Find the most Jitsu area first and then feel for a connection: The Jitsu area might sink or shrink while the Kyo area rises or expands; an electrical pulse might be transmitted from one hand to the other; a sense of a closed circuit might arise, or the practitioner might intuit that the two areas are energetically related.
68. Firm pressure is used in back diagnosis.
69. Tenderness or sharp pain in a Shu/Yu point on the inner Bladder Meridian indicates a Qi imbalance that manifests physically in the corresponding organ or organ system.

70. Tenderness or sharp pain in a Shu/Yu point on the outer Bladder Meridian corresponds to a Qi imbalance that manifests psychologically in the corresponding mental/emotional capacity.
71. Hara diagnosis tends to reflect short-term imbalances, while back diagnosis reflects long-term imbalances.
72. To tonify Kyo, apply pressure gradually at a light to medium depth and sustain for a long period of time to attract Qi to the area to warm it.
73. The Mother/Son hand technique is the standard method for tonifying Kyo.
74. Traction and Meridian stretch positions are gentle enough to be tonifying.
75. To disperse Jitsu, apply pressure smoothly but relatively quickly at a medium to deep depth and combine with movement to disperse stagnant or blocked Qi.
76. Kenbiki means "pushing and pulling." It is a stimulating technique used to disperse Jitsu. Examples include cross-fiber friction, torsion wringing, and compression plus rocking.
77. Jostling, vibrating, and pummeling are also Jitsu dispersal techniques.
78. BMTs that move a limb through a full range of motion and facilitated stretches that move a limb to its outer limit are stimulating.
79. Move from superior to inferior (top to bottom) and from proximal to distal (core to extremities) to disperse Jitsu; or move against the current of the Meridian, from the last or highest-numbered point to the first or lowest-numbered point.
80. Move from inferior to superior (bottom to top) and from distal to proximal (extremities to core) to tonify Kyo; or move with the current of the Meridian, from the first point to the last point.
81. Circle counterclockwise from the practitioner's perspective to release Jitsu.
82. Circle clockwise from the practitioner's perspective to draw in energy toward Kyo.

CHAPTER 7 ACUPOINTS

1. Acupoints are portals into the body's energy system; they are points where vital energy flow is more accessible.
2. An Ahshi point is painful, either spontaneously or upon palpation; such sensitivity or irritability usually indicates congestion and stagnation.
3. Acupoints transmit energy readily; they are points of low electrical resistance and high electrical conductivity.
4. Energy flow near acupoints tends to slow down or stop.
5. Acupoints are numbered in consecutive order from the beginning to the end of a Meridian.
6. Acupoints are also identified by poetic names that indicate their location or function.
7. Acupoints are generally located on knots or ropes of tense muscle or in hollow indentations of joints.
8. A cun is a unit of measurement unique to the individual: the breadth of the thumb or the space between the creases of the middle joint of the middle finger.
9. The cun is better than a standard unit of measurement, since it is proportional to the individual.

10. The nerve reflex arc theory is premised on the concept that the inside and outside of the body communicate with and affect one another; hence, one can discern organ problems by examining the associated reflex zones, and one can treat those problems by treating the reflex zones.
11. Distortions in superficial tissues may indicate a problem with the associated organ.
12. Acupressure can benefit the organs and organ systems.
13. In the sympathetic mode, the body is in a state of excitation (increased heart rate, respiration, and blood volume flow, and heightened sensory awareness).
14. In the parasympathetic mode, the body is in a state of relaxation (with emphasis on housekeeping functions of digestion, assimilation, elimination, regeneration, and reproduction).
15. To induce the relaxation response, apply acupressure to the inner Bladder Meridian beside the spinal column in the neck and back, as well as the sacrum.
16. According to the gate theory, the sensory input of acupressure interferes with the transmission of pain signals to the brain.
17. According to the biochemical theory, acupressure stimulates the release of endorphins, which are naturally produced opiates.
18. Acupressure points, especially Ahshi points, correspond to trigger points.
19. A trigger point is a hyperirritable spot in a muscle that refers sensation to a distant location. Trigger points are caused by muscle tension.
20. A hypertonic (tense, spastic) muscle is ischemic (blood deficient) because its contracture restricts blood flow to the tissues.
21. Ischemia results not only in poor cell nutrition, but also in poor waste removal; ischemic tissues are saturated by their own waste products.
22. Acupressure releases the muscle spasm.
23. The Golgi tendon organ monitors the load or tension on the muscle (detects overload or overstretch).
24. If there is an excessive load, the Golgi tendon organ will induce the muscle to relax to prevent the muscle fibers from tearing.
25. Stretching also triggers the Golgi tendon organ.
26. No; TCM is theoretically distinct and different from Western anatomy and physiology; Qi flow is a mechanism in its own right; it is not just another term for blood and lymph flow or nerve conduction.
27. The body's Qi system affects and is affected by the other bodily systems (their influence is mutual).
28. The two main ways of selecting acupoints are local selection (choosing a point on or near the affected site) and distal selection (choosing a point far from the affected site based on its therapeutic property or Meridian function).
29. Stimulating point combinations (rather than isolated points) intensifies and balances the treatment.
30. Combine a point near the affected site (local) with a point far from the affected site (distal) but having a salutary influence on the affected site.
31. Combine a point on the torso or head (local) with a point on the limbs (distal).
32. Stimulate distal points first to clear blockages caused by the invasion of climatic agents or blood or Qi stagnation.
33. Distal points on the feet are more intense and powerful than distal points on the hands.

34. Stimulate distal points on the feet if strong energy is needed to clear blockages and disperse stagnation, as in cases of acute injury.
35. Stimulate distal points on the hand if the client is weak, depleted, or frail.
36. The principle of correspondence between joints pairs similar joints: ankle and wrist, knee and elbow, hip and shoulder. Joint problems can be treated not only with acupressure points on the troubled joint, but also with acupressure points on the corresponding joint.
37. The principle of correspondence between Meridians pairs Meridians of the same polarity (those that are located on the same aspect of a limb): St/LI, GB/TH, Bl/SI, Sp/Lu, Lr/PC, Ki/Ht.
38. Combine a point or points above the waist (superior) with a point or points below the waist (inferior).
39. Usually, points on the upper half of the body are balanced with points on the lower half. However, sometimes, as in the case of Liver Yang rising, too much energy is in the upper half, in which case one should stimulate points on the lower half of the body (especially the lower legs and feet) to draw energy downward.
40. Sometimes, as in the case of sinking Qi, too much energy is in the lower half, in which case one should stimulate points on the upper half of the body (especially the head) to raise energy upward.
41. Combine a point or points on the front of the body (anterior) with a point or points on the back of the body (posterior).
42. Shu/Yu points are on the back of the torso.
43. Mu/Bo points are on the front of the torso.
44. The inner Bladder Meridian is used to treat physical dysfunctions of the organs, while the outer Bladder Meridian is used to treat psychological dysfunctions associated with the organs.
45. Back transporting points are indicated in cases of chronic organ maladies or problems with the associated sense organs.
46. Front collecting points are indicated in cases of acute organ maladies.
47. The right/left point combination is based on the bilateral structure of Meridians and points.
48. Unilateral point stimulation is required when one side of the body cannot be treated (perhaps because it is recuperating from injury or surgery or because of an artificial joint). The other side is then treated for a reflexive effect. Similarly, if a disparity in energy exists—too much on one side but not enough on the other—more time is spent tonifying the weak or depleted side.
49. If only Yang points are used, a client may feel wired and edgy.
50. If only Yin points are used, a client may feel enervated and drowsy.

CHAPTER 8 COMPLEMENTARY HEALING MODALITIES

1. Moxabustion is a type of heat therapy that penetrates an acupoint with Yang energy; typically, smoldering mugwort is held over a point to penetrate it with heat.
2. Moxabustion is indicated for Cold Damp conditions.
3. Moxabustion is contraindicated for Heat conditions such as inflammation, since the application of heat would only aggravate them.

4. Moxabustion stimulates the flow of Qi, blood, and vital substances in the body.
5. Aside from the benefits of heat energy, the moxa itself enters the body, triggering the immune response and alkalizing the blood.
6. In the direct method, loose moxa punk is set on the skin, lit, and allowed to burn down to the skin, blistering and scarring it.
7. Blistering and scarring are not typically done in the West.
8. Types of bases include a slice of perforated ginger, onion, or garlic; a flat piece of chives; a dab of miso paste; and a pinch of salt.
9. There are several indirect methods, the most popular of which is the cylindrically shaped moxa cigar.
10. Aside from the client's verbal feedback, the practitioner can gauge the intensity of heat by placing a finger near the point being stimulated.
11. Good ventilation is important because of the profuse quantity of smoke produced by the moxa.
12. Moxabustion entails the risk of accidental burning.
13. One alternative to administering moxa to a client is to instruct the client how to self-administer moxa.
14. Moxa is well suited for self-administration because the person applying the moxa also experiences the heat and knows when to withdraw the applicator.
15. The arms and legs are especially accessible to self-administration.
16. Seeds and pellets provide continual acupressure to points over a period of several days.
17. A practitioner can give a client a plaster of seeds or pellets to wear or can refer the client to a business that supplies seeds and pellets.
18. A practitioner can place a magnetic mat or pad on top of the futon so that the client receives magnetic therapy during Shiatsu. After Shiatsu, the practitioner can give the client a plaster of magnets to wear over key acupressure points to prolong the therapeutic effect of the treatment; or can refer the client to a business that supplies magnets.
19. The client should not be exposed to magnets in excess of 2,500 gauss for longer than the duration of a Shiatsu session.
20. Weaker magnets may be left on for several days.
21. The bionorth side of the magnet calms, relaxes, and reduces symptoms of pain; it is indicated for Jitsu/Yang conditions.
22. The biosouth side of the magnet stimulates and energizes; it is indicated for Kyo/Yin conditions.
23. Gua Sha is a skin-scraping technique that is popular in China.
24. Sha refers to (1) the pathogen afflicting the body and (2) its manifestation as petechiae (red speckles) in the surface membrane after friction rubbing.
25. Almost any oil, liniment, or balm may be used to lubricate the skin.
26. The active ingredient eucalyptus makes Vicks® VapoRub® particularly good for Heat conditions because it is cooling.
27. The active ingredient clove makes Tiger Balm particularly good for Cold conditions because it is warming.
28. In the West, the lid of a Tiger Balm container (but not a Vicks® VapoRub® container) or a Chinese soup spoon (available at Asian markets) is often used to scrape.
29. Traditionally, Gua Sha is applied at the onset of an illness to prevent a full-blown case from developing.

30. Gua Sha is also indicated for Heat conditions, sore muscles, and stiff joints.
31. Gua Sha is adaptogenic in that the treatment effects adjust to the client's needs; for example, a hot client will feel cooler after Gua Sha, while a cold client will feel warmer after Gua Sha.
32. From a TCM perspective, Gua Sha expels pathogens and propels the movement of Qi, blood, and other vital substances that promote internal organ function.
33. From a Western perspective, Gua Sha extravasates (forces out) stagnant blood, fluids, and metabolic wastes congesting the subcutaneous tissues and muscles, thereby restoring normal circulation and cell respiration (nutrient delivery and waste removal), which promote good health.
34. Obtaining the client's informed consent before doing Gua Sha is important because of the petechiae that arise; this temporary skin blemishing looks a bit like road rash or patches of hickeys.
35. With normal circulation, the petechiae should resolve in 2 to 4 days.
36. To determine the presence of Sha, press the skin with your fingers and remove them quickly. If you see the pale afterimages of your fingerprints fading slowly, that indicates Sha.
37. Hold the instrument at a 10 to 15 degree angle to the skin's surface; lead the stroke with your fingers or thumb; press firmly into the fascia in a unilateral direction, taking care not to backstroke; on the back, direct the strokes downward toward the feet; on the shoulders and hips, direct the stroke outward toward the extremities; strokes should be 4 to 6 inches in length and repeated 7 to 11 times in overlapping swaths or until the Sha surfaces.
38. For frozen shoulder, Gua Sha the neck, back (Governing Vessel, inner and outer Bladder Meridian), shoulder, and down the arm, if necessary.
39. For hip pain, Gua Sha the lower back, sacrum, hip, and down the leg, if necessary.
40. The treatment should be tailored to resolve the client's unique pain pattern, which is not fixed, but mobile. Following the shifting path of pain with Gua Sha treatment is called chasing the dragon.
41. Contraindications to Gua Sha include any skin disruption or disorder such as a bruise, scrape, cut, open wound, rash, or burn. A pregnant woman's abdomen is also contraindicated.
42. Work around a pimple or mole by covering it with your finger to protect it. If the back is covered with pimples or moles, do not Gua Sha.
43. Gua Sha can be done once every 2 weeks.
44. Red Sha indicates Heat. Brown or dark Sha indicates Heat and deficiency of Yin in the blood. Blue or purple Sha indicates long-term blood stagnation. Light Sha indicates deficiency of blood.
45. The client should immediately cover up after Gua Sha to protect against invasion of Cold Wind or Cold Damp or Wind Heat.
46. The client should avoid all excesses, including drugs, alcohol, sex, fasting, overeating, and strenuous physical exertion. The client should wear a shirt to bed at night.
47. If the client's tissues harbor Sha again soon after treatment, the client's lifestyle is probably causing or contributing to Sha. Permanent improvement cannot be expected apart from lifestyle reform.
48. Liniments contain essential oils that have antiseptic properties and promote circulation.

49. Liniments are beneficial for sore, achy muscles; stiff joints; sprains; and strains. Some even promote the healing of minor wounds such as cuts and scrapes, through cell regeneration.

CHAPTER 9 PRACTICE PRELIMINARIES

1. A contraindication is any condition for which Shiatsu is inappropriate, either because Shiatsu could exacerbate it or because it poses a health hazard.
2. Most contraindications apply to clients, but some apply to practitioners as well—for example, practitioners should not give Shiatsu if they have a cold or other contagious illness or a break in the skin of their hands, such as a cut.
3. Abstaining from Shiatsu when contraindications are present protects the client and the practitioner from physical harm and litigation.
4. Colds, flu, strep throat, bronchitis, and pneumonia are contraindications.
5. It may be possible to work around a skin disorder if it is isolated or to work through clothing in some cases, as when the client has poison oak or poison ivy. Nevertheless, caution is advisable.
6. Lacerations (cuts), abrasions (scrapes), ulcers (open wounds), and burns are contraindications.
7. Work around the injury or anomaly or work on the opposite side to promote a sympathetic healing response.
8. Contusions (bruises), hematomas (blood tumors), strains (ruptured muscles or tendons), sprains (ruptured ligaments), any abnormal lumps and hypersensitive operation scars are contraindications.
9. Work above and below the fracture or on the opposite side to promote a sympathetic healing response.
10. The risk factors for cardiovascular disease are an overweight body type, a sedentary lifestyle, stress, and smoker status. Additionally, men over age 40 are at greater risk.
11. On clients at risk for cardiovascular disease, ischemic compression—deep, sustained pressure—should be avoided, as should ampuku.
12. Manual manipulation could dislodge a thrombus (blood clot), which could then enter the bloodstream and eventually block an artery, causing a heart attack, stroke, or death.
13. Yes; one can work around the site of a varicose vein.
14. Manual manipulation would aggravate inflammation by promoting blood and lymph flow to an area that is already under fluid pressure.
15. Thermal disorders, extreme debility or exhaustion, intoxication, and social phobia are contraindications.
16. Previously, any kind of massage therapy, including Shiatsu, was regarded as contraindicated for cancer patients due to an unfounded concern that manual manipulation could facilitate or expedite the spread of cancer. Now, however, Shiatsu and other massage modalities are regarded as beneficial, promoting normal functions, easing pain and anxiety, and comforting the patient.
17. Obtain permission from the cancer patient's oncologist.
18. Use lighter pressure on cancer patients, as they may bruise or fracture easily. Avoid the site of tumors, radiation burns, or attached medical devices.
19. Use lighter pressure on an elderly client; increase comfort with pillows and bolsters.

20. Use light pressure on a client who has osteoporosis, as the bones are brittle and could break.
21. Avoid BMTs and passive stretches on an artificial joint (it could become dislocated).
22. The following conditions are contraindications to Shiatsu during pregnancy: a positive sign on the homen test (the client experiences radiating pain when the foot is passively dorsiflexed, which indicates the presence of thrombi); a positive sign on the pitted edema test, which indicates pre-eclampsia; and placenta previa.
23. LI 4, Sp 6, and GB 21 are acupressure points contraindicated for pregnancy, especially during the first trimester, because they draw energy downward and could induce a miscarriage (for the same reason, these acupoints are used to facilitate delivery).
24. Avoid deep pressure anywhere below the knees during pregnancy. An ultraconservative approach is to do only very light work on the legs, due to increased fibrogenic activity, which increases the risk of thrombi (blood clots).
25. The prone position usually becomes uncomfortable during the second trimester because of the mother's protruding abdomen.
26. A client should wear loose, comfortable clothing, preferably made of natural fiber that absorbs sweat and doesn't create static electricity.
27. A healing response is a detoxification process; a client may feel worse before feeling better.
28. Signs of toxicity include dry skin; skin that feels cemented to the tissues underneath it (that can't be plucked up); hard, resistant flesh; and stiff, rigid joints.
29. A healing response typically lasts 24 hours.
30. Some symptoms of a healing response include fatigue, general malaise, headache, upset stomach, increased urination, and a bout of irritability or mild depression.
31. The client should drink lots of water, take an Epsom salt bath, rest, and later, if desired, do light exercise or stretching.
32. Having a low center of gravity means having a broad, bottom-heavy base of support.
33. A low center of gravity is stable.
34. Kneeling lunges and squats have a low center of gravity.
35. Hara is the Japanese word for abdomen, which refers to the body's center of power and gravity.
36. The hara (abdomen and hips) should face the target area being worked.
37. Facing the target area with one's hara increases power, reduces effort, and eliminates any strain caused by twisting.
38. One can gain leverage in the prone and supine positions by rising up and over the client and sinking one's body weight into the client (thereby harnessing the power of gravity).
39. The hara should initiate movements.
40. Moving from the hara is more powerful, stable, and less strenuous.
41. Apply pressure at a 90 degree (perpendicular) angle.
42. Apply and release pressure gradually to give the tissues time to adapt to changes in tension load.

43. Ideally, a point should be held for a count of three.
44. Apply pressure "through" rather than "on" or "to" the client; this is more penetrating.
45. Exhale during the work phase when applying pressure; inhale during the release phase when letting go of pressure.
46. Progressing from general to specific is desirable because general techniques using broad, flat surfaces and light to moderate pressure warm and loosen the tissues and prepare them for specific techniques using focused, pointed surfaces and deeper pressure.
47. Examples of general techniques include those using the palms, the heels of the hands, all four fingerpads, and the forearms. Examples of specific techniques include those using the thumbs, knuckles, and elbows.
48. In two-hand connectedness, the practitioner forms a closed circuit of energy between the client and himself.
49. The Mother hand applies static pressure on or near the torso while the Son hand applies dynamic pressure along the length of a limb.
50. The Mother/Son hand technique is preferable for clients whose tissues are hypersensitive and for low-energy clients whose energy needs to be recharged.
51. Two-handed compression produces a more intense sensation and stronger effect; it is preferable for clients who enjoy deeper pressure or whose energy needs to be discharged.
52. In general, the palm should mold to the contours of the body.
53. Use the pad of the thumb (not the tip).
54. Avoid applying pressure with the thumb in a hyperextended position (with the thumb pulled away from the rest of the hand).
55. The sharpness of the elbow tip can be softened by extending and increasing the angle of the elbow joint (straightening the arm slightly).
56. The sharpness of the elbow tip can be intensified by flexing and decreasing the angle of the elbow joint (bending the arm).
57. Firm, fleshy parts of the body, such as shoulders and hips, are suitable for elbow pressure.
58. Delicate, bony parts of the body are contraindicated for elbow techniques.
59. Depending on how one is positioned in relation to the client, one can stabilize oneself when using the knees by supporting some of one's body weight on the balls of the feet or on the hands.
60. Firm, fleshy parts of the body, such as shoulders, hips, and the backs of the legs, are suitable for knee pressure.
61. Delicate, bony parts of the body are contraindicated for knee techniques.
62. Firm, fleshy parts of the body—shoulders, hips, the backs of the legs, and even the soles of the feet—are suitable for foot techniques.
63. The Bladder Meridian is especially accessible in the prone position.
64. Neck and lower back issues, large breasts and abdomen, and tight, dorsiflexed ankles (feet that can't point) can make the prone position uncomfortable.
65. Client comfort in the prone position can be improved by placing a pillow under the chest and abdomen, placing a bolster under the ankles, and rotating the head from left to right periodically.
66. The supine position is best for BMTs and passive stretches.

67. The Stomach and Spleen Meridians are especially accessible in the supine position.
68. Client comfort in the supine position can be improved by placing a bolster under the knees.
69. The supine position is contraindicated for women in advanced stages of pregnancy because the weight of the fetus compresses the inferior vena cava, restricting or blocking blood flow back to the Heart.
70. The sidelying position is best for pregnant women.
71. The Gallbladder Meridian is especially accessible in the sidelying position.
72. Client alignment and comfort in the sidelying position can be improved by placing a pillow under the head, a pillow under the uppermost arm, and a pillow under the uppermost leg.
73. Facilitated stretches should be administered after compression techniques because then the tissues will be warmed and loosened and prepared to adapt to the elastic tension of a stretch.
74. Facilitated stretches should be administered slowly, smoothly, and carefully, noting the condition of the client's soft tissues and the quality of the client's energy and respecting the level of resistance encountered. Forcing, jerking, and bouncing should be avoided.

Appendix 3: Answers to Tests

Chapter 1 History of Shiatsu (20 points)

1. finger pressure
2. Traditional Chinese Medicine
3. China
4. TCM is at least 4,000 years old; it predates 2000 B.C.
5. E (Qi Massage)
6. B (Acupuncture)
7. A (Moxabustion)
8. D (Qi Gong)
9. G (Ampuku)
10. H (Tsubo Therapy)
11. C (Herbalism)
12. F (An Mo, Tui Na, Dian Xue)
13. D (Serizawa)
14. B (Namikoshi)
15. C (Masunaga)
16. D (Serizawa)
17. B (Namikoshi)
18. C (Masunaga)
19. D (Serizawa)
20. A (Tempaku)

Chapter 2 Qi and Meridians (45 points)

1. vital energy, life force, bioelectricity
2. Ki
3. matter, energy
4. No. Qi simply transforms from one thing to another.
5. Qi animates and empowers all physiological and psychological processes.
6. The three primary sources of Qi in humans are one's parents (prenatal ancestral source), air (postnatal source), and food (postnatal source).
7. Movement includes voluntary activities of skeletal muscles and involuntary activities such as heart beat, respiration, and intestinal motility.
8. Transformation involves the conversion of air and food into bodily substances and functions and physical and mental activities.
9. Protection concerns the body's defense against External Pernicious Influences and pathogens through various means such as a skin barrier, an energetic barrier, or an immune response.

10. Stabilization involves the maintenance of structural integrity and the retention of things in their proper place, such as organs in their respective locations and blood within vessels.
11. Warmth entails the regulation of body temperature.
12. Jing refers to one's genetic makeup, ancestral inheritance, and general constitution.
13. Jing governs vitality, fertility, and longevity, especially long-term processes of development over a lifetime.
14. As a nonrenewable resource with limited reserve, Jing is depletable; however, it can be conserved through a healthy lifestyle and moderation.
15. Shen refers to various aspects of the psyche, including consciousness, awareness, psychological disposition, and social interaction.
16. Shen governs personality and social dynamics.
17. Mental and emotional states affect the body.
18. True
19. False (Shiatsu recognizes the role of the psyche in health.)
20. False (the listed examples describe rebellious Stomach Qi. A reversal of Lung Qi manifests as sneezing and coughing.)
21. True
22. True
23. True
24. False (Meridians have no physical structure in the body; they are an invisible concentrations of Qi flow.)
25. True
26. False (Like blood and lymph flow, Meridians are an aspect and sign of life; hence, Meridians do not exist in a corpse.)
27. True
28. True
29. False (Except for the Conception and Governing Vessels, which run along the midline of the torso, the 12 main Meridians are structured in bilateral (two-sided) pairs that mirror one another.)
30. False (Meridians are coupled in Yin Yang pairs.)
31. True (The Triple Heater does not correspond to a single organ; rather, it corresponds to an organ complex or interrelated system of organs.)
32. False (Meridians are associated with both physiological and psychological functions.)
33. False (Yang Meridians are located on the back and outside of the body, whereas Yin Meridians are located on the front and inside of the body.)
34. True
35. True
36. True
37. False (Sanjaio corresponds to an organ complex or interrelated system of organs rather than a single organ.)
38. True

CHAPTER 3 YIN YANG (40 POINTS)

1. Taoist (*Note:* The answer "Chinese" is too general because Chinese philosophy could refer to Taoism, Buddhism, or Confucianism.)
2. shady, sunny
3. Yin, Yang
4. Yin, Yang
5. change, transformation, flux.
6. Yang
7. Yin
8. Yin
9. Yang
10. Yang
11. Yin
12. Yin
13. Yang
14. Yang
15. Yin
16. Yin
17. Yang
18. Yin
19. Yang
20. Yang
21. Yin
22. Yin
23. Yang
24. False (Yin and Yang are relative qualities.)
25. False (Everything contains both Yin and Yang.)
26. False (Yin and Yang arise simultaneously, concurrently.)
27. False (Yin and Yang are determined in context, in relation to other things.)
28. True
29. True
30. True
31. False (Yin and Yang are in dynamic flux; they wax, wane, and metamorphose into each other).
32. True
33. False (The transformation of Yin to Yang can also occur gradually and smoothly.)
34. True
35. False (The chest is more Yang than the abdomen because it is superior.)
36. True
37. True

CHAPTER 4 THE FIVE ELEMENTS (50 POINTS)

1. the Five Processes, Stages, Phases, Transitions, Transformations, or Metamorphoses
2. Ki/Chi/Qi/energy
3. Shen refers to the Creative Cycle. (*Note:* This differs from the concept of Shen as spirit or mind.)
4. In Shen, the elements are in nurturing, fostering, promoting, supportive relationships.
5. The Mother (the element that promotes or generates)
6. The Child (the element that is fostered or produced)
7. To remedy a deficiency, the practitioner should tonify the deficient element, tonify its deficient Mother (if indicated), and sedate its excessive controller (if indicated).
8. Ko refers to the Control Cycle.
9. In Ko, the elements are in limiting, regulatory relationships.
10. Insult is one possible element reaction to overregulation. Insult occurs when the regulated element rebels against and "insults" its regulator, inhibiting or incapacitating it. This can be likened to a teenager rebelling against and insulting an overly strict or authoritarian parent.
11. Sedate the rebellious element, and tonify the controller.
12. Humiliation is another possible element response to overregulation. Humiliation occurs when the regulated element is "humiliated" by its regulator—that is, compromised or debilitated in its function. This can be likened to a teenager whose personality is meek, timid, shy, and withdrawn on account of a harsh, overbearing parent.
13. Tonify the humiliated element, and sedate the controller.
14. E (Water)
15. C (Earth)
16. A (Wood)
17. D (Metal)
18. B (Fire)
19. A (Wood)
20. B (Fire)
21. C (Earth)
22. D (Metal)
23. E (Water)
24. E (Water)
25. C (Earth)
26. B (Fire)
27. E (Water)
28. A (Wood)
29. D (Metal)
30. C (Earth)
31. B (Fire)
32. A (Wood)
33. C (Earth)

34. D (Metal)
35. E (Water)
36. E (Water)
37. C (Earth)
38. B (Fire)
39. D (Metal)
40. A (Wood)
41. True
42. True
43. True
44. False (Metal is the Mother of Water.)
45. True
46. Earth
47. Wood
48. Water
49. Metal
50. Fire

CHAPTER 5 THE ZANG FU ORGAN SYSTEM (50 POINTS)

1. E (PC/TH)
2. C (Ht/SI)
3. A (Lu/LI)
4. B (Sp/St)
5. F (Lr, GB)
6. D (Ki/Bl)
7. Pericardium
8. Small Intestine
9. Liver
10. Gallbladder
11. Bladder
12. Heart
13. Triple Heater
14. Stomach
15. Lungs
16. Spleen
17. Large Intestine
18. Kidneys
19. E (Ki/Bl)
20. A (Lu/LI)
21. B (Sp/St)
22. F (PC/TH)
23. C (Ht)
24. G (Lr/GB)

25. D (SI)
26. G (Lr/GB)
27. C (Ht)
28. D (SI)
29. F (PC/TH)
30. B (Sp/St)
31. A (Lu/LI)
32. E (Ki/Bl)
33. C (Fire)
34. E (Metal)
35. D (Earth)
36. C (Fire disharmony)
37. E (Metal disharmony)
38. B (Wood)
39. B (Wood disharmony)
40. A (Water: Yang type)
41. A (Water: Yin type)
42. D (Earth)
43. A (Water: Yang type)
44. D (Earth)
45. A (Water: Yin type)
46. E (Metal)
47. B (Wood)
48. C (Fire)
49. D (Earth)
50. B (Wood)

CHAPTER 6 THE EIGHT PRINCIPLE PATTERNS AND KYO JITSU (60 POINTS)

1. G (Excess)
2. A (Interior/Exterior)
3. G (Excess)
4. B (Deficiency/Excess)
5. F (Deficiency)
6. C (Cold/Heat)
7. H (Cold)
8. I (Heat)
9. F (Deficiency)
10. D (Interior)
11. G (Excess)
12. H (Cold)
13. E (Exterior)
14. I (Heat)
15. E (Exterior)

16. G (Excess)
17. Jitsu
18. Kyo
19. Jitsu
20. Kyo
21. Kyo
22. Kyo
23. Jitsu
24. Kyo
25. Kyo
26. Jitsu
27. Kyo
28. Jitsu
29. Jitsu
30. Kyo
31. Jitsu
32. Kyo
33. Kyo
34. Jitsu
35. Jitsu
36. Kyo
37. Kyo
38. Jitsu
39. Jitsu
40. Kyo
41. Jitsu
42. Jitsu
43. Jitsu
44. Kyo
45. Kyo
46. Jitsu
47. True
48. False (Kyo Jitsu imbalances can arise from normal fluctuations in energy levels, such as cycles of hunger and satisfaction or work and rest.)
49. True
50. False (Imbalances due to unhealthy lifestyle habits can be resolved only by lifestyle reform.)
51. False (Whether to begin by sedating Jitsu or tonifying Kyo depends on the client.)
52. False (Starting a session with gentle techniques on a Yang client will most likely make the client uneasy, fidgety, restless, and disgruntled; Yang types need to be tranquilized first through sedating techniques before they can lie still and enjoy the subtler moves.)
53. False (Yin clients tend to prefer gentle work and might find dispersal techniques too aggressive and even injurious to their low or depleted Qi.)
54. True

55. False (Right/left disparity implicates the Gallbladder and Liver Meridians.)
56. False (Although dispersal techniques should be used on a Jitsu chest, they should not be used on the vulnerable abdomen.)
57. False (Firm pressure is applied to the back and light pressure to the abdomen.)
58. True (This is the "search for the connection" technique.)
59. True
60. False (Hara diagnosis reflects short-term conditions, whereas back diagnosis reflects long-term conditions.)

CHAPTER 7 ACUPOINTS (60 POINTS)

1. An acupoint is an entry into the body's energy system, where the flow of vital energy is more accessible.
2. Tsubo is the Japanese term for acupoint.
3. Ahshi ("ouch" point) emphasizes the hypersensitivity, tenderness, or pain of a point.
4. Acupoints transmit electrical currents readily; they are points of low electrical resistance and high electrical conductivity.
5. Distortions in superficial tissues indicate a problem in the associated organ.
6. Energy flow tends to slow down, stagnate, or get blocked near acupoints.
7. Acupoints are found on or near knots of tense muscle and in the hollows of joints.
8. One cun equals the width of the thumb or the width between the creases of the middle joint of the middle finger.
9. A cun is preferable to a standard unit of measurement because it is relative to the proportions of the individual.
10. D (biochemical theory)
11. A (nerve reflex arc theory)
12. E (trigger point theory)
13. B (relaxation response theory)
14. C (gate theory)
15. G (TCM theory)
16. F (Golgi tendon organ theory)
17. E (trigger point theory)
18. A (nerve reflex arc theory)
19. B (relaxation response theory)
20. C (gate theory)
21. G (TCM theory)
22. F (Golgi tendon organ theory)
23. A (nerve reflex arc theory)
24. G (TCM theory)
25. H (right/left point combo)
26. F (superior/inferior point combo)
27. H (right/left point combo)

28. G (posterior/anterior point combo)
29. H (right/left point combo)
30. I (Yin/Yang point combo)
31. E (local/distal point combo)
32. G (posterior/anterior point combo)
33. A (local point)
34. B (distal point)
35. D (posterior point)
36. C (anterior point)
37. True
38. True
39. False (Distal points on the feet are more intense than distal points on the hands.)
40. False (When the client is infirm, stimulate distal points on the hands because they are milder in sensation and effect.)
41. False (When the client feels lethargic, stimulate distal points on the feet because they are stronger in effect and will revitalize and invigorate the client.)
42. True
43. True
44. False (In cases of sinking Qi, stimulate points on the upper half of the body to elevate energy.)
45. True
46. True
47. True
48. False (working too many Yang points will overstimulate a client).
49. False (working too many Yin points will overrelax or drain a client.)
50. I (anxiety/emotional upset)
51. C (low back and hip pain)
52. J (pregnancy and labor)
53. A (headaches)
54. D (knee pain)
55. B (shoulder and arm pain)
56. H (lower burner disorders)
57. G (digestive disorders)
58. F (colds; flus; sinus disorders)
59. E (ankle pain)

CHAPTER 8 COMPLEMENTARY HEALING MODALITIES (45 POINTS)

1. E (liniments and balms)
2. A (moxabustion)
3. B (seeds and pellets)
4. D (Gua Sha)
5. C (magnets)

6. D (Gua Sha)
7. E (liniments and balms)
8. E (liniments and balms)
9. D (Gua Sha)
10. B (seeds and pellets)
11. D (Gua Sha)
12. A (moxabustion)
13. D (Gua Sha)
14. A (moxabustion) and/or D (Gua Sha)
15. C (magnets)
16. A (moxabustion)
17. E (liniments and balms)
18. A (moxabustion)
19. D (Gua Sha)
20. C (magnets)
21. True
22. False (The herb used for moxa is a member of the sage family but smells like hemp.)
23. True
24. False (Do not blister and scar.)
25. False (Withdraw the moxa before inflicting pain.)
26. True
27. False (Do not place the biosouth side on a spastic area, since the biosouth side stimulates and energizes and may therefore aggravate tension. Instead, place the bionorth side on a spastic area, since the bionorth side calms, relaxes, and reduces symptoms.)
28. False (Do not place a magnet near a malignancy, not even the bionorth side, which is reputed to reduce biological activity.)
29. False (Do not place a magnet on the abdomen of a pregnant woman, not even the biosouth side, which is reputed to increase biological activity.)
30. True (Weaker magnets can be left on for days, but stronger magnets—2,500 to 9,000 gauss—should be left on only for a few hours.)
31. False (A magnet can interfere with the functioning of a cardiac pacemaker and is therefore contraindicated.)
32. True (Sha also refers to the petechiae that occur upon friction rubbing.)
33. False (A pale—not red—afterimage that is slow to fade indicates the presence of Sha.)
34. False (Strokes are always performed downward toward the feet and outward toward the extremities to facilitate the expulsion of pathogens.)
35. False (Strokes are unidirectional—only downward or outward—to facilitate the expulsion of pathogens; at the end of a stroke, the instrument is lifted and reset at the starting point.)
36. False (Chasing the dragon means following the path of pain with Gua Sha whereever it migrates; stop Gua Sha as soon as Sha surfaces or the area begins to sting.)
37. False (A bruise is a local contraindication for Gua Sha: even light scraping could exacerbate tissue trauma.)

38. False (Following Gua Sha, the client should rest and allow the body to detoxify and heal.)
39. False (Gua Sha should not be done more than once every 2 weeks. Doing Gua Sha 3 days in a row on the same location would be very abrasive and traumatize the skin and subcutaneous tissues.)
40. No. The petechiae that result from Gua Sha would interfere with her plans to wear a low-cut evening dress that night and a bikini the following day.
41. No, at least not in that enclosed space, because of the smoke produced. If feasible, one could moxa the client elsewhere, even outside, weather permitting.
42. Advise the client to buy an antinausea wristband (a type of magnetic therapy) available at most pharmacies.
43. First, the treatment period is too long, especially for a magnet of that strength. One should apply magnets of 2,500 gauss or more only for a limited duration, such as a couple of hours, not an entire week. Second, the client should place the bionorth side toward his tense muscles since the bionorth side calms (the biosouth side energizes and might aggravate his condition.)

CHAPTER 9 PRACTICE PRELIMINARIES (35 POINTS)

1. A contraindication is any condition for which Shiatsu is inadvisable.
2. Work around the site or on the opposite side of the body.
3. Cardiovascular disorders that require localized abstention from Shiatsu include phlebitis or inflammation of the deep veins, usually affecting the legs; varicose veins, also usually affecting the legs; and the presence of risk factors for cardiovascular disease (an overweight body type, a sedentary lifestyle, stress, smoker status), which requires one to refrain from ischemic compression near major arteries and ampuku, or abdominal massage.
4. Take extra precautions to protect the cancer patient from exposure to germs by washing up to the elbows and postponing treatment if anyone in one's household is feeling unwell; use lighter pressure and gentler techniques because of the risk of bruising and fracturing; avoid the site of tumors, radiation burns, catheters and ports, and surgical incisions.
5. On an elderly client, especially one who is frail or presents signs of osteoporosis, use lighter pressure because of the risk of fracturing the bones; avoid traction, BMTs, and facilitated stretches on artificial joints.
6. Abstain from applying heavy pressure below the knees because of the risk of thrombi from increased fibrogenic activity during pregnancy. An ultraconservative approach would be to use only very light pressure on the legs.
7. Acupressure points that are contraindicated during pregnancy because they draw energy downward and could induce a miscarriage are LI 4, GB 21, and Sp 6.
8. C (leverage)
9. D (general to specific)
10. C (leverage)
11. A (low center of gravity)
12. B (hara)
13. A (low center of gravity)
14. B (hara)
15. B (Mother/Son hand technique)

16. A (two-hand connectedness)
17. C (two-handed compression)
18. C (two-handed compression)
19. B (Mother/Son hand technique)
20. False (Apply pressure at a perpendicular or 90 degree angle.)
21. False (Apply pressure slowly and sustain for a few counts.)
22. False (Exhale when applying pressure; inhale when releasing.)
23. True
24. True
25. False (Facilitated stretches are best applied after compression techniques have warmed and loosened the tissues.)
26. False (Stretches should be administered slowly, smoothly, and carefully; swift, thrusting, and rhythmically bouncing stretches increase the risk of pain and injury.)
27. B (supine)
28. A (prone)
29. B (supine)
30. C (sidelying)
31. A (prone)
32. C (sidelying)
33. C (sidelying)
34. A (prone)
35. B (supine)

Appendix 4: Resources

Books (TCM and Other Asian Healing Arts)

Redwing Book Company
44 Linden Street, Brookline, MA 02445
or
202 Bendix Drive, Taos, NM 87571
1-800-873-3946 (orders/catalog)
1-505-758-7768
info@redwingbooks.com (e-mail)
www.redwingbooks.com (website)
orders@redwingbooks.com (orders)

Ceramic Wall Sculptures (Featured in Chapter 4 on Five Element Theory)

Diane Husson
9415 Sturgis Street
Norfolk, VA 23503
1-757-587-4342 (orders/commissions)
dianehusson@cox.net (e-mail)
newrelics.com (website)

Futons, Bolsters, Room Ambiance

Gaiam Living Arts (mats, bolsters)
360 Interlocken Boulevard
Broomfield, CO 80021
1-800-254-8464 (orders/catalog)
www.gaiam.com (website)

Hugger-Mugger Yoga Products (mats, bolsters)
3937 South 500 West
Salt Lake City, UT 84123
1-800-473-4888 (orders/catalog)
1-801-268-9642
www.huggermugger.com (website)

Japanese Gifts (home decor)
www.japanesegifts.com (website)

Haiku Designs (home decor)
P.O. Box 4673
Boulder, CO 80306
1-800-736-7614
www.haikudesigns.com (website)

Lotus Palm School (mats)
5870 Waverly Street
Montreal, Quebec, Canada H2T 2Y3
1-514-270-5713
www.lotuspalm.com (website)

MAGNETS, MOXABUSTION, AND GUA SHA SUPPLIES

Lhasa-OMS (formerly OMS)
230 Libbey Parkway
Weymouth, MA 02189
1-800-722-8775 (orders/catalog)
1-781-340-1071
www.LhasaOMS.com (website)

MUSIC

CHINESE

Horn, Paul, & Mingue Liang, David. (1987). *China*. Celestial Harmonies.

Rong, Shao. (2000). *Orchid*. Pacific Moon/Chapter One.

Shanghai Chinese Traditional Orchestra. (1995). *Tortoise: Chinese Feng Shui Music*. Wind Records.

Shanghai Chinese Traditional Orchestra. (1997). *Yin Music: Chinese Regimen Music for Better Health*. Wind Records.

JAPANESE

Hoo, Kavin. (2004). *Lifescapes: Just Relax, The Orient*. Compass Productions.

Lee, Riley. (1984). *Sanctuary: Music from a Zen Garden*. Narada Productions.

Lee, Riley. (1991). *Oriental Sunrise: Music for Shakuhachi and Koto*. Enso Records.

Lee, Riley. (1993). *Rainforest Reverie*. New World Productions.

Miyata, Kohachiro. (1991). *Shakuhachi: The Japanese Flute*. Elektra Nonesuch.

Richardson, Stan. (1997). *Shakuhachi Meditation Music*. Sounds True Records.

Yoshizawa, Masakazu & Gumi, Kokin. (2000). *Zen Garden*. Avalon Music.

MISCELLANEOUS

Ackerman, Will. (1998). *Sound of Wind Driven Rain*. Windham Hill Records. (guitar)

Anuvida & Tyndall, Nik. (1995). *Reiki: Healing Hands*. New Earth Records.

Eno, Brian. (1978). *Ambient 1: Music for Airports*. EG Records. (ambient)

Eno, Brian. (1985). *Thursday Afternoon*. Virgin Records. (ambient)

Frantzich, Paul & Frantzich, Tim. (1999). *Lifescapes: Calming Massage*. Compass Productions.

Jones, Wayne. *Lifescapes: Yoga*. Compass Productions.

Shastro. (1999). *Shanay: Mystic Trance*. Malimba Records. (Sufi)

Shastro. (2000). *Tantric Heart: Music for Lovers*. Malimba Records. (Indian)

Shastro & Nadama. (1999). *Zen Notes*. Malimba Records. (sax and piano)

Yogafit. (2002). *Music for a Peaceful Paradise*. New World Music.

NATIVE AMERICAN

Allen, Michael, & Stramp, Barry. (1997). *In Beauty I Walk: The Best of Coyote Oldman.* Hearts of Space.

Anugama. (2000). *Shamanic Dream.* Nightingale/Meistersinger.

Nakai, Carlos, & Eaton, William. (1988). *Carry the Gift.* Canyon Records.

Raye, Marina, & Olabayo. (2000). *Drumming into Paradise.* Native Heart Music.

PROFESSIONAL ASSOCIATIONS AND/OR PURVEYORS OF MALPRACTICE LIABILITY INSURANCE

American Massage Therapy Association (AMTA)
500 Davis Street, Suite 900
Evanston, IL 60201
1-877-905-2700
info@amtamassage.org (e-mail)
www.amtamassage.org (website)

American Organization for Bodywork Therapies of Asia (AOBTA)
1010 Haddonfield-Berlin Road, Suite 408
Voorhees, NJ 08043
1-856-782-1616
office@aobta.org (e-mail)
www.aobta.org (website)

Associated Bodywork and Massage Professionals (ABMP)
1271 Sugarbush Drive
Evergreen, CO 80439
1-800-458-2267
expectmore@eabmp.com (e-mail)
www.abmp.com (website)

International Massage Association (IMA)
P.O. Box 421
25 South Fourth Street
Warrenton, VA 20188
1-540-351-0800
info@imagroup.com (e-mail)
www.holisticbenefits.com/ima (website)

PROFESSIONAL ONLINE JOURNALS

Journal of Alternative and Complementary Medicine
Mary Ann Liebert, Inc. Publishing
140 Huguenot Street, 3rd Floor
New Rochelle, NY 10801
1-914-740-2100
www.liebertpub.com/acm (website)
Note: Articles are available online at cost.

***Massage & Bodywork Magazine* (published by ABMP)**
1271 Sugarbush Drive
Evergreen, CO 80439
1-800-458-2267
www.massageandbodywork.com (website)
Note: Major articles in the most recent issue are available free online.

Massage Magazine
5150 Palm Valley Road, Suite 103
Ponte Vedra Beach, FL 32082
1-800-533-4263
www.massagemag.com (website)
Note: Selected articles are available free online.

***Massage Therapy Journal* (published by AMTA)**
500 Davis Street, Suite 900
Evanston, IL 60201
1-877-905-2700
www.amtamassage.org/journal/home.html (website)
Note: The entire text of the most recent issue is available free online. Major articles in archival issues dating back five years are also available free online. Articles on topics of interest, such as Shiatsu, may be found by conducting a journal index search.

***Massage Today* (published by MPAmedia)**
P.O. Box 4139
Huntington Beach, CA 92605
1-800-752-6012 (circulation)
1-714-230-3150 (editorial)
www.massagetoday.com (website)
Note: Articles in the most recent issue and archival issues dating back five years are available free online. Articles on topics of interest, such as Asian bodywork, may be found by conducting a topic search. A subscription to the periodical is free to massage therapists.

Merck Manual
Merck & Co., Inc.
One Merck Drive
P.O. Box 100
Whitehouse Station, N.J. 08889–0100
908–423–1000
www.merck.com/mmhe/index.html (website)
Note: Free information on medical disorders and diseases compiled by medical experts.

MULTI MEDIA (INSTRUCTIONAL VIDEOS, DVDS)

Amma
By Shogo Mochizuki
Demonstrates Japanese massage
Available through the Acupressure Institute
http://www.acupressure.com
or
http://www.stressreliefproducts.com

Do In
By Cindy Banker
Demonstrates Meridian stretches, breathing exercises, and bodywork
Available through Redwing Reviews
http://www.redwingbooks.com

Gua Sha Step by Step: A Visual Guide to a Traditional Technique for Modern Practice
By Arya Nielsen
Demonstrates Gua Sha

Available in the U.S. through Redwing Reviews
http://www.redwingbooks.com
or
http://www.guasha.com (website)
iatramea@aol.com (email)
Distribution elsewhere:
Verlag fuer Ganzheitliche Medizin
Dr. Erich Wuehr GmbH, Muellerstr. 7, D-93444 Koetzting, Germany
http://www.vgm-portal.de (website)
info@vgm-portal.de (email)

Fundamentals of Acupressure
Zen Shiatsu
By Michael Gach
Demonstrates acupressure and stretches
Available through Redwing Reviews
http://www.redwingbooks.com
or
Acupressure Institute
http://www.acupressure.com
info@acupressure.com

The Stretching Process
By Michael Alicia
Demonstrates Shiatsu stretches and BMTs
Available through
The Body Break Company
259 Seventh Ave. Suite #4,
New York, NY 10001
212-229-1529 (phone)
http://members.aol.com/bodybreaks (website)

Qigong Massage: Self and Partner
By Yang Jwing Ming
Demonstrates Chinese massage
Available through Redwing Reviews
http://www.redwingbooks.com

INDEX